The Asymmetrical Brain

The Asymmetrical Brain

edited by Kenneth Hugdahl and Richard J. Davidson

A Bradford Book
The MIT Press
Cambridge, Massachusetts
London, England

© 2003 Massachusetts Institute of Technology

This book was set in Palatino on 3B2 by Asco Typesetters, Hong Kong and was printed and bound in the United States of America.

Library of Congress Cataloging-in-Publication Data

The asymmetrical brain / edited by Kenneth Hugdahl and Richard J. Davidson.
   p.; cm.
 Rev. ed. of: Brain asymmetry / edited by Richard J. Davidson and Kenneth Hugdahl. c1995.
 "A Bradford book."
 Includes bibliographical references and index.
 ISBN 0-262-08309-4 (alk. paper)
 1. Cerebral dominance. 2. Laterality. I. Hugdahl, Kenneth. II. Davidson, Richard J. III. Brain asymmetry.
 [DNLM: 1. Dominance, Cerebral. 2. Brain—physiology. 3. Laterality. WL 335 A8608 2003]
 QP385.5 .B725   2003
 612.8′2—dc21   2002025092

10 9 8 7 6 5 4 3 2 1

Contents

Preface

In April 1999, at the Cognitive Neuroscience Meeting in Washington, D.C., MIT Press representative Michael Rutter asked one of us (KH) if it was not about time to publish a second edition of *Brain Asymmetry*, which had been published by MIT Press in 1995. Had not the field progressed since 1995, so that it was now time for an update, or even a new book based on the most recent research in the field of brain asymmetry? On his way home to Bergen, Norway, Kenneth Hugdahl stopped over in Madison, Wisconsin, to meet with Richard Davidson, the other editor of the first book. Davidson agreed that indeed the field had progressed during the years since the first volume; thus a new volume could be an important update of the most recent findings in the field. That was the start of this volume, which is a completely new book on brain asymmetry, with 21 original chapters.

In the preface to the 1995 volume we wrote, "We cannot identify any other construct that forms the focus of such a diverse array of behavioral processes. The study of brain asymmetry continues to attract unique forms of integration in the biobehavioral sciences." The mysteries of the two hemispheres of the brain, how they differ functionally and structurally, how they communicate, and how they participate in the cortical and subcortical circuitry underlying complex cognition and affect still fascinate and interest young and old neuroscientists. What we wrote in 1995 about the diverse array of behavioral processes being reflected in the asymmetry construct is no less relevant today than it was in 1995. To mention just one example, the development of new neuroimaging techniques—functional magnetic resonance imaging (fMRI), positron emission tomography (PET), and magnetoence-paholograpy (MEG)—have revealed how neuronal activation is asymmetrically organized and distributed across the hemispheres, providing evidence for how the asymmetry construct becomes ever more refined and detailed. This topic was not included in the 1995 volume but has a part of its own in the present volume. Another topic that has been the focus of much recent research is the use of high-resolution structural MR imaging to reveal subtle morphological differences between the hemispheres. Thus, it has become possible to look for correspondences of structural and functional asymmetries between the hemispheres. Most of the interest has been in the upper posterior parts of the temporal lobe and adjacent areas in the parietal lobe. Both the planum temporale and the planum parietale, in the temporal and parietal lobes, respectively, have attracted much interest, relating structural-functional asymmetries in these areas to such diverse clinical syndromes as dyslexia and schizophrenia. This is covered in several chapters in the present volume.

A goal of the present volume has been to show the international interest in brain asymmetry and related concepts. We hope this is reflected in the various contributions, with authors from the United States, Canada, United Kingdom, Germany, France, and Norway.

Folk psychology statements like "The left hemisphere is specialized, or dominant, for language, and the right hemisphere is specialized, or dominant, for visuospatial functions, or space orientation" obviously tell an incomplete, and sometimes inaccurate, story. First of all, such statements imply that the brain basically is specialized only for two functions, language and the ability to orient in the environment. Second, they imply that half the brain does only language and the other half does only visual processing. This also is obviously wrong. On the contrary, a prevailing aspect of research throughout the history of brain asymmetry is the notion that asymmetries exist at all levels of the nervous system, including also the peripheral and autonomic nervous systems. Another prevailing idea is that asymmetries exist not only for higher cognitive processes, like language and visuospatial processing, but also for emotional processes. A third aspect is that recent advances in methods have made it possible to quantify structural asymmetries with much greater precision and resolution than was available previously. This has resulted in new theories and models of how functional asymmetries may have their structural correlates in brain anatomy. A fourth aspect is the development of the new neuroimaging techniques, both hemodynamic techniques (e.g., PET and fMRI) and other techniques (ERP [event-related potential], MEG, and transcranial magnetic stimulation [TMS]). A fifth aspect of recent asymmetry research is its application to clinical areas with regard to psychiatric, neurological, and developmental disorders. It is our intention to cover all these ideas and developments as a reflection of the current status of the field, from both a basic research and a clinical perspective.

In selecting the contributors, it was our intention to focus on relatively recent and new topics as well as a few older topics where there have been new developments since 1995. Selecting the contributors therefore meant, as always, that not all prominent researchers in the field could be invited. This would have made the volume unwieldy. We have therefore chosen to present the field through a mixed selection of chapters ranging from basic physiological processes on the neuronal level to major clinical disorders like schizophrenia and depression. When inviting the selected authors, it was our intention to include promising and novel ideas in the field, with potential for possible breakthroughs in the near future. For these reasons the book is divided into seven major parts that include animal models of asymmetry and basic asymmetrical functions (e.g., handedness), neuroimaging studies, visual asymmetry, auditory asymmetry, emotional asymmetry, and applications for neurological and psychiatric disorders. Each part has two or more chapters that are intended to illustrate the range of methods and research topics within each area that is represented.

In part I, on animal models and basic functions, Onur Güntürkün provides a review of studies on the lateralization of the visual system in various species of birds, thus providing an animal model for the understanding of the neuronal substrates of visual asymmetry. This is followed by the chapter by Akaysha Tang, who presents a new theory of asymmetry based on the role played by left and right nuclei complexes in the hippocampus, taking a bottom-up approach to asymmetry and laterality. In the third chapter, Craig Berridge and coworkers show how stress and coping are related to the asymmetry of the dopamine system within the prefrontal cortex. The final chapter in part I, by Alan Beaton, provides an updated and comprehensive review of handedness effects in research on brain asymmetry.

Part II, which deals with brain imaging and brain stimulation, starts with a chapter by Karl Friston on experimental design and statistical analysis of functional brain imaging studies, focusing on issues related to asymmetry and lateralization in functional brain architecture. Next,

Lutz Jäncke and Helmut Steinmetz review their extensive research on anatomical brain asymmetry, particularly research on the role of the planum temporale area in the upper posterior temporal lobe. This is followed by a chapter by Alvaro Pascual-Leone and Vincent Walsh on the new transcranial magnetic stimulation (TMS) technique and what this method will contribute to an enhanced understanding of the functions of the cerebral hemispheres.

Part III is devoted to studies on visual asymmetry and laterality, starting with the contribution by Marie Banich on hemispheric interactions, and implications for theories of information processing and processing capacity in the brain and in the left and right hemispheres. Bruno Laeng and collaborators review studies on asymmetries in encoding of spatial relations, providing evidence for different kinds of spatial encoding properties in the left and right hemispheres. Next, Clifford Saron and coworkers present an extensive review of ERP work with visual half-field stimulus presentations, focusing on the complexities of interhemispheric communication.

Part IV consists of three chapters, are devoted to auditory laterality. Robert Zatorre reviews work related to hemispheric asymmetries in the processing of tonal stimuli, including asymmetries for musical stimuli and music. Kenneth Hugdahl presents an update on dichotic listening studies with speech sounds, including a new database containing dichotic listening performances from more than 1000 subjects. Finally, Daniel O'Leary shows the effects of attention on the asymmetry for speech and nonspeech sounds, with applications to schizophrenia.

Part V, on emotional laterality, opens with a chapter by Diego Pizzagalli, Alexander J. Shackman, and Richard Davidson on how the two hemispheres of the brain differ in their contributions to emotions and emotional behavior, focusing on functional neuroimaging data. Next, Wendy Heller and collaborators present a model of anxiety and emotional functioning with a focus on the asymmetrical contributions of the left and right hemispheres to the understanding of the neural implementation of emotions and emotional disorders. James Coan and John Allen close the part with a comprehensive review of studies of frontal EEG asymmetry as a measure of state and trait indices of positive and negative emotions, and the interactions with the functioning of the left and right cerebral hemispheres.

Part VI deals with studies of asymmetry in relation to neurological disorders. Maryse Lassonde and Hannelore Sauerwein present their work on patients with agenesis of the corpus callosum and implications for understanding the nature of both specialization and integration of the hemispheres. Next, Mark Eckert and Christiana Leonard review data and theories of dyslexia, one of the most common developmental disorders, and its neurobiological substrates from the perspective of brain asymmetry. This is followed by a chapter by Michel Habib and Fabrice Robichon, who also focus on the brain mechanisms of dyslexia, presenting evidence for the importance of structures outside of those brain regions traditionally believed to be important for the understanding of dyslexia.

In part VII, on psychiatric disorders, Gerard Bruder presents behavioral, electrophysiological, and hemodynamic brain imaging data showing functional asymmetries in depression and depressive disorders, and how this relates to, for example, clinical features. In the final chapter, Michael Green and coworkers present an overview of theoretical models of and empirical evidence for a view of schizophrenia as being related to impaired asymmetry and laterality, and possibly having neuroanatomical substrates as well.

It is our sincere hope that this volume will contribute to a continued interest in one of the most fascinating aspects of the mammalian brain, its division into left and right halves along the neuroaxis. We further hope that it will contribute to better integration of the neurosciences, with different subdisciplines—psychology, psychiatry, neurophysiology, neurology, and neurosurgery, to mention a few examples—working together to unravel the great mystery of the brain.

In addition to thanking the authors of the chapters, we would like to acknowledge the contributions of several other people without whose help and assistance this volume would not have been published. Our thanks go first to Mette Thomassen at the Department of Biological and Medical Psychology, University of Bergen, Norway, for assisting in all stages of the editorial process, and Hilde Gundersen for assistance with the proofreading. Second, we would like to thank the staff at MIT Press, who have helped and advised us throughout the editorial process.

I Animal Models/Basic Functions

1   Hemispheric Asymmetry in the Visual System of Birds

Onur Güntürkün

The quest for the biological foundations of functional cerebral asymmetries has dominated lateralization research since the days of Broca (1865). Meanwhile, several anatomical asymmetries correlating with certain lateralized functions have been described in man. However, our knowledge of the ontogenetic variables that shape these structural asymmetries is still limited to an important extent (Previc, 1991). Likewise, we have few clues to how these asymmetries are translated into the lateralized functioning of a whole brain. Animal models can provide a powerful tool to permit detailed insights into the neuronal processes governing lateralized function. Avian visual lateralization is a particularly useful model because it not only allows experimental investigation of the interplay of neurobiological substrate and behavioral functions, but also provides an opportunity to study the ontogenetic events leading to asymmetries. Therefore the main emphasis of the following account is threefold. First, the behavioral framework of visual lateralization will be recapitulated in various species of birds. Then, the neuronal substrate of visual asymmetry will be outlined. Finally, the ontogentic scenario that ultimately results in a lateralized functional architecture will be described. The picture emerging from this overview will show that visual asymmetries in birds develop due to a tight interplay of genetic and epigenetic factors that finally, during a short critical period, mold ascending visual pathways into a lateralized status. Once the neuronal substrate is wired in this lateralized fashion, perceptual, cognitive, and motor systems start to function asymmetrically for the rest of the individual's lifetime.

VISUAL LATERALIZATION IN BIRDS—A BEHAVIORAL ANALYSIS

Tasks Favoring the Left Hemisphere

Birds are the most visually dependent class of vertebrates, and the statement of Rochon-Duvigneaud (1943) that a pigeon is nothing but two eyes with wings is probably valid for most avian species. Man, a highly visual primate, sees the world with the information transmitted by about 1 million fibers within each optic nerve. This is only 40% of the number of retinal axons counted in a single optic nerve of pigeons and chicks (Binggeli & Paule, 1969; Rager & Rager, 1978). The acuity of many birds of prey surpasses that of other living beings (Fox et al., 1976), and even the unspecialized pigeon excels relative to humans in its ability to discriminate luminances (Hodos et al., 1985) and to discern subtle color differences (Emmerton & Delius, 1980). However, the most important advantage of the avian model for asymmetry research is not its visual specialization, but the ease with which each hemisphere can be tested virtually separately. The optic nerves in birds decussate nearly completely, and only less than 0.1% of the fibers proceed to the ipsilateral side (Weidner et al., 1985). Since only limited numbers of axons recross via mesencephalic and thalamic commissures, the avian visual system is remarkably crossed.

This anatomical condition enables the use of eyecaps to study the performance of the animals with sight restricted to one eye, and thus mainly the contralateral hemisphere. With this procedure, visual lateralization can be demonstrated using a wide range of techniques. Using the right eye, adult pigeons are superior in discriminating two-dimensional artificial patterns (Güntürkün, 1985) and three-dimensional natural objects (Güntürkün & Kesch, 1987). These results are very similar to experiments with zebra finches (Alonso, 1998) and with chicks tested with the pebble-floor task. Here, young chicks peck food grains from a background of small pebbles that are stuck to the floor. The animals usually learn to discriminate food from pebbles within 60 pecks. Under either left- or right-eye learning conditions, their performance is higher with the right eye/left hemisphere (Hambley & Rogers, 1979; Mench & Andrew, 1986). In pigeons this greater visual processing capacity of the right eye system in pattern discrimination also leads to a higher degree of illusion of this side when being confronted with geometrical optic illusions (Güntürkün, 1997b).

All experiments summarized up to now employed a positive and a negative stimulus that had to be distinguished. A new aspect of avian visual lateralization emerges if more than two stimuli are used to induce a memory load. In a visual memory task pigeons learned under binocular conditions to discriminate between 100 negative (S−) and 625 positive (S+) artificial patterns. The stimuli had been randomly assigned to these two categories (figure 1.1). After reaching criterion, the birds were tested alternately with their left or right eye seeing. The pigeons were able to remember most of the 725 patterns with their right eye, but were barely above chance level with their left (Fersen & Güntürkün, 1990). This experiment suggests that visual engrams learned during training were stored, at least in part, unilaterally in the dominant left hemisphere, although both eyes had equal access to the patterns during acquisition.

Indeed, the existence of such unilateral memory stores with limited access by the other hemisphere could be shown in another complex task in which pigeons had to distinguish symmetric from asymmetric patterns. In this study they faced two vertically arranged pecking keys on which the same patterns were displayed. If these two identical patterns were symmetric, the animals had to peck the lower key; if they were asymmetric, the upper key was correct. Pigeons needed about five months to learn this conjunction of stimulus class and location. Up to that point they did not wear eyecaps. Then they were to proceed with the left or the right eye open, alternately. This new condition revealed that most animals had learned the task with their right eye/left hemisphere. The other side was completely naive, and in some birds needed an additional five months to catch up with the "knowing" hemisphere (Güntürkün, 1997a). This experiment is a very dramatic demonstration of unilaterality of engrams.

Such unilateral storage is not restricted to pigeons but has also been demonstrated, albeit for shorter time spans, with chicks (Gaston & Gaston, 1984), macaques (Doty et al., 1973), and even humans (Risse & Gazzaniga, 1978). Thus, it is likely that the avian left hemisphere stores large amounts of acquired pattern information to which the right hemisphere has only limited access.

It is probably this asymmetry in memorizing visual stimuli that results in a significant right eye advantage when homing from a distant release site over known territory to the loft (Ulrich et al., 1999). Homing makes great demands on spatial orientation. To find a left hemisphere

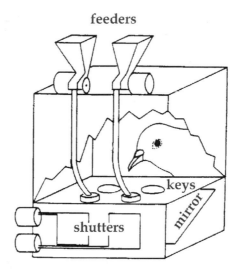

feeders

keys

mirror

shutters

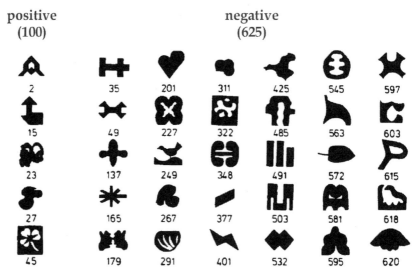

positive
(100)

negative
(625)

2	35	201	311	425	545	597
15	49	227	322	485	563	603
23	137	249	348	491	572	615
27	165	267	377	503	581	618
45	179	291	401	532	595	620

Figure 1.1 Setup and some of the stimuli used in the study of Fersen and Güntürkün (1990). Two out of 725 stimuli (100 positive [S+], 625 negative [S−]) were backprojected onto the vertical pecking keys with S+ and S− randomly changing between left and right. (Adapted from Fersen & Güntürkün, 1990.)

advantage during homing is therefore astonishing, considering the large body of data showing a right hemisphere dominance for visuospatial tasks. However, spatial orientation is a multicomponent feature in which several cognitive processes with diverse cerebral asymmetries interact (Hellige, 1995). It is therefore conceivable that the pigeons used a cognitive strategy that is more left-hemisphere based. As discussed by Ulrich et al. (1999), it is likely that the birds utilized visual memory-based snapshot tracking to pursue visual features along their pre-learned route. Due to their left-hemisphere dominance for memorizing and discriminating visual features, the homing task was therefore probably performed by a succession of visual feature discriminations. If pigeons are tested in a maze where they cannot utilize this strategy, the left hemisphere advantage vanishes (Prior & Güntürkün, 2001).

Visual lateralization also affects cognitive processes of the animals. Diekamp et al. (1999) tested pigeons under monocular conditions in successive color reversals. The animals learned to favor green (S+) over red (S−) until reaching learning criterion. Then the conditions were changed; red was now rewarded (S+) and green was not (S−). As soon as the pigeons successfully learned the reversal, conditions were altered again, and so on. One group of animals performed 30 reversals under right-eye-seeing, and the other group under left-eye-seeing, conditions. After a couple of reversals both groups showed a "learning-to-learn" effect such that each reversal was achieved with fewer trials. Reversal learning can be described best on a mathematical basis by an exponential function of the type $y = a + \exp^{(b-cx)}$ with a representing the asymptote (i.e., the error rate around which the performance oscillates after several reversals), b determining the starting value of the function for the first reversal, and c representing the steepness of the curve (i.e., the rate of error reduction over successive reversals). For both a and c, Diekamp et al. (1999) could reveal a right eye superiority. Thus, using the right eye/left hemisphere, the animals were faster in understanding the basic principle of this experiment (c) and exhibited a higher level of performance after reaching asymptote (a). Visual lateralization in birds, therefore, not only consists of asymmetries in simple pattern recognition and memorization processes, but also affects "cognitive" systems that extract general properties of the visual world.

The behavioral asymmetry summarized in these studies is very likely not due to simple psychophysical differences between the eyes (but see Hart et al., 2000, in starlings), but involves differences in "higher" functions that affect hemisphere-specific performances in cognitively demanding tasks. This conclusion is supported by studies showing no left-right differences in purely psychophysical tasks: There are no asymmetries in acuity (Güntürkün & Hahmann, 1994), in depth resolution (Martinoya et al., 1988), or in wavelength discrimination (Remy & Emmerton, 1991). That visual lateralization is generated by central mechanisms is additionally shown by experiments revealing asymmetrical effects of unilateral lesions or pharmaceutical insults of the left or the right hemisphere (Howard et al., 1980; Güntürkün & Hoferichter, 1985; Güntürkün & Hahmann, 1999; Deng & Rogers, 1998a).

Interim Summary   When distinct features of visual objects have to be identified, memorized, and/or categorized, a right eye/left hemisphere dominance arises in all avian species studied up to now (Andrew, 1991). This right eye superiority is valid for the majority of individuals of a population (65–79%, Güntürkün, 1997b; Güntürkün et al., 2000), indicating a clear population asymmetry.

Tasks Favoring the Right Hemisphere

None of the avian hemispheres completely dominates visual analysis, but cerebral asymmetries are organized in complementary specializations for different kinds of stimuli within the visual scenery. If birds have to encode spatial configurations, a left eye/right hemisphere superiority can be demonstrated (but see the discussion above for homing data from Ulrich et al., 1999). This was clearly shown by Rashid and Andrew (1989). They trained chicks to find food buried under sawdust in an arena. When the chicks were tested monocularly without food, birds under monocular left conditions searched from posthatch day 9 onward in the two areas specified by cues, while chicks in the monocular right condition searched randomly over the complete arena.

The lateralized role of different spatial and nonspatial cues can be beautifully studied in food-storing birds during cache localization. Marsh tits store food in large numbers of caches scattered over the home range that they can retrieve many days later with astounding accuracy (Shettleworth, 1990). It is possible to study lateralization of food storing and cache retrieval under controlled conditions, using a room with artificial trees, perches, and small holes for caching. In one of these studies (Clayton & Krebs, 1994) four feeders were used that were distinguishable by their specific location and by markings that made them visually unique. Under monocular conditions birds were given parts of a nut in one out of four feeders and were then removed for 5 min. During this interval the location of the correct feeder was swapped with an empty one so that spatial and object cues could be dissociated. Then the animals reentered and were allowed to retrieve the rest of the nut with the same eyecap condition. With the left eye, marsh tits looked for the seed at the correct spatial location, while they relied on object-specific cues when using the right eye. Thus, the right hemisphere used spatial cues, while the left half of the brain utilized object cues to locate the nut.

Vallortigara and colleagues were able to design a variety of ingenious tasks that demonstrate a similar pattern of results in chicks. In one of these experiments (Vallortigara, 2000; Tommasi & Vallortigara, 2001), chicks were trained to find food under sawdust by scratching ground in the center of a square arena. The position of the food was indicated by its geometric position (arena center) and by a conspicuous landmark, which also was placed centrally (figure 1.2). After learning attainment, the landmark was displaced to a novel position so as to generate conflicting local (the landmark) and global (the center of the arena) information. Chicks viewing with their left eye (right hemisphere) still searched in the center, completely ignoring the new location of the landmark. Right-eye chicks (left hemisphere) did exactly the opposite, searching close to the landmark and ignoring the global spatial information provided by the environment. Binocular-seeing chicks were mainly relying on right hemisphere mechanisms and scratched in the arena's center. Thus, different species of birds utilize left hemisphere mechanisms if relying on object cues and right hemisphere functions if using spatial cues. Chicks also scrutinize the stimuli mainly with their right eye when object-specific cues are to be used, but look mainly with their left eye when spatial cues have to utilized (Vallortigara et al., 1996).

Besides spatial tasks, visually guided social recognition also seems to be a domain of the right hemisphere. If chicks have to choose in a runway between a cagemate and an unfamiliar chick, male animals decide for the stranger, while females take the cagemate (Vallortigara & Andrew, 1994). Under monocular conditions these sex-dependent choice patterns persist when using the left eye, whereas the animals behave at random when using the right (Vallortigara, 1992). This has also been shown with the social pecking test, which takes advantage of

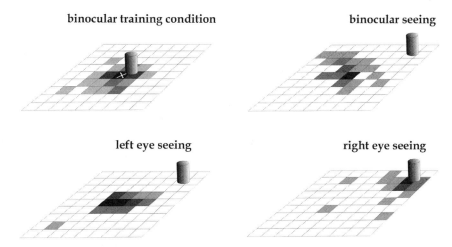

binocular training condition   binocular seeing

left eye seeing   right eye seeing

Figure 1.2 Search behavior of chicks trained to find food in the center of a square arena next to a conspicuous object. The upper left picture depicts areas of searching intensity under binocular conditions after initial training. The darker the areas, the more often the chicks searched under sawdust. The other three pictures show the results after displacement of the landmark to a novel position, inducing a conflict between geometry-based and object-based spatial codings. After landmark displacement, chicks were tested under binocular, left-eye, and right-eye seeing conditions. Right and left hemispheres seem to code for geometry- and object-specific cues, respectively. (Adapted from Vallortigara, 2000.)

the marked xenophobia exhibited by young socially reared chicks toward unfamiliar conspecifics, which become the target of aggressive pecking bouts. If young chicks wearing eyecaps are confronted with both a familar and an unfamiliar bird, they mainly peck the stranger when viewing with the left eye, while their aggressive encounters against the other two animals are random under monocular right conditions (Vallortigara, 1992). These data indicate that right hemisphere processes are of prime importance for social recognition. Up to now this has been demonstrated only in preference tests where it is up to the animal to behave in a certain way. Whether the results of these preference tests will reveal the same data pattern as in forced discrimination studies is presently an open question.

Interim Summary When birds have to locate food in a complex environment, they rely on object-specific cues when seeing with the right eye and on geometric information when seeing with the left. In preference tests it can be shown that visually guided social recognition also seems to be a right hemisphere domain. However, it is at present unclear how the pattern of right hemisphere dominances for social recognition and the previously reviewed data on a left hemisphere superiority in visual feature categorization can be matched, since a social companion first has to be recognized as a visual object, which is a typical left hemisphere task. It is conceivable that social cues are rich in emotional (Vallortigara & Andrew, 1994) or movement information, and thus may be treated differently from static visual cues (Dittrich & Lea, 1993).

ANATOMICAL SUBSTRATES FOR VISUAL LATERALIZATION

In birds, retinal information to the forebrain is processed by two parallel pathways: the tectofugal system and the thalamofugal system, suggested to be equivalent to the extrageniculo-cortical and the geniculo-cortical visual pathways of mammals, respectively (Shimizu & Karten, 1993). The avian tectofugal pathway is composed of optic nerve fibers projecting to the contralateral optic tectum, from which fibers lead bilaterally to the thalamic n. rotundus (Rt) and n. triangularis (T), which themselves project to the ipsilateral ectostriatum (E) of the forebrain (figure 1.3). The thalamofugal pathway projects from the retina via the contralateral n. geniculatus lateralis, pars dorsalis (GLd) bilaterally to the visual Wulst in the telencephalon (see figure 1.5) (Güntürkün, 2000). The tectofugal and thalamofugal pathways have been shown to constitute structural asymmetries related to lateralized visual behavior in pigeons and chicks, respectively.

The Tectofugal Pathway

In the asymmetry experiments with pigeons, the stimuli fell into the frontal binocular visual field of the animals. Since this portion of the visual field is mainly represented within the tectofugal pathway in pigeons (Hellmann & Güntürkün, 1999; Güntürkün & Hahmann, 1999), it is conceivable that it is mainly the tectofugal system which generates visual lateralization in this species (figure 1.3).

About 90% of all retinal ganglion cells project to the tectum in pigeons (Remy & Güntürkün, 1991). The optic tectum is a highly complex neural entity in which even simple histological techniques visualize

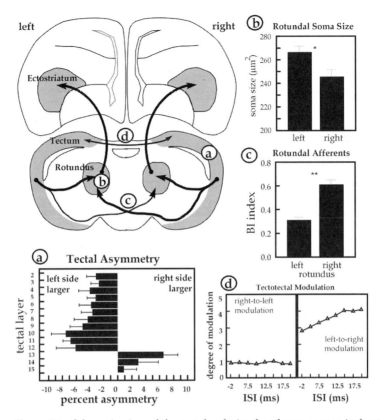

Figure 1.3 Schematic view of the tectofugal visual pathway as seen in frontal sections. Letters within the figure indicate areas or connections for which asymmetries were described. (*a*) Morphological asymmetries of neuronal somata in different tectal layers. Layer 1 is not shown because it consists of fibers. Left or right skews of histograms depict larger somata on the left or right tectal side for this layer, respectively. Note consistent left skews in layers 2–12, which are mostly visual. (Based on Güntürkün, 1997c.) (*b*) Average soma size of rotundal neurons on the left or the right side. (Based on Manns & Güntürkün, 1999b.) (*c*) Bilaterality of rotundal afferents from the ipsilateral and the contralateral tectum. An index of 0 decribes absolute symmetry, while 1 constitutes a system that is characterized by ipsilateral afferents only. The significant difference in the bilaterality index points to a larger proportion of contralateral tectal afferents in the left rotundus. (Based on Güntürkün et al., 1998.) (*d*) Asymmetries of tectotectal modulation. Electrical stimulation of the right tectum was unable to substantially modulate the amplitude of a visual evoked potential recorded within the left tectum (right-to-left modulation), regardless of different interstimulus intervals (ISI). However, electrical stimulation of the visually dominant left tectum resulted in much higher modulations of visually evoked potentials within the right tectum (left-to-right modulation). (Based on Keysers et al., 2000.)

15 laminae (Ramón y Cajal, 1911). In pigeons, a morphometric study of tectal perikarya sizes revealed morphological asymmetries with the superficially located retinorecipient cells being larger on the left side, contralateral to the dominant eye (Güntürkün, 1997c). This is also the case for the n. rotundus, the next tectofugal entity (Manns & Güntürkün, 1999b). Thus, the pigeon's tectofugal system displays significant morphological asymmetries that might be related to the behavioral lateralization of the animals.

Tectal lamina 13 neurons project bilaterally onto the n. rotundus (Hellmann & Güntürkün, 1999). The bilaterality of this projection should lead to representations of both the ipsi- and the contralateral eye in the tectofugal system of each hemisphere. Indeed, Engelage and Bischof (1993) were able to show that binocular input is represented in the ectostriatum. In pigeons, Güntürkün et al. (1998) demonstrated with anterograde and retrograde tracers that the ratio of ipsi- to contralateral tectorotundal projections is asymmetrically composed. While the number of ipsilateral tectorotundal projections is about equal, the number of neurons projecting contralaterally from the right tectum to the left rotundus is about twice the number in the opposite direction (Güntürkün et al., 1998). As a result, the n. rotundus on the left side receives, beside a massive ipsilateral tectal input, a large number of afferents from the contralateral tectum. Consequently, the visual input of the n. rotundus that projects to the left hemisphere is bilaterally organized to a significantly higher degree than its counterpart in the right halfbrain. Functionally, this anatomical condition could enable the left rotundus to integrate and process visual inputs from both eyes, and thus from both sides of the bird's visual world. Indeed, a study has shown that left rotundal processes are significantly related to acuity performance with the right and the left eye, whereas right rotundus participates only in binocular acuity (Güntürkün & Hahmann, 1999).

These data on the tectofugal system suggest that visual asymmetry is anatomically wired, and thus probably "static" and unmodifiable over the lifetime. However, several lines of evidence suggest this assumption is incomplete. If the tectal and the posterior commissures, which connect the tecta of both hemispheres, are transsected, visual lateralization reverses to a left eye dominance; this laterality reversal is proportional to the number of transsected fibers (Güntürkün & Böhringer, 1987) (figure 1.4). If hemispheric asymmetry is reversed by tectal commissurotomy, it is likely that this asymmetry was maintained pre-

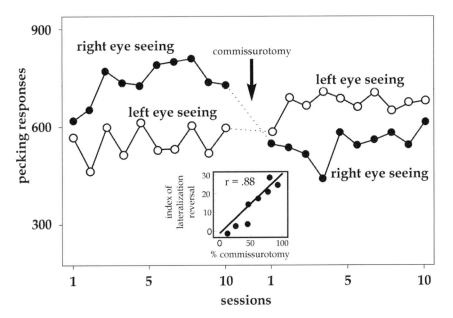

Figure 1.4 Lateralization reversal after tectal commissurotomy in pigeons. Pigeons performed a pattern discrimination with right eye or left eye seeing. Preoperatively, significantly more pecks on the correct pattern were made with the right eye seeing; this lateralization changed after commissurotomy. The inset shows that the degree of asymmetry change, as expressed with an index, was significantly related to the extent of the commissurotomy. (Based on Güntürkün & Böhringer, 1987.)

viously, at least partly, by asymmetrical interactions between the tecta (see also Parsons & Rogers, 1993) that are known to be primarily inhibitory (Robert & Cuénod, 1969; Hardy et al., 1984). Keysers et al. (2000) tested this hypothesis by recording field potentials from left or right intratectal electrodes in response to a stroboscope flash to the contralateral eye and an electrical stimulation of the contralateral tectum. They found that the left tectum was able to modulate the flash-evoked potential of the right tectum to a larger extent than vice versa. This lateralized interhemispheric cross talk thus could constitute an important "dynamic" component of asymmetric visual processing (figure 1.3).

This result makes it likely that the emergence of visual asymmetry in pigeons is related to a dual coding of left-right differences. Thus, visual lateralization cannot be explained entirely by the anatomical differences between left and right components of the tectofugal pathway. Obviously a second, more dynamic component exists that is able to modulate neural processes of the optic tecta in an asymmetrical manner. Altering this second dynamic component, as in the commissurotomy experiment of Güntürkün and Böhringer (1987), results in an important alteration of visual asymmetry.

Interim Summary   The pigeon's tectofugal pathway displays numerous morphological asymmetries that are probably related to the visual lateralization at the behavioral level. On the left side of the brain, which dominates object recognition mechanisms, soma sizes of most visual cells are larger. In addition, the left n. rotundus integrates input from both eyes to a greater extent than the right rotundus. In addition to these structural left-right differences, the tecta inhibit each other differently, with the left tectum modulating visual processes of the contralateral side to a greater degree than vice versa. Thus, visual asymmetry within the tectofugal pathway is dually coded by structural and by dynamic properties.

The Thalamofugal Pathway

At first glance the general organization of the thalamofugal pathway seems to be similar in pigeons and chicks. However, in contrast to pigeons (Hodos et al., 1984), thalamofugal lesions affect frontal viewing in chicks importantly (Deng & Rogers, 1997). This suggests that, unlike pigeons, the frontal field is represented within the thalamofugal system in chicks. But this is not the only difference between chicks and pigeons. As will be outlined below, the organization of tecto- and thalamofugal pathways also seems to be different with respect to asymmetry in chicks and pigeons.

   With unilateral injections of retrograde tracers into the Wulst label cells in the GLd of both sides (figure 1.5), the ratio of contralaterally to ipsilaterally labeled GLd neurons is higher after right-sided than after left-sided Wulst injections in 2-day-old chicks (Rogers & Sink, 1988). As shown by Rogers and Deng (1998), this lateralized ratio difference is due to a higher number of fibers from the left thalamus to the contralateral right forebrain than vice versa. The asymmetry of the crossed thalamotelencephalic projection is pronounced in young males but disappears at about three weeks of age, consistent with the behavioral

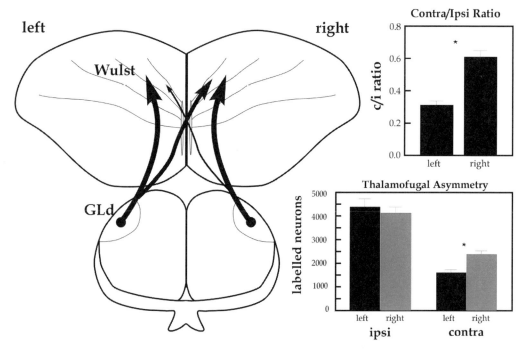

Figure 1.5 Schematic view of the chick's thalamofugal visual pathway in frontal sections. The crossed projections from the left nucleus geniculatus lateralis pars dorsalis (GLd) to the right Wulst are more numerous than vice versa. The upper right histogram shows that the ratio of contralateral to ipsilateral fibers (c/i ratio) is significantly higher in the right Wulst. The lower right histograms depict that this asymmetry is mainly due to the number of contralateral afferents to the Wulst. (Based on Rogers & Deng, 1999.)

data on lateralized performance in the pebble-floor task (Adret & Rogers, 1989; Rogers, 1996). The asymmetry of the contralateral thalamofugal projections of female chicks is lower, but present and in the same direction as in males (Rajendra & Rogers, 1993). This sex difference in the degree of this connectional asymmetry could be an explanation for the gender difference in lateralized performance, which is more pronounced in male chicks (Zappia & Rogers, 1987).

The sex difference in visual asymmetry of chicks indicates a role of steroids. Indeed, injections of 17β-estradiol (E_2) in unhatched male embryos increases the number of forebrain-projecting GLd neurons and thus abolishes thalamofugal asymmetry, probably due to a ceiling effect (Rogers & Rajendra, 1993). Thus, the reduced behavioral asymmetry in females (Zappia & Rogers, 1987) might be due to their higher levels of circulating estradiol during a sensitive period and the subsequent increase in the number of GLd relay cells, which overshadow the projectional asymmetry observed in males. Injection of testosterone also reduces structural asymmetry in the thalamofugal projection in females and even reverses the thalamofugal asymmetry of males (Schwarz & Rogers, 1992). The reversal in male chicks is accompanied by a reversal of eye dominance in visual discrimination (Zappia & Rogers, 1987). Thus, the development of visual lateralization in chicks is fundamentally influenced by circulating sex steroids.

Interim Summary   The thalamofugal pathway of chicks was shown to be asymmetrically organized with respect to the contralaterally ascending thalamotelencephalic components. Changes in the degree of this asymmetry correlate with alterations of visual lateralization. This pattern is sex-dependent, with males having more pronounced left-right differences.

Species Differences in Asymmetrical Organization of Visual Pathways

Since visual lateralization in pigeons and chicks is similar at the behavioral level, a comparable organization of their neural asymmetries would be expected. Studies, however, have shown this not to be the case. While the thalamofugal pathway of pigeons is "frontally blind" (Remy & Güntürkün, 1991), there is strong evidence in chicks that this pathway receives input from the frontal visual field (Wilson, 1980; Deng & Rogers, 1997). Therefore, at the level of the retinothalamic projections, the thalamofugal system already seems to be organized differently in these two species.

A further point of divergence is the asymmetrical projections within the thalamo- and the tectofugal systems. In pigeons, the number of projections from the right tectum to the left rotundus is larger than from the left tectum to the right rotundus (Güntürkün et al., 1998). This condition creates a higher degree of bilateral representation in the left tectofugal pathway, which is functionally dominant for object discriminations (Güntürkün & Hahmann, 1999). The case is different with chicks, in which no asymmetry can be found in the overall tectorotundal projections (Deng & Rogers, 1998b; Rogers & Deng, 1999). Thus, the organization of the tectofugal pathway differs markedly in chicks and pigeons.

The same applies to the thalamofugal pathway. While in chicks there is a significantly higher number of contralateral fibers from the left GLd to the right Wulst (Rogers & Deng, 1999), a comparable asymmetry is absent in pigeons (Hellmann et al., in preparation). These species differences in asymmetry are accompanied by differences in the detailed composition of ascending projections: In pigeons the crossed projection from the GLd onto the contralateral Wulst is constituted by a large number of bilaterally projecting neurons (Miceli et al., 1990). In chicks, however, ipsi- and contralaterally projecting GLD cells come from different neuronal populations (Deng & Rogers, 1998a). In addition, the asymmetry of the thalamofugal system is sex-different in chicks (Rogers & Rajendra, 1993), while in pigeons there is, at least at the behavioral level, no evidence for a sex dependency of visual asymmetry (Güntürkün & Kischkel, 1992).

These differences between chicks and pigeons could reflect a simple species effect in the anatomy of the ascending systems. However, it is also possible that they result from age differences, since the data have been collected from adult pigeons and young chicks. In fact, age is known to affect the thalamofugal projections, with GLd-Wulst asymmetries disappearing by the time the animals are three weeks old (Rogers & Sink, 1988). Therefore, the species effect might arise due to the differences between the developmental speed of chicks and pigeons. Chicks are precocial animals that are active directly after hatch. Consequently, both visual systems seem to be functional at hatch in chicks (Mey & Thanos, 1992). This is remarkably different in the altricial pigeon, where the embryonic visual pathways are far less functional. There is evidence that retinotectal projections become functional shortly before hatch (Manns & Güntürkün, 1997), but the animals hatch with their lids closed and are initially unable to perform complex visuomotor behaviors. Up to now any information on the maturation of the thalamofugal system is lacking in pigeons. Since prehatch light input is of decisive importance for the maturation of the ascending visual pathways (see below), it is conceivable that the species differences between chicks and pigeons are triggered by their different maturational speed.

Interim Summary Although seemingly similar, visual lateralization in chicks and pigeons is generated by different visual systems. In both animals the contralateral components of the ascending projections are asymmetrically organized, with the thalamofugal and the tectofugal systems being the critical pathways in chicks and pigeons, respectively. These differences in neuronal wiring might be due to the maturational speed being slower in pigeons than in chicks. This could generate species-specific differences of the ontogenetic conditions that affect the developing visual systems of chicks and pigeons.

Asymmetries of Associative Forebrain Structures: Imprinting

The important role of left hemispheric forebrain structures becomes especially evident when using stimuli for which chicks have a predisposition, as in imprinting studies. When young chicks are exposed to a visually conspicuous object, they approach it, learn its characteristics, and form a social attachment to it. In natural conditions the object is usually the hen, but it need not to be; a wide range of objects will do, though some are more effective than others. Given a choice between a stimulus to which it was exposed and a different object, a chick will prefer the training stimulus and will actively avoid the other one.

Evidence from autoradiographic and lesion studies suggests that the intermediate part of the hyperstriatum ventrale (IMHV), an associative forebrain structure, is part of a memory system in which the representation of the imprinting stimulus is at least partly stored (Horn, 1991). The IMHV partly overlaps with the more ventrally located mediorostral neostriatum/hyperstriatum ventrale (MNH), which is especially involved in processing auditory imprinting stimuli (Bredenkötter & Braun, 2000). Neurons in the left and right IMHV are active during imprinting learning, as judged by the number of neurons expressing Fos-like immunoreactivity about 1 h after the end of training, and expression of this protein increases with the strength of learning (McCabe & Horn, 1994). At about 60 min after imprinting, however, the changes that can be detected in the right IMHV diverge from those in the left. The protein kinase C mediated phosphorylation of proteins that have the capacity to contribute to synaptic plasticity increases in left IMHV (Meberg et al., 1996). Consequently, strongly imprinted animals develop, on the average, 10% larger postsynaptic densities in the left IMHV than in the right, with the values of the right IMHV not being different from controls (Bradley et al., 1981). The amount of binding to NMDA receptors in the left, but not in the right, IMHV correlates significantly with the behavioral preference scores of the chicks for the imprinting stimulus (McCabe et al., 1982). Since morphological changes are a prerequisite for long-term synaptic plasticity, Solomonia et al. (1997, 1998) studied clathrin proteins and neural cell adhesion molecules (N-CAMs), which are both involved in synaptic remodeling. They found higher amounts of clathrin and N-CAM in the left IMHV 24 h after learning, with both clathrin and N-CAM amounts correlating with learning strength of imprinting.

Bilateral IMHV lesions impair imprinting but have no effect on visual associative learning in general (Johnson & Horn, 1986). These lesions also impair sexual imprinting, so that lesioned adult females no longer show clear preferences for males that are selected by control females (Bolhuis et al., 1989). The neurobiological differences between left and right IMHV suggests that the two hemispheres participate differently in the imprinting process. Indeed, studies in which the IMHV of the left and the right side were lesioned sequentially support this assumption. These experiments suggest that the left IMHV is important for the first acquisition and also can act as long-term store. The right IMHV acts as a buffer store, passing information out to further, probably distributed, long-term stores over a period of about 6 h (Horn & Johnson, 1989). Due to this sequence of processes, a chick that receives a left IMHV lesion 3 h after imprinting, followed 26 h later by lesioning of the right IMHV, can recall the memory on retest because in this case the engram could successfully be transferred to structures outside the IMHV (Cipolla-Neto et al., 1982).

Thus, both IMHVs contribute to imprinting (Johnston & Rogers, 1998), albeit with functional differences. These differences are reflected in the single unit properties of left and right IMHV neurons. About 30% of cells within this structure respond highly selectively to the familiar imprinting object, irrespective of left or right (Brown & Horn, 1994; Nicol et al., 1995). The difference between the hemispheres seems not to be related to the training stimulus but to the stimuli that were *not* used for imprinting training. While for the left IMHV, training results in an increase of cells responding to the training stimulus without affecting responses to the other stimuli (Brown & Horn, 1994), the same increase occurs in the right IMHV, but is associated with a decrease in sites responding to the alternative stimuli (Nicol et al., 1995). These alterations should result in an overall higher signal-to-noise ratio in the right IMHV. Taking these single unit data into account, Nicol et al. (1995) assume that the lack of ultrastructural and molecular changes observed in the right IMHV after imprinting is not due to an absence of changes, but to the presence of two contrary events, one increasing synaptic efficiency for the trained stimulus, and one decreasing efficiency for the untrained stimulus. Obviously the simpler changes in the left IMHV suffice for recognition in the context of imprinting tests of animals with right IMHV lesions. However, these chicks are unable to utilize the training stimulus as an S+ in subsequent visual discrimination tasks (Honey et al., 1995). Only chicks with an elaborate representation in different forebrain areas manage this transfer, and the differentiated alterations in right IMHV synaptic structure seem to be a prerequisite for the formation of a distributed memory store with widespread effects for the adult animal.

Interim Summary Young chicks very quickly form an attachment to a conspicuous object. This imprinting learning requires the forebrain IMHV to be intact. Left and right IMHV contribute differently to this learning process. While the left IMHV seems to be essential during initial learning, the right IMHV is essential to induce processes that subsequently stabilize and elaborate the imprinting engram.

Asymmetries of Associative Forebrain Structures: One-Trial Avoidance Learning

Young chicks peck spontaneously at small, conspicuous objects, and thus learn to discriminate between unpleasant and tasty items. If they are confronted with a small, bright bead coated with the bitter-tasting substance methylanthranilate (MeA), their pecking behavior is followed by an intense disgust response. Subsequent tests with the same bead lead to avoidance. This highly discrete passive avoidance learning (PAL) is accompanied by a number of lateralized events in the forebrain.

If chicks acquire PAL under binocular conditions with a bead of a certain color and are subsequently tested monocularly, they avoid all beads, irrespective of their color, with the left eye, but are selective for the color used during training with their right eye (Andrew, 1988). Thus, it is conceivable that the more specific memory trace has been laid down in the left hemisphere. This assumption is supported by 2-[^{14}C] deoxyglucose (2-DG) experiments which demonstrate that 2-DG injected shortly before training leads to higher radioactivity scores in the left IMHV and the left lobus parolfactorius (LPO) (Rose & Csillag, 1985). The early phase of memory consolidation involves a cascade of synaptic events that seem to hold the trace briefly and simultaneously initiate the gene activation processes required for long-term memory (Rose, 1995). In brief, these steps first require an increased glutamate receptor binding in the left, but not the right, IMHV (Stewart et al., 1992); a concomitant upregulation of NMDA (Steele et al., 1995); then a pre- and postsynaptic Ca^{2+} flux (Salinska et al., 1999). The increased opening of Ca^{2+} channels, combined with further molecular events, leads to an activation of the immediate early genes c-fos and c-jun (Anokhin & Rose, 1991), which probably initiate pre- and postsynaptic structure alterations.

These asymmetric morphological alterations are generally more pronounced in the left IMHV and have been analyzed at the ultrastructural level. Some of these lateralized changes show up within the first hour after PAL: the number of synapses per volume neuropil are significantly larger in the left but not in the right IMHV after training; similarly, posttraining vesicles per synapse are about 60% more numerous in the left IMHV (Stewart et al., 1984). Some other asymmetries exist before training, but are subsequently abolished or even reversed: The number of synaptic vesicles per volume neuropil are larger on the right in control animals, while this asymmetry is reversed after PAL (Stewart et al., 1984). These synaptic changes are accompanied by a reversal in the number of dendritic spines on large multipolar projection neurons. These were found to be more numerous in the right IMHV of unlearned animals, but subsequent to training there was an increase in number on the left such that this hemispheric asymmetry disappeared (Patel et al., 1988a,b).

Morphological changes after PAL are not restricted to the IMHV, but are also observed in the LPO and the paleostriatum augmentatum (PA), two structures that correspond to the dorsal corpus striatum of mammals. While the initial acquisition of memory involved largely transient changes in the spatial organization of synapses in the left IMHV, longer-term changes are more prominent in the LPO and involve a bilateral, albeit predominantly left-sided, increase in synaptic density and height (Stewart & Rusakov, 1995; Rose & Stewart, 1999).

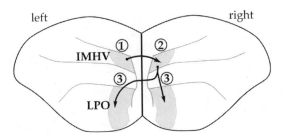

Figure 1.6 Schematic frontal section through the forebrain of a chick showing the position of the intermediate medial hyperstriatum ventrale (IMHV) and the lobus parolfactorius (LPO). According to the "memory flow" model of Rose (1991), the engram for passive avoidance learning is first held in the left IMHV (1), then moves to the right IMHV (2), and then is further transmitted to the LPO of both hemispheres (3).

Lesion studies demonstrated asymmetric effects of unilateral IMHV and LPO lesions, and in addition support a model in which the memory trace after training is not fixed to a certain area but "flows" from one structure to the other (Rose, 1991; figure 1.6). The presence of an intact left IMHV seems to be a necessity for a long-term acquisition of PAL, and consequently pretraining lesions of this area make the animals amnesic shortly after the learning session. However, if the animals have learned the task and the left IMHV is lesioned 1 h after training, the chick is not amnesic (Patterson et al., 1990). The engram seems to have left the IMHV of the left hemisphere for yet another store, and it is likely that this second store is the right IMHV, followed, within about an hour, by the third store, which is LPO (Gilbert et al., 1991). It is yet to be determined what this "flow" actually is. Probably the engrams are not translocated from one store to another, but memory consolidation or mechanisms of retrieval require different forebrain areas to be activated successively.

Interim Summary After a single exposure, chicks learn to avoid pecking a bead with a bitter substance. IMHV, the forebrain structure that is of prime importance for imprinting, also seems to be essential for this kind of one-trial avoidance learning. The first and most prominent cellular changes after the first peck seem to occur in the left IMHV, but the right IMHV and, most important, both sides of the LPO (parts of the basal ganglia) are subsequently involved. Thus, the trace seems to "flow" from one area to the next in a lateralized fashion.

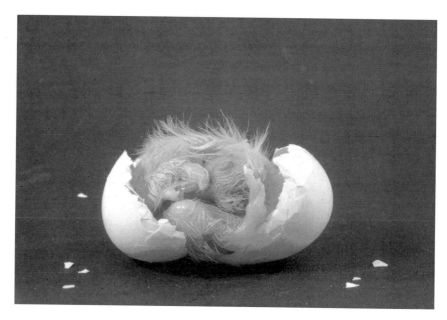

Figure 1.7 A pigeon embryo during hatching. Note the position of the head, which is bent forward and points to the right. The right wingbud rests on the beak.

THE DEVELOPMENT OF AVIAN VISUAL LATERALIZATION

Embryos of virtually all avian species keep the head turned so that the right eye is exposed to light shining through the translucent shell while the left eye is occluded by the body (Kuo, 1932) (figure 1.7). Since brooding parents regularly turn their eggs and often leave their nests for short time periods, the embryo's right eye has a high probability of being stimulated by light before hatching. Thus, it is conceivable that asymmetry of light stimulation is the key event leading to visual lateralization. Indeed, dark incubation of chick and pigeon eggs prevents the establishment of visual lateralization in grain-grit discriminations (Rogers, 1982; Güntürkün, 1993), and a mere 2 h of light exposure with 400 lux within the last days before hatch suffices to establish visual lateralization in dark-incubated chicken eggs (Rogers, 1982). It is even possible to reverse the direction of the behavioral and the thalamofugal asymmetry by withdrawing the head of the chicken embryo from the egg before hatch, occluding the right eye and exposing the left to light (Rogers & Sink, 1988; Rogers, 1990).

Since pigeons are altricial animals, the developmental plasticity of their visual pathways is prolonged and extends far into posthatching time (Manns & Güntürkün, 1997). Therefore, covering the right eye of newly hatched pigeons for 10 days reverses the anatomical asymmetry of tectal soma sizes and the behavioral visual lateralization of these animals as tested up to three years later (Manns & Güntürkün, 1999a). Thus, light stimulation asymmetry during a critical ontogenetic time span seems to be the trigger for visual asymmetry in pigeons, as it is in chicks.

In principle, these results are in accordance with findings from monocular deprivation studies in mammals. These experiments reported smaller soma sizes of neurons receiving afferents from the deprived eye (Sherman & Spear, 1982). This is similar to pigeons, where the right retinorecipient tectal neurons contralateral to the eye with the "natural monocular deprivation" are smaller.

However, different mechanisms must be involved. Morphological soma size effects of monocular deprivation in mammals are regarded as secondary consequences of synaptic competition at the cortical level between geniculate fibers representing the deprived eye and the nondeprived eye (Rauschecker, 1991). However, a detailed analysis in pigeons shows that "natural monocular deprivation" effects also occur in those neural structures in which a comparable competition is absent (Güntürkün, 2001). This suggests that visual deprivation effects in birds are mediated through activity-correlated, and eventually trophic, deprivation effects within one hemisphere, and that they possibly operate without direct synaptic competition between neurons representing the deprived eye and the nondeprived eye.

In addition, only the unilateral absence of contoured visual patterns induces significant deprivation effects in the mammalian geniculocortical system. Asymmetries of luminance alone do not lead to alterations (Movshon & Van Sluyters, 1981). This supports the assumption that fiber competition is mediated by a Hebbian mechanism which requires correlated activity of pre- and postsynaptic cells for stabilization or retraction of synapses (Rauschecker, 1991). In chicks and pigeons, the situation must be different, since light has to shine through the eggshell and the closed lid of the embryo to induce cerebral asymmetries. Therefore, avian asymmetry triggered by "natural monocular deprivation" has to be induced by brightness and not by contoured visual pattern differences. Brightness differences are probably coded by mere activity differences between the eyes, and could induce asymmetries by activity-dependent cellular effects.

Prehatch light stimulation asymmetry seems to be the *conditio sine qua non* to induce visual lateralization of object discrimination. It is, however, not essential for other forms of visually guided behavior. Dark-incubated chicks have functional asymmetries in imprinting (Johnston & Rogers, 1998) and display biochemical left-right differences in IMHV (Johnston et al., 1995). These asymmetries can, however, be altered by a lateralized light input (Johnston et al., 1997; Johnston & Rogers, 1999). Therefore, for some asymmetries (visual discriminations) a lateralized light input is critical to induce neural left-right differences. In other lateralizations (imprinting), asymmetries are prewired but can be altered by a biased light input.

ASYMMETRY PAYS

This overview has shown that visual lateralization in birds depends on an interaction of genetic factors that induce a torsion of the embryo's head to the right and the epigenetic factor light that subsequently induces higher levels of activity in the right eye system. As a consequence, neuronal systems are altered during a critical developmental period in a lateralized way such that multiple aspects of visually guided behavior of the animals are asymmetrically organized. Is all this *l'art pour l'art*, an epiphenomenon without costs but also without benefits for the animal? Or does visual lateralization pay? To seek an answer, Güntürkün et al. (2000) determined the individual asymmetry index of 108 pigeons by separately analyzing their left- and right-eye performances in grain-grit discrimination. Then the animals were tested on the same task binocularly, and their discrimination success was correlated with their asymmetry index. Animals with higher asymmetries were significantly more successful in discriminating grain from grit. This means that a rise in asymmetry resulted in a concomitant rise of food reward (figure 1.8). Thus, asymmetry pays.

LESSONS FROM THE AVIAN BRAIN

Birds heavily rely on vision. If asymmetry pays, it is understandable that it is their visual system which is lateralized. Likewise, it is possible that asymmetries of language or manual skills improve human performance. According to the studies on avian lateralization, it might even be conceivable that these and other human asymmetries emerge during

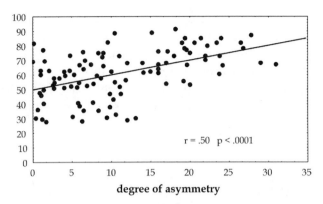

Figure 1.8 Relationship between the degree of lateralization and binocular discrimination performance. Pearson's product moment correlation (scatter plot) reveals higher performance in more lateralized individuals. (Adapted from Güntürkün et al., 2000.)

ontogeny due to subtle left-right differences that in the beginning affect only subcortical mechanisms.

Indeed, as shown by Hepper et al. (1991), fetuses from 15 weeks of gestational age to term have a strong lateralized bias of thumb sucking on the right side. The corticospinal tract cannot mediate this asymmetry because it reaches cervical to thoracic segments much later and even at term is myelinated only as far caudally as the cerebral peduncles (Stanfield, 1992). Even in the adult the rubrospinal tract reaches only as far as the uppermost cervical segments, and the olivospinal pathway known from studies in rats seems not to exist in man (Nathan & Smith, 1982). The lateral subcorticospinal pathway, which encompasses a variety of descending tracts crucial for distal limb and hand movements, myelinates only at 28–34 weeks of gestational age (Sarnat, 1984). Thus, thumb sucking in the early fetus is mediated virtually only by spinal mechanisms without relay through cortical relays (Sarnat, 1989). In addition, asymmetrical gene expression mechanisms in early neuro-ontogeny result in a slight torsion of the embryo with the forehead turning to the right (Ramsdell & Yost, 1998).

This last point is probably common to all vertebrates, and could result in a higher probability of mouth-hand contacts on the right side. The rightward spinal torsion could also be the reason why most newborns still have a preference for a right turn of their head when in a supine position (Michel, 1981)—a preference that correlates with subsequent handedness (Michel & Harkins, 1986). Therefore, a lateralization of hand-mouth and hand-eye contacts in humans probably depends on spinal asymmetries. If they are manifested in early neuro-ontogeny, they may bias the processing mode of cortical structures that later connect to those motoneurons which innervate the hands and which are known to be significantly larger on the right side (Melsbach et al., 1996). Therefore, the initial bias for handedness might start subcortically, then be controlled much later by cortical structures. Thus, at least some human asymmetries might display a developmental pattern comparable with that outlined for birds.

CONCLUSIONS

1. In birds, visual information is treated in a lateralized fashion. While object discrimination is left-hemisphere based, geometrical aspects of spatial encoding and social recognition are primarily processed in the right hemisphere.

2. This visual lateralization is also reflected in tasks, like imprinting and one-trial-avoidance learning, in which the animal very quickly forms a mental trace of the visual characteristics of a biologically relevant object.

3. The lateralized behavior corresponds to asymmetries in the morphology and connectivity of the ascending visual pathways. These anatomical asymmetries can vary between species. Thus, seemingly similar asymmetries of behavior can be generated by different lateralized neural systems.

4. At least in pigeons, visual lateralization seems to be dually coded; anatomically, by morphological and connectional differences of ascending visual pathways, and physiologically, by asymmetrical commissural interactions that result in a lateralized modulation of visual processing.

5. In the last days before hatching, avian embryos bend forward and keep their head turned to the right in such a way that the right eye is exposed to light which is shining through the translucent eggshell, while the left eye is occluded by the body. Ontogenetically, visual lateralization of object discriminations is triggered by the subsequently stronger light input to the right eye. This lateralized stimulation induces asymmetrical morphological effects within the developing visual system, and thereby establishes left-right differences at the behavioral level.

6. Birds with higher visual asymmetries are superior in visual discriminations. Thus, asymmetry increases efficiency of processing within the visual system.

REFERENCES

Adret, P., & Rogers, L. J. (1989). Sex difference in the visual projections of young chicks: A quantitative study of the thalamofugal pathway. *Brain Research, 478,* 59–73.

Alonso, Y. (1998). Lateralization of visual guided behaviour during feeding in zebra finches (*Taeniopygia guttata*). *Behavioural Processes, 43,* 257–263.

Andrew, R. J. (1988). The development of visual lateralization in the domestic chick. *Behavioural Brain Research, 29,* 201–209.

Andrew, R. J. (1991). The nature of behavioural lateralization in the chick. In R. J. Andrew (Ed.), *Neural and Behavioural Plasticity* (pp. 536–554). Oxford: Oxford University Press.

Anokhin, K. V., & Rose, S. P. R. (1991). Learning-induced increase of immediate early gene messenger RNA in the chick forebrain. *European Journal of Neuroscience, 3,* 162–167.

Binggeli, R. L., & Paule, W. J. (1969). The pigeon retina: Quantitative aspects of the optic nerve and ganglion cell layer. *Journal of Comparative Neurology, 137,* 1–18.

Bolhuis, J., Johnson, M., Horn, G., & Bateson, P. (1989). Long-lasting effects of IMHV lesions on social preferences in domestic fowl. *Behavioral Neuroscience, 103,* 438–441.

Bradley, P. M., Horn, G., & Bateson, P. (1981). Imprinting: An electron microscopic study of chick hyperstriatum ventrale. *Experimental Brain Research, 41,* 115–120.

Bredenkötter, M., & Braun, K. (2000). Development of neuronal responsiveness in the mediorostral neostriatum/hyperstriatum ventrale during auditory filial imprinting in domestic chicks. *Neurobiology of Learning and Memory, 73,* 114–126.

Broca, P. (1865). Sur le siège de la faculté du langage articulé. *Bulletin de la Société de Anthropologie* (Paris), *6,* 377–393.

Brown, M. W., & Horn, G. (1994). Learning-related alterations in the visual responsiveness of neurons in a memory system of the chick. *European Journal of Neuroscience, 6,* 1479–1490.

Cipolla-Neto, J., Horn, G., & McCabe, B. J. (1982). Hemispheric asymmetry and imprinting: The effect of sequential lesions to the hyperstriatum ventrale. *Experimental Brain Research, 48,* 22–27.

Clayton, N. S., & Krebs, J. R. (1994). Memory for spatial and object-specific cues in food-storing and non-storing birds. *Journal of Comparative Physiology A, 174,* 371–379.

Deng, C., & Rogers, L. J. (1997). Differential contributions of the two visual pathways to functional lateralization in chicks. *Behavioural Brain Research, 87,* 173–182.

Deng, C., & Rogers, L. J. (1998a). Bilaterally projecting neurons in the two visual pathways of chicks. *Brain Research, 794*, 281–290.

Deng, C., & Rogers, L. J. (1998b). Organisation of the tectorotundal and SP/IPS-rotundal projections in the chick. *Journal of Comparative Neurology, 394*, 171–185.

Diekamp, B., Prior, H., & Güntürkün, O. (1999). Lateralization of serial color reversal learning in pigeons (*Columba livia*). *Animal Cognition, 2*, 187–196.

Dittrich, W. H., & Lea, S. E. G. (1993). Motion as a natural category for pigeons: Generalization and a feature-positive effect. *Journal of Experimental Analysis of Behaviour, 59*, 115–129.

Doty, R. W., Negrao, N., & Yamaga, K. (1973). The unilateral engram. *Acta Neurobiologica Experimentalis, 33*, 711–728.

Emmerton, J., & Delius, J. D. (1980). Wavelength discrimination in the "visible" and ultraviolet spectrum by pigeons. *Journal of Comparative Physiology, 141*, 47–52.

Engelage, J., & Bischof, H. J. (1993). The organization of the tectofugal pathway in birds: A comparative review. In H. P. Zeigler & H.-J. Bischof (Eds.), *Vision, brain, and behavior in birds* (pp. 137–158). Cambridge, Mass.: MIT Press.

Fersen, L., & Güntürkün, O. (1990). Visual memory lateralization in pigeons. *Neuropsychologia, 28*, 1–7.

Fox, R., Lehmkuhle, S. W., & Westendorf, D. H. (1976). Falcon visual acuity. *Science, 192*, 263–265.

Gaston, K. E., & Gaston, M. G. (1984). Unilateral memory after binocular discrimination training: Left hemisphere dominance in the chick. *Brain Research, 303*, 190–193.

Gilbert, D. B., Patterson, T. A., & Rose, S. P. R. (1991). Dissociation of brain sites necessary for registration and storage of memory for a one-trial passive avoidance task in the chick. *Behavioral Neuroscience, 105*, 553–561.

Güntürkün, O. (1985). Lateralization of visually controlled behavior in pigeons. *Physiology and Behavior, 34*, 575–577.

Güntürkün, O. (1993). The ontogeny of visual lateralization in pigeons. *German Journal of Psychology, 17*, 276–287.

Güntürkün, O. (1997a). Avian visual lateralization—a review. *NeuroReport, 6*, iii–xi.

Güntürkün, O. (1997b). Visual lateralization in birds: From neurotrophins to cognition? *European Journal of Morphology, 35*, 290–302.

Güntürkün, O. (1997c). Morphological asymmetries of the tectum opticum in the pigeon. *Experimental Brain Research, 116*, 561–566.

Güntürkün, O. (2000). Sensory physiology: Vision. In G. C. Whittow (Ed.), *Sturkie's avian physiology* (pp. 1–19). Orlando, Fla.: Academic Press.

Güntürkün, O. (in press). Ontogeny of visual asymmetry in pigeons. In L. J. Rogers & R. Andrew (Eds.), *Lateralization, learning and memory*. Cambridge, U.K.: Cambridge University Press.

Güntürkün, O., & Böhringer, P. G. (1987). Reversal of visual lateralization after midbrain commissurotomy in pigeons. *Brain Research, 408*, 1–5.

Güntürkün, O., Diekamp, B., Manns, M., Nottelmann, F., Prior, H., Schwarz, A., & Skiba, M. (2000). Asymmetry pays: Visual lateralization improves discrimination success in pigeons. *Current Biology, 10*, 1079–1081.

Güntürkün, O., & Hahmann, U. (1994). Visual acuity and hemispheric asymmetries in pigeons. *Behavioural Brain Research, 60*, 171–175.

Güntürkün, O., & Hahmann, U. (1999). Functional subdivisions of the ascending visual pathways in the pigeon. *Behavioural Brain Research, 98*, 193–201.

Güntürkün, O., Hellmann, B., Melsbach, G., & Prior, H. (1998). Asymmetries of representation in the visual system of pigeons. *NeuroReport, 9*, 4127–4130.

Güntürkün, O., & Hoferichter, H. H. (1985). Neglect after section of a left telencephalo-tectal tract in the pigeon. *Behavioural Brain Research, 18*, 1–9.

Güntürkün, O., & Kesch, S. (1987). Visual lateralization during feeding in pigeons. *Behavioral Neuroscience, 101*, 433–435.

Güntürkün, O., & Kischkel, K. F. (1992). Is visual lateralization sex-dependent in pigeons? *Behavioural Brain Research, 47*, 83–87.

Hambley, J. W., & Rogers, L. J. (1979). Retarded learning induced by intracerebral administration of amino acids in the neonatal chick. *Neuroscience, 4*, 677–684.

Hardy, O., Leresche, N., & Jassik-Gerschenfeld, D. (1984). Postsynaptic potentials in neurons of the pigeon's optic tectum in response to afferent stimulation from the retina and other visual structures. *Brain Research, 311*, 65–74.

Hart, N. S., Partridge, J. C., & Cuthill, I. C. (2000). Retinal asymmetry in birds. *Current Biology, 10*, 115–117.

Hellige, J. B. (1995). Hemispheric asymmetry for components of visual information processing. In R. J. Davidson & K. Hugdahl (Eds.), *Brain asymmetry* (pp. 99–121). Cambridge, Mass.: MIT Press.

Hellmann, B., & Güntürkün, O. (1999). Visual field specific heterogeneity within the tectofugal projection of the pigeon. *European Journal of Neuroscience, 11*, 1–18.

Hepper, P. G., Shahidullah, S., & White, R. (1991). Handedness in the human fetus. *Neuropsychologia, 29*, 1107–1111.

Hodos, W., Bessette, B. B., Macko, K. A., & Weiss, S. R. B. (1985). Normative data for pigeon vision. *Vision Research, 25*, 1525–1527.

Hodos, W., Macko, K. A., & Bessette, B. B. (1984). Near-field acuity changes after visual system lesions in pigeons. II. Telencephalon. *Behavioural Brain Research, 13*, 15–30.

Honey, R. C., Horn, G., Bateson, P., & Walpole, M. (1995). Functionally distinct memories for imprinting stimuli: Behavioral and neural dissociations. *Behavioral Neuroscience, 109*, 689–698.

Horn, G. (1991). Imprinting and recognition memory: A review of neural mechanisms. In R. J. Andrews (Ed.), *Neural and behavioural plasticity* (pp. 219–261). Oxford: Oxford University Press.

Horn, G., & Johnson, M. H. (1989). Memory systems in the chick: Dissociations and neuronal analysis. *Neuropsychologia, 27,* 1–22.

Howard, K. J., Rogers L. J., & Boura, A. L. A. (1980). Functional lateralisation of the chicken forebrain revealed by use of intracranial glutamate treatment. *Brain Research, 188,* 369–382.

Johnson, M. H., & Horn, G. (1986). Dissociation of recognition memory and associative learning by a restricted lesion of the chick forebrain. *Neuropsychologia, 24,* 329–340.

Johnston, A. N. B., Bourne, R. C., Stewart, M. G., Rogers, L. J., & Rose, S. P. R. (1997). Exposure to light prior to hatching induces asymmetry of receptor binding in specific regions of the chick forebrain. *Developmental Brain Research, 103,* 83–90.

Johnston, A. N. B., & Rogers, L. J. (1998). Right hemisphere involvement in imprinting memory revealed by glutamate treatment. *Pharmacology, Biochemistry and Behavior, 60,* 863–871.

Johnston, A. N. B., & Rogers, L. J. (1999). Light exposure of chick embryo influences lateralized recall of imprinting memory. *Behavioral Neuroscience, 113,* 1267–1273.

Johnston, A. N. B., Rogers, L. J., & Dodd, P. R. (1995). [3H]MK-801 binding asymmetry in the IMHV region of dark-reared chicks is reversed by imprinting. *Brain Research Bulletin, 37,* 5–8.

Keysers, C., Diekamp, B., & Güntürkün, O. (2000). Evidence for asymmetries in the phasic intertectal interactions in the pigeon (*Columba livia*) and their potential role in brain lateralisation. *Brain Research, 852,* 406–413.

Kuo, Z. Y. (1932). Ontogeny of embryonic behavior in aves. III. The structural and environmental factors in embryonic behavior. *Journal of Comparative Psychology, 13,* 245–271.

Manns, M., & Güntürkün, O. (1997). Development of the retinotectal system in the pigeon: A choleratoxin study. *Anatomy and Embryology, 195,* 539–555.

Manns, M., & Güntürkün, O. (1999a). Monocular deprivation alters the direction of functional and morphological asymmetries in the pigeon's visual system. *Behavioral Neuroscience, 113,* 1–10.

Manns, M., & Güntürkün, O. (1999b). "Natural" and artificial monocular deprivation effects on thalamic soma sizes in pigeons. *NeuroReport, 10,* 3223–3228.

Martinoya, C., Le Houezec, J., & Bloch, S. (1988). Depth resolution in the pigeon. *Journal of Comparative Physiology, 163,* 33–42.

McCabe, B. J., Cipolla-Neto, J., Horn, G., & Bateson, P. (1982). Amnestic effects of bilateral lesions placed in the hyperstriatum ventrale of the chick after imprinting. *Experimental Brain Research, 48,* 13–21.

McCabe, B. J., & Horn, G. (1994). Learning-related changes in Fos-like immunoreactivity in the chick forebrain after imprinting. *Proceedings of the National Academy of Sciences, USA, 91*, 11417–11421.

Meberg, P. J., McCabe, B. J., & Routtenberg, A. (1996). MARCKS and protein F1/GAP-43 mRNA in chick brain: Effects of imprinting. *Brain Research and Molecular Brain Research, 35*, 149–156.

Melsbach, G., Spiess, M., Wohlschläger, A., & Güntürkün, O. (1996). Morphological asymmetries of motoneurons innervating upper extremities—clues to the anatomical foundations of handedness? *International Journal of Neuroscience, 86*, 217–224.

Mench, J. A., & Andrew, R. J. (1986). Lateralization of a food search task in the domestic chick. *Behavioral and Neural Biology, 46*, 107–114.

Mey, J., & Thanos, S. (1992). Development of the visual system of the chick. A review. *Journal für Hirnforschung, 33*, 673–702.

Michel, G. F. (1981). Right-handedness. A consequence of infant supine head-orientation preference? *Science, 212*, 685–687.

Michel, G. F., & Harkins, D. A. (1986). Postural and lateral asymmetries in the ontogeny of handedness during infancy. *Developmental Psychobiology, 19*, 247–258.

Miceli, D., Marchand, L., Repérant, J., & Rio, J. P. (1990). Projections of the dorsolateral anterior complex and adjacent thalamic nuclei upon the visual Wulst in the pigeon. *Brain Research, 518*, 1–7.

Movshon, J. A., & Van Sluyters, R. C. (1981). Visual neural development. *Annual Review of Psychology, 32*, 477–522.

Nathan, P. W., & Smith, M. C. (1982). The rubrospinal and central tegmental tracts in man. *Brain, 105*, 233–269.

Nicol, A. U., Brown, M. W., & Horn, G. (1995). Neurophysiological investigations of a recognition memory system for imprinting in the domestic chick. *European Journal of Neuroscience, 7*, 766–776.

Parsons, C. H., & Rogers, L. J. (1993). Role of the tectal and posterior commissures in lateralization of the avian brain. *Behavioural Brain Research, 54*, 153–164.

Patel, S. N., Rose, S. P. R., & Stewart, M. G. (1988a). Training induced dendritic spine density changes are specifically related to memory formation processes in the chick, *Gallus domesticus. Brain Research, 463*, 168–173.

Patel, S. N., Rose, S. P. R., & Stewart, M. G. (1988b). Changes in the number and structure of dendritic spines 25 hours after passive avoidance training in the domestic chick, *Gallus domesticus. Brain Research, 449*, 34–46.

Patterson, T. A., Gilbert, D. B., & Rose, S. P. R. (1990). Pre- and post-training lesions of the intermediate medial hyperstriatum ventrale and passive avoidance learning in the chick. *Experimental Brain Research, 80*, 189–195.

Previc, F. H. (1991). A general theory concerning the prenatal origins of cerebral laterali-sation in humans. *Psychological Review, 98*, 299–334.

Prior, H., & Güntürkün, O. (2001). Parallel working memory for spatial location and object-cues in foraging pigeons. Binocular and lateralized monocular performance. *Learning and Memory, 8*, 44–51.

Rager, G., & Rager, U. (1978). Systems-matching by degeneration. I. A quantitative electron-microscopic study of the generation and degeneration of retinal ganglion cells in the chicken. *Experimental Brain Research, 33*, 65–78.

Rajendra, S., & Rogers, L. J. (1993). Asymmetry is present in the thalamofugal visual pro-jections of female chicks. *Experimental Brain Research, 92*, 542–544.

Ramón y Cajal, S. (1911). *Histologie du système nerveux de l'homme et des vertébrés.* Paris: Maloine.

Ramsdell, A. F., & Yost, H. J. (1998). Molecular mechanisms of vertebrate left-right de-velopment. *Trends in Genetics, 14*, 459–465.

Rashid, N., & Andrew, R. J. (1989). Right hemisphere advantage for topographic orienta-tion in the domestic chick. *Neuropsychologia, 27*, 937–948.

Rauschecker, J. P. (1991). Mechanisms of visual plasticity: Hebb synapses, NMDA recep-tors, and beyond. *Physiological Reviews, 71*, 587–613.

Remy, M., & Emmerton, J. (1991). Directional dependence of intraocular transfer of stim-ulus detection in pigeons (*Columba livia*). *Behavioral Neuroscience, 105*, 647–652.

Remy, M., & Güntürkün, O. (1991). Retinal afferents of the tectum opticum and the nu-cleus opticus principalis thalami in the pigeon. *Journal of Comparative Neurology, 305*, 57–70.

Risse, G. L., & Gazzaniga, M. S. (1978). Well-kept secrets of the right hemisphere: A ca-rotid amytal study of restricted memory transfer. *Neurology, 28*, 950–953.

Robert, F., & Cuénod, M. (1969). Electrophysiology of the intertectal commissures in the pigeon. II. Inhibitory interaction. *Experimental Brain Research, 9*, 123–136.

Rochon-Duvigneaud, A. (1943). *Les yeux et la vision des vertébrés.* Paris: Masson.

Rogers, L. (1996). Behavioral, structural and neurochemical asymmetries in the avian brain: A model system for studying visual development and processing. *Neuroscience and Biobehavioral Reviews, 20*, 487–503.

Rogers, L. J. (1982). Light experience and asymmetry of brain function in chickens. *Nature, 297*, 223–225.

Rogers, L. J. (1990). Light input and the reversal of functional lateralization in the chicken brain. *Behavioural Brain Research, 38*, 211–221.

Rogers, L. J., & Deng, C. (1998). Light experience and lateralization of the two visual pathways in the chick. *Behavioural Brain Research, 98*, 1–15.

Rogers, L. J., & Rajendra, S. (1993). Modulation of the development of light-initiated asymmetry in the chick thalamofugal visual projections by oestradiol. *Experimental Brain Research, 93*, 89–94.

Rogers, L. J., & Sink, H. S. (1988). Transient asymmetry in the projections of the rostral thalamus to the visual hyperstriatum of the chicken, and reversal of its direction by light exposure. *Experimental Brain Research, 70*, 378–384.

Rose, S. P. R. (1991). How chicks make memories: The cellular cascade from c-fos to dendritic remodelling. *Trends in Neuroscience, 14*, 390–397.

Rose, S. P. R. (1995). Cell adhesion molecules, glucocorticoids and memory. *Trends in Neuroscience, 18*, 502–506.

Rose, S. P. R., & Csillag, A. (1985). Passive avoidance training results in lasting changes in deoxyglucose metabolism in left hemisphere regions of chick brain. *Behavioural and Neural Biology, 44*, 315–324.

Rose, S. P. R., & Stewart, M. G. (1999). Cellular correlates of stages of memory formation in the chick following passive avoidance training. *Behavioural Brain Research, 98*, 237–243.

Salinska, E. J., Chaudhury, D., Bourne, R. C., & Rose, S. P. (1999). Passive avoidance training results in increased responsiveness of voltage- and ligand-gated calcium channels in chick brain synaptoneurosomes. *Neuroscience, 93*, 1507–1514.

Sarnat, H. B. (1984). Anatomic and physiologic correlates of neurologic development in prematurity. In H. B. Sarnat (Ed.), *Topics in neonatal neurology* (pp. 1–25). Orlando, Fla.: Grune and Stratton.

Sarnat, H. B. (1989). Do the corticospinal and corticobulbar tracts mediate functions in the human newborn? *Journal of Canadian Science and Neurology, 16*, 157–160.

Schwarz, I. M., & Rogers, L. J. (1992). Testosterone: A role in the development of brain asymmetry in the chick. *Neuroscience Letter, 146*, 167–170.

Sherman, S. M., & Spear, P. D. (1982). Organization of visual pathways in normal and visually deprived cats. *Physiological Reviews, 62*, 738–855.

Shettleworth, S. J. (1990). Spatial memory in food-storing birds. *Philosophical Transactions of the Royal Society of London, B329*, 143–151.

Shimizu, T., & Karten, H. J. (1993). The avian visual system and the evolution of the neocortex. In H. P. Zeigler & H.-J. Bischof (Eds.), *Vision, brain and behavior in birds* (pp. 103–114). Cambridge, Mass.: MIT Press.

Solomonia, R. O., McCabe, B. J., & Horn, G. (1998). Neural cell adhesion molecules, learning, and memory in the domestic chick. *Behavioral Neuroscience, 112*, 646–655.

Solomonia, R. O., McCabe, B. J., Jackson, A. P., & Horn, G. (1997). Clathrin proteins and recognition memory. *Neuroscience, 80*, 59–67.

Stanfield, B. B. (1992). The development of the corticospinal projection. *Progress in Neurobiology, 38*, 169–202.

Steele, R. J., Stewart, M. G., & Rose, S. P. (1995). Increases in NMDA receptor binding are specifically related to memory formation for a passive avoidance task in the chick: A quantitative autoradiographic study. *Brain Research, 674,* 352–356.

Stewart, M. G., Bourne, R. C., & Steele, R. J. (1992). Quantitative autoradiographic demonstration of changes to binding in NMDA sensitive ^{3}H-MK801, but not ^{3}H-AMPA receptors in chick forebrain 30 min after passive avoidance training. *European Journal of Neuroscience, 4,* 936–943.

Stewart, M. G., Rose, S. P. R., King, T. S., Gabbott, M., & Bourne, R. C. (1984). Hemispheric asymmetry of synapses in chick medial hyperstriatum ventrale following passive avoidance training: A stereological investigation. *Developmental Brain Research, 12,* 261–269.

Stewart, M. G., & Rusakov, D. A. (1995). Morphological changes associated with stages of memory formation in the chick following passive avoidance training. *Behavioural Brain Research, 66,* 21–28.

Tommasi, L., & Vallortigara, G. (2001). Encoding of geometric and landmark information in the left and right hemispheres of the avian brain. *Behavioral Neuroscience, 115,* 602–619.

Ulrich, C., Prior, H., Duka, T., Leshchins'ka, I., Valenti, P., Güntürkün, O., & Lipp, H.-P. (1999). Left-hemispheric superiority for visuospatial orientation in homing pigeons. *Behavioural Brain Research, 104,* 169–178.

Vallortigara, G. (1992). Right hemisphere advantage for social recognition in the chick. *Neuropsychologia, 30,* 761–768.

Vallortigara, G. (2000). Comparative neuropsychology of the dual brain: A stroll through animals' left and right perceptual worlds. *Brain and Language, 73,* 189–219.

Vallortigara, G., & Andrew, R. J. (1994). Differential involvement of right and left hemisphere in individual recognition in the domestic chick. *Behavioural Processes, 33,* 41–58.

Vallortigara, G., Regolin, L., Bortolomiol, G., & Tommasi, L. (1996). Lateral asymmetries due to preferences in eye use during visual discrimination learning in chicks. *Behavioural Brain Research, 74,* 135–143.

Weidner, C., Reperant, J., Miceli, D., Haby, M., & Rio, J. P. (1985). An anatomical study of ipsilateral retinal projections in the quail using autoradiographic, horseradish peroxidase, fluorescence and degeneration techniques. *Brain Research, 340,* 99–108.

Wilson, P. (1980). The organisation of the visual hyperstriatum in the domestic chick: I. Topology of the visual projections. *Brain Research, 188,* 319–332.

Zappia, J. V., & Rogers, L. J. (1987). Sex differences and reversal of brain asymmetry by testosterone in chickens. *Behavioural Brain Research, 23,* 261–267.

2   A Hippocampal Theory of Cerebral Lateralization

Akaysha C. Tang

A new theory of cerebral lateralization that centers on the role of the hippocampus and experience-dependent synaptic modification is proposed. In contrast to top-down cognitive approaches to cerebral lateralization (Kosslyn et al., 1989; van Kleek & Kosslyn, 1991), but similar in its conceptual framework to neural network models (Levitan & Reggia, 2000; Reggia et al., 1998; Shevtsova & Reggia, 1999), this theory takes a bottom-up, learning-based (Rumelhart et al., 1986) approach. It builds upon findings at the level of neurons and synapses, and their modulation by neurochemicals. It considers the influence of experience or learning on the development of cerebral asymmetry (Denenberg, 1981; Kosslyn, 1987), and attempts to bring the hippocampus—a more primitive cortical structure and an extensively studied brain region (Amaral & Witter, 1995; Johnston & Amaral, 1998)—into the foreground of cerebral lateralization.

The chapter is conceptually divided into two parts. The first part discusses findings and ideas that led to the conception of the hippocampal theory of cerebral lateralization. Key components of the theory will be developed through these findings. Because the goal of this chapter is to develop a new conceptual framework, I will emphasize potential relations among seemingly unrelated or loosely related areas instead of providing extensive reviews of each of the component areas. Thus, regrettably, many important works in each of the areas will not be discussed. To compensate for the selectivity, references for reviews are given.

The second part focuses on behavioral, neuroanatomical, and neurophysiological data collected in my own laboratory to offer support for a subset of the hypotheses that constitute the hippocampal theory of cerebral lateralization. Specifically, I will present results demonstrating that exposing neonatal rats to a novel environment can lead to long-term changes in the symmetry of the hippocampus, and that the nature of the change is an increase in the right hippocampal dominance manifested in the size of the structure, its synaptic plasticity, and the modulation of this plasticity by the stress hormone corticosterone. Finally, I will present behavioral data from a rodent "handedness" study to demonstrate that the same neonatal novelty manipulation which led to an increase in the right hippocampal dominance also leads to an increase in left-paw dominance. The opposite direction of shift in this peripherally and centrally measured asymmetry is consistent with a hippocampal contribution to lateralization of cerebral function.

EXPERIENCE-DEPENDENT MODIFICATION OF BRAIN ASYMMETRY: A COMPUTATIONAL FRAMEWORK

It has been known for some time that cerebral lateralization is sensitive not only to asymmetric sensory stimulation or damage from lesions (Rogers, 1982; Whishaw & Kolb, 1988), but also to apparently unbiased stimulations, such as neonatal handling and prenatal maternal stress (Anderson et al., 1986; Denenberg et al., 1978; Fitch et al., 1993; A. Tang & Verstynen, 2002). The first evidence came from a cortical lesion study in rats in which the effects of left and right unilateral lesions on open field activity were measured (Denenberg et al., 1978). Left and right cortical lesions produced different effects, but only for the rats that had experienced the neonatal handling treatment (Denenberg, 1964; Levine, 1957). This "handling" treatment consisted of three components: separation of the pup from the dam and its litter mates, exposure to a novel cage, and handling by the experimenter during the transfer between the home and novel cages. The treatment typically lasts 3–10 min per day for the first 3 postnatal weeks. This seemingly unbiased early life stimulation altered patterns of brain asymmetry indexed by a lesion effect on behavioral activity (Denenberg et al., 1978). More recently, asymmetric effect on auditory processing (Fitch et al., 1993) and on "handedness" (A. Tang & Verstynen, 2002) in rodents have been found, using similar methods of neonatal stimulation.

Such demonstrations of experience-dependent asymmetry beg the question of how and where the seemingly unbiased early life experience could be encoded in the brain to allow behavioral manifestations of functional asymmetry. In the following text, I will adopt a neural network approach (Rumelhart et al., 1986) providing a minimal conceptual framework in which experience, learning, and cerebral dominance are discussed. The brain is considered as a network of interconnected neurons that receive inputs from various sensory organs. In such a model, the connection strengths among the neurons, or the synaptic strength of the neurons, is modified by experience through two classes of learning rules. Under the unsupervised learning rules (Hebbian learning rules), the connection strengths between two neurons increase with their simultaneous activations. Under the supervised learning rules, error feedback is used to adjust the connection strength. A combination of both learning rules can be used. Given this simple model of the brain, the development of cerebral lateralization can be viewed as the development of dominance in neuronal activations and synaptic connections within a bilaterally symmetric neural network. To understand the development of cerebral dominance is to understand how patterns of dominance develop through appropriate modification in sets of synaptic connections.

Using this general framework, Reggia et al. (1998) studied functional lateralization in a neural network that learned to generate sequences of phonemes using supervised learning rules. In this model, learning leads to lateralization under a variety of parameter conditions. Having a larger size, a higher neuronal excitability, or a higher learning rate (plasticity) in one of the two "hemispheres" readily leads to lateralization. Many of the network behaviors are best interpreted as a result of a "race to learn" between the model's two hemispheres. It is suggested that besides larger size and higher neuronal excitability, asymmetric hemispheric plasticity is one of the critical causative factors in lateralization. Functional lateralization was also studied within the context of letter identification, using a combination of supervised and unsupervised learning rules (Shevtsova & Reggia, 1999), and within the context of cortical map formation, using unsupervised learning rules (Levitan & Reggia, 2000). Although the choice of learning rules under which each of the three factors influencing lateralization differed, the size of the hemisphere, neuronal excitability, and synaptic plasticity remain the major factors affecting lateralization. These findings offer insight into potential mechanisms that mediate the development of cerebral lateralization. They also make theoretical predictions about how lateralization of function and lateralization of various cellular mechanisms are related.

NEUROCHEMICALS AS SOURCES OF CEREBRAL LATERALIZATION

A critical dimension that remains unexplored in the neural network models of lateralization is the function of the neuromodulators and hormones. Neuromodulators and hormones are known to influence neuronal excitability and synaptic plasticity (de Kloet et al., 1999; Hasselmo, 1995; Joels & de Kloet, 1992; Kaczmarek & Levitan, 1987; Marder, 1998; McEwen & Sapolsky, 1995) and to alter the effective connectivity of the neural network (Hasselmo & Bower, 1993; Marder et al., 1996). Because lateralization of a function corresponds to a particular pattern of neuronal activation and connectivity, neuromodulators and hormones can play a crucial role in the formation of such patterns, thus influencing the development of cerebral lateralization.

Several properties make neurochemicals potential *sources*, or driving forces, for the development of lateralization and for transiently modulating patterns of lateralization. The first property is their ability to enhance or inhibit neuronal activation in major cortical structures. These structures include the neocortex subserving various higher-level cognitive functions, and the hippocampus, a structure critical for acquiring new declarative memory and spatial and nonspatial relational learning (Eichenbaum, 1997; O'Keefe & Nadel, 1978; Squire, 1982, 1992; Sutherland & Rudy, 1987). When combined with activity-dependent synaptic modification, this property allows the neurochemical to influence long-term reorganization of the cortical networks necessary for functional lateralization.

The second property of neurochemicals is that they are a part of an evolutionarily more primitive system. This property maximizes the chance that the source for initiating the lateralization process can function under a wide range of biological conditions and in diverse species. Because functional lateralization is widely distributed phylogenetically (Hiscock & Kinsbourne, 1995), the fact that sources of lateralization are part of the primitive system provides for a more parsimonious unifying theory of lateralization.

The third property of neurochemicals is their asymmetric distribution in terms of their concentration or of their receptor distributions. Asymmetric distributions of neuromodulators and hormones have been found in both human and animals (Tucker & Williamson, 1984; Wittling, 1995). These asymmetries are typically measured as asymmetric control of release (e.g., Sullivan & Gratton, 1999; Wittling & Pfluger, 1990) or asymmetric receptor distributions between the two hemispheres (e.g., Barneoud et al., 1990; Oke et al. 1978). In contrast, the asymmetry in the stress hormone corticosterone observed in my own laboratory is a *functional* asymmetry, measured by corticosterone's dynamic effect on hippocampal synaptic plasticity. This neurochemical asymmetry can serve as a powerful source to drive asymmetric neuronal activation and asymmetric synaptic modification.

The final property of neurochemicals is their diffuse influence over many regions throughout the entire hemisphere despite their rather focal origin. For example, cholinergic innervation of the hippocampus and neocortex is provided by clusters of cholinergic neurons in the medial septum and nucleus basalis, respectively; noradrenergic inputs to the hippocampus and neocortex originate from the locus caeruleus; serotonergic inputs, from the rapheal nuclei; and dopaminergic inputs, from the ventral tegmental areas (figure 2.1c). This property is particularly important when one considers the problem of how to genetically code for multiple functional expressions in cerebral lateralization.

Barneoud and Vanderloos (1993) bred left- and right-pawed mice and found that the paw preference could be predicted by a genetically expressed structural asymmetry in a sensory system, the whisker-to-barrel pathway. In their speculation regarding a possible connection between the "whiskeredness" and "handedness," they suggested that the two asymmetries are associated either through links at the level of a neural circuit between the two sensory pathways or through two linked gene sets, one for each asymmetry. Because of their diffuse influence, asymmetric neuromodulatory inputs can provide such links not only between the sensory systems underlying "whiskeredness" and "handedness" but also among other systems of asymmetry. Nature may take advantage of this diffuse influence by using only a few gene sets to code modulatory asymmetries and let these asymmetries interact with environmental factors in creating the ultimate functional asymmetry.

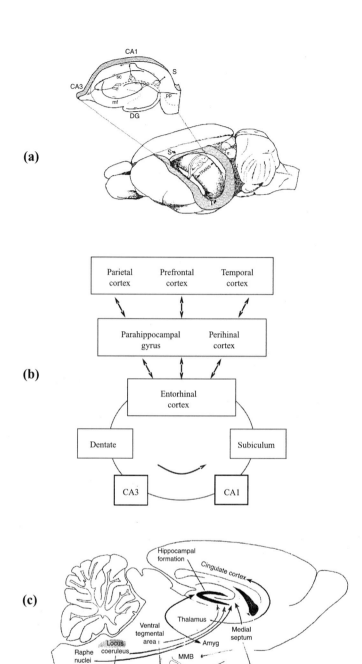

Akaysha C. Tang

HIPPOCAMPUS AS A CANDIDATE FOR EXPERIENCE-DEPENDENT LATERALIZATION

Because many of the highly lateralized functions, such as language and spatial processing, do not exist at birth, in order to understand the adult form of their lateralization, one must consider the process via which new experience can be encoded. The hippocampus (figure 2.1a), one of the most extensively studied brain regions of the mammalian central nervous system (Amaral & Witter, 1995; Johnston & Amaral, 1998), is an ideal candidate for such experience-dependent modification because of its critical role in learning and memory (O'Keefe & Nadel, 1978; Squire, 1982, 1992). Although theories differ in precisely how the hippocampus contributes to the process of memory consolidation (Eichenbaum, 1996; Morgan & Squire, 1990; Squire & Alvarez, 1995; Sutherland & Rudy, 1987; Sutherland et al., 2001; Wallenstein et al., 1998), the essential and definitive role in memory consolidation is undisputed—destruction of the hippocampus prevents the formation of new declarative memory.

A great deal of what is known today concerning experience-dependent synaptic plasticity (Bliss & Collingridge, 1993; Malenka & Nicoll, 1999; Martin et al., 2000) was derived from studies of long-term potentiation (LTP), a form of synaptic plasticity in subregions of the hippocampus (figure 2.1a). The relationship between synaptic plasticity and memory, a central issue in neuroscience (Barnes, 1995; Malenka & Nicoll, 1999; Martin et al., 2000; Stevens, 1996, 1998), has been explored mainly in the hippocampus, using genetic (Aiba et al., 1994; Y. Tang et al., 1999; Tsien et al., 1996) and environmental (Duffy et al., 2001; van Praag et al., 1999) manipulations that affected both LTP and learning, and through a demonstration that LTP induction affected subsequent learning (Barnes et al., 1994; Moser et al., 1998).

Figure 2.1 The hippocampus and its relation to the neocortex. (*a*) The location of the hippocampus in the rat and the typical brain slice preparation for in vitro electrophysiological studies. (Reprinted from Amaral & Witter, 1989.) (*b*) The anatomical connections between the hippocampus and other cortical areas. (Reprinted from Rolls, 2000.) The backprojections from the hippocampus allow the hippocampus to influence neuronal excitability, synaptic transmission, and plasticity between the hippocampus and neocortex and among the neocortical regions. By assuming a relatively faster rate of synaptic modification within the hippocampus than within the neocortex, a hippocampal-cortical model of memory consolidation accounts for a wide range of existing experimental and clinical data. (*c*) The hippocampus receives multiple neuromodulatory inputs.

In recent years the neuroanatomical connections between the hippocampal formation and the neocortex have received a great deal of attention (O'Mara, 2000). As shown in figure 2.1b, the hippocampus assumes a central position in integrating sensory inputs from various sensory cortices and polymodal association cortex, including the frontal cortex (Lavenex & Amaral, 2000; Rolls, 2000; Thierry et al., 2000). Currently, dominating theories for memory consolidation consider these hippocampal-cortical connections to be a central mechanism that accounts for a wide range of experimental and clinical data (McClelland et al., 1995; Nadel et al., 2000; Squire, 1992). Computational models of memory consolidation (McClelland et al., 1995; O'Reilly, 1998; O'Reilly & Rudy, 2000; Squire & Alvarez, 1995) place additional emphasis on properties of synaptic plasticity among and between hippocampal and cortical neurons. The importance of hippocampal-cortical interactions has also been emphasized in the study of asymmetric limbic regulation of cognition (Liotti & Tucker, 1995).

These hippocampal-cortical connections suggest that asymmetry in the hippocampal neuronal activity may directly influence the formation of synaptic connections among cortical neurons, thus affecting the development of cortical functional asymmetry in sensory (Hellige, 1995; Hugdahl, 1995) and emotional (Davidson, 1995) processing. A recent functional brain imaging study revealed significant correlations between the left hippocampal volume and recall of verbal information, and between the right hippocampal volume and recall of spatial locations (de Toledo-Morrell et al., 2000). These correlations are consistent with the notion that the left and right hippocampi can each modulate its corresponding neocortices that subserve the higher-level cognitive functions.

While the hippocampal-cortical connections allow the hippocampus to potentially propagate its asymmetry to other regions of the neocortex, the converging neuromodulatory (Hasselmo, 1995) and hormonal influences (McEwen, 2000) on the hippocampus can serve to initiate or potentiate hippocampal asymmetry via their own asymmetric distributions (Wittling, 1995). While hormones can affect hippocampal function through the circulatory system, major neuromodulatory systems, such as the cholinergic, the noradrenergic, and the serotonergic systems, affect hippocampal function via their projections to the hippocampus (figure 2.1c). Therefore, neurochemical asymmetry can set the initial asymmetry in neuronal activity within the hippocampus by providing a direct asymmetric excitation or an inhibition of neuronal excitability. This asymmetric activation may further allow asymmetries within the hippocampus to be potentiated through asymmetric modulation of synaptic plasticity. The resulting asymmetric activation can be further propagated to other cortical as well as subcortical structures through their reciprocal connections with the hippocampus.

A final reason to consider is that the hippocampus appears to play a similar role in animals and in humans (McEwen, 2000). This similarity permits better generalization from findings and theories based on animal models to the understanding of human cerebral lateralization.

A HIPPOCAMPAL THEORY OF CEREBRAL LATERALIZATION

The convergence of sensory information to the hippocampus and the backprojections from the hippocampus to various uni- and polysensory neocortices, the frontal cortex, and other subcortical regions place the hippocampus in a unique position to broadly influence neuronal activation patterns throughout the brain. The presence of receptors for major neuromodulators and hormones and their asymmetric distribution provide a potential source for hippocampal asymmetry. The sensitivity of the hippocampus to experience and its associated asymmetric changes allows the hippocampus to modify its symmetry through the process of learning, defined as modifications of the synaptic strengths according to patterns of neuronal activation due to sensory inputs. The asymmetric sensitivity of synaptic plasticity to neuromodulation can further potentiate and maintain existing asymmetry. Through the hippocampal-cortical network and learning, hippocampal asymmetry can be propagated to cortical areas responsible for high-level functions. Thus, the key components of this hippocampal theory of cerebral lateralization can be summarized below:

1. Hippocampal neuroanatomical, neurophysiological, and neurochemical asymmetries exist.

2. Experience-dependent learning contributes to hippocampal asymmetry.

3. Asymmetry in neuromodulatory systems can serve as a source for the development of hippocampal and cortical asymmetry.

4. Hippocampal asymmetry, particularly hippocampal synaptic plasticity, modulates and interacts with cortical asymmetry.

It is my hope that each of these components is clearly stated in such a way that critical experiments can be designed to test and modify the theory. The objective of this hippocampal theory is to provide a framework in which several previously unrelated research areas or topics can be integrated to offer new perspectives for the understanding of cerebral asymmetry. These areas include the interaction between experience and cerebral lateralization, the computational role of the hippocampus in memory consolidation, electrophysiological study of synaptic plasticity in the hippocampus, and the hormonal modulation of hippocampal synaptic plasticity. In the rest of the chapter, I will focus on offering empirical evidence for the existence of hippocampal asymmetry in volume, synaptic plasticity, and sensitivity to corticosterone modulation, and its relation to behaviorally measured functional asymmetry in rodent "handedness."

TESTING THE HIPPOCAMPAL THEORY USING NEONATAL NOVELTY EXPOSURE

Neonatal novelty exposure (A. Tang, 2001), an early life environmental manipulation, is similar to the well-known neonatal handling method (Denenberg, 1964; Levine, 1957) in its enhancing effects on hippocampal-dependent learning (Meaney et al., 1988; A. Tang, 2001) and in its induction of lateralized functional and anatomical changes (Denenberg et al., 1978; Fitch et al., 1993; A. Tang & Verstynen, 2002; Verstynen et al., in press). The handling method involves removing entire litters of pups from the dams and siblings, and exposing them to a novel non-home cage for 3 min daily during the first 3 weeks of life.

Because the handling procedure introduces differences in maternal separation, exposure to a novel environment, and handling by the experimenter, this method is considered multicomponent (figure 2.2a). From this multicomponent manipulation, one can only conclude that the cause for any handling-induced change is one of the three or any combination of the three components. For example, one could argue that exposure to a novel nonhome environment, or maternal separation, or simply being handled by the experimenter leads to enhanced learning and hippocampal function. The practical implications of these three attributions are very different.

In contrast, the neonatal novelty procedure consists of only the exposure to a novel nonhome cage (figure 2.2b). This is achieved by using

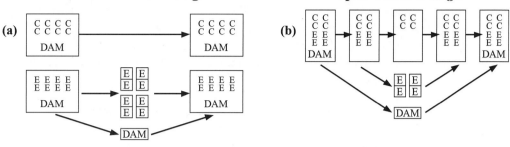

Between–Litter Design **Split–Litter Design**

Figure 2.2 Neonatal handling (*a*) and neonatal novelty (*b*) procedures. Each box represents a separate cage.

a split-litter design and by matching the amount of experimenter handling between the experimental (E, Novel) and control (C, Home) groups (for details, see A. Tang, 2001). By isolating a single component, the neonatal novelty method permits more precise control for the causal factors involved. With this tighter control, one can draw definitive conclusions that neonatal novelty exposure is sufficient, and that maternal separation or experimenter handling is not necessary for the enhanced hippocampal functions. My choice of the neonatal novelty exposure was motivated by these methodological considerations.

The reason for using the neonatal novelty manipulation, as opposed to the environmental enrichment method (Rosenzweig, 1996)—which typically involves more toys and a more complex housing environment—is that longer-lasting changes in hippocampal function have been reported for neonatal handling and neonatal novelty treatment (Meaney et al., 1988; A. Tang, in press; A. Tang & Zou, in press; Zou et al., 2001) than for the enrichment treatment (Duffy et al., 2001; van Praag et al., 1999). Hippocampal-dependent learning in the standard fixed-platform Morris water task (Morris, 1981) and hippocampal receptor binding for the stress hormone corticosterone were enhanced during senescence, long after the initial neonatal handling (Meaney et al., 1985, 1988, 1991, 1996).

Parallel and complementary to the handling results, neonatal novelty exposure has been shown to enhance hippocampal-dependent learning during both infancy and adulthood (A. Tang, 2001) in the working memory version of the Morris water task (Whishaw, 1985) and in a nonspatial, nonaversive two-odor discrimination task. In addition,

Hippocampal Theory of Lateralization

neonatal exposure has been shown to enhance hippocampal synaptic plasticity (A. Tang & Zou, 2002) and to enhance the sensitivity of hippocampal synaptic transmission and plasticity to corticosterone modulation in adult rats (Zou et al., 2001). All these changes in synaptic functions were observed many months after the initial neonatal novelty manipulation.

ASYMMETRIC CHANGES IN HIPPOCAMPAL VOLUMES

The hypothesis that experience, specifically neonatal novelty exposure, can induce asymmetric changes in hippocampal volume has been evaluated (Verstynen et al., 2001). Following the daily 3-min exposure to a novel environment for the first 3 weeks of life, rats were sacrificed at 8 months of age, and their hippocampal volumes were measured histologically, using a cresyl violet stain (figure 2.3a). We measured subfields CA1–CA3, the dentate gyrus, and alveus of the hippocampus, the fornix, the fimbria, and the subicular complex. We excluded the entorhinal cortex (EC) from our analysis because the precise boundary between the EC and the rest of the cortex was not clearly delineated.

Hippocampal asymmetry was measured by a directional lateralization score (L score), defined as $(V_{left} - V_{right})/(V_{left} + V_{right}) * 100\%$, where V = volume (Rosen et al., 1992). The volumetric difference $(V_{left} - V_{right})$ is first normalized by the total hippocampal volume of that individual $(V_{left} + V_{right})$ via division. This normalization removes the variance in the total hippocampal volume from the asymmetry measure. To express asymmetry in proportion (percentage) to the total hippocampal volume, the normalized asymmetry measure is multiplied by 100%. The resulting L score can be interpreted as hippocampal volumetric asymmetry expressed as a percentage of the total hippocampal volume. The absolute lateralization score, defined as *abs* (L), measures the magnitude of asymmetry regardless of the direction of asymmetry.

To test for a neonatal novelty effect on hippocampal volumetric asymmetry, average L scores were first computed for the Novel and Home rats from each litter. The difference score for each litter, $D_L = L_{Novel} - L_{Home}$, was computed as an index for the effect of novelty exposure. If neonatal novelty exposure does have an effect on hippocampal asymmetry, one would expect D_L to be significantly different from 0. A one-sample t-test performed on D_L revealed that D_L was significantly smaller than 0 ($p < .005$), indicating that the neonatal novelty exposure led to a significant reduction in the directional L scores. This effect is

Akaysha C. Tang

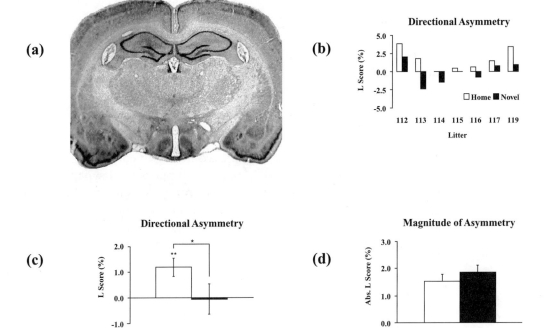

Figure 2.3 Neonatal novelty exposures induced a right shift in hippocampal volumetric dominance in adult rats (7–8 months old). (*a*) A coronal section through the hippocampus. (*b*) Neonatal novelty exposure induced a right shift in hippocampal volumetric asymmetry (Home: open bars; Novel: filled bars), shown in average directional L scores of the Novel and Home rats for each litter. (*c*) The directional L score of the Home rats was significantly greater than 0, indicating left dominance, and the directional L score of the Novel rats was not. (*d*) Magnitude of the directional L score (absolute value) of the Novel and Home rats did not differ significantly.

consistent across litters because, as shown in figure 2.3b, within every litter the average L score of the Home group was greater than that of the Novel group. Since a positive L score indicates a left dominance, this reduction in L score suggests a possible right shift in hippocampal dominance.

Because this reduction in directional L scores could be due to a reduction in the magnitude of asymmetry or to a right shift in hippocampal asymmetry (see figure 2.3c), one must distinguish between the two possibilities. To rule out the possibility of a reduction in the magnitude of asymmetry, a paired t-test was performed on the magnitude of directional L scores between the Novel and Home groups. We found no significant difference between the Novel and Home groups in their magnitude of asymmetry ($p > .20$, figure 2.3d). Therefore, the reduction in the directional L scores is best explained by a right shift in hippocampal volumetric asymmetry rather than a reduction in the magnitude of such asymmetry.

ASYMMETRIC ENHANCEMENT OF HIPPOCAMPAL LONG-TERM POTENTIATION

The hypothesis that early life experience through neonatal novelty exposure can lead to asymmetric changes in hippocampal synaptic plasticity was evaluated using an in vitro electrophysiological method (Zou & Tang, 2001). Following a daily 3-min exposure to a novel environment for the first 3 weeks of life, at the age of 7–8 months, LTP of population spikes and excitatory postsynaptic potentials (EPSPs) were evaluated double-blind, using a brain slice preparation (figure 2.4a). Novel and Home rats were tested in pairs, one animal per day on 2 consecutive days. The order of testing within each pair was randomized, with the Novel rats tested before the Home rats in half of the pairs. All rats were sacrificed at a set time of day (approximately 11 A.M.). For afferent stimulation, constant current pulses (0.1–0.2 mA, 0.2 ms duration) were delivered at 0.1 Hz (test pulses) to the CA1 stratum radiatum. Field potentials were recorded from the stratum pyramidale layer of CA1 for the population spike measure and from the stratum radiatum layer for the EPSP measure (figure 2.4a). Population spike LTP (figure 2.4b) and EPSP LTP (figure 2.4d) were induced by high-frequency stimulations (10 trains of 20 test pulses at 200 Hz, one each 2 s).

Particular care was taken to remove any potential procedural artifacts that might confound the difference between the left and right hippocampi. The left and right hippocampal slices were cut simultaneously, with the blade moving in an anterior-to-posterior direction. This cut was symmetric with respect to the midline, thus preventing potential systematic asymmetry introduced by the cutting process. Slices from the two hippocampi were incubated in the same chamber to ensure similar incubation conditions. The only systematic procedural asymmetry was the angle of the electrodes relative to the direction of the dendritic tree. As will be shown below, left and right differences were found only in slices from the Novel rats and not in those from the

Akaysha C. Tang

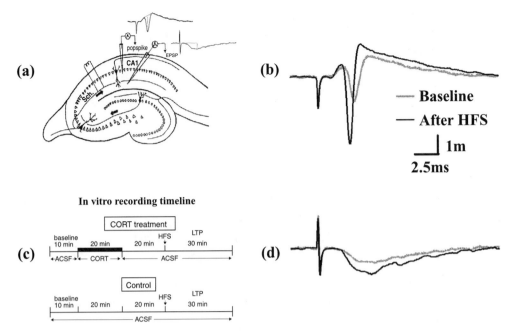

Figure 2.4 (*a*) A schematic diagram of a coronal slice of the hippocampus showing the stimulation and recording sites. (*c*) A time line for in vitro electrophysiological recordings in CORT-treated and control slices. Note that the time delay to LTP induction was matched between the CORT and ACSF conditions, and the acute inhibitory effect was washed out with the perfusion of ACSF before induction. (*b, d*) Examples of population spike and EPSP LTP, respectively.

Home rats. Therefore, the Home slices served as a control for the lateralized effects found for the Novel rats.

In the absence of significant between-group differences in the baseline amplitude, latency, and width of the evoked potentials, for the right hippocampus, the population spike LTP recorded from the Novel slices was significantly greater than that from the Home slices (Novel: $238.97 \pm 21.88\%$; Home: $180.99 \pm 15.41\%$; $p < .05$, figure 2.5a). In contrast, for the left hippocampus there was no significant difference between LTP in the Novel and Home slices (Novel: $189.87 \pm 12.53\%$; Home: $191.84 \pm 13.86\%$; $p > .20$, figure 2.5b). EPSP LTP showed a similar pattern of results. For the right hippocampus, EPSP LTP recorded from the Novel slices was significantly greater than that from the Home slices (Novel: $171.05 \pm 6.80\%$; Home: $141.21 \pm 3.51\%$; $p <$

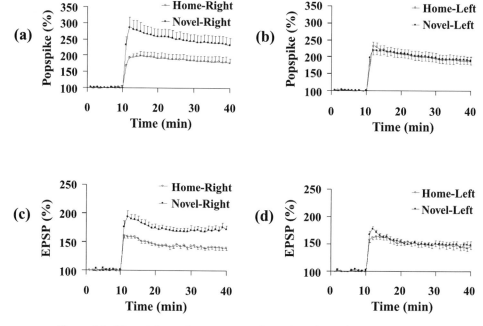

Figure 2.5 Neonatal novelty exposure selectively enhanced long-term potentiation of population spikes (*a, b*) and excitatory postsynaptic potentials (EPSPs; *c, d*) in the right (*a, c*), but not the left (*b, d*), CA1 of the rat hippocampi. LTP is expressed in percent of baseline. Data shown in mean ± sem.

.001, figure 2.5c). In contrast, for the left hippocampus, there was no significant difference between LTP in the Novel and Home slices (Novel: 148.85 ± 4.86%; Home: 148.80 ± 5.61%, $p > .20$, figure 2.5d).

ASYMMETRIC ENHANCEMENT OF CORTICOSTERONE (CORT) EFFECT ON HIPPOCAMPAL LTP

The hypothesis that early life experience through neonatal novelty exposure can lead to asymmetric changes in the sensitivity of hippocampal synaptic plasticity to corticosterone has been evaluated (A. Tang & Zou 2002). Similar in vitro electrophysiological methods and procedures were used. Before the LTP induction, the slices were perfused with corticosterone (100 nM CORT in artificial cerebrol spinal fluid (ACSF) and 0.009% ethanol) for 20 min. The slices were allowed to recover from the acute inhibitory effect by a 20–30 min wash with

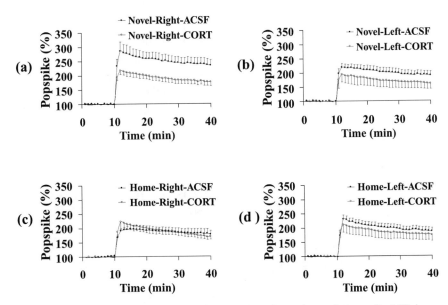

Figure 2.6 Neonatal novelty exposure selectively enhanced population spike LTPs' sensitivity to corticosterone modulation in the right, but not the left, CA1 of the hippocampi (compare *a* to *c* and *a*, *c* to *b*, *d*).

ACSF (Zou et al., 2001). This perfusion sequence (figure 2.4c) differs from typical pharmacological treatment in that it allows the separation of CORT's acute inhibitory effect on neuronal excitability from delayed effect on plasticity. In addition, the time lines for CORT and ACSF perfusions were matched to remove the delay time to LTP induction as a confounding factor.

LTP of population spikes was induced under four conditions: with CORT or ACSF perfusion and in Novel or Home slices (figure 2.6). For the Novel rats, CORT preexposure reduced population spike LTP in the right hippocampal slices by approximately 60% of baseline (ACSF: 238.97 ± 21.88%; CORT: 180.39 ± 13.76%, $p < .05$, figure 2.6a). In contrast, for the left hippocampus, CORT preexposure reduced population spike LTP by approximately 30% of the baseline without reaching statistical significance (ACSF: 191.84 ± 13.86%; CORT: 164.35 ± 20.66%, $p = 0.152$, figure 2.6b). For the Home rats, CORT preexposure did not affect population spike LTP in slices from either side (figure 2.6c, d).

We also assessed CORT effect on a shorter-term plasticity, post tetanic potentiation (PTP) measured 3 min after LTP induction (as opposed to 30 min after induction). For the Novel rats, CORT preexposure reduced population spike PTP in the right hippocampal slices by approximately 60% of baseline (ACSF: 269.83 ± 27.61%; CORT: 208.67 ± 15.79%, $p < .05$, figure 2.6a). In contrast, for the left hippocampus, CORT preexposure reduced population spike LTP by approximately 26% of baseline without reaching statistical significance (ACSF: 213.81 ± 12.42%; CORT: 187.42 ± 27.96%, $p > .20$, figure 2.6b). For the Home rats, CORT preexposure did not affect PTP in slices from either side (figure 2.6c, d).

NEONATAL NOVELTY EXPOSURE INCREASED RIGHT HIPPOCAMPAL DOMINANCE

The issue of whether the hippocampus can be a site for long-term, experience-dependent *asymmetric* modification was addressed in the above-described three experiments. In the first experiment, after neonatal rats were briefly exposed to a novel nonhome environment (3 min daily during the first 3 weeks of life), we histologically measured the volumes of the hippocampus at adulthood (8 months of age). We investigated whether the left and right hippocampi were preferentially modified by the neonatal novelty exposure. We found that the neonatal novelty exposure led to a relative increase of the right hippocampal volume. In the second experiment, following the same neonatal novelty exposure procedure, we examined in vitro synaptic plasticity in the CA1 subfield of the hippocampus at adulthood (7–8 months of age), using the brain slice electrophysiological method. We investigated whether neonatal novelty exposure affects synaptic plasticity symmetrically in the two hippocampi. We found that the early life experience selectively enhanced LTP in the right hippocampus. In the third experiment, using the same methods, we investigated whether sensitivity of hippocampal plasticity to the stress hormone corticosterone is modified asymmetrically by the neonatal novelty exposure (13–14 months of age). We found that early life experience preferentially enhances the effect of the stress hormone on synaptic plasticity in the right hippocampus.

Collectively, these experiments demonstrated that the size of the hippocampus, the magnitude of synaptic plasticity, and the sensitivity to corticosterone modulation are asymmetrically modified by the neonatal novelty exposure. In all three measures, the asymmetric changes correspond to an increased dominance of the right hippocampus. This

Akaysha C. Tang

increased right dominance is consistent in direction with Denenberg's finding that early life stimulation resulted in an increased influence of a right hemisphere lesion on behavior (Denenberg et al., 1978). A right shift in hippocampal volumetric asymmetry can suggest increases in the number of neurons or in the number of synapses, both of which afford increased computation capacity. A right-sided enhancement in long-term potentiation suggests a greater potential for synaptic modification necessary for the encoding of new information in the right hippocampus. A right-sided enhancement in the sensitivity to corticosterone modulation allows the activity and plasticity within the right hippocampus to be more effectively regulated by corticosterone during stress. Inhibition of both excessive excitation and long-term potentiation by corticosterone during stress can minimize the potentiation of synaptic strength due to non-task-related, stress-triggered activation, thus preventing stress from interfering with task learning (de Kloet et al., 1999). Asymmetric protection from the detrimental effect of excessive stress could potentially be the cause of enhanced memory functions subserved by the right hippocampus.

So far, the findings from the neonatal novelty exposure studies have provided direct support for the first two components of the hippocampal theory of lateralization: hippocampal neuroanatomical, neurophysiological, and neurochemical asymmetries exist (component one), and experience-dependent learning contributes to hippocampal asymmetry (component two). To directly test components three and four—that neuromodulatory asymmetry serves as a source for other forms of asymmetry and that hippocampal asymmetry serves as a source for cortical asymmetry—new experiments are called for. In the next section, I will present a behavioral and functional asymmetry study that may be used to verify the hippocampal theory of lateralization. Tighter experiments than the one provided below should be designed to offer more direct tests.

NEONATAL NOVELTY EXPOSURE INCREASED "LEFT-HANDEDNESS"

To study a form of functional asymmetry that has a greater relevance to human laterality and to which the sensorimotor cortex makes a definitive contribution, to avoid the use of invasive methods in detecting the hemispherical difference (e.g., using lesions, as in Denenberg et al.,

1978), and to obtain a behavioral laterality index that corresponds to a more clearly defined neural system than open field activity, we examined paw preference in rats. By examining the paw preference at both infancy (6 weeks of age) and adulthood (7.5 months of age), we established the stability in both short-term and long-term experience-dependent modification of functional lateralization. Using a custom-made reaching apparatus designed to minimize extrinsic influences on paw preference (figure 2.7a–c), we were able to obtain efficient and stable measurement of paw preference with daily testing sessions of as few as 8 trials (A. Tang & Verstynen, 2002).

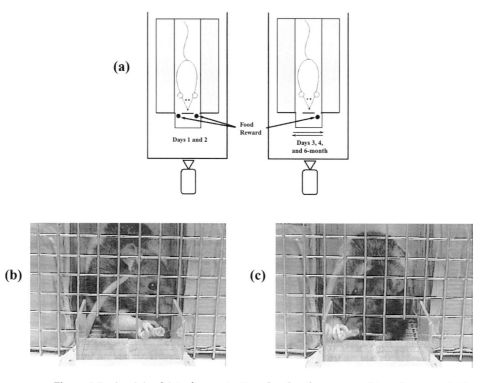

Figure 2.7 A minimal interference testing chamber for paw reaching allows a reliable measurement of paw preference with as few as eight trials per day. (*a*) An aerial view of the testing chamber. The gray areas were blocked with cardboard to reduce the variances in the angle of approach to the openings, where food rewards were presented. (*b, c*) Examples of reaches made by a right-pawed rat through the left and right openings of the reaching apparatus.

Akaysha C. Tang

During the first 3 weeks of life, rat pups experienced the neonatal novelty exposure. At 6 weeks of age, the rats were tested on 4 consecutive days. To control for the influence of potential asymmetric cues in the environment, we varied the localization of the food reward and the presentation sequence across the 4 days (for details, see A. Tang & Verstynen, 2002). At 7.5 months of age, the rats were tested again on a single day. The direction of paw preference was measured by a daily directional lateralization score (directional L score) computed as $(L - R)/(R + L)$, where R and L are the number of reaches made by the right and left paws, respectively. Scores of $+1$ and -1 correspond to perfect left- and right-paw preferences, respectively. A score of 0 indicates ambidexterity (i.e., a lack of either left or right preference). A change from a more negative to a more positive score indicates a right-to-left shift in paw preference, and vice versa.

The measures of the lateralization scores are reliable across multiple days (table 2.1). The Spearman's correlations ranged between 0.734 and 0.876 for any two days of comparison. Despite a 6-month delay between the last two days of testing, strongly left- and right-pawed rats remained left- and right-pawed, and ambidextrous remained ambidextrous (figure 2.8b, c). These results indicate that the paw preference was also stable at the level of individuals across different testing conditions and different developmental stages. In the control (Home) rats, there was a population-level right paw preference based on the average of the direction L scores for all 5 days of performance (figure 2.8a; $p < .05$, df $= 25$). This right-paw population bias is consistent with a number of rodent paw-preference studies (Glick & Ross, 1981; Tsai & Maurer, 1930; Waters & Denenberg, 1994).

Let us consider possible outcomes from this neonatal novelty manipulation: We could have found no effect of early experience on paw

Table 2.1 Correlations of lateralization scores across 5 days of testing

	Day 1	Day 2	Day 3	Day 4	6 months later
Day 1	1.000	0.792	0.757	0.737	0.734
Day 2		1.000	0.824	0.823	0.788
Day 3			1.000	0.876	0.844
Day 4				1.000	0.844
6 months later					1.000

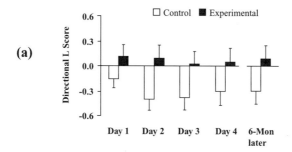

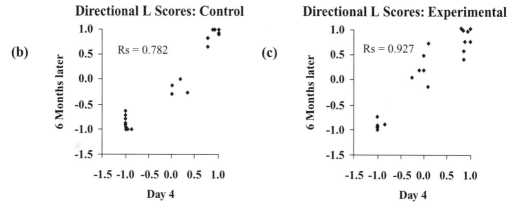

Figure 2.8 Neonatal novelty exposure induced a left shift in paw preference in both juvenile (6 weeks old) and adult (7.5 months old) rats. (*a*) The control rats showed a clear population-level right paw preference, and the neonatal novelty exposure caused a left shift in paw preference (there was no significant difference in magnitudes of paw preference). (*b, c*) The paw preference was stable over a 6-month delay, shown in the scatter plots of lateralization scores before and the delay for the Home (*b*) and Novel (*c*) rats.

preference; we could have found a left shift or a right shift in paw preference. If the right hippocampal dominance does influence the dominance of cortical areas underlying paw preference, one would predict a left shift in paw preference. The results showed that (Novel) rats differed significantly from the control (Home) rats in that they showed a reduction in their directional L scores ($p < .05$, df $= 50$, figure 2.8a). This reduction was found in the absence of a significant difference in the magnitude of asymmetry. Thus, the reduction in directional

L scores is best explained by a left shift in paw preference among the Novel rats, as predicted by a right hippocampal dominance. Therefore, the data offer support for the hippocampal modulation hypothesis (component four).

DISCUSSION

I have proposed a hippocampal theory of cerebral lateralization and have provided behavioral, neuroanatomical, neurophysiological, and pharmacological data to evaluate a subset of hypotheses that constitute the theory. This theory emphasizes the contribution of the hippocampus, the role of experience-dependent learning (as in synaptic modification), and neurochemical asymmetry as a primitive driving force for the development of cerebral lateralization. This theory is a global theory of lateralization in the sense that it considers interactions between cortical and subcortical structures, and interactions between the cellular mechanisms that support the lateralization of functions and the neurochemicals that modulate these mechanisms.

In evaluating the hippocampal theory of lateralization, we found, in adult rats, a right shift in the hippocampal volumetric asymmetry, an increase in right hippocampal synaptic plasticity, and an increase in hippocampal sensitivity to the stress hormone corticosterone as a result of a brief and transient neonatal novelty exposure. We have discovered that this early life experience can also induce changes in rodent "handedness," a functional asymmetry in sensorimotor function analogous to human handedness (Whishaw et al., 1992). Consistent with the hypothesis that hippocampal asymmetry can modulate cortical asymmetry, the direction of changes in paw preference (leftward) can be predicted by the complementary rightward changes observed in the hippocampus following the same neonatal stimulation.

It is tempting to speculate about which behavioral and cognitive consequences are likely to follow these neonatal novelty exposure-induced increases in right hippocampal dominance. The most direct prediction is that functions preferentially served by the right hippocampus, and the right hemisphere in general, might be preferentially enhanced. In humans, the right hemisphere is known to dominate in spatial and emotional processing. One would expect that early life experience, equivalent to that created by our neonatal novelty exposure, would enhance spatial learning and memory as a result of enhanced hippocampal synaptic plasticity and enhanced sensitivity to the stress hormone corticosterone. We would also expect a reduction in emotional reactivity and fear responses due to the enhanced negative feedback mechanism for controlling neuronal excitability within the limbic structures that is mediated by the increased sensitivity to corticosterone. In rodents, both enhanced spatial learning and reduced fear responses were observed as a result of neonatal novelty exposure (A. Tang, 2001).

While the existence of experience-induced increase in right hippocampal dominance offers evidence for the hippocampal theory of cerebral lateralization, the current formulation of the theory does not require that all experience-induced neurochemical, neurophysiological, and neuroanatomical changes must be rightward. As more neuroscientists begin to take separate left and right measures and to perform the statistical analysis that is appropriate for testing changes in lateralization, we may find both leftward and rightward shifts in the symmetry of basic neural mechanisms. We may also find parallel leftward and rightward shifts in various functional asymmetries. The initial, perhaps also very small, asymmetry in the neurochemicals is more likely to be genetically determined. The amplification and the expression of this initial asymmetry in other cellular mechanisms are highly likely to interact with a particular sequence of experiences and environments, and so will the resulting expression and direction of functional asymmetry.

The in vitro electrophysiological evidence provided in the chapter is at a lower level of analysis than most of the previous functional lateralization studies, in that it describes how the behavior of a population of neurons and synapses shows hemispherical asymmetry. These electrophysiological studies are motivated by a fundamental assumption that functional lateralization at higher levels, such as the level of different cognitive functions, must be mediated by some forms of functional asymmetry in the underlying neuronal and synaptic mechanisms. In the sense that the proposed hippocampal theory of cerebral lateralization is formulated at the level of neurons and synapses, and is formulated in an attempt to explain higher-level functional asymmetry, this theory is considered bottom-up.

Such a "bottom-up" theory does not preclude the contribution of top-down influence. In fact, top-down influences can play a critical role during the performance of tasks through which lateralized functions at the behavioral level are demonstrated. Two forms of top-down influences can easily be formulated within the framework of the hippocampal theory. The first is top-down influence via prior experience, as in the example of more rapidly recognizing an object in an ambiguous figure after seeing that object in that ambiguous picture once before. The cortical representation for the previously seen object can be used as top-down inputs or feedback inputs to other processing areas, including the hippocampus. The second is the effect of reward or punishment as a consequence of behavior. The neuromodulator dopamine has been considered a major mediator of this form of top-down influence, and is considered part of the initial driving force for the development of cerebral lateralization by the hippocampal theory of cerebral lateralization.

The degree and direction of changes induced by such neonatal stimulation may vary, depending on the level of stress incurred during the neonatal manipulation and the stress history or stress context before and after the manipulation, similar to the effects induced by neonatal handling within the hypothalamic-pituitary-adrenal (HPA) axis and its target structures (Denenberg, 1977; Levine, 1960; Meaney et al., 1996) and similar to the effects of corticosterone on neuronal excitability and synaptic plasticity as an inverted-U-shaped dose-response curve (de Kloet et al., 1999). This contextual effect may offer an explanation for the comment made by Lewis and Diamond (1995) that in some studies, experience did not result in changes in lateralization.

Due to the limited space, I am unable to evaluate the hippocampal theory against other theories of lateralization. Instead, I will point to references for theories and models that are relevant to the understanding of cerebral lateralization. The learning-centered hippocampal theory should be contrasted with theories that focus on the genetic contribution to cerebral lateralization (Annett, 1985; McManus & Bryden, 1993) and theories that focus on early fetal development (Yeo & Gangestad, 1993). The general hippocampal-cortical interaction and neurochemical modulation-based theory should be compared with specific theories of lateralization or approaches to lateralization that focus on either a particular region or a particular connection in the brain (Anninos et al., 1984; Cook & Beech, 1990; Ringo et al., 1994), or particular lateralized functions (Brown & Kosslyn, 1995). Finally, because cerebral lateralization can be viewed as a special case of modularity (Fodor, 1989), the hippocampal theory of lateralization can also be contrasted with models that are motivated by the idea of modularity in information processing (Jacobs et al., 1991).

ACKNOWLEDGMENTS

I am grateful to all my students who have participated in the studies summarized above and to Robert Sutherland, whose presence undoubtedly influenced my thinking. I thank Bethany Reeb for her comments and tireless help with the preparation of the chapter. I thank George Cowan and Michael Dougher for their financial and moral support.

REFERENCES

Aiba, A., Chen, C., Herrup, K., Rosenmund, C., Stevens, C., & Tonegawa, S. (1994). Reduced hippocampal long-term potentiation and context-specific deficit in associative learning in mglur1 mutant mice. *Cell, 79*, 365–375.

Amaral, D., & Witter, M. (1989). The three-dimensional organization of the hippocampal formation: A review of anatomical data. *Neuroscience, 31*(3), 571–591.

Amaral, D., & Witter, M. (1995). Hippocampal formation. In G. Paxinos (Ed.), *The rat nervous system*. Second edition (pp. 443–486). San Diego: Academic Press.

Anderson, R., Fleming, D., Rhees, R., & Kinghorn, E. (1986). Relationships between sexual activity, plasma testosterone, and the volume of the sexually dimorphic nucleus of the preoptic area in prenatally stressed and nonstressed rats. *Brain Research, 370*(1), 1–10.

Annett, M. (1985). *Left, right, hand and brain: The right shift theory*. Hillsdale, NJ: Lawrence Erlbaum Associates.

Anninos, P., Argyrakis, P., & Skouras, A. (1984). A computer model for learning processes and the role of the cerebral commissures. *Biological Cybernetics, 50*(5), 329–336.

Barneoud, P., Lemoal, M., & Neveu, P. (1990). Asymmetric distribution of brain monoamines in left-handed and right-handed mice. *Brain Research, 520*(1–2), 317–321.

Barneoud, P., & Vanderloos, H. (1993). Direction of handedness linked to hereditary asymmetry of a sensory system. *Proceedings of the National Academy of Sciences, USA, 90*(8), 3246–3250.

Barnes, C. (1995). Involvement of LTP in memory: Are we searching under the street light? *Neuron, 15*(4), 751–754.

Barnes, C., Jung, M., McNaughton, B., Korol, D., Andreasson, K., & Worley, P. (1994). LTP saturation and spatial-learning disruption: Effects of task variables and saturation levels. *Journal of Neuroscience, 14*(10), 5793–5806.

Bliss, T., & Collingridge, G. (1993). A synaptic model of memory: Long-term potentiation in the hippocampus. *Nature, 363*, 31–39.

Brown, H., & Kosslyn, S. (1995). Hemispheric differences in visual object processing: structural versus allocation theories. In R. Davidson & K. Hugdahl (Eds.). *Brain asymmetry* (pp. 78–98). Cambridge, MA: MIT Press.

Cook, N., & Beech, A. (1990). The cerebral hemispheres and bilateral neural nets. *International Journal of Neuroscience, 52*(3–4), 201–210.

Davidson, R. (1995). Cerebral asymmetry, emotion, and affective style. In R. Davidson & K. Hugdahl (Eds.), *Brain asymmetry.* (pp. 361–387). Cambridge, MA: MIT Press.

de Kloet, E., Oitzl, M., & Joels, M. (1999). Stress and cognition: Are corticosteroids good or bad guys? *Trends in Neuroscience, 22*(10), 422–426.

de Toledo-Morrell, L., Dickerson, B., Sullivan, M., Spanovic, C., Wilson, R., & Bennett, D. (2000). Hemispheric differences in hippocampal volume predict verbal and spatial memory performance in patients with Alzheimer's disease. *Hippocampus, 10*, 136–142.

Denenberg, V. (1964). Critical periods, stimulus input, and emotional reactivity: A theory of infantile stimulation. *Psychological Review, 71*, 335–351.

Denenberg, V. (1977). Assessing the effects of early experience. In R. Myers (Ed.), *Methods in psychobiology.* Vol. 3 (pp. 127–147). Academic Press.

Denenberg, V. (1981). Hemispheric laterality in animals and the effects of early experience. *Behavioural Brain Science, 4*(1): 1–21.

Denenberg, V., Garbanati, J., Sherman, G., Yutzey, D., & Kaplan, R. (1978). Infantile stimulation induces brain lateralization in rats. *Science, 201*(4361), 1150–1152.

Duffy, S., Craddock, K., Abel, T., & Nguyen, P. (2001). Environmental enrichment modifies the PKA-dependence of hippocampal LTP and improves hippocampus-dependent memory. *Learning and Memory, 8*(1), 26–34.

Eichenbaum, H. (1996). Is the rodent hippocampus just for "place"? *Current Opinions in Neurobiology, 6*(2), 187–195.

Eichenbaum, H. (1997). Declarative memory: Insights from cognitive neurobiology. *Annual Review of Psychology, 48*, 547–572.

Fitch, R., Brown, C., Oconnor, K., & Tallal, P. (1993). Functional lateralization for auditory temporal processing in male and female rats. *Behavioral Neuroscience, 107*(5), 844–850.

Fodor, J. (1989). *The modularity of mind.* Cambridge, MA: MIT Press.

Glick, S., & Ross, D. (1981). Right-sided population bias and lateralization of activity in normal rats. *Brain Research, 205*(1), 222–225.

Hasselmo, M. (1995). Neuromodulation and cortical function: Modeling the physiological basis of behavior. *Behavioural Brain Research, 67*(1), 1–27.

Hasselmo, M., & Bower, J. (1993). Acetylcholine and memory. *Trends in Neuroscience, 16*(6), 218–222.

Hellige, J. (1995). Hemispheric asymmetry for components of visual information processing. In R. Davidson & K. Hugdahl (Eds.), *Brain asymmetry* (pp. 99–121). Cambridge, MA: MIT Press.

Hiscock, M., & Kinsbourne, M. (1995). Phylogeny and ontogeny of cerebral lateralization. In R. Davidson & K. Hugdahl (Eds.), *Brain asymmetry* (pp. 535–578). Cambridge, MA: MIT Press.

Hugdahl, K. (1995). Dichotic listening: Probing temporal lobe functional integrity. In R. Davidson & K. Hugdahl (Eds.), *Brain asymmetry* (pp. 123–156). Cambridge, MA: MIT Press.

Jacobs, R., Jordan, M., Nowlan, S., & Hinton, G. (1991). Adaptive mixtures of local experts. *Neural Computation, 3,* 79–87.

Joels, M., & de Kloet, E. (1992). Control of neuronal excitability by corticosteroid hormones. *Trends in Neuroscience, 15*(1), 25–30.

Johnston, D., & Amaral, D. (1998). Hippocampus. In G. M. Shepherd (Ed.), *The synaptic organization of the brain.* Fourth edition (pp. 417–458). New York and Oxford: Oxford University Press.

Kaczmarek, L., & Levitan, I. (1987). *Neuromodulation: The biochemical control of neuronal excitability.* New York: Oxford University Press.

Kosslyn, S., Sokolov, M., & Chen, J. (1989). The lateralization of BRIAN: A computational theory and model of visual hemispheric specialization. In D. Klahr & K. Kotovsky (Eds.), *Complex information processing comes of age* (pp. 3–29). Hillsdale, NJ: Lawrence Erlbaum Associates.

Kosslyn, S. (1987). Seeing and imagining in the cerebral hemispheres: A computational approach. *Psychological Review, 94*(2), 148–175.

Lavenex, P., & Amaral, D. (2000). Hippocampal-neocortical interaction: A hierarchy of associativity. *Hippocampus, 10*(4), 420–430.

Levine, S. (1957). Infantile experience and resistance to physiological stress. *Science, 126,* 405.

Levine, S. (1960). Stimulation in infancy. *Scientific American, 202,* 80–86.

Levitan, S., & Reggia, J. (2000). A computational model of lateralization and asymmetries in cortical maps. *Neural Computation, 12*(9), 2037–2062.

Lewis, D., & Diamond, M. (1995). The influence of gonadal steroids on the asymmetry of the cerebral cortex. In R. Davidson & K. Hugdahl (Eds.). *Brain asymmetry* (pp. 31–50). Cambridge, MA: MIT Press.

Liotti, M., & Tucker, D. (1995). Emotion in asymmetric corticolimbic networks. In R. Davidson & K. Hugdahl (Eds.), *Brain asymmetry* (pp. 389–423). Cambridge, MA: MIT Press.

Malenka, R., & Nicoll, R. (1999). Long-term potentiation—a decade of progress? *Science, 285,* 1870–1874.

Marder, E. (1998). From biophysics to models of network function. *Annual Review of Neuroscience, 21,* 25–45.

Marder, E., Abbott, L., Turrigiano, G., Liu, Z., & Golowasch, J. (1996). Memory from the dynamics of intrinsic membrane currents. *Proceedings of the National Academy of Sciences, USA, 93*(24), 13481–13486.

Martin, S., Grimwood, P., & Morris, R. (2000). Synaptic plasticity and memory: An evaluation of the hypothesis. *Annual Review of Neuroscience, 23,* 649–711.

McClelland, J., McNaughton, B., & O'Reilly, R. (1995). Why there are complementary learning systems in the hippocampus and neocortex: Insights from the successes and failures of connectionist models of learning and memory. *Psychological Review, 102*(3), 419–457.

McEwen, B. (2000). Stress, sex, and the structural and functional plasticity of hippocampus. In M. Gazzaniga (Ed.), *The new cognitive neurosciences.* Second edition (pp. 171–198). Cambridge, MA: MIT Press.

McEwen, B., & Sapolsky, R. (1995). Stress and cognitive function. *Current Opinions in Neurobiology, 5,* 205–216.

McManus, I. C., & Bryden, M. P. (1993). The neurobiology of handedness, language, and cerebral dominance: A model for the molecular genetics of behavior. In M. Johnson (Ed.), *Brain development and cognition* (pp. 679–702). Cambridge, U.K.: Basil Blackwell.

Meaney, M., Aitken, D., Bhatnagar, S., Vanberkel, C., & Sapolsky, R. (1988). Effect of neonatal handling on age-related impairments associated with the hippocampus. *Science, 239,* 766–769.

Meaney, M., Aitken, D., Bodnoff, S., Iny, L., & Sapolsky, R. (1985). The effects of postnatal handling on the development of the glucocorticoid receptor systems and stress recovery in the rat. *Progress in Neuropsychopharmacological and Biological Psychiatry, 7,* 731–734.

Meaney, M., Diorio, J., Francis, D., Widdowson, J., Laplante, P., Caldji, C., Sharma, S., Seckl, J., & Plotsky, P. (1996). Early environmental regulation of forebrain glucocorticoid receptor gene expression: Implications for adrenocortical responses to stress. *Developmental Neuroscience, 18*(1–2), 49–72.

Meaney, M., Mitchell, J., Aitken, D., Bhatnagar, D., Bodnoff, S., Iny, L., & Sarrieau, A. (1991). The effects of neonatal handling on the development of the adrenocortical response to stress: Implications for neuropathology and cognitive deficits in later life. *Psychoneuroendocrinology, 16*(1–3), 85–103.

Morgan, S., & Squire, L. (1990). The primate hippocampal formation: Evidence for a time-limited role in memory storage. *Science, 250*(4978), 288–290.

Morris, R. (1981). Spatial localization does not require the presence of local cues. *Learning and Motivation, 12,* 239–260.

Moser, E., Krobert, K., Moser, M., & Morris, R. (1998). Impaired spatial learning after saturation of long-term potentiation. *Science, 281*(5385), 2038–2042.

Nadel, L., Samsonovich, A., Ryan, L., & Moscovitch, M. (2000). Multiple trace theory of human memory: Computational, neuroimaging, and neuropsychological results. *Hippocampus, 10*(4), 352–368.

Oke, A., Keller, R., Mefford, I., & Adams, R. (1978). Lateralization of norepinephrine in human thalamus. *Science, 200*(4348), 1411–1413.

O'Keefe, J., & Nadel, L. (1978). *The hippocampus as a cognitive map.* Oxford: Oxford University Press.

O'Mara, S. (2000). Introduction to the special issue on the nature of hippocampal-cortical interaction: Theoretical and experimental perspectives. *Hippocampus, 10,* 351.

O'Reilly, R. (1998). Six principles for biologically based computational models of cortical cognition. *Trends in Neuroscience, 2*(11), 455–462.

O'Reilly, R., & Rudy, J. (2000). Computational principles of learning in the neocortex and hippocampus. *Hippocampus, 10*(4), 389–397.

Reggia, S., Goodall, S., & Shkuro, Y. (1998). Computational studies of lateralization of phoneme sequence generation. *Neural Computation, 10*(5), 1277–1297.

Ringo, J., Doty, R., Demeter, S., & Simard, P. (1994). Time is of the essence: A conjecture that hemispheric specialization arises from interhemispheric conduction delay. *Cerebral Cortex, 4*(4), 331–343.

Rogers, L. (1982). Light experience and asymmetry of brain function in chickens. *Nature, 297*(5863), 223–225.

Rolls, E. (2000). Hippocampo-cortical and cortico-cortical backprojections. *Hippocampus, 10*(4), 380–388.

Rosen, G., Sherman, G., & Galaburda, A. (1992). Biological substrates of anatomic asymmetry. *Progress in Neurobiology, 39*(5), 507–515.

Rosenzweig, M. (1996). Aspects of the search for neural mechanisms of memory. *Annual Review of Psychology, 47,* 1–32.

Rumelhart, D., McClelland, J., & P. R. Group. (1986). *Parallel distributed processing: Explorations in the microstructure of cognition.* Vol. 1 (pp. 51–59). Cambridge, MA: MIT Press.

Shevtsova, M., & Reggia, J. (1999). A neural network model of lateralization during letter identification. *Journal of Cognitive Neuroscience, 11*(2), 167–181.

Squire, L. (1982). *Memory and brain.* New York: Oxford University Press.

Squire, L. (1992). Memory and the hippocampus: A synthesis from findings with rats, monkeys and humans. *Psychological Review, 99,* 195–231.

Squire, L., & Alvarez, P. (1995). Retrograde amnesia and memory consolidation: A neurobiological perspective. *Current Opinions in Neurobiology, 5,* 169–177.

Stevens, C. (1996). Spatial learning and memory: The beginning of a dream. *Cell, 87,* 1147–1148.

Stevens, C. (1998). A million dollar question: Does LTP = memory? *Neuron, 20,* 1–2.

Sullivan, R., & Gratton, A. (1999). Lateralized effects of medial prefrontal cortex lesions on neuroendocrine and autonomic stress responses in rats. *Journal of Neuroscience, 19,* 2834–2840.

Sutherland, R., & Rudy, J. (1987). Configural association theory: The role of the hippocampal formation in learning, memory, and amnesia. *Psychobiology, 17,* 129–144.

Sutherland, R., Weisend, M., Mumby, D., Astur, R., Hanlon, F., Koerner, A., Thomas, M., Wu, Y., Moses, S., Cole, C., Hamilton, D., & Hoesing, J. (2001). Retrograde amnesia after hippocampal damage: Recent vs. remote memories in two tasks. *Hippocampus, 11*(1), 27–42.

Tang, A. (2001). Neonatal exposure to novel environment enhanced hippocampal-dependent memory function during infancy and adulthood. *Learning and Memory, 8,* 257–264.

Tang, A., & Verstynen, T. (2002). Early life exposure to a novel environment modulates "handedness" in rats. *Behavioural Brain Research, 131,* 1–7.

Tang, A., & Zou, B. (2002). Neonatal exposure to novelty enhanced long-term potentiation in CA1 region of the rat hippocampus. *Hippocampus, 13,* 398–404.

Tang, Y., Shimizu, E., Dube, G., Rampon, C., Kerchner, G., Zhuo, M., Liu, G., & Tsien, J. (1999). Genetic enhancement of learning and memory in mice. *Nature, 401*(6748), 63–69.

Thierry, A., Gioanni, Y., Degenetais, E., & Glowinski, J. (2000). Hippocampo-prefrontal cortex pathway: Anatomical and electrophysiological characteristics. *Hippocampus, 10*(4), 411–419.

Tsai, L. S., & Maurer, S. (1930). Right-handedness in white rats. *Science, 72,* 436–438.

Tsien, J., Huerta, P., & Tonegawa, S. (1996). The essential role of hippocampal CA1 NMDA receptor-dependent synaptic plasticity in spatial memory. *Cell, 87,* 1327–1338.

Tucker, C., & Williamson, P. (1984). Asymmetric neural control systems in human self-regulation. *Psychological Review, 91*(2), 185–215.

van Kleek, M., & Kosslyn, S. (1991). Use of computer models to study cerebral lateralization. In F. Kitterle (Ed.), *Cerebral laterality: Theory and research.* Hillsdale, NJ: Lawrence Erlbaum Associates.

van Praag, G., Christie, B., Sejnowski, T., & Gage, F. (1999). Running enhances neurogenesis, learning, and long-term potentiation in mice. *Proceedings of the National Academy of Sciences, USA, 96*(23), 13427–13431.

Verstynen, T., Tierney, R., Urbanski, T., & Tang, A. (2001). Neonatal novelty exposure modulates hippocampal volumetric asymmetry in the rat. *NeuroReport, 12,* 3019–3022.

Wallenstein, G., Eichenbaum, H., & Hasselmo, M. (1998). The hippocampus as an associator of discontiguous events. *Trends in Neuroscience, 21*(8), 317–323.

Waters, N., & Denenberg, V. (1994). Analysis of 2 measures of paw preference in a large population of inbred mice. *Behavioural Brain Research, 63*(2), 195–204.

Whishaw, I. (1985). Formation of a place learning-set by the rat: A new paradigm for neurobehavioral studies. *Physiological Behavior, 35,* 139–143.

Whishaw, I., & Kolb, B. (1988). Sparing of skilled forelimb reaching and corticospinal projections after neonatal motor cortex removal or hemidecortication in the rat: Support for the Kennard doctrine. *Brain Research, 451*(1–2), 97–114.

Whishaw, I., Pellis, S., & Gorny, B. (1992). Skilled reaching in rats and humans: Evidence for parallel development or homology. *Behavioural Brain Research, 47*(1), 59–70.

Wittling, W. (1995). Brain asymmetry in the control of autonomic-physiologic activity. In R. Davidson & K. Hugdahl (Eds.), *Brain asymmetry* (pp. 305–357). Cambridge, MA: MIT Press.

Wittling, W., & Pfluger, M. (1990). Neuroendocrine hemisphere asymmetries: Salivary cortisol secretion during lateralized viewing of emotion-related and neutral films. *Brain and Cognition, 14*(2), 243–265.

Yeo, R., & Gangestad, S. (1993). Developmental origins of variation in human hand preference. *Genetica, 89*, 281–296.

Zou, B., Golarai, G., Connor, J. A., & Tang, A. (2001). Neonatal exposure to a novel environment enhances the effects of corticosterone on neuronal excitability and plasticity in adult hippocampus. *Developmental Brain Research, 130*, 1–7.

Zou, B., & Tang, A. C. (2001). Neonatal exposure to novel environment selectively enhanced LTP in the ca1 of the right hippocampus in rats. *Journal of Cognitive Neuroscience,* (Abstract, p. 72).

3 Stress and Coping: Asymmetry of Dopamine Efferents within the Prefrontal Cortex

Craig W. Berridge, Rodrigo A. España, and Thomas A. Stalnaker

The rise to prominence of the concept of stress within modern society is a relatively recent development, arising from scientific observations made since the early twentieth century. These studies identified two important principles. First, they identified a sensitivity of physiological systems to challenging environmental conditions. Second, later studies demonstrated a strong association between stress (and anxiety) and a wide variety of physiological, cognitive, and affective dysfunctions. Much effort been devoted to elucidating the neural mechanisms underlying stress and anxiety, and the contribution of stress-related neural circuits to cognitive and affective dysfunction. The vast majority of this work has utilized animal models and these studies have yielded substantial insight into the neurobiology of stress and anxiety. One early observation was that a robust activation of cerebral dopamine (DA) and other monoamines occurs in stress, including within the prefrontal cortex (PFC).

These and other observations indicate that a relatively widespread network of cortical and subcortical limbic and autonomic structures plays a prominent role in the regulation of behavior and physiology in stress. Included in this network is the central nucleus of the amygdala (CeA), which via extensive efferent and afferent projections appears to modulate a variety of stress-related physiological and behavioral processes, including stress-related activation of DA efferents to PFC. The PFC plays a pivotal role in a variety of cognitive, affective, and physiological processes. At least some PFC-dependent functions display a hemispheric asymmetry, with left and right PFC associated with qualitatively distinct affect-related processes. DA efferents to PFC also display hemispheric lateralization, with those projecting to the right hemisphere displaying an enhanced sensitivity to both uncontrollable stressors and behavioral coping responses.

Currently, the extent to which stress- and coping-related alterations in DA neurotransmission contribute to behavioral and physiological responding in stress remains unclear. However, recent observations indicate a prominent role of PFC DA in stress-related alterations in cognitive and physiological functions and significant effects of coping on PFC neural activity. Combined, these observations suggest an important role of PFC DA and asymmetry within both PFC and DA efferents to PFC in cognitive, affective, and physiological processes associated with stress and coping.

NEUROCHEMICAL CORRELATES OF STRESS: PREFRONTAL CORTICAL DOPAMINE

The current conceptualization of stress as a behavioral state elicited by challenging or threatening events arises from nearly a century of research starting with the seminal work of Cannon (1914) and Selye (1946). In these studies, various physiological systems were observed to be affected similarly by disparate environmental events that had in common a potential to disrupt homeostasis or threaten animal well-being. Although generation of a universally accepted definition of stress has proved difficult, the above-described definition has wide acceptance and has proved useful heuristically. Initially, emphasis was placed on stressor-induced activation of peripheral systems, primarily endocrine systems. In these studies it was determined that stressors elicit activation of both peripheral catecholamine systems and the pituitary-adrenal axis, and the consequent increase in levels of circulating glucocorticoids. The activation of these systems results in enhanced ability of the animal to physically contend with the challenging situation. More recently, substantial effort has been devoted to elucidating the central nervous system mechanisms underlying affective and cognitive components of stress-related behavior. Much of this work is, in part, motivated by a need to better understand the neural mechanisms of stress-related affective and cognitive dysfunctions.

One early observation regarding central responses in stress was that, similar to the periphery, an activation of central monoaminergic systems is a hallmark feature of the constellation of physiological responses that define the state of stress. Initially, it was demonstrated

C. W. Berridge, R. A. España, and T. A. Stalnaker

that stressors increase the release of DA within PFC of rats (Thierry et al., 1976). Subsequent studies demonstrated that in addition to an activation of DA systems, stressors reliably increase release and turnover of norepinephrine (NE) and serotonin (5-HT). The activation of DA, NE, and 5-HT systems in stress has been observed within a variety of cortical and subcortical structures (Abercrombie et al., 1989; Abercrombie et al., 1992; Dunn et al., 1986; Dunn, 1988; Goldstein et al., 1996; Roth et al., 1988; Tam & Roth, 1985; Thierry et al., 1976). The extent to which activation of these systems is observed is dependent on the type of stressor, stressor intensity, and experience of the animal.

Despite this generally global activation across multiple transmitter systems, there is substantial regional and chemical specificity to stressor-induced alterations in rates of brain monoaminergic neurotransmission. Thus, across DA systems, there is a differential sensitivity to the activational effects of stressors, with DA efferents projecting to the PFC demonstrating the greatest sensitivity, in terms of both response threshold and magnitude (see figure 3.1, No-Chew group; Abercrombie et al., 1989; Dunn, 1988; Roth et al., 1988; Thierry et al., 1976). Within PFC, the magnitude of the stressor-induced increase in DA release is comparable to that of NE, whereas a lesser magnitude increase in 5-HT utilization is typically observed (figure 3.2, No-Chew group; Kirby et al., 1995; Berridge et al., 1999). Within subcortical structures, a lesser magnitude activation of the mesoaccumbens and mesostriatal DA systems is often observed in stress, relative to PFC DA efferents (figure 3.1; Abercrombie et al., 1989; Dunn, 1988; Goldstein et al., 1996). The degree to which stressors elicit activation of extra-PFC DA systems is dependent on the magnitude of stressor intensity: mild stressors can produce a selective activation of the PFC DA system (for review, see Horger & Roth, 1996). The nearly obligatory nature of the PFC DA response in stress has made this response a primary index of stress.

The nucleus accumbens is associated with motivational and reinforcement processes. Historically, the nucleus accumbens has been viewed as a ventral extension of the neostriatum, with a distinctive limbic afferentation distinguishing it from the overlying caudate-putamen (Heimer & Wilson, 1975). However, more recent studies suggest that the nucleus accumbens is, in fact, a heterogeneous collection of distinct subfields, delineated on the basis of the organization of afferent and efferent projections, as well as by the distribution of immunohistochemical markers (Groenewegen & Russchen, 1984; Heimer et al., 1991; Zahm

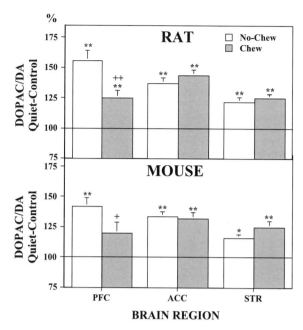

Figure 3.1 Effects of novelty and chewing on DOPAC/DA in PFC, accumbens (ACC), and striatum (STR) in rats (*top*) and mice (*bottom*). Shown are mean ± SEM DOPAC/DA ratios, expressed as a percentage of Quiet-Controls. Novelty-exposed animals were placed in the testing chamber in the absence (No-Chew) or in the presence (Chew) of inedible objects. Shown in top panel are combined results from three experiments. Novelty increased DOPAC/DA levels in PFC, ACC, and STR. The PFC DOPAC/DA response to novelty was significantly smaller in Chew animals than in No-Chew animals. In these studies left and right PFC hemispheres were not analyzed separately. In contrast to the effect observed within PFC, chewing had no significant effects on the DOPAC/DA response to novelty in either ACC or STR. Nearly identical effects of both novelty exposure and chewing were observed in mice. $*p < .05$, $**p < .01$ vs. Quiet-Controls; $^+p < .05$, $^{++}p < .01$ vs. No-Chew.

& Brog, 1992; Brog et al., 1993; Berridge et al., 1997). Within the caudal three-fourths of the nucleus accumbens, a "shell" region located along its medial and ventral aspects can be differentiated from the more centrally situated "core" subregion.

Anatomical, neurochemical, and pharmacological, as well as recent behavioral, studies (Maldonado-Irizarry et al., 1995; Pulvirenti et al., 1994; Pierce & Kalivas, 1995; Pontieri et al., 1995) suggest that the accumbens core represents a ventral extension of the striatum that is closely linked to the extrapyramidal motor system. In contrast, the

C. W. Berridge, R. A. España, and T. A. Stalnaker

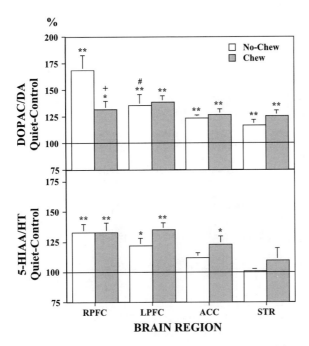

Figure 3.2 Effects of novelty and chewing on DOPAC/DA and 5-HIAA/5-HT levels in left (LPFC) and right (RPFC) hemispheres of PFC, nucleus accumbens (ACC), and striatum (STR). Shown are mean ± SEM DOPAC/DA and 5-HIAA/5-HT ratios, expressed as a percentage of Quiet-Controls. In No-Chew animals, a significantly greater novelty-induced increase in DOPAC/DA was observed in RPFC than in LPFC. In this experiment, chewing resulted in a significantly lower DOPAC/DA response in the RPFC, but not in the LPFC. Novelty exposure also increased 5-HIAA/5-HT levels in RPFC and LPFC. Chewing did not significantly alter the 5-HIAA/5-HT response in these two regions. Although a trend for increased 5-HIAA/5-HT was observed in ACC, this was statistically significant only in the Chew group. $*p < .05$, $**p < .01$ vs. Quiet-Controls; $+p < .05$ vs. No-Chew; $\#p < .05$ vs. No-Chew RPFC.

accumbens shell is heavily allied with limbic circuitry (Alheid & Heimer, 1988; Deutch & Cameron, 1992; Zahm & Brog, 1992). Thus, the core subregion preferentially sends efferent projections to motor-related structures, such as the globus pallidus, substantia nigra, and dorso-lateral ventral pallidum, whereas the shell projects selectively to more limbic-related structures, such as the ventral tegmental area, lateral hypothalamus, ventromedial ventral pallidum, and brain stem auto-nomic centers (Heimer et al., 1991). Within the nucleus accumbens, DA efferents projecting to the shell subdivision display greater reactivity to

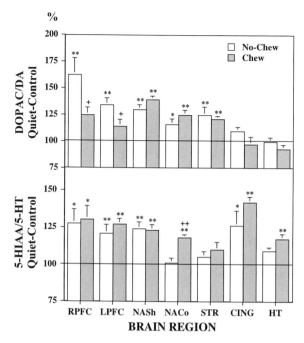

Figure 3.3 Effects of novelty and chewing on DOPAC/DA and 5-HIAA/5-HT levels in left (LPFC) and right (RPFC) hemispheres of PFC, shell (NASh) and core (NACo) subregions of the nucleus accumbens, striatum (STR), cingulate cortex (CING), and hypothalamus (HT). Shown are mean ± SEM DOPAC/DA and 5-HIAA/5-HT ratios, expressed as a percentage of Quiet-Controls. Similar to that shown in figure 3.2, a greater (though not statistically significant) novelty-induced increase in DOPAC/DA was observed in RPFC of No-Chew animals than in LPFC. Chew animals displayed a significantly lower DOPAC/DA response in RPFC. In contrast to that observed in the experiment of figure 3.2, chewing also significantly suppressed the novelty-induced DOPAC/DA response in LPFC in this experiment. Novelty exposure increased 5-HIAA/5-HT levels in RPFC, LPFC, NASh, and CING. Chewing did not alter these increases in 5-HIAA/5-HT. Chewing resulted in a significant increase in 5-HIAA/5-HT in NACo as well as in HT. A nonsignificant trend for greater 5-HIAA/5-HT responses in Chew animals was also observed in CING. $^{*}p < .05$, $^{**}p < .01$ vs. Quiet-Controls; $^{+}p < .05$, $^{++}p < .01$ vs. No-Chew.

stressors than DA efferents within the core subdivision (figure 3.3; Deutch & Cameron, 1992; Kalivas & Duffy, 1995; Berridge et al., 1999).

Interestingly, anxiolytic benzodiazepines decrease basal levels of PFC DA and attenuate stressor-induced increases in DA release in PFC (Lavielle et al., 1978; Finlay et al., 1995). Conversely, the potently anxiogenic benzodiazepine inverse agonists (e.g., β-carbolines) increase

C. W. Berridge, R. A. España, and T. A. Stalnaker

PFC DA utilization (Lavielle et al., 1978; Tam & Roth, 1985; Tam & Roth, 1990). Thus, both pharmacological and environmental manipulations that elicit stress and/or anxiety elicit a robust activation of PFC DA efferent, whereas treatments that reduce anxiety suppress DA neurotransmission within PFC. Combined, these observations have suggested a critical role of PFC DA efferents in stress and/or anxiety-related behavioral and physiological processes.

THE PFC AND DA

Often described as serving "executive functions," the PFC plays a pivotal role in memory, attention, and intentional motor function. These actions of PFC are superimposed upon affective- and motivation-related functions of PFC that are essential components of goal-directed behavior. Dysfunction of PFC circuitry has been implicated in a variety of affective disorders, including stress-related disorders such as depression and anxiety. In primates, there is substantial anatomical and functional heterogeneity within PFC, with distinct regions receiving specific sensory information and serving distinct cognitive and/or affective functions (Diorio et al., 1993; Goldman-Rakic, 1987; Neafsey, 1990; Sutton & Davidson, 1997). In rodents, there appears to be less of an anatomically defined specialization of PFC, raising the question of whether rodent PFC (anterior cingulate) is actually homologous to primate PFC (Preuss, 1995). Nonetheless, recent observations indicate a certain degree of anatomical heterogeneity within rodent PFC (Tzschentke & Schmidt, 1999). Further, similar to that of primate, rodent PFC appears to exert a prominent influence on cognitive, affective, and autonomic and endocrine processes, many of which are associated with fear, stress, and anxiety (Burns & Wyss, 1985; Diorio et al., 1993; Neafsey, 1990; Murphy, Arnsten, Jentsch, et al., 1996; Miner et al., 1997; Zahrt et al., 1997). In both primates and rodents, actions of the PFC are dependent on a diverse array of PFC efferents that target cortical, limbic, and brain stem structures (Reep, 1984; Sesack et al., 1989).

DA-synthesizing neurons located within the ventral tegmental area (VTA, A10) and substantia nigra (A9) provide a relatively high-density DA innervation to neocortex (Fallon, 1981; Swanson, 1982; S. M. Williams & Goldman-Rakic, 1998). Although this innervation is generally widespread, targeting most cortical regions, there is substantial regional and laminar specificity in the distribution of DA cortical projections (for review, see Foote & Morrison, 1987). For example, primary somatosensory, auditory, and visual cortices receive a sparse DA innervation, whereas primary motor cortex and PFC receive a relatively dense DA innervation. Within PFC, the densest DA innervation is found in layers I/II and V/VI (Gaspar et al., 1989; Berger et al., 1991; S. M. Williams & Goldman-Rakic, 1993). This anatomical organization positions DA axons for prominent modulation of neocortical pyramidal neurons via synaptic contacts with pyramidal dendrites and soma.

Currently, at least five different DA receptors are believed to exist, distributed across two receptor families. The D1 receptor family consists of D1 and D5 receptors, and the D2 receptor family is comprised of the D2, D3, and D4 receptors. The distribution of these different receptors, including the identification of cell type and efferent/afferent connections of DA receptor-expressing cells, remains to be described fully. However, evidence indicates that there is both laminar and subcellular specialization in the distribution of DA receptor subtypes. For example, within primate layer V, mRNA for all DA receptor subtypes is found, and this layer contains the highest density of DA receptor mRNA and D2 binding sites (Goldman-Rakic et al., 1990; Lidow et al., 1991, 1998). At the subcellular level, D1 receptors are preferentially localized to dendritic spines of pyramidal cells, whereas D5 receptors are found more commonly in dendritic shafts of these neurons (Bergson et al., 1995). These observations are consistent with additional observations indicating a preferential DA innervation of dendritic shafts and spines of PFC pyramidal neurons (Goldman-Rakic et al., 1989; Carr & Sesack, 1996). This latter observation is of interest because previous studies demonstrate that pyramidal cell dendritic shafts and spines each receive qualitatively distinct afferent information (for review, see Yang et al., 1999). In addition to direct DA modulation of pyramidal neurons, DA terminals synapse onto select local circuit neurons, including GABAergic interneurons (Sesack et al., 1995, 1998).

Combined, these observations suggest an anatomically organized and receptor subtype-selective modulation of functionally specific information arriving in PFC. To complicate the matter further, some DA receptors are not in direct opposition to presynaptic release sites, suggesting the occurrence of extrasynaptic synaptic (or volume) neurotransmission (Garris & Wightman, 1994; Smiley et al., 1994; Yung et al., 1995; Caille et al., 1996; Gonon, 1997). Presumably, distance from the

C. W. Berridge, R. A. España, and T. A. Stalnaker

release site will influence the extent to which a receptor is sensitive to small differences in temporal patterns and quantity of transmitter release. Thus, actions of DA within PFC may occur across a variety of temporal domains, each of which is sensitive to different firing patterns and absolute activity levels of DA neurons. This becomes of interest when discussing alterations in rates of DA release and whether they are sustained in nature, such as that observed in stress or appetitive states (for review, see Berridge & Robinson, 1998) or brief (e.g., phasic fluctuations), such as that observed in response to brief presentation of sensory information guiding reward-acquisition behavior (Schultz et al., 1993).

Consistent with the above-described anatomical observations, actions of DA on PFC electrophysiological activity are complex, being dependent on layer, cell type (e.g., inhibitory GABAergic interneuron vs. pyramidal cells), and activity state of the target neuron (for review, see Yang et al., 1999). The complexity of these interactions appears to stem, in part, from the differential distribution of receptor subtypes across multiple neuronal classes and the actions of DA on a variety of Na^+, K^+, and Ca^{2+} ionic conductances (for review, see Yang et al., 1999). Based on these observations, it is inappropriate to categorize DA as primarily an inhibitory or excitatory neurotransmitter. Rather, DA acts within PFC to modulate information processing, the exact influence being dependent on the activity state of PFC neurons and, presumably, both quantitative and qualitative aspects of incoming information.

LATERALIZATION OF DA RESPONSES WITHIN PFC

Previous studies indicate a lateralization of cerebral DA systems within both cortical and subcortical structures. For example, it has long been known that lesion-induced asymmetry in striatal DA neurotransmission elicits rotational locomotor activity, with rotation observed in the direction away from the hemisphere with greater rates of DA neurotransmission (Pycock, 1980). In intact rats, individual differences in spontaneous and systemic amphetamine-induced turning behavior are observed, suggesting potential individual differences in lateralization of DA neurotransmission within the striatum (for review, see Carlson & Glick, 1989). Further, this behavioral asymmetry has been associated with a variety of additional behavioral processes, including baseline locomotor activity and susceptibility to self-administration of drugs of abuse (Carlson & Glick, 1989; Nielsen et al., 1999). These observations are consistent with extensive evidence indicating a role of DA neurotransmission within subcortical and cortical structures in locomotor activity and self-administration of drugs of abuse (for review, see Berridge & Robinson, 1998).

Previous studies demonstrate lateralization of stress-related activation of PFC DA systems. However, the pattern of the lateralization (left > right, right > left) varies, depending on the nature and duration of the stressor (Carlson et al., 1988, 1991, 1993). For example, 15-min restraint stress produced a preferential increase in DA utilization in the left hemisphere, as indicated by increases in the ratios of concentrations of the primary DA catabolites to DA (e.g., HVA/DA and DOPAC/DA). However, at 30 min, restraint elicited a comparable activation of both left and right DA PFC systems (Carlson et al., 1991). Similarly, food deprivation elicited a greater PFC DA response in the left hemisphere than that observed in the right. In contrast to that observed with food deprivation and 15-min restraint, a greater responsivity of the right hemisphere PFC DA system was observed in animals exposed to uncontrollable footshock, delivered in a learned helplessness paradigm (Carlson et al., 1993). In this paradigm, animals that controlled shock delivery displayed comparable DA activation in both left and right hemispheres, the magnitude of which was comparable to the left hemisphere of yoked animals.

Similar to that of inescapable footshock, we observed greater reactivity of right hemisphere PFC DA efferents during novelty stress (Berridge et al., 1999). In these studies, mice and rats were exposed to a brightly lit novel environment in the presence of 80dB white noise for approximately 20 min. These conditions had previously been demonstrated to elicit neuroendocrine indices of stress (Hennessy & Foy, 1987). Immediately following this, the animals were removed and their brains were dissected. DA and 5-HT utilization were assessed by calculating the ratio of the concentration of primary catabolite (DOPAC and 5-HIAA, respectively) to parent amine. In these studies it was observed that novelty stress consistently produced greater increases in DOPAC/DA levels in the right hemisphere PFC than those observed in the left hemisphere (see figures 3.2, 3.3). These observations were made in both rats and mice, across a number of experiments. Thus, DA efferents to the right hemisphere PFC display an enhanced sensitivity to novelty stress. However, consistent with results described above, in

C. W. Berridge, R. A. España, and T. A. Stalnaker

pilot studies, an activation of the left PFC DA system was occasionally observed in quiet controls, relative to both the right hemisphere of these animals as well as the left hemisphere of quiet controls of previous studies (Berridge et al., 1999).

These observations suggest that DA efferents within the left hemisphere may be more sensitive to currently ill-defined environmental/physiological variables (e.g., fluctuations in temperature or humidity, viral infection, etc.). The lateralization of PFC DA responsivity in novelty stress is neurochemically selective in that lateralization of PFC 5-HT responses are not observed. Thus, although novelty stress elicits a moderate increase in 5-HT utilization within the PFC, comparable responses are observed in the left and right hemispheres (figures 3.2, 3.3). The currently available observations do not permit a simple distinction between stressors that preferentially affect the left hemisphere vs. right hemisphere DA efferents. However, the results obtained with controllable and uncontrollable shock delivery suggest the possibility that right PFC DA efferents are sensitive to conditions permitting or not permitting controllability or some other aspect of coping with stress.

COPING WITH STRESS: LATERALIZATION OF PFC DA ACTIVITY

Recent observations support the hypothesis that DA efferents to the right hemisphere of PFC are preferentially sensitive to coping. Although preferential activation of PFC DA efferents is generally observed in response to a variety of stressors, limited exceptions to this have been observed. For example, enhanced release of PFC DA was not observed following tail-pinch stress, despite an increase in DA release within the nucleus accumbens (D'Angio et al., 1987). Similarly, Berridge and Dunn (1989) observed that mice exposed to a complex novel environment display a variety of physiological indices of stress, including activation of the hypothalamic-pituitary-adrenal axis and enhanced DA utilization within the nucleus accumbens and striatum. However, an activation of the PFC DA system was not observed in these animals. Thus, in both cases minimal increases in DA utilization within the PFC were observed despite the presence of multiple physiological indices of stress.

Interestingly, in both the tail-pinch and novelty exposure paradigms described above, animals readily engage in chewing, or gnawing, of inedible objects during exposure to these stressors (Antelman et al.,

1975; Berridge & Dunn, 1989). Chewing has been demonstrated to attenuate a variety of physiological indices of stress, including activation of the hypothalamic-pituitary-adrenal axis (a primary index of stress) and activation of cerebral noradrenergic systems (Hennessy & Foy, 1987; Mason, 1968; Levine, 1985; Tsuda et al., 1988). Given that chewing, a nonescape behavior, attenuates physiological indices of stress, this behavior can be considered a coping response.

Based on the above described observations, we posited that the lack of activation of PFC DA efferents observed in the tail-pinch and novelty exposure studies described above may have resulted from engagement in chewing on inedible objects (Berridge et al., 1999). This hypothesis was tested in both rats and mice, using the paradigm of Hennessey and Foy (1987), described above, in which animals are exposed to a brightly lit novel environment and provided or not provided the opportunity to chew on inedible objects (wood, Styrofoam, foil). Animals were exposed to the novel environment for 18–22 min, immediately following which they were removed, their brains were dissected, and DOPAC/DA and 5-HIAA/5-HT ratios were calculated in a variety of cortical and subcortical structures.

As described by Hennessy and Foy (1987), most animals provided the opportunity engaged in a substantial amount of chewing. Time spent chewing increased with increasing time spent in the novel environment (figure 3.4). Typically, animals spent approximately 100–120 s chewing during the testing period, representing approximately 10% of the testing period. Although not explicitly measured, the animals did not appear to ingest the material, consistent with previous observations (Hennessey & Foy, 1987). Excluding time spent chewing, animals permitted or not permitted the opportunity to chew displayed comparable behavioral activity in the novel environment. The one exception to this was that animals which chewed spent significantly less time grooming than animals that did not chew (134 ± 25 vs. 258 ± 54 s, $p < .05$).

The neurochemical results indicated that the PFC DA system is uniquely sensitive to actions of this coping behavior: in both rats and mice, engagement in chewing selectively attenuates the stressor-induced increase in DA utilization within PFC (figures 3.1, 3.2). This effect was neurochemically specific in that chewing did not alter novelty-induced activation of PFC 5-HT systems (figure 3.2). Further, the effect of chewing on stressor-induced PFC DA activation was regionally specific in

C. W. Berridge, R. A. España, and T. A. Stalnaker

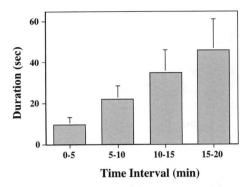

Figure 3.4 Time spent chewing during exposure to a novel environment. Shown are the mean total time (s) ± SEM spent chewing on inedible objects per 5-min epoch of a 20-min exposure period. Similar to that previously reported (Hennessy & Foy, 1987), time spent chewing increased during subsequent 5-min epochs. Results shown here are comparable to those observed in all experiments, in that animals spent approximately 10% (mean: 112 s) of the testing period engaged in chewing inedible objects.

that chewing did not alter DOPAC/DA ratios in other brain regions in novelty-exposed animals (figures 3.1, 3.2, 3.3).

The sensitivity of PFC DA efferents to this coping behavior is partially lateralized, being observed consistently in the right hemisphere in all three of the experiments in which this was examined (figures 3.2, 3.3). In contrast, chewing did not alter PFC DOPAC/DA measures in the left hemisphere in two of these studies (figure 3.2). In the third, chewing resulted in a reduction in left hemisphere DOPAC/DA comparable to that observed in the right hemisphere (figure 3.3). Thus, for reasons currently unclear, although the left hemisphere PFC DA system is not entirely insensitive to chewing, it is less consistently affected by this coping behavior during exposure to novelty stress.

Chewing and other relatively stereotyped behaviors have long been noted to occur under behaviorally activating, or stressful, conditions. Examples of these behaviors include chewing, grooming, fighting, and stimulant-induced oral stereotypy. These so-called displacement behaviors were originally noted because they appeared to occur out of context, elicited by environmental stimuli not "normally" associated with that specific behavioral response (e.g., fighting while being shocked; for review, see McFarland, 1966; Tinbergen, 1952). At least two of these, chewing and fighting, have been demonstrated to attenuate certain physiological measures of stress/arousal (Dantzer & Mormede, 1985; Hennessy & Foy, 1987; Stolk et al., 1974; Tsuda et al., 1988). Thus, although they originally were identified solely on the basis of behavioral observations, current evidence suggests that at least some displacement behaviors may not, in fact, be inappropriate. Rather, these behaviors may serve to modify certain physiological responses in stress. The above-described observations demonstrate that at least one of these behaviors has a substantial influence on dopaminergic utilization within PFC in stress.

This raises the question of whether all previously identified displacement or coping behaviors also suppress DA neurotransmission within PFC. We sought to test this hypothesis in preliminary studies in which we prevented animals from engaging in grooming behavior (using plastic Elizabethan collars) when exposed to a novel environment in the absence of inedible objects. It was hypothesized that if grooming also attenuates DA utilization in stress, animals prevented from grooming will have higher rates of DA utilization than animals permitted to groom. In these studies, preventing animals the opportunity to groom in novelty stress did not increase DA utilization, compared to animals permitted to groom. Thus, assuming grooming is in fact a coping and/or displacement behavior, not all of these behaviors have the same effect on PFC DA neurotransmission. It is possible that different displacement behaviors target different physiological systems. In this case, the most effective response to an inescapable stressor may involve engagement in multiple nonescape behavioral responses.

Currently, it is not clear how engagement in chewing selectively suppresses stressor-induced increases in DA utilization in the PFC. However, certain of the above-described observations appear to rule out further consideration of certain potential mechanisms/hypotheses. For example, it could be proposed that chewing results in a less stressed, or aroused, animal through some unidentified mechanism. In this case, the attenuated PFC DA response could reflect this lower level of arousal or stress. However, this does not appear to be the case, because other physiological indices of arousal or stress, including 5-HT utilization in PFC, indicate that animals which chew are at least as responsive to the novel environment as animals that do not chew. For example, animals that chew have consistently higher rates of 5-HT utilization in accumbens core, striatum, and hypothalamus than animals that do not chew (figures 3.2, 3.3).

C. W. Berridge, R. A. España, and T. A. Stalnaker

Alternatively, evidence suggests that excitatory and inhibitory amino acids may influence rates of monoamine release through actions within the terminal field (Cheramy et al., 1986; Peoples et al., 1991; Raiteri et al., 1991; Jones et al., 1993; Verma & Moghaddam, 1998). Further, stressors elicit large increases in excitatory amino acid neurotransmission, and excitatory amino acids, acting within PFC, modulate rates of DA release in stress (Moghaddam, 1993; Takahata & Moghaddam, 1998). These observations suggest the possibility that coping may selectively target excitatory (or inhibitory) amino acid neurotransmitters within PFC, and that this may contribute to coping-induced suppression of PFC DA release.

The attenuation of the stressor-induced increase in PFC utilization is similar to that observed following administration of benzodiazepine anxiolytics (Lavielle et al., 1978; Tam & Roth, 1990), and opposite to that observed following administration of the anxiogenic β-carbolines (Horger & Roth, 1996; Tam & Roth, 1985). This suggests that chewing-induced suppression of PFC DA utilization may serve an anxiolytic function. In addition, behavioral modulation of PFC DA utilization may contribute to behavior-dependent modulation of the hypothalamic-pituitary-adrenal axis, described previously (Dantzer & Mormede, 1985; Hennessy & Foy, 1987; Neafsey, 1990).

AMYGDALA REGULATION OF DA RELEASE IN STRESS

The neural mechanisms regulating DA utilization in stress remain to be elucidated. Substantial evidence indicates a role of the amygdala, particularly the central nucleus of the amygdala (CeA), in stress and in stress-related behavioral and physiological processes. For example, lesions of the CeA block stressor-conditioned changes in heart rate, startle response, and freezing as well as unconditioned activation of the hypothalamic-pituitary-adrenal axis (Beaulieu et al., 1986; Davis, 1992; Le Doux, 1995; Kapp et al., 1998). Further, CeA sends efferent projections to mesencephalic DA cell bodies (Gonzales & Chesselet, 1990; Zahm et al., 1999; Fudge & Haber, 2000). In combination, these observations suggest the possibility that CeA participates in stressor-induced activation of DA systems projecting to PFC. Supporting this hypothesis, bilateral lesions of CeA block both footshock and novelty-induced PFC DA activation as well as activation of cortical and subcortical DA systems to a conditioned stressor (Davis et al., 1994; Goldstein et al.,

1996). These observations indicate that actions of CeA neurons are necessary for stressor-induced increases in cortical and subcortical DA neurotransmission. However, the extent to which CeA neuronal activity elicits activation of DA efferents in the absence of a stressor and contributes to asymmetrical activation of PFC DA efferents in stress remains unclear.

To better understand the extent to which CeA regulates DA neurotransmission within cortical and subcortical structures, we recently examined the effects of CeA activation, via infusions of a glutamate agonist, AMPA, on tissue indices of DA utilization. In these studies, animals received two bilateral infusions (250 nl/60 s) of either vehicle or AMPA (5 ng/infusion) into CeA. Infusions were separated by 2 min. Following the last infusion, animals were placed back into their home cage and removed 30 min later. They were decapitated and the brains were removed, dissected, and frozen for later analyses of DA, 5-HT, and their catabolites. AMPA infusions elicited a stresslike pattern of activation of DA efferents: A robust activation was observed within PFC and a lesser magnitude activation was observed within the nucleus accumbens (figure 3.5). AMPA infusions into the basolateral nucleus do not alter DA utilization in either cortical or subcortical structures (data not shown). The magnitude of AMPA-induced increases in PFC DA utilization was comparable in the left and right hemispheres.

Further, in a small number of additional animals, the effects of unilateral AMPA infusions into CeA were examined. In these preliminary studies, unilateral AMPA infusions into either the left or the right CeA did not elicit noticeable alterations in DA utilization in either the left or the right PFC or subcortical structures. These observations, combined with those from previous amygdala lesion studies, indicate that bilateral CeA neuronal activity is both sufficient and necessary for stress-related increases in DA utilization. However, because an asymmetrical activation of PFC DA efferents was not observed with either bilateral or unilateral AMPA infusions into CeA, it appears that CeA does not contribute to lateralization of PFC DA activity observed in stress.

FUNCTIONAL CONSEQUENCES OF STRESSOR-INDUCED ALTERATIONS IN RATES OF PFC DA NEUROTRANSMISSION

The observations that stressors increase, whereas coping and anxiolytic drugs attenuate, DA release in PFC raises the question of what are

C. W. Berridge, R. A. España, and T. A. Stalnaker

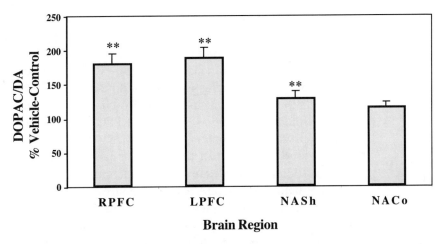

Figure 3.5 Effects of bilateral AMPA infusions (total of 10 ng per hemisphere) into the central nucleus of the amygdala (CeA) on DOPAC/DA ratios in the left (LPFC) and right (RPFC) hemispheres of PFC, as well as the shell (NASh) and core (NACo) subregions of the nucleus accumbens. Shown are mean ± SEM DOPAC/DA ratios, expressed as a percentage of vehicle controls. Rats were cannulated bilaterally over CeA. On the day of testing, they received either bilateral vehicle (artificial extracellular fluid) or bilateral 10 ng AMPA in vehicle, using an infusion procedure consisting of two 250 nl infusions. Each infusion was performed over a 1-min period, and infusions were separated by 2 min (5 ng/hemisphere/infusion). 30 min following infusions, rats were decapitated and brain regions were collected, frozen, and later analyzed for DA and DOPAC levels, using HPLC and electrochemical detection. Infusion sites were verified histologically. Bilateral AMPA infusions into CeA elicited a robust increase in DA utilization in both the left and right hemispheres of PFC and a lesser magnitude increase in DA utilization within NASh. **$p < .05$ vs. vehicle-controls.

the functional consequence of alterations in PFC DA release in stress. Unfortunately, currently, little is known concerning the role of DA within PFC in stress. In part, this stems from an incomplete understanding of the cognitive, affective, and physiological processes subserved by PFC combined with an incomplete understanding of the neuromodulatory actions of DA within PFC. Nonetheless, current evidence indicates that PFC is a critical component in the neural infrastructure supporting cognitive, affective, and physiological processes. In terms of affective function, previous observations suggest a role of PFC in appetitive and avoidance behavior, and that at least some of these functions are partially asymmetrically distributed across the hemispheres: Neuronal activity within the right hemisphere PFC is associated with higher levels of anxiety and withdrawal in humans, whereas left PFC activity is associated with approach-related behavior (Davidson, 1992; Rauch et al., 1995; Sutton & Davidson, 1997). Current evidence indicates that, via actions within PFC, DA modulates at least a subset of cognitive, affective, and autonomic/endocrine-related processes. Although any discussion of the actions of DA within PFC needs to take into account the asymmetry of PFC DA efferents as well as the asymmetry of PFC function, this has rarely been explicitly examined in animal studies of the function of DA efferents within PFC. Certainly, future studies need to examine the functional significance of asymmetrical activation of PFC DA efferents in stress.

Perhaps the best-characterized relationship between DA, stress, and PFC function concerns working memory. There is an extensive body of work documenting a critical role of the PFC in working memory (for review, see Goldman-Rakic, 1999). Further, DA modulates PFC neuronal activity, and these actions have been observed during performance of a working memory task (G. V. Williams & Goldman-Rakic, 1995). Pharmacological and lesion studies demonstrate that DA, acting within PFC, modulates working memory. The relationship between DA neurotransmission and performance in tests of working memory is nonmonotonic, with both deficits in and excess DA neurotransmission producing impairment on tests of working memory (an inverted-U dose-response relationship). For example, depletions of DA within PFC impair performance in a delayed-response test in monkeys and rats, and these deficits can be reversed with administration of DA receptor agonists (Brozoski et al., 1979; Bubser & Schmidt, 1990).

Further, systemic and intra-PFC infusions of pharmacological treatments that increase rates of DA neurotransmission impair working memory in both rats and monkeys (Murphy, Arnsten, et al., 1996; Jentsch, Tran, et al., 1997; Jentsch, Redmond, et al., 1997; Zahrt et al., 1997; Arnsten & Goldman-Rakic, 1998). This includes treatment with direct-acting D1 receptor agonists as well as indirect agonists, including the anxiogenic so-called GABAergic inverse agonist, FG-7412. Consistent with these observations, stressors, which increase PFC DA utilization, also impair working memory of rats and monkeys and this deficit in working memory is reversed by pretreatment with DA antagonists (Murphy, Arnsten, Jentsch, et al., 1996; Arnsten & Goldman-Rakic, 1998). The extent to which PFC modulation of working memory is lateralized and the extent to which stressor-induced impairment of

C. W. Berridge, R. A. España, and T. A. Stalnaker

working memory involves asymmetry of PFC DA systems currently remain to be determined.

In addition to the role of PFC in stressor-induced alterations of working memory, existing evidence indicates that PFC modulates a variety of physiological processes which are associated with stress and arousal. For example, PFC innervates regions associated with autonomic regulation, and fluctuations in PFC neuronal activity elicit alterations in blood pressure and heart rate (for review, see Neafsey, 1990). Further, PFC lesions block certain conditioned responses in heart rate to an aversive stimulus (for review, see Neafsey, 1990). The extent to which DA participates in stressor-conditioned changes in heart rate remains unknown.

The PFC also appears to modulate stress-related alterations in corticosterone secretion in rats. Further, manipulations of DA neurotransmission globally within the brain demonstrate a positive relationship between rates of DA neurotransmission and rates of corticosterone secretion (Fuller & Snoddy, 1981; Kitchen et al., 1988; Borowsky & Kuhn, 1992; Casolini et al., 1993). The extent to which DA, acting within PFC, modulates PFC-dependent autonomic and endocrine function remains to be determined, although limited evidence suggests a role of PFC DA in the modulation of stress-related increases in corticosterone secretion (Diorio et al., 1993; Sullivan & Gratton, 1997).

Finally, existing evidence indicates that PFC DA modulates cold-stress-related ulcer development (Sullivan & Szechtman, 1995). In these studies 6-OHDA lesions of PFC DA fibers increased ulcer development in rats exposed to cold stress. Although both bilateral lesions and left hemisphere lesions tended to increase ulcer development, a significant increase in ulceration was observed only following lesions confined to the right hemisphere. A sensitivity of the right hemisphere in these studies is similar to the enhanced sensitivity of the right PFC DA utilization in stress and coping described above.

Aside from stress-related physiology and behavior, asymmetry of PFC DA activity has also been linked to alcohol consumption (Nielsen et al., 1999). Thus, DA lesions within the left PFC increased, whereas right PFC DA lesions decreased, alcohol consumption. Both of these effects were most robust in those animals that displayed low levels of spontaneous locomotor activity prior to the lesions. The extent to which these actions of PFC DA are affected in stress and contribute to any stress-related alterations in alcohol- or other drug-seeking behavior remains to be examined. Related to these latter observations, subcortical DA has been implicated in both self-administration of drugs of abuse as well as spontaneous and amphetamine-induced locomotor activity (for review, see Berridge & Robinson, 1998). Current evidence suggests that PFC may modulate subcortical DA neurotransmission. For example, pharmacologically induced decreases in PFC neuronal activity increases DA release in the contralateral striatum in rats (Karreman & Moghaddam, 1996). Conversely, activation of PFC neuronal activity decreases striatal DA release (Karreman & Moghaddam, 1996). Similarly, the stressor-induced increase in DA release within the nucleus accumbens is attenuated by intra-PFC infusions of a GABA$_B$-receptor agonist (Doherty & Gratton, 1999).

Evidence indicates that the PFC-dependent regulation of subcortical DA neurotransmission may be modulated by actions of DA within PFC. For example, PFC DA lesions increased DA utilization in both accumbens and striatum (Pycock et al., 1980; Haroutunian et al., 1988). Further, PFC DA lesions enhance the responsivity of subcortical DA systems in stress (Deutch et al., 1990). The left PFC hemisphere may play a larger role in these effects, given that left, but not right, hemisphere PFC DA lesions increased stressor-induced DA utilization within the nucleus accumbens, an effect greater in left-turning animals (Carlson et al., 1996). Further, in this latter study, left-turning rats displayed disrupted escape behavior to footshock. These observations indicate a potential asymmetry in the DA-sensitive regulation by PFC of both subcortical DA utilization and behavior in stress. The extent to which PFC, in general, and PFC DA, specifically, contribute to individual differences in behavior and physiology, both related to and independent of stress, remains to be determined. For example, differences in basal PFC-subcortical DA interactions could contribute to the above-mentioned correlation between baseline locomotor activity and alcohol intake.

Interpretation of many of the above-described studies is confounded by the use of DA lesions and the well-documented, lesion-induced compensatory responses observed following catecholamine lesions. These compensatory responses are observed at the levels of release, postsynaptic number, and second-messenger systems (Skolnick et al., 1978; Harik et al., 1981; Logue et al., 1985; Robinson et al., 1994; Venator et al., 1999). Compensation can occur to such a degree as to produce a system

C. W. Berridge, R. A. España, and T. A. Stalnaker

that appears hyperactive relative to the prelesion state (Diaz et al., 1978; Mogilnicka, 1986; Berridge & Dunn, 1990). Thus, it remains to be determined unambiguously whether PFC DA lesion-induced disruption of behavior and physiology reflects the consequences of hypoactive dopaminergic neurotransmission. Nonetheless, the fact that PFC DA lesions alter stress-related behavioral and physiological responses indicates a functional role of PFC DA in stress-related behavioral and physiological processes.

An additional caveat to interpretation of the above-described studies concerns indices of DA utilization used in these studies. Much of the work on DA asymmetry within PFC in stress and coping has utilized relatively indirect postmortem measures of DA release (e.g., measurement of DA and DA catabolites). Extensive evidence indicates that these measures generally reflect alterations in DA neuronal discharge rates (Elchisak, et al., 1976; Roth et al., 1976; Wood & Altar, 1988). Further, upon examination, a surprising degree of cohesion has been observed across studies examining the effects of stressors and anxiolytics on DA neurotransmission using postmortem measures and studies using more direct measures of extracellular levels of DA, such as microdialysis (Abercrombie et al., 1989, 1992). Thus, it is likely that the above-described effects of stressors and coping on DOPAC/DA measures reflect alterations in extracellular DA levels. Nonetheless, it is important that future studies confirm the lateralization of DA systems in stress and coping by using more direct measures of extracellular levels of DA than have been used previously.

FUNCTIONAL CONSEQUENCES OF COPING-INDUCED ALTERATIONS IN RATES OF PFC DA NEUROTRANSMISSION IN STRESS

Our previous studies indicated that performance of a coping response (e.g., chewing) in the presence of an inescapable stressor (novelty) reduces PFC DA release and that this is more consistently observed in the right hemisphere. An important question raised by this observation is the extent to which coping-induced decreases in PFC DA neurotransmission exert physiologically relevant alterations in PFC activity and/or function. Given the widespread PFC efferent projection system to limbic and brain stem regulatory systems, it is predicted that coping-induced alterations in stress-related PFC DA neurotransmission will have a significant impact on stress-related behavior and physiology. Currently, this question remains largely unaddressed.

However, in preliminary studies, we examined the effects of coping on PFC neuronal activity in stress, using immunohistochemical measures of the transcription factor, Fos, as an index of neuronal activity. Fos is the protein product of c-fos, a member of the immediate-early gene family. Production of Fos and other immediate-early gene products increases with neuronal activation. We compared immunoreactive Fos-like levels in PFC of animals exposed to a novel environment for 20 min that did or did not engage in the coping response of chewing. It was observed that chewing resulted in greater number of Fos-like immunoreactive cells in the right hemisphere PFC compared to animals that did not chew (figure 3.6). Given that this coping response suppresses DA release in stress in the right PFC, these results suggest that stressor-induced increases in DA release within PFC provide an inhibitory tone, on at least a subpopulation of PFC neurons. The extent to which this behavior-induced alteration in PFC neuronal activity is beneficial to the animal, and identification of the physiological, cognitive, and affective processes affected by this remain to be determined.

DOES DA PLAY A CAUSAL ROLE IN THE INDUCTION OF STRESS AND/OR ANXIETY STATES?

The ability of environmental and pharmacological stressors to increase rates of DA neurotransmission within PFC suggests the possibility that PFC DA may provide a unique and critical contribution to the induction of anxiety and/or stress states (for review, see Horger & Roth, 1996). Consistent with this hypothesis is the suppression of PFC DA neurotransmission by anxiolytic benzodiazepines. However, there are a few important additional observations that call into question either the extent to which the actions of DA within PFC in stress are truly unique or, more important, the extent to which PFC DA plays a causal role in the induction of stress-related behavioral states. First, the qualitative effects of stressors and anxiogenics are not necessarily unique to DA: A similar activation of PFC projecting noradrenergic efferents by stressors is observed, and benzodiazepines also suppress PFC noradrenergic neurotransmission (Finlay et al., 1995). Thus, an argument can be made

C. W. Berridge, R. A. España, and T. A. Stalnaker

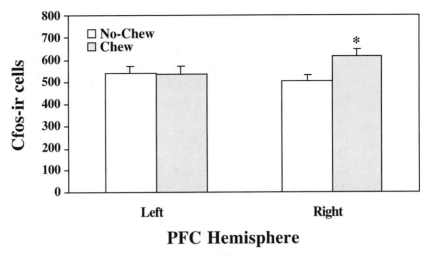

Figure 3.6 Effects of chewing on novelty-associated increases in Fos-like immunoreactivity in left and right hemisphere PFC. Shown are mean ± SEM number of Fos-positive nuclei within dorsal PFC. Cell counts were calculated from two horizontally oriented 750 × 1000 μm fields collected within dorsal PFC at a 100X magnification. The boundaries of the first field were defined by placing the dorsalmost and medialmost aspects of the field at the dorsalmost and medialmost aspects of PFC, respectively. The dorsal border of the second field was even with the dorsal border of the genu of the corpus callosum, and the medial edge of this region contained layer I. Animals were housed in pairs for 10 days prior to testing. On the day of testing, animals were removed from their home tubs and placed into a brightly lit plastic chamber in the presence of 80 dB white noise. Twelve rats had access to inedible objects (wood, Styrofoam, foil) during novelty exposure (Chew). An additional 8 rats did not have access to inedible material during novelty exposure (No Chew). 70–75 min after introduction to novelty exposure animals were anesthetized and perfused, and the brains were processed for immunohistochemical visualization of Fos. Chewing resulted in a significant increase in the number of Fos-positive nuclei within the right hemisphere PFC. *$p < .05$, significantly different from No-Chew animals.

for a role of PFC NE in stress and anxiety similar to that of a role of PFC DA in stress.

Further, the benzodiazepine-induced reduction of basal and stressor-induced PFC DA and NE release appears to occur only at doses that are higher than those required to decrease behavioral indices of anxiety in the rat (Finlay et al., 1995). This could result in part from a lack of sensitivity of the neurochemical measures, which only indirectly assess rates of release. Alternatively, it is possible that PFC DA may not participate in anxiety per se, but may be related to state-dependent cognitive or affective processes that covary to some degree with stress and/or anxiety. The nature of these processes remains to be determined.

Importantly, increases in DA neurotransmission are not associated only with aversive or stressful environmental stimuli. There is a large literature demonstrating a robust activation of cerebral DA systems by both pharmacological and environmental stimuli that are reinforcing (Damsma et al., 1992; Cenci et al., 1992; Phillips et al., 1993; Ahn & Phillips, 1999; Berridge & Robinson, 1998). The rewarding/reinforcing nature of these stimuli would suggest that increased DA release per se does not produce subjective, aversive aspects of stress and/or anxiety. At least superficially, the magnitude and time course of stressor- and food-induced increases in DA release are comparable, suggesting that differences between rewarding and aversive states cannot be explained by differing levels of DA or temporal profiles of DA neurotransmission across rewarding and aversive conditions. Further, manipulations of accumbens DA neurotransmission exert pronounced and similar effects on conditioned responses to both aversive and reinforcing stimuli (for review, see Salamone, 1994; Berridge & Robinson, 1998). This has suggested the hypothesis that accumbens DA may not underlie pleasure or distress per se, but rather, actions of DA within the nucleus accumbens may serve an important role in the process through which sensory stimuli elicit motivated behavior (Berridge & Robinson, 1998). Similar arguments can be made for DA actions within PFC.

Aversive and appetitive behaviors have in common that an animal attends to specific stimuli in the environment and engages in specific goal-directed behaviors. Thus, appetitive and avoidance behaviors involve at least a subset of similar, if not identical, attention- and/or motivation-related processes. It is possible that enhanced DA release within PFC modulates either of these processes to permit the animal to better contend with the environmental situation at hand. None of these hypothesized functions of PFC DA need be exclusive. If PFC serves multiple cognitive and affective processes, it is expected that DA acting within PFC will modulate multiple cognitive and affective processes. Given the interdependence of affective, attentional, arousal, and motivational processes, it is unlikely that animal studies alone, which generally rely on motoric responses to environmental situations, will be able to elucidate completely the affective functions of PFC DA efferents.

C. W. Berridge, R. A. España, and T. A. Stalnaker

Additional pharmacological studies in humans are needed to better address these questions.

SUMMARY

The PFC plays a pivotal role in the coordination of behavioral and autonomic processes associated with interacting with the environment and adapting to challenging situations. Combined, the above-described observations indicate that stressors induce physiologically relevant alterations in DA release within PFC. Anatomically, DA is well positioned to influence a variety of PFC-dependent motor, cognitive, and affective processes that presumably are essential for effectively contending with challenging environmental situations. Further, manipulations of DA neurotransmission within PFC elicit alterations in autonomic and behavioral functions. Some of these actions display a lateralization, with manipulations of right and left hemisphere DA neurotransmission associated with different patterns of effects on behavior and physiology. Further, engagement in a coping behavior suppresses rates of DA release within PFC in stress and impacts stress-related PFC neuronal activity.

Much of the previous work on the functional role of DA within PFC has been conducted in rodent medial PFC (anterior cingulate), which appears to be anatomically and functionally heterogeneous (e.g., it supports both working memory and affect-related autonomic functions). A currently large lacuna in our understanding of PFC is the lack of information concerning the role of DA within the major subdivisions of primate PFC, particularly orbitomedial PFC.

Lateralization of PFC DA response properties in stress is interesting in light of evidence suggesting lateralization of PFC function in humans, especially in terms of affective processes, including anxiety and depression. Of particular interest is the association of right PFC activity with anxiety and withdrawal. These observations suggest that the right hemisphere of the PFC may play a unique role in anxiety and/ or anxiety-related processes. Combined, these observations suggest that (1) DA efferents to the right hemisphere may play a unique role in affective and cognitive processes in stress, and (2) engagement in certain nonescape, coping behaviors may have a significant impact on anxiety-related cognitive and/or affective processes.

REFERENCES

Abercrombie, E. D., Keffe, K. A., DiFrischia, D. S., & Zigmond, M. J. (1989). Differential effect of stress on in vivo dopamine release in striatum, nucleus accumbens, and medial frontal cortex. *Journal of Neurochemistry, 52*, 1655–1658.

Abercrombie, E. D., Nisenbaum, L. K., & Zigmond, M. J. (1992). Impact of acute and chronic stress on the release and synthesis of norepinephrine in brain: Microdialysis studies in behaving animals. In R. Kvetnansky, R. McCarty, & J. Axelrod (Eds.), *Stress: Neuroendocrine and molecular approaches* (pp. 29–42). New York: Gordon and Breach.

Ahn, S., & Phillips, A. G. (1999). Dopaminergic correlates of sensory-specific satiety in the medial prefrontal cortex and nucleus accumbens of the rat. *Journal of Neuroscience, 19*, 1–6.

Alheid, G. F., & Heimer, L. (1988). New perspectives in basal forebrain organization of special relevance for neuropsychiatric disorders: The striatopallidal, amygdaloid, and corticopetal components of substantia innominata. *Neuroscience, 27*, 1–39.

Antelman, S. M., Szechtman, H., Chin, P., & Fisher, A. E. (1975). Tail pinch-induced eating, gnawing and licking behavior in rats: Dependence on the nigrostriatal dopamine system. *Brain Research, 99*, 319–337.

Arnsten, A. F., & Goldman-Rakic, P. S. (1998). Noise stress impairs prefrontal cortical cognitive function in monkeys: Evidence for a hyperdopaminergic mechanism. *Archives of General Psychiatry, 55*, 362–368.

Beaulieu, S., Di Paolo, T., & Barden, N. (1986). Control of ACTH secretion by the central nucleus of the amygdala: Implication of the serotonergic system and its relevance to the glucocorticoid delayed negative feedback mechanism. *Neuroendocrinology, 44*, 247–254.

Berger, B., Gaspar, P., & Verney, C. (1991). Dopaminergic innervation of the cerebral cortex: Unexpected differences between rodents and primates. *Trends in Neuroscience, 14*, 21–27.

Bergson, C., Mrzljak, L., Smiley, J. F., Pappy, M., Levenson, R., & Goldman-Rakic, P. S. (1995). Regional, cellular, and subcellular variations in the distribution of D1 and D5 dopamine receptors in primate brain. *Journal of Neuroscience, 15*, 7821–7836.

Berridge, C. W., & Dunn, A. J. (1989). Restraint-stress-induced changes in exploratory behavior appear to be mediated by norepinephrine-stimulated release of CRF. *Journal of Neuroscience, 9*, 3513–3521.

Berridge, C. W., & Dunn, A. J. (1990). DSP-4-induced depletion of brain norepinephrine produces opposite effects on exploratory behavior 3 and 14 days after treatment. *Psychopharmacology, 100*, 504–508.

Berridge, C. W., Mitton, E., & Roth, R. H. (1999). Selective suppression of the stressor-induced activation of the prefrontal cortical dopamine system by engagement in a behavioral coping response. *Synapse, 32*, 187–197.

Berridge, K. C., & Robinson, T. E. (1998). What is the role of dopamine in reward: Hedonic impact, reward learning, or incentive salience? *Brain Research Reviews, 28*, 309–369.

Berridge, C. W., Stratford, T. L., Foote, S. L., & Kelley, A. E. (1997). Distribution of dopamine β-hydroxylase-like immunoreactive fibers within the shell subregion of the nucleus accumbens. *Synapse, 27,* 230–241.

Borowsky, B., & Kuhn, C. M. (1992). D1 and D2 dopamine receptors stimulate hypothalamo-pituitary-adrenal activity in rats. *Neuropharmacology, 31,* 671–678.

Brog, J. S., Salyapongse, A., Deutch, A. Y., & Zahm, D. S. (1993). The patterns of afferent innervation of the core and shell in the "accumbens" part of the rat ventral striatum: Immunohistochemical detection of retrogradely transported fluoro-gold. *Journal of Comparative Neurology, 338,* 255–278.

Brozoski, T. J., Brown, R. M., Rosvold, H. E., & Goldman, P. S. (1979). Cognitive deficit caused by regional depletion of dopamine in prefrontal cortex of rhesus monkey. *Science, 205,* 929–932.

Bubser, M., & Schmidt, W. J. (1990). 6-hydroxydopamine lesions of the rat prefrontal cortex increase locomotor activity, impair acquisition of delayed alternation tasks, but do not affect uninterrupted tasks in the radial maze. *Behavioural Brain Research, 37,* 157–168.

Burns, S. M., & Wyss, W. (1985). The involvement of the anterior cingulate cortex in blood pressure control. *Brain Research, 340,* 71–77.

Caille, I., Dumartin, B., & Bloch, B. (1996). Ultrastructural localization of D1 dopamine receptor immunoreactivity in rat striatonigral neurons and its relation with dopaminergic innervation. *Brain Research, 730,* 17–31.

Cannon, W. B. (1914). The emergency function of the adrenal medulla in pain and the major emotions. *American Journal of Physiology, 33,* 356–372.

Carlson, J. N., Fitzgerald, L. W., Keller, R. W., & Glick, S. D. (1991). Side and region dependent changes in dopamine activation with various durations of restraint stress. *Brain Research, 550,* 313–318.

Carlson, J. N., Fitzgerald, L. W., Keller, R. W., & Glick, S. D. (1993). Lateralized changes in prefrontal cortical dopamine activity induced by controllable and uncontrollable stress in the rat. *Brain Research, 630,* 178–187.

Carlson, J. N., & Glick, S. D. (1989). Cerebral lateralization as a source of interindividual differences in behavior. *Experientia, 45,* 788–798.

Carlson, J. N., Glick, S. D., Hinds, P. A., & Baird, J. L. (1988). Food deprivation alters dopamine utilization in the rat prefrontal cortex and asymmetrically alters amphetamine-induced rotational behavior. *Brain Research, 454,* 373–377.

Carlson, J. N., Visker, K. E., Keller, R. W., & Glick, S. D. (1996). Left and right 6-hydroxydopamine lesions of the medial prefrontal cortex differentially alter subcortical dopamine utilization and the behavioral response to stress. *Brain Research, 711,* 1–9.

Carr, D. B., & Sesack, S. R. (1996). Hippocampal afferents to the rat prefrontal cortex: Synaptic targets and relation to dopamine terminals. *Journal of Comparative Neurology, 369,* 1–15.

Casolini, P., Kabbaj, M., Leprat, F., Piazza, P. V., Rougé-Pont, F., Angelucci, L., Simon, H., Le Moal, M., & Maccari, S. (1993). Basal and stress-induced corticosterone secretion is decreased by lesion of mesencephalic dopaminergic neurons. *Brain Research, 622,* 311–314.

Cenci, M. A., Kalen, P., Mandel, R. J., & Bjorklund, A. (1992). Regional differences in the regulation of dopamine and noradrenaline release in medial frontal cortex, nucleus accumbens and caudate-putamen: A microdialysis study in the rat. *Brain Research, 581,* 217–228.

Cheramy, A., Romo, R., Godeheu, G., Baruch, P., & Glowinski, J. (1986). In vivo pre-synaptic control of dopamine release in the cat caudate nucleus-II. Facilitatory or inhibitory influence of l-glutamate. *Neuroscience, 19,* 1081–1090.

Damsma, G., Pfaus, J. G., Wenkstern, D., Phillips, A. G., & Fibiger, H. C. (1992). Sexual behavior increases dopamine transmission in the nucleus accumbens and striatum of male rats: Comparison with novelty and locomotion. *Behavioral Neuroscience, 106,* 181–191.

D'Angio, M., Serrano, A., Rivy, J. P., & Scatton, B. (1987). Tail-pinch stress increases extracellular DOPAC levels (as measured by in vivo voltammetry) in the rat nucleus accumbens but not frontal cortex: Antagonism by diazepam and zolpidem. *Brain Research, 409,* 169–174.

Dantzer, R., & Mormede, P. (1985). Stress in domestic animals: A psychoneuroendocrine approach. In G. Moberg (Ed.), *Animal stress* (pp. 81–95). Baltimore: Waverly Press.

Davidson, R. J. (1992). Anterior cerebral asymmetry and the nature of emotion. *Brain and Cognition, 20,* 125–151.

Davis, M. (1992). The role of the amygdala in fear and anxiety. *Annual Review of Neuroscience, 15,* 353–375.

Davis, M., Hitchcock, J. M., Bowers, M. B., Berridge, C. W., Melia, K. R., & Roth, R. H. (1994). Stress-induced activation of prefrontal cortex dopamine turnover: Blockade by lesions of the amygdala. *Brain Research, 664,* 207–210.

Deutch, A. Y., & Cameron, D. S. (1992). Pharmacological characterization of dopamine systems in the nucleus accumbens core and shell. *Neuroscience, 46,* 49–56.

Deutch, A. Y., Clark, W. A., & Roth, R. H. (1990). Prefrontal cortical dopamine depletion enhances the responsiveness of mesolimbic dopamine neurons to stress. *Brain Research, 521,* 311–315.

Diaz, J., Elison, G., & Masouka, D. (1978). Stages of recovery from central norepinephrine lesions in enriched and impoverished environments: A behavioral and biochemical study. *Experimental Brain Research, 31,* 117–130.

Diorio, D., Viau, V., & Meaney, M. J. (1993). The role of the medial prefrontal cortex (cingulate gyrus) in the regulation of hypothalamic-pituitary-adrenal responses to stress. *Journal of Neuroscience, 13,* 3839–3847.

Doherty, M. D., & Gratton, A. (1999). Effects of medial prefrontal cortical injections of GABA receptor agonists and antagonists on the local and nucleus accumbens dopamine responses to stress. *Synapse, 32,* 288–300.

C. W. Berridge, R. A. España, and T. A. Stalnaker

Dunn, A. J. (1988). Stress-related activation of cerebral dopaminergic systems. In P. W. Kalivas & C. B. Nemeroff (Eds.), *The mesocorticolimbic dopamine system* (pp. 188–205). New York: New York Academy of Sciences.

Dunn, A. J., Elfvin, K., & Berridge, C. W. (1986). Changes in plasma corticosterone and cerebral biogenic amine catabolites during training and testing of mice in passive avoidance behavior. *Behavioral and Neural Biology, 46*, 410–423.

Elchisak, M. A., Murrin, C. L., Roth, R. H., & Maas, J. W. (1976). Free and conjugated dihydroxyphenylacetic acid: Effect of alterations in impulse flow in rat neostriatum and frontal cortex. *Psychopharmacology Communications, 2*, 411–420.

Fallon, J. H. (1981). Collateralization of monoamine neurons: Mesotelencephalic dopamine projections to caudate, septum, and frontal cortex. *Journal of Neuroscience, 1*, 1361–1368.

Finlay, J. M., Zigmond, M. J., & Abercrombie, E. D. (1995). Increased dopamine and norepinephrine release in medial prefrontal cortex induced by acute and chronic stress: Effects of diazepam. *Neuroscience, 64(3)*, 619–628.

Foote, S. L., & Morrison, J. H. (1987). Extrathalamic modulation of cortical function. *Annual Review of Neuroscience, 10*, 67–95.

Fudge, J. L., & Haber, S. N. (2000). The central nucleus of the amygdala projection to dopamine subpopulations in primates. *Neuroscience, 97*, 479–494.

Fuller, R. W., & Snoddy, H. D. (1981). Repeated administration of pergolide to rats attenuates the acute elevation of serum corticosterone by pergolide. *Pharmacology, Biochemistry and Behavior, 15*, 933–936.

Garris, P. A., & Wightman, R. M. (1994). Different kinetics govern dopaminergic transmission in the amygdala, prefrontal cortex, and striatum: An in vivo voltammetric study. *Journal of Neuroscience, 14*, 442–450.

Gaspar, P., Berger, B., Febvret, A., Vigny, A., & Henry, J. P. (1989). Catecholamine innervation of the human cerebral cortex as revealed by comparative immunohistochemistry of tyrosine hydroxylase and dopamine-beta-hydroxylase. *Journal of Comparative Neurology, 279*, 249–271.

Goldman-Rakic, P. S. (1987). Circuitry of the primate prefrontal cortex and the regulation of the behavior by representational memory. In F. Plum (Ed.), *Handbook of physiology. The nervous system: Higher functions of the brain*, Vol. 5, pt. 1 (pp. 373–417). Bethesda, MD: American Physiological Society.

Goldman-Rakic, P. S. (1999). The physiological approach: Functional architecture of working memory and disordered cognition in schizophrenia. *Biological Psychiatry, 46*, 650–661.

Goldman-Rakic, P. S., Leranth, C., Williams, S. M., Mons, N., & Geffard, M. (1989). Dopamine synaptic complex with pyramidal neurons in primate cerebral cortex. *Proceedings of the National Academy of Sciences, USA, 86*, 9015–9019.

Goldman-Rakic, P. S., Lidow, M. S., & Gallager, D. W. (1990). Overlap of dopaminergic, adrenergic, and serotonergic receptors and complementarity of their subtypes in primate prefrontal cortex. *Journal of Neuroscience, 10*, 2125–2138.

Goldstein, L. E., Rasmusson, A. M., Bunney, B. S., & Roth, R. H. (1996). Role of the amygdala in the coordination of behavioral, neuroendocrine, and prefrontal cortical mono-amine responses to psychological stress in the rat. *Journal of Neuroscience, 16*, 4787–4798.

Gonon, F. (1997). Prolonged and extrasynaptic excitatory action of dopamine mediated by D1 receptors in the rat striatum in vivo. *Journal of Neuroscience, 17*, 5972–5978.

Gonzales, C., & Chesselet, M. F. (1990). Amygdalonigral pathway: An anterograde study in the rat with *Phaseolus vulgaris* leucoagglutinin (PHA-L). *Journal of Comparative Neurology, 297*, 182–200.

Groenewegen, H. J., & Russchen, F. T. (1984). Organization of the efferent projections of the nucleus accumbens to pallidal, hypothalamic, and mesencephalic structures: A tracing and immunohistochemical study in the cat. *Journal of Comparative Neurology, 223*, 347–367.

Harik, S. I., Duckrow, R. B., LaManna, J. C., Rosenthal, M., Sharma, V. K., & Banerjee, S. P. (1981). Cerebral compensation for chronic noradrenergic denervation induced by locus ceruleus lesion: Recovery of receptor binding, isoproterenol-induced adenylate cy-clase activity, and oxidative metabolism. *Journal of Neuroscience, 1*, 641–649.

Haroutunian, V., Knott, P., & Davis, K. L. (1988). Effects of mesocortical dopaminergic lesions upon subcortical dopaminergic function. *Psychopharmacology Bulletin, 24*, 341–344.

Heimer, L., & Wilson, R. D. (1975). The subcortical projections of allocortex: Similarities in the nerual associations of the hippocampus, the piriform cortex and the neocortex. In M. Santini (Ed.), *Golgi Centennial Symposium Proceedings* (pp. 177–193). New York: Raven Press.

Heimer, L., Zahm, D. S., Churchill, L., Kalivas, P. W., & Wohltmann, C. (1991). Specificity in the projection patterns of accumbal core and shell in the rat. *Neuroscience, 41*, 89–125.

Hennessy, M. B., & Foy, T. (1987). Nonedible material elicits chewing and reduces the plasma corticosterone response during novelty exposure in mice. *Behavioral Neuroscience, 101*, 237–245.

Horger, B. A., & Roth, R. H. (1996). The role of mesoprefrontal dopamine neurons in stress. *Critical Reviews in Neurobiology, 10*, 395–418.

Jentsch, J. D., Redmond, D. E., Elsworth, J. D., Taylor, J. R., Youngren, K. D., & Roth, R. H. (1997). Enduring cognitive deficits and cortical dopamine dysfunction in monkeys after long-term administration of phencyclidine. *Science, 277*, 953–955.

Jentsch, J. D., Tran, A., Lee, D., Youngren, K. D., & Roth, R. H. (1997). Subchronic phen-cyclidine administration reduces mesoprefrontal dopamine utilization and impairs pre-frontal cortical-dependent cognition in rat. *Neuropsychopharmacology, 17*, 92–99.

Jones, C. A., Zempleni, E., & Reynolds, G. P. (1993). Glutamate stimulates dopamine re-lease from cortical and limbic rat brain in vitro. *European Journal of Pharmacology, 242*, 183–187.

Kalivas, P. W., & Duffy, P. (1995). Selective activation of dopamine transmission in the nucleus accumbens by stress. *Brain Research, 675,* 325–328.

Kapp, B. S., Silvestri, A. J., & Guarraci, F. A. (1998). Vertebrate models of learning and memory. In J. L. Martinez and R. Kessner (Eds.), *Neurobiology of learning and memory* (pp. 289–332). San Diego: Academic Press.

Karreman, M., & Moghaddam, B. (1996). The prefrontal cortex regulates the basal release of dopamine in the limbic striatum: An effect mediated by ventral tegmental area. *Journal of Neurochemistry, 66,* 589–598.

Kirby, L. G., Allen, A. R., & Lucki, I. (1995). Regional differences in the effects of forced swimming on extracellular levels of 5-hydroxytryptamine and 5-hydroxyindoleacetic acid. *Brain Research, 682,* 189–196.

Kitchen, I., Kelly, M., & Turner, M. (1988). Dopamine receptor modulation of corticosterone secretion in neonatal and adult rats. *Journal of Pharmacy and Pharmacology, 40,* 580–581.

Lavielle, S., Tassin, J. P., Thierry, A. M., Blanc, G., Herve, D., Barthelemy, C., & Glowinski, J. (1978). Blockade by benzodiazepines of the selective high increase in dopamine turnover induced by stress in mesocortical dopaminergic neurons of the rat. *Brain Research, 168,* 585–594.

LeDoux, J. E. (1995). Emotion: Clues from the brain. *Annual Review of Psychology, 46,* 209–235.

Levine, S. (1985). A definition of stress? In G. Moberg (Ed.), *Animal stress* (pp. 51–69). Baltimore: Waverly Press.

Lidow, M. S., Goldman-Rakic, P. S., Gallager, D. W., & Rakic, P. (1991). Distribution of dopaminergic receptors in the primate cerebral cortex: Quantitative autoradiographic analysis using [^{3}H]raclopride, [^{3}H]spiperone and [^{3}H]SCH23390. *Neuroscience, 40,* 657–671.

Lidow, M. S., Wang, F., Cao, Y., & Goldman-Rakic, P. S. (1998). Layer V neurons bear the majority of mRNAs encoding the five distinct dopamine receptor subtypes in the primate prefrontal cortex. *Synapse, 28,* 10–20.

Logue, M. P., Growdon, J. H., Coviella, I. L. G., & Wurtman, R. J. (1985). Differential effects of DSP-4 administration on regional brain norepinephrine turnover in rats. *Life Sciences, 37,* 403–409.

Maldonado-Irizzary, C. S., Swanson, C. J., & Kelley, A. E. (1995). Glutamate receptors in the nucleus accumbens shell control feeding behavior via the lateral hypothalamus. *Journal of Neuroscience, 15,* 6779–6788.

Mason, J. W. (1968). The scope of psychoendocrine research. *Psychosomatic Medicine, 30,* 565–575.

McFarland, D. J. (1966). On the causal and functional significance of displacement activities. *Zeitschrift für Tierpsychologie, 23,* 217–235.

Miner, L. A. H., Ostrander, M., & Sarter, M. (1997). Effects of ibotenic acid-induced loss of neurons in the medial prefrontal cortex of rats on behavioral vigilance: Evidence for executive dysfunction. *Journal of Psychopharmacology, 11*, 169–178.

Moghaddam, B. (1993). Stress preferentially increases extraneuronal levels of excitatory amino acids in the prefrontal cortex: Comparison to hippocampus and basal ganglia. *Journal of Neurochemistry, 60*, 1650–1657.

Mogilnicka, E. (1986). Increase in β- and α_1-adrenoceptor binding sites in the rat brain and in the α_1-adrenoceptor functional sensitivity after the DSP-4-induced noradrenergic denervation. *Pharmacology, Biochemistry and Behavior, 25*, 743–746.

Murphy, B. L., Arnsten, A. F. T., & Goldman-Rakic, P. S. (1996). Increased dopamine turnover in the prefrontal cortex impairs spatial working memory performance in rats and monkeys. *Proceedings of the National Academy of Sciences, USA, 93*, 1325–1329.

Murphy, B. L., Arnsten, A. F. T., Jentsch, J. D., & Roth, R. H. (1996). Dopamine and spatial working memory in rats and monkeys: Pharmacological reversal of stress-induced impairment. *Journal of Neuroscience, 16*, 7768–7775.

Neafsey, E. J. (1990). Prefrontal cortical control of the autonomic nervous system: Anatomical and physiological observations. *Progress in Brain Research, 85*, 147–166.

Nielsen, D. M., Crosley, K. J., Keller, R. W., Glick, S. D., & Carlson, J. N. (1999). Rotation, locomotor activity and individual differences in voluntary ethanol consumption. *Brain Research, 823*, 80–87.

Peoples, R. W., Giridhar, J., & Isom, G. E. (1991). γ-aminobutyric acid enhancement of potassium-stimulated release of [3H]norepinephrine by multiple mechanisms in rat cortical slices. *Biochemical Pharmacology, 41*, 119–123.

Phillips, A. G., Atkinson, L. J., Blackburn, J. R., & Blaha, C. D. (1993). Increased extracellular dopamine in the nucleus accumbens of the rat elicited by a conditional stimulus for food: An electrochemical study. *Canadian Journal of Physiology and Pharmacology, 71*, 387–393.

Pierce, R. C., & Kalivas, P. W. (1995). Amphetamine produces sensitized increases in locomotion and extracellular dopamine preferentially in the nucleus accumbens shell of rats administered repeated cocaine. *Journal of Pharmacology and Experimental Therapeutics, 275*, 1019–1029.

Pontieri, F. E., Tanda, G., & Di Chiara, G. (1995). Intravenous cocaine, morphine, and amphetmaine preferentially increase extracellular dopamine in the "shell" as compared with the "core" of the rat nucleus accumbens. *Proceedings of the National Academy of Sciences, USA, 92*, 12304–12308.

Preuss, T. M. (1995). Do rats have prefrontal cortex? The Rose-Woolsey-Akert program reconsidered. *Journal of Cognitive Neuroscience, 7*, 1–24.

Pulvirenti, L., Berrier, R., Kriefeldt, M., & Koob, G. F. (1994). Modulation of locomotor activity by NMDA receptors in the nucleus accumbens core and shell regions of the rat. *Brain Research, 664*, 231–236.

Pycock, C. J. (1980). Turning behaviour in animals. *Neuroscience, 5*, 461–514.

Pycock, C. J., Carter, C. J., & Kerwin, R. W. (1980). Effect of 6-hydroxydopamine lesions of the medial prefrontal cortex on neurotransmitter systems in subcortical sites in the rat. *Journal of Neurochemistry, 34*, 91–99.

Raiteri, M., Garrone, B., & Pittaluga, A. (1991). *N*-methyl-D-aspartic acid (NMDA) and non-NMDA receptors regulating hippocampal norepinephrine release. II. Evidence for functional cooperation and for coexistence on the same axon terminal. *Journal of Pharmacology and Experimental Therapeutics, 260*, 238–242.

Ramos, A., & Mormede, P. (1998). Stress and emotionality: A multidimensional and genetic approach. *Neuroscience and Biobehavioral Reviews, 22*, 33–57.

Rauch, S. L., Savage, C. R., Alpert, N. M., Euripedes, C. M., Baer, L., Breiter, H. C., Fischman, A. J., Manzo, P. A., Moretti, C., & Janike, M. A. (1995). A positron emission tomographic study of simple phobic symptom. *Archives of General Psychiatry, 52*, 20–28.

Ravard, S., Carnoy, P., Hervé, D., Tassin, J., Thiébot, M., & Soubrié, P. (1990). Involvement of prefrontal dopamine neurones in behavioural blockade induced by controllable vs. uncontrollable negative events in rats. *Behavioural Brain Research, 37*, 9–18.

Reep, R. L. (1984). Relationship between prefrontal and limbic cortex: A comparative anatomical review. *Brain, Behavior and Evolution, 25*, 1–80.

Robinson, T. E., Mocsary, Z., Camp, D. M., & Whishaw, I. Q. (1994). Time course of recovery of extracellular dopamine following partial damage to the nigrostriatal dopamine system. *Journal of Neuroscience, 14*, 2687–2696.

Roth, R. H., Murrin, C. L., & Walters, J. R. (1976). Central dopaminergic neurons: Effects of alterations in impulse flow on the accumulation of dihydroxyphenylacetic acid. *European Journal of Pharmacology, 36*, 163–171.

Roth, R. H., Tam, S., Ida, Y., Yang, J., & Deutch, A. Y. (1988). Stress and the mesocorticolimbic dopamine systems. In P. W. Kalivas & C. B. Nemeroff (Eds.), *The mesocorticolimbic dopamine system* (pp. 138–147). New York: New York Academy of Sciences.

Salamone, J. D. (1994). The involvement of nucleus accumbens dopamine in appetitive and aversive motivation. *Behavioural Brain Reseach, 61*, 117–133.

Schultz, W., Apicella, P., & Ljungberg, T. (1993). Responses of monkey dopamine neurons to reward and conditioned stimuli during successive steps of learning a delayed response task. *Journal of Neuroscience, 13*, 900–913.

Selye, H. (1946). The general adaptation syndrome and the diseases of adaptation. *Journal of Clinical Endocrinology, 6*, 117–230.

Sesack, S. R., Deutch, A. Y., Roth, R. H., & Bunney, B. S. (1989). Topographical organization of the efferent projections of the medial prefrontal cortex in the rat: An anterograde tract-tracing study with *Phaseolus vulgaris* leucoagglutinin. *Journal of Comparative Neurology, 290*, 213–242.

Sesack, S. R., Hawrylak, V. A., Melchitzky, D. S., & Lewis, D. A. (1998). Dopamine innervation of a subclass of local circuit neurons in monkey prefrontal cortex: Ultrastructural analysis of tyrosine hydroxylase and parvalbumin immunoreactive structures. *Cerebral Cortex, 8,* 614–622.

Sesack, S. R., Snyder, C. L., & Lewis, D. A. (1995). Axon terminals immunolabeled for dopamine or tyrosine hydroxylase synapse on GABA-immunoreactive dendrites in rat and monkey cortex. *Journal of Comparative Neurology, 363,* 264–280.

Skolnick, P., Stalvey, L. P., Daly, J. W., Hoyler, E., & Davis, J. N. (1978). Binding of alpha and beta adrenergic ligands to cerebral cortical membranes. Effect of 6-hydroxydopamine treatment and relationship to the responsiveness of cyclic AMP generating systems in two rat strains. *European Journal of Pharmacology, 47,* 201–210.

Smiley, J. F., Levey, A. I., Ciliax, B. J., & Goldman-Rakic, P. S. (1994). D1 dopamine receptor immunoreactivity in human and monkey cerebral cortex: Predominant and extrasynaptic localization in dendritic spines. *Proceedings of the National Academy of Sciences, USA, 91,* 5720–5724.

Stolk, J. M., Conner, R. L., Levine, S., & Barchas, J. D. (1974). Brain norepinephrine metabolism and shock-induced fighting behavior in rats: Differential effects of shock and fighting on the neurochemical response to a common footshock stimulus. *Journal of Pharmacology and Experimental Therapeutics, 190,* 193–209.

Sullivan, R. M., & Gratton, A. (1997). Relationships between stress-induced increases in medial prefrontal cortical dopamine and plasma corticosterone levels in rats: Role of cerebral laterality. *Neuroscience, 83,* 81–91.

Sullivan, R. M., & Szechtman, H. (1995). Asymmetrical influence of mesocortical dopamine depletion on stress ulcer development and subcortical dopamine systems in rats: Implications for psychopathology. *Neuroscience, 65,* 757–766.

Sutton, S. K., & Davidson, R. J. (1997). Prefrontal brain asymmetry: A biological substrate of the behavioral approach and inhibition systems. *Psychological Science, 8,* 204–210.

Swanson, L. W. (1982). The projections of the ventral tegmental area and adjacent regions: A combined fluorescent retrograde tracer and immunofluorescence study in the rat. *Brain Research Bulletin, 9,* 321–353.

Takahata, R., & Moghaddam, B. (1998). Glutamatergic regulation of basal and stimulus-activated dopamine release in the prefrontal cortex. *Journal of Neurochemistry, 71,* 1443–1449.

Tam, S. Y., & Roth, R. H. (1985). Selective increases in dopamine metabolism in the prefrontal cortex by the anxiogenic beta-carboline FG7142. *Biochemical Pharmacology, 34,* 1595–1598.

Tam, S. Y., & Roth, R. H. (1990). Modulation of mesoprefrontal dopamine neurons by central benzodiazepine receptors. I. Pharmacological characterization. *Journal of Pharmacology and Experimental Therapeutics, 252,* 989–996.

Thierry, A. M., Tassin, J. P., Blanc, G., & Glowinski, J. (1976). Selective activation of the mesocortical DA system by stress. *Nature, 263,* 242–243.

Tinbergen, N. (1952). "Derived" activities: Their causation, biological significance, origin, and emancipation during evolution. *Quarterly Review of Biology, 27*, 1–32.

Tsuda, A., Tanaka, M., Ida, Y., Shirao, I., Gondoh, Y., Oguchi, M., & Yoshida, M. (1988). Expression of aggression attenuates stress-induced increases in rat brain noradrenaline turnover. *Brain Research, 474*, 174–180.

Tzschentke, T. M., & Schmidt W. J. (1999). Functional heterogeneity of the rat medial prefrontal cortex: Effects of discrete subarea-specific lesions on drug-induced conditioned place preference and behavioural sensitization. *European Journal of Neuroscience, 11*, 4099–4109.

Venator, D. K., Lewis, D. A., & Finlay, J. M. (1999). Effects of partial dopamine loss in the medial prefrontal cortex on local baseline and stress-evoked extracellular dopamine concentrations. *Neuroscience, 93*, 497–505.

Verma, A., & Moghaddam, B. (1998). Regulation of striatal dopamine release by metabotropic glutamate receptors. *Synapse, 28*, 220–226.

Williams, G. V., & Goldman-Rakic, P. S. (1995). Modulation of memory fields by dopamine D1 receptors in prefrontal cortex. *Nature, 376*, 572–575.

Williams, S. M., & Goldman-Rakic, P. S. (1993). Characterization of the dopaminergic innervation of the primate frontal cortex using a dopamine-specific antibody. *Cerebral Cortex, 3*, 199–222.

Williams, S. M., & Goldman-Rakic, P. S. (1998). Widespread origin of the primate mesofrontal dopamine system. *Cerebral Cortex, 8*, 321–345.

Wood, P. L., & Altar, C. A. (1988). Dopamine release in vivo from nigrostriatal, mesolimbic, and mesocortical neurons: Utility of 3-methoxytryamine measurements. *Pharmacology Review, 40*, 163–187.

Yang, C. R., Seamans, J. K., & Gorelova, N. (1999). Developing a neuronal model for the pathophysiology of schizophrenia based on the nature of electrophysiological actions of dopamine in the prefrontal cortex. *Neuropsychopharmacology, 21*, 161–194.

Yung, K. K., Bolam, J. P., Smith, A. D., Hersch, S. M., Ciliax, B. J., & Levey, A. I. (1995). Immunocytochemical localization of D1 and D2 dopamine receptors in the basal ganglia of the rat: Light and electron microscopy. *Neuroscience, 65*, 709–730.

Zahm, D. S., & Brog, J. S. (1992). On the significance of subterritories in the "accumbens" part of the rat ventral striatum. *Neuroscience, 50*, 741–767.

Zahm, D. S., Jensen, S. L., Williams, E. S., & Martin, J. R. (1999). Direct comparison of projections from the central amygdaloid region and nucleus accumbens shell. *European Journal of Neuroscience, 11*, 1119–1126.

Zahrt, J., Taylor, J. R., Rex, G. M., & Arnsten, A. F. T. (1997). Supranormal stimulation of D1 dopamine receptors in the rodent prefrontal cortex impairs spatial working memory performance. *Journal of Neuroscience, 17*, 8528–8535.

4 The Nature and Determinants of Handedness

Alan A. Beaton

The large area of the human cortex devoted to representation of the hands attests to the importance of manual skill in the course of evolution, yet the two hands are rarely used with equal facility. Although right-handedness is the dominant tendency among all societies that have been studied (Harris, 1980, 1990; Peters, 1995), a proportion of the population has always preferred the left hand. Variation in this proportion in different regions of the world may be due to cultural (see Payne, 1987; Connolly & Bishop, 1992; De Agostini et al., 1997) and/or biological factors (see Bryden et al., 1997).

Despite a long history of speculation and investigation, the cause(s) of handedness remain(s) elusive (Snyder, 2000). The question of causation arises at a number of different levels. At the population level, Bol et al. (1997) suggested that the evolution of handedness may have been influenced by bacterial meningitis. They adduced evidence showing that severe forms of the disease are more often localized to the right hemisphere. On the assumption that cortical control of movements of the hands is largely contralateral, they argued that left-handers, more often than right-handers, may have died before reproductive age or, if they survived, suffered from sequelae that affected their reproductive fitness.

At the level of the individual, genetic (and other mechanisms) are undoubtedly implicated in handedness (see Levy, 1976). There is a higher incidence of left-handedness among the relatives of left-handed than of right-handed propositi, and a higher incidence of left-handedness among offspring when one parent is, or both are, left-handed (e.g., Chamberlain, 1928; Ashton, 1982; Annett, 1983, 1999a; Speigler & Yeni-Komishan, 1983; Curt et al., 1995; McKeever, 2000).

These facts on their own do not establish that handedness is genetically transmitted, but they make a search for a genetic factor worthwhile. Adoption studies can provide compelling evidence of a genetic contribution to a phenotypic characteristic. Unfortunately, there are few studies of adoption, and most concern children adopted after the age at which handedness is thought to be established or before it has become firmly fixed, and thus they contribute little, if anything, to the argument. The most satisfactory study to date (Carter-Saltzman, 1980) concluded that handedness of children is more closely related to that of their biological parents than to that of their adoptive parents. However, the distribution of children's handedness as a function of parental handedness was not computed for biological parents and their own adopted children, only for adoptive and nonadoptive families.

Traditional genetic theories have been couched in terms of genes coding for direction of handedness, but as has long been recognized (e.g., Pye-Smith, 1871; Koch, 1933), handedness is not absolute; there are different degrees of handedness. Collins suggested, on the basis of experiments with mice, that the degree, but not the direction, to which lateral preference is expressed is under genetic control (Collins, 1985).

It is in relation to language lateralization that handedness has been of greatest interest. Dominance of the right cerebral hemisphere for speech in right-handers has been considered so rare that intensive investigations have been devoted to individual cases of so-called crossed aphasia. However, Annett (1975) demonstrated that the proportion of individuals with right hemisphere speech dominance is a function of the criterion used to define left-handedness. In fact, unless the criterion is very generous, the majority of individuals with right hemisphere speech are expected to be right-handed (Annett & Alexander, 1996). At one time it was anticipated that the manner in which a pen was held in the hand would indicate which hemisphere was dominant for language (Levy & Reid, 1976). The results of Wada testing of neurosurgical patients (Volpe et al., 1981) and findings from laboratory studies (see Weber & Bradshaw, 1981) rather dashed that hope. Interest in hand posture has therefore declined despite the possibility that this variable may have some relation to familial sinistrality (McKeever & VanEys, 1989), and hence to mechanisms of inheritance. However, findings on familial sinistrality itself have been inconsistent (see McKeever, Cerone, & Chase-Carmichael, 2000), and doubts have been expressed as to their usefulness in laterality research (Bishop, 1990a; see also McManus, 1995).

It used to be thought (see Koch, 1933), and is still argued by some, that handedness falls into one of two, or perhaps three, distinct biological types corresponding to right-, left-, and mixed-handers. For example, McManus (1985a) favors the writing hand as the basis of a categorical classification, partly on the ground that the writing hand "has the strongest laterality score and is probably the most reliable of laterality measures (with the usual provisos being made about individuals who have been forced to change their writing hand as a result of social pressure)" (p. 14). An alternative view holds that handedness should be regarded as a continuously distributed variable (see Annett, 1970, 1985; Peters & Durding, 1978).

Hand preference is usually measured by questionnaire, although behavioral methods of assessing preference have been proposed by some researchers (Bryden et al., 1994; Calvert & Bishop, 1998). How to classify individuals on the basis of questionnaire data is a problematic issue (see, e.g., Peters, 1990a, 1990b, 1992, 1998; Bryden & Steenhuis, 1991; Steenhuis & Bryden, 1999), since the nature of the preference distribution obtained depends upon the questionnaire that is administered. The extent to which a particular hand is preferred varies for different tasks, being more marked for some activities than for others (e.g., Annett, 1970, 1985; Gilbert & Wysocki, 1992; Steenhuis & Bryden, 1989) even in preliterate cultures (Marchant et al., 1995). Classification of a person's handedness therefore can vary considerably depending upon the type and number of questions asked, which clearly has important theoretical implications (see Peters, 1990a). A particularly thorny issue concerns whether each item on a questionnaire should be given equal weighting in the assessment of overall handedness, an approach that has been criticized by some workers (Annett, 1985, 1995; Beaton & Moseley, 1984; Beaton, 1985).

Despite the fact that questionnaires are intended to reflect a continuum of handedness, most investigators use a cutoff score to categorize respondents into two handedness classes: right- versus left-handers or right- versus non-right-handers. If handedness is indeed a continuous distribution, then the point at which the distribution is bisected is purely arbitrary. Much of the inconsistency in the literature can be put down to different criteria of left-handedness being adopted by different investigators. As Annett (1991) points out, "There are no absolute answers to questions about left-handers; the reply must always begin with, 'It depends on who you call left handed'" (p. 339).

Inman (1924) remarked that "A curious feature about left-handedness is that it is rarely as complete as right-handedness" (p. 212), a view that was echoed by others (Humphrey, 1951; Benton et al., 1962) and is still prevalent (e.g., Rigal, 1992; Steenhuis & Bryden, 1999). However, the extent to which left-handers are less lateralized than right-handers has quite possibly been exaggerated. My own data show that approximately 60% of British students report carrying out all 12 items of Annett's questionnaire with their right hand (see also Annett, 1985). The corresponding proportion who do everything with their left hand is very much smaller, approximately 4%. When researchers want to compare groups of right- and left-handers, it is highly likely that they end up with or choose extremely strong or consistent right-handers but are forced to accept a more homogeneous group of left-handers. The upshot is that strong or consistent right-handers are compared on some performance measure of laterality with people who are less strongly or consistently handed. Thus the belief persists that "left-handers" are less lateralized than "right-handers." Data collected by my students and me show that if strong right-handers are compared with equally strong left-handers, the latter are almost as strongly "lateralized" as the former.

The preferred or dominant hand or wrist is usually but not invariably stronger than its partner (e.g., Koch, 1933; Chau et al., 1998). The right hand (of dextrals) is also usually faster and more accurate than the left on tasks requiring speeded actions such as aiming at a target, placing pegs in holes, or finger-tapping. The source of the right-hand advantage, however, has proved difficult to identify (for review, see Elliott & Chua, 1996). On peg-moving and finger-tapping tasks, right-handed adults and children (e.g., Peters & Durding, 1978, 1979; Todor et al., 1982; Carlier et al., 1993) tend to show greater variability of the left than of the right hand. Indeed, Schmidt et al. (2000) suggested that variability in hand performance might be regarded as a better index of asymmetry between the hands than performance measured in terms of speed or number of taps.

Notwithstanding the usual superiority of the right hand, the left has often been found to *initiate* aimed movements slightly but consistently faster than the right hand (e.g., Guiard et al., 1983; Helsen et al., 1998; Velay & Benoit-Dubrocard, 1999). The left hand may be quicker also in tasks that emphasize accurate spatial localization, such as intercepting a projectile (Watson & Kimura, 1989) or in reproducing the position of the fingers (Kimura & Vanderwolf, 1970; Ingram, 1975).

There has been some debate as to whether handedness is a unidimensional or multidimensional characteristic (see, e.g., Fleishman & Hempel, 1954; Healey et al., 1986; Bryden & Steenhuis, 1991). At one level the argument is unproductive, since the number of dimensions discovered depends on the nature and amount of data entered into a factor analysis. More interestingly, it does not seem that the two hands reflect different dimensions of handedness. Barnsley and Rabinovitch (1970) claimed, on the basis of a factor-analytic approach, that "although the same skills are to be found for either hand, the preferred hand is characterized by better performance in each skill" (p. 359).

Ogle (1871) pointed out that females were less likely than males to be left-handed, an observation that has been amply confirmed both in modern Western societies (see, e.g., Annett, 1985; Porac & Coren, 1981; Gilbert & Wysocki, 1992) and in cultures said to have a lower frequency of left-handedness (e.g., Hatta & Nakatsuka, 1976; Hoosain, 1990). Of course, a sex difference may not be found for every manual activity (Rigal, 1992).

On experimental tasks such as finger-tapping (King et al., 1978; Dodrill, 1979; Rigal, 1992) males tend to be faster overall than females, perhaps because the latter tend to be more cautious in their responses, emphasizing accuracy rather than speed (Kauranen & Vanharanta, 1996). Conversely, females may be quicker than males in tasks requiring fine dexterity, such as moving a ring along a bent wire without touching it (Sanders et al., 1989). Examination of the normative data provided by Gardner and Broman (1979) for performance on the Purdue peg board shows that at most ages, the superiority shown by girls is greater for the preferred compared with the nonpreferred hand (see also Rigal, 1992), consistent with adult findings of a wider difference between the hands of females than of males (e.g., King et al., 1978; Rigal, 1992; Curt et al., 1995). The age of participants and the nature of the task appear to be crucial to the direction of any sex-by-hand interaction (Kilshaw & Annett, 1983; Carlier et al., 1993).

The frequency distribution for hand preference is usually J-shaped (e.g., Curt et al., 1997), the precise form of the curve depending on the questions asked and the method of scoring the responses. Steenhuis and Bryden (1989) distinguished between skilled and unskilled manual activities, and found that while the preference distribution for skilled activities was J-shaped, that for less skilled activities was normal (while still showing a right bias). Unlike the J-shaped preference curve, the distribution for differences between the left and right hand in performance or skill is approximately normal for tasks such as peg-moving (Annett, 1970; Curt et al., 1992) or finger-tapping (Peters & Durding, 1978; Ingram, 1975).

For some tasks, such as placing a dot in a series of small circles (Falek, 1958; Tapley & Bryden, 1985; Curt et al., 1992; Annett, 1992a; Crow et al., 1998), the distribution of skill asymmetry is bimodal rather than unimodal, though this may not become evident with fairly small samples. Thus the distribution obtained depends upon the task used for assessment, and in particular on whether it is a well-practiced one (Dellatolas & Curt, 1995). McManus (1985a) argues that a second (left-handers') mode will sometimes be hidden in the main distribution according to the extent to which the task under consideration shares mechanisms with writing. More generally, whether there is evidence of bimodality will, of course, depend upon the separation between scores for the putative subpopulations, the relative size of these subpopulations, and the variance about their own mean, regardless of the actual task used.

Self-reported handedness does not always correspond with handedness measured objectively, especially for self-classified left-handers (Humphrey, 1951; Steenhuis & Bryden, 1999). Provins (1997a) argued that "Because hand preferences are inconsistent across tasks, and relative proficiency is also task specific, comparisons between the two measures can be valid only if they relate to the same activity or range of activities" (p. 187). However (at a group level), asymmetry between the hands in peg-moving or finger-tapping is systematically related to hand preference as determined by questionnnaire (e.g., Benton et al., 1962; Annett, 1970, 1976; Bishop, 1989; Peters & Durding, 1978; Triggs et al., 2000), despite the fact that the questionnaire items relate to tasks other than peg-moving or finger-tapping. In my own laboratory, we have found that the size of the correlation between preference and skill depends on whether preference is measured using the Edinburgh Handedness Inventory (Oldfield, 1971) or Annett's (1970) questionnaire, and on whether skill is measured by peg-moving or finger-tapping.

The causal relationship between preference and skill is not self-evident (Morgan & McManus, 1988). That there is a relationship cannot be doubted, although there is some dispute (see Bishop, 1989) as to which (if either) determines the other. Some authors see differences in skill between the hands as fundamental (Koch, 1933; Hildreth, 1950; Annett, 1985). Others (e.g., McManus, 1985a, 1985b) regard preference as primary. McManus and his collaborators claim support for this position from their finding that some autistic children show no skill asymmetry, yet have a clear preference for the right hand (McManus et al., 1992).

It might be thought that as one hand becomes more skilled, the other becomes less so. This is not, in fact, the case. Among right-handers, degrees of right hand preference are related to the performance of one hand only, the left. Performance of the right hand remains relatively constant across different hand preference categories; performance of the left hand declines with increasing right hand preference. This has been shown (e.g., Annett, 1995a; McManus et al., 1993; Beaton, 1995; Palmer & Corballis, 1996; Leask & Crow, 1997) for both peg-moving and finger-tapping tasks. My colleagues and I have found that the same pattern applies to left-handers. Thus the general picture appears to be that the level of skill is relatively constant for the preferred hand; what determines asymmetry between the hands is the level of skill of the nonpreferred hand. This general pattern seems to me to have important implications for the etiology of handedness.

Summarizing the main points of this chapter so far: (a) the majority of the population has a stronger, faster, and more accurate right hand; (b) handedness has a familial component; (c) males tend to be more frequently left-handed than females; (d) handedness is a continuum; (e) relative differences in skill between preferred and nonpreferred hand depend upon variation in level of skill of the nonpreferred hand. These are the minimal observations that any complete theory of handedness needs to address.

THEORIES OF HANDEDNESS

Theories of handedness fall into a number of categories, not all of which are mutually exclusive.

Historical Theories

One well-known view is that right-handedness arose because the left hand protected the heart with a shield, thus leaving the right hand free for wielding a weapon. Natural selection would lead to this arrangement being favored over the opposite arrangement, whereby the shield is held in the right hand. Although the this view has been attributed to Thomas Carlyle, and Pye-Smith (1871) thought himself the originator, neither appears to have been the first to think of it (see Wilson, 1886). According to Wile (1934), the theory is in fact "as old as Homer" (p. 123). Wile himself attributed right-handedness to the direction of rotation of the Earth. Other early theories include the ideas that right-handedness arose as a counterbalance to the body's center of gravity on the left side (Buchanan, 1862); that there is a better blood-supply to the left hemisphere (O'Connor, 1890); and that right-handedness is a consequence of a dominant right eye (Parson, 1924). Such early theories have been discussed by a number of authors since the beginning of the twentieth century, most recently by Harris (1990).

Genetic Theories

Alongside the more fanciful theories there was a growing belief that handedness is inherited. Early genetic theories that treated handedness in terms of classic Mendelian theory were abandoned when it became clear that predictions of family inheritance made by these theories were not supported by the data. In particular, if left-handedness were indeed determined by a recessive gene, then the children of two left-handed parents should not be right-handed. Data collected by Chamberlain (1928) and Annett (1983) show the prediction to be false. Attempts to rescue the hypothesis, according to which expression of the recessive gene was said to be incomplete (Trankell, 1955), were made.

Levy and Nagylaki (1972) proposed a two-gene model in which alleles at one locus coded for left or right hemispheric language lateralization, and at a second locus determined whether handedness was ipsilateral or contralateral to the language-dominant hemisphere. However, following publication of the influential paper by Morgan and Corballis (1978), in which it was pointed out that (being simply linear strings of base pairs) genes are essentially "left-right agnosic," it increasingly came to be realized that lateral asymmetries of various kinds may be determined by essentially random processes or chance, a principle embodied in several recent models of handedness.

Annett (e.g., 1985, 1995a) has consistently argued that (given the systematic relationship between hand preference and skill) what has to be explained about human handedness is that the frequency distribution of skill differences between the two hands is shifted to the right relative to a hypothetical distribution which has a mean of 0 (i.e., no mean difference between left and right sides). This is why her model is termed the right-shift (RS) theory.

Annett's model posits two alleles, rs^+ and rs^-, at a single locus. The rs^+ allele (gene) ensures that speech processes are lateralized to the left hemisphere and coincidentally leads its possessor to be more likely to become right-handed. This influence is over and above those random factors which otherwise determine handedness. The distribution of differences between the hands in skill is conceived as being made up of a subdistribution of individuals who lack the right-shift gene (i.e., are of genotype rs^{--}) and one or two subdistributions of individuals who possess the rs^+ gene in single or double dose. In her earlier publications Annett considered only two subdistributions (rs^{--} versus rs^{+-} and rs^{++} combined), but more recently she has favored an additive model (see Annett & Kilshaw, 1983) in which the subdistributions of rs^{+-} and rs^{++} are separated.

Annett's is a threshold model in the sense that the proportion of left-handers used for genetic calculations depends upon where on the overall distribution of differences in skill between the hands (the laterality distribution) a cutoff is made. This is a most powerful aspect of Annett's theory because it enabled her to predict (Annett, 1979) the proportion of left-handed children in families as a function of parental left-handedness (ranging from 4% to 24%) and filial incidences (ranging from 5% to 40%), according to different criteria of left-handedness adopted by different investigators. The ability to successfully predict handedness in families (see also Annett, 1999a; McManus, 1985b) must be regarded as strong evidence for any genetic model on which the predictions are based, and thereby constitutes a convincing argument that handedness is to some extent genetically determined.

Annett has argued that her hypothesized right-shift gene works by handicapping the right hemisphere in some way. Although formulated in part as a result of findings showing that right-handers have a weak left hand in comparison with the right hand of left-handers (Kilshaw & Annett, 1983) , this proposal can explain the fact that in right-handers, differences in degree of asymmetry in hand skill are related to variation in performance of the left hand but not of the right hand. The effect of the gene is expected to be over and above chance differences between the hands. This means that in individuals of rs^{--} genotype (of whom close to 50% are expected to be left-handed), chance would be the only systematic determinant of left-right differences in hand skill. The majority of right-handers would, on Annett's theory, be expected to carry the rs⁺ gene, and thus to show a greater degree of asymmetry between the hands than noncarriers. (An analogous argument applies to a sex difference in skill asymmetry, if the gene is expressed more strongly in males). However, in my laboratory Karen Thomas and I have noticed that the extent of the difference among left-handers is not very different from that for right-handers, provided we compare subgroups of each handedness category whose degree of preference is approximately similar.

Klar (1996) claimed to offer a new genetic theory of handedness, but it is in virtually all crucial respects identical to Annett's right-shift theory. Klar acknowledges certain similarities between his own model and that of McManus (1985b, 1991). Like Annett's model, McManus's model incorporates the idea of randomness or chance (which is not to dismiss the differences [Annett, 1995a, 1995b] between Annett's and McManus's models in this regard). McManus's model has two alleles (at a single autosomal locus; but see below). One allele (C) is conceptually similar to Annett's rs⁻ gene in that it allows handedness to vary according to chance. In the model handedness is explicitly regarded as being discrete rather than continuous, this postulate deriving from the observation that the distribution of skill asymmetry for some tasks is bimodal rather than unimodal (see above).

The model (McManus, 1985b) holds that there is a gene (D) which codes for dextrality and one (C) which codes for chance (or fluctuating asymmetry). The homozygote DD is always dextral; in the case of the CC homozygote, right-handedness occurs on 50% of occasions and left-handedness on the other 50%. McManus proposes that in the case of the heterozygote DC, D is expressed half the time and C the other half of the time; when C is expressed, the outcome is dextral 50% of the time and sinistral on the remainder. Dextral and sinistral are regarded as discrete biological types. The D gene is regarded as a gene for left-hemisphere speech as well as a handedness gene. Thus all those of DD genotype would be expected to be right-handed and left-dominant for speech. Among CC genotypes, handedness and brainedness are independent, and each is dermined by separate chance events. Among those of DC genotype, one quarter are expected to be right-brained (in the same way that one-quarter are expected to be left-handed) but the asymmetries of hand and brain are independent.

The genetic models of Annett and McManus are currently the most widely quoted in the laterality literature. They differ from previous models in not postulating a gene specifically for left-handedness. According to both Annett and McManus, chance plays a major role in the determination of handedness. Annett's model has a postulate that the expression of the right-shift gene is greater in females than in males (and is reduced in twins compared with singletons). McManus's model (see McManus & Bryden, 1992) has a sex-linked "modifier gene," which explains the excess number of male compared with female left-handers.

Crow has posited that a gene for laterality is located in homologous regions of the X and Y chromosomes (e.g., Crow, 1995, 1998). Consistent with this view, Corballis et al. (1996) reported that concordance for sex is significantly higher among siblings of the same handedness than among those whose handedness is discordant. Subsequently, Corballis (1997) argued that there are serious difficulties for this hypothesis. In particular, the difference in the incidence of left-handedness in males and females predicted by the theory is much larger than the observed difference (see also McKeever, 2000). Corballis (1997) proposed that while "evolutionary considerations must weigh against the location of a single handedness gene in homologous regions of the sex chromosomes" (p. 722), it is possible that an autosomal gene for laterality is modified by a sex-linked modifier gene, as suggested by McManus and Bryden (1992). In reply, Jones and Martin (2000) argued that if left-handedness is considered to be "genetically recessive rather than additive," then the sex-chromosome hypothesis provides a parsimonious account not only of sex differences but also of twin and generational effects. The hypothesis of an X-linked effect on handedness was rejected by Tambs et al. (1987) in their study of handedness in the families of twins, but evidence in favor of linkage to the X chromosome was more recently obtained by McKeever (2000) in a study of family handedness in students.

Laland et al. (1995) published what they called a gene-culture model of handedness that incorporates certain of the assumptions of the McManus model. In particular, it assumes that handedness is categorical rather than continuous, and that there is a "true" incidence of left-handedness. Laland et al. assume that an individual's handedness is a function of that person's genotype (with alleles labeled D and C, as in the McManus model) and the phenotypic handedness of his or her parents. They do not imply that children directly copy their parents or that the latter deliberately teach their children; rather, the probability of a child becoming right-/left-handed as a function of parental handedness being both right, both left, or mixed is specifically accounted for by separate parameters of the model. A central assumption of this model is that selection has eliminated all genetic variation contributing to handedness. Laland et al. argue that "Variation in handedness among humans is generated by accidents of early development, which by chance give greater skill or strength to one side or the other. All our genes do is simply load the handedness die to favor the right" (p. 441). This, of course, is precisely Annett's view!

Peters (1990b) obtained data to show that among student volunteers, the majority of right-handers were consistently right-sided in terms of preference, performance, and strength. A group termed consistent left-handers preferred their left hand for writing and throwing; they were faster at finger-tapping with this hand; and the left hand was stronger and wider than the right hand. A group classified as inconsistent left-handers preferred the left hand for writing and tapped faster with this hand, but threw with the right hand, which was slightly larger and stronger than the left hand. Peters argued that this posed problems for single-gene theories of handedness, which can not "deal with the systematic dissociation between fine manual skill and strength seen in the ICL's" (p. 287). Risch and Pringle (1985) concluded, on the basis of a segregation analysis of handedness in 1564 families, that their data were consistent with either a single-locus or a polygenic model of inheritance.

THE DEVELOPMENTAL INSTABILITY MODEL

Deviations from perfect symmetry in the two sides of an organism can be classified in one of three ways: directional asymmetry, where there is a consistent asymmetry in favor of one side; anti-symmetry, where an asymmetry is usually present but is variable as to which side is more developed; and fluctuating asymmetry, which refers to small deviations in length or conformation at the left and right sides (see A. R. Palmer & Strobeck, 1986). On average, for any given bilateral trait, such as ear breadth or finger length, one side will be the larger or more developed as often as the other. Since the two sides of an organism are produced by the same combinations of genes, fluctuating asymmetry is seen as the result of an inability to resist the various environmental and other perturbations that beset the organism during its early development. In the absence of such perturbations, the organism would develop as perfectly bilaterally symmetrical. The ability of an organism to precisely express its developmental design in the face of various environmental and genetic perturbations is referred to as developmental stability.

Under normal circumstances, the eyes gradually move toward each other and the ears move up the neckline during the first trimester of pregnancy. Widely spaced eyes or low-set ears, referred to as minor physical anomalies, are said to result from disruption of normal developmental processes. That is, they are signs of developmental instability. Yeo and Gangestad (1993) reported that, in comparison with more weakly lateralized individuals, both strong left-handers and strong right-handers showed greater developmental instability, as reflected in a composite score involving both minor physical anomalies and fluctuating asymmetry. Yeo et al. (1997) confirmed that a composite DI score correlated with hand preference as well as with asymmetry of performance.

Assuming an association between fluctuating asymmetry and polygenic inheritance, Yeo et al. (1993) argued that their data are incompatible with the single-gene models of Annett and McManus. Further, their finding that both left-handers and right-handers have an elevated proportion of left-handed parents (Gangestad & Yeo, 1994) also would not be predicted by these models. In reply, Annett (1996) pointed out that, using the same criterion as Yeo et al. (1993), her own data (see also McKeever et al., 2000) fail to show the (counterintuitive) increase in left-handed parents of strongly right-handed students reported by Yeo et al.

Gangestad et al. (1996) claimed to find an association between handedness and certain human leukocyte antigens (HLA) that constitute part of the major histocompatibility complex of genes. Gangestad et al. argued that HLA may influence handedness through one of two ways. One way is directly, through one or more of the alleles affecting prenatal hormone levels or through an influence on the immune response of mother or fetus (see below). Another way is indirectly, by virtue of an association between an unidentified allele linked with the HLA cluster of alleles that they identified. Either way, Gangestad et al. conclude that if there is a single gene influencing handedness, then it must be somewhere on chromosome 6 (since the relevant alleles have been located on this chromosome).

Gangestad et al. (1996) also found that left-handers produced fewer offspring than right-handers, a result reported by some other authors (see McManus & Bryden, 1992; McKeever et al., 2000) but not replicated in Annett's data. Their finding was regarded by Gangestad et al. (1996) as representing a "serious challenge to any genetic model of handedness." However, the possibility that individuals of exclusively homosexual orientation are less biased toward the right than the general population (see Annett, 1988; Lalumière et al., 2000) might explain any reduction in fertility attributed to left-handers.

The concept of fluctuating asymmetry as related to developmental instability actually refers to asymmetry of morphological characters, not to behavioral phenomena. Thus proponents of the developmental instability model presumably regard handedness as being isomorphic with structural asymmetry of the brain. The theory proposes that extreme handedness in either direction represents deviation from the norm of moderate (modal) right-handedness. Saying this does not explain why right-handedness is the norm; the bias toward the right still has to be explained. Degrees of handedness can be readily accommodated by the theory as it incorporates the notion of fluctuating asymmetry. The theory requires little in the way of additional postulates to explain the sex difference in handedness, if it is accepted that an HLA allele may influence prenatal testosterone levels (Gangestad et al., 1996). What is less clear is that it can explain the observation that variation in hand skill concerns mainly the nonpreferred hand. Nor is it clear what quantitative predictions the theory makes with regard to the distribution of handedness in families. This contrasts with the ability of both the right-shift theory of Annett and the symmetric bimodal model of McManus. For further comparisons of the theories see Annett (1996).

THE ROLE OF LEARNING

There seems to be little doubt that the relative frequency of left-handedness (e.g., Tambs et al., 1987; Gilbert & Wysocki, 1992; Davis & Annett, 1994; Hugdahl et al., 1996) and left-footedness (Porac, 1996; Bell & Gabbard, 2000) declines with age and now is less than it was a century ago. The reason for this is much debated, but one theory is that it represents a relaxation in recent years of cultural pressure toward obligatory use of the right hand for certain tasks (Brackenridge, 1981). Implicit in this view is the notion that handedness is modifiable through cultural or environmental factors. If that is so, might not such factors explain handedness in the first place?

The idea that handedness is a learned characteristic has a long history. Some authors, though admitting a congenital bias toward right-handedness in some or all children, have concluded that learning is the major determinant (e.g., Humphry, 1861; Perelle et al., 1981; Provins, 1997a, 1997b), while some have strongly opposed this view (Buchanan, 1862; Annett, 1985; McManus & Bryden, 1993). Other writers have been more cautious. Heilman, Coyle et al. (1973), for example, note that "although dexterity is normally greater in the dominant hand, one must keep in mind the possibility that dexterity is the result of preferred use, rather than vice versa" (p. 25).

Provins (1997b) reiterated his belief that handedness derives from practice effects. Briefly, he contends that "What is genetically determined is a neural substrate that has significantly increased its functional plasticity in the course of evolution.... What is fine-tuned is the relative motor proficiency or skills achieved by the two sides in any given task according to their use and the demands made on them as a result of social pressure, other environmental influences or habit" (p. 556).

An alternative opinion was expressed by McManus et al., (1986), who argued that practice is unlikely to be the cause of performance differences between the hands, since degree of improvement in a simple tapping task was similar for both preferred and nonpreferred hands (and for typists and piano players as well as for nonspecialist participants).

The view that handedness is learned leaves unanswered the question of why the cultural bias should always lead to the majority being right-handed. Nor does this argument explain why approximately 80% of left-handers have two right-handed parents, or why two left-handed parents do not have a majority of left-handed offspring (Annett, 1983; McKeever, 2000). More generally, it is difficult to see how genetic models can predict family handedness data so successfully if learning is the major cause of hand differences.

A further objection to a purely learning-based account of handedness is that it cannot easily explain those findings on fetal thumb-sucking (Hepper et al., 1991) or arm movements (Hepper et al., 1998) which suggest that some manual functions are lateralized prior to birth. (Of course it remains to be shown that these early manifestations of asymmetry relate to adult handedness).

Finally (but not exhaustively), handedness has been related (frequently if not convincingly) not only to physical features connected with, for example, the nose, (Sutton, 1963), testicles (Chang et al., 1960), and handprints and fingerprints (Newman, 1934), but also to behavioral phenomena such as eye dominance (McManus et al., 1999; Annett, 1999b, 2000) and laterality of jaw movements (Koch, 1933), which are difficult to reconcile with an effect of learning. The fact that anatomical brain asymmetry has been related to a familial as well as a personal history of left-handedness (Steinmetz et al., 1991) is particularly problematic for a learning account.

No one would deny that a change of handedness may be brought about by early cerebral damage (see Satz, 1972) or unilateral upper limb injury (Dellatolas et al., 1993). However, it is also true that individuals appear to differ considerably in the extent to which their nervous system "resists" attempts at retraining after loss of one hand (Smith, 1927, p. 189) or temporary injury (Porac, 1995; see also Beaton et al., 1994). It is also undeniable that parts of the brain concerned with manual dexterity can undergo considerable functional and even structural modification through extensive training (e.g., Wang et al., 1995; Elbert et al., 1995). However, it is difficult to see on a purely learning-based account why performance levels of the preferred hand should be approximately constant across different subgroups while that of the nonpreferred hand varies. It is also difficult to accept that the sex difference in handedness is entirely attributable to learning, though it may contribute to some extent (see Porac et al., 1986).

In view of all the arguments against a learning theory of hand preference and skill, it seems reasonable to conclude that biology plays the major role but that learning may play some part in helping to "fix" the magnitude of handedness within a given direction, left or right.

THE TESTOSTERONE THEORY

Geschwind and Behan (1982) proposed that at a critical stage of prenatal brain maturation, excessively high levels of fetal male hormone, for example, testosterone, cause a slowing down in development of the left cerebral hemisphere relative to the right hemisphere in a region known as the planum temporale, part of the superior surface of the temporal lobe. The homologous region on the right side was said to grow larger to compensate for the reduction in growth of the left side. Since the planum on the left side was thought normally to be larger than that on the right (Geschwind & Levitsky, 1968), excess testosterone will lead to a symmetrical brain or reduced asymmetry. The reduction in left hemisphere development was considered responsible for an increase in probability of developmental language disorders and left-handedness. In addition, it was argued that by suppressing maturation of the thymus gland, testosterone influenced the immune system. These two postulates were considered to explain associations reported by Geschwind and Behan (on the basis of not very strong evidence) between left-handedness and elevated frequencies both of certain disorders of the immune system and of developmental learning disorders such as dyslexia. For a critique of this paper, see Satz and Soper (1986).

The theory was developed in a series of papers (combined as Geschwind & Galaburda, 1987) in which high levels of fetal testosterone were said to be associated not with left-handedness, per se, but with "anomalous dominance" or shifts in lateralization (cerebral or manual) away from the standard or typical pattern of left lateralization for language, right-handedness, or both. (Right hemisphere functions were also included but are not relevant in the present context, and will be ignored). The theory provides no obvious account of the standard pattern of lateralization, only of deviations from it. Geschwind and Galaburda (1985) simply accept that "in most humans there is an innate bias toward left-hemisphere dominance [for language and handedness] and that certain influences during fetal life act to diminish this innate bias" (p. 447).

Research by Galaburda and his colleagues suggested that the planum temporale was symmetrical in four autopsied cases of dyslexia (see Beaton, 1997 for critique and review). Subsequent reanalysis of brains first studied by Geschwind and Levitsky (1968) revealed that symmetrical brains were characterized by two relatively large plana rather than two small or two medium-sized plana. The implication was that a symmetrical brain is due not to a smaller left hemisphere but to a larger right hemisphere. The theory was therefore modified (Galaburda et al., 1987) to suggest that excess testosterone in some way interfered with or arrested the process (epigenetic involution) whereby one hemisphere (usually the right) is reduced in size relative to the other.

An attempt to formalize the major postulates of the Geschwind-Behan-Galaburda (GBG) theory was made by McManus and Bryden (1991), and an evaluation of the evidence in its favor was published by

Bryden et al. (1994a) as a major target article (for replies to peer commentaries, see Bryden et al., 1994b), and will therefore be dealt with only briefly here. The theory is considered in the context of hormonal and other intrauterine influences by Habib et al. (1990).

Indirect support for the GBG hypothesis comes from research with people whose mothers during pregnancy received a drug known as diethylstilbestrol (DES) to prevent miscarriage. Geschwind and Galaburda suggested that this drug resembles testosterone in its actions on the central nervous system. Subsequently Schacter (1994) reported that in 77 daughters of women who had been given DES, the distribution of handedness was shifted away from strong toward moderate right-handedness. Similar findings were reported by Scheirs and Vingerhoets (1995).

Congenital adrenal hyperplasia (CAH) is a genetic disorder in which male hormone levels are elevated. Reports that females with CAH are more often left- or mixed-handed (Nass et al., 1987), and that CAH children (and their siblings) more frequently show atypical patterns of planum temporale asymmetry (Plante et al., 1996) might be seen as consistent with the GBG hypothesis. However, there have been failures to find any difference in handedness (or cerebral lateralization as determined by dichotic listening) between CAH participants and controls (e.g., Helleday et al., 1994).

Most work carried out within the framework of the GBG hypothesis has looked at two- or three-way associations between handedness, dyslexia, and immune disorders (see Bryden et al., 1994a). It was not until ten years after its initial proposal that the major postulate was directly tested. Amniotic testosterone levels measured at 16 weeks gestational age were found by Grimshaw et al. (1995) to predict handedness in girls and language lateralization (assessed by dichotic listening) in boys at age 10 years. However, the results were in the opposite direction to that predicted by the GBG hypothesis (and thus in the direction proposed by Witelson, 1991; see below). That is, higher levels of prenatal testosterone were associated with stronger right-handedness and stronger left language lateralization. It has also been found (Moffat & Hampson, 1996) that adult right-handers show higher levels of salivary testosterone than left-handers. This, too, contradicts the GBG hypothesis unless low levels of fetal testosterone are associated with high levels of salivary testosterone in adulthood, which intuitively seems unlikely.

Hormonal and genetic theories of cerebral lateralization and handedness are not necessarily incompatible (Geschwind & Behan, 1982; Habib et al., 1990); indeed, they might well be complementary. The GBG hypothesis (at least in its modified form) does not conflict with the observation that degrees of preferred hand advantage are associated with variation only in skill of the nonpreferred hand (see also Annett, 1992b). The sex difference in handedness, too, can be handled by the theory, although given that so much store is placed on the role of the male hormone testosterone, one might have expected that the handedness distributions for males and females would overlap far less than in fact they do. However, the theory fails to explain why the majority of the population is right-handed.

THE LIEPMANN HYPOTHESIS

The most common "explanation" of right-handedness is that it has something to do with a superiority of the left over the right hemisphere in motor control, as was argued by Ogle (1871) over 100 years ago. The contrary position, that development of the left hemisphere is due to preferential use of the right hand, has also been proposed (Wharton, 1884).

Apraxia (or dyspraxia) is a term used (somewhat loosely and confusingly) to refer to disorders in planning, remembering, or executing voluntary, purposeful movements or sequences of movement, including those involved in tool use (Heilman & Rothi, 1993). Two main categories of apraxia traditionally have been identified—ideational and ideomotor—but these terms no more indicate the precise nature and functional locus of the praxic difficulty than the word "aphasia" specifies the nature of a language difficulty. More recent cognitive neuropsychological approaches (e.g., Riddoch et al., 1989; Rothi et al., 1991; Roy, 1996) therefore represent an improvement on earlier descriptions of apraxia. The disorder was brought to prominence in the early years of the twentieth century by Liepmann and Maas (1907) who believed that manual dominance is a reflection of the ability of one hemisphere to learn and retain the "engrams" or "movement formulae" for motor tasks more readily than the other hemisphere, a view for which there is considerable evidence (see Kimura, 1993).

Although rare, apraxia is sometimes seen after cortical damage on the right side in right-handed patients (e.g., De Renzi et al., 1980; Marchetti & Della Sala, 1997; Raymer et al., 1999). Among left-handers, apraxia is seen more frequently after left-sided than right-sided lesions, and is uncommon following a right hemisphere lesion (Archibald, 1987; see Rapcsack et al., 1987). Cases of apraxia following a lesion on the same side as the preferred hand, so called crossed apraxia, raise a problem for Liepmann's hypothesis that handedness is due to the superior motor prowess of the contralateral hemisphere (but see Marchetti & Della Sala, 1997). The hypothesis can be maintained by proposing that in such cases the preferred hand is controlled from the hemisphere dominant for praxis via a transcallosal and/or a subcortical route.

The fact that destruction of primary motor cortex does not necessarily produce apraxia (Kimura, 1982), despite producing weakness or paralysis of the contralateral hand, led Liepmann to emphasize the role of the corpus callosum in the control of hand and arm movements of both left and right limbs. Liepmann and Maas (1907) reported a now celebrated case of a right-handed patient with a lesion of the anterior corpus callosum who exhibited apraxia and agraphia of the left hand. Similar cases in right-handers were reported more recently by Geschwind and Kaplan (1962) and by Goldenberg et al. (1985). The location of the lesions in these different cases points to the anterior callosum as being involved in left hemisphere control of the left hand, although it may be that the pattern of symptoms seen in cases of callosal apraxia depends upon the precise locus of the lesion (see Gersh & Damasio 1981).

Patients in whom the interhemispheric commissures have been surgically sectioned would appear to provide an excellent test of Liepmann's hypothesis. Data on nine commissurotomized patients were summarized by Gazzaniga et al. (1967). Left-hand apraxia in response to a verbal command was seen initially in all patients, and persisted chronically in at least some (Zaidel & Sperry, 1977). However, the required movements could generally be imitated (see also Milner & Kolb, 1985) if demonstrated by an examiner, thereby undermining the generality of Liepmann's hypothesis.

Lausberg et al. (1999) reported the case of a left-handed patient who sustained a lesion of the anterior four-fifths of the left side of the corpus callosum together with both sides of the splenium. This patient had no preexisting brain damage or seizures, and did not come to surgery. Nonethelesss, the patient showed the classic signs of disconnection syndrome as seen after commissurotomy, thereby confirming that the effects are genuinely attributable to separation of the hemispheres. Of particular interest in the present context is the fact that the patient exhibited ideomotor apraxia of the left hand both to verbal command and to imitation. There was no apraxia evident for the right hand, which implies that a general difficulty in comprehending instructions cannot explain the apraxia for the left hand (and leg). The case is similar to the classic case reported by Liepmann and Maas (1907) in showing apraxia limited to the left hand.

Liepmann's patient was right-handed. If his explanation of the left-hand apraxia is accepted, then it is clear from the case of the left-hander reported by Lausberg et al. (1999) that hand preference and motor dominance need not reside within the same cerebral hemisphere. It further follows that manual preference is not determined by "motor dominance" in the sense intended by Liepmann. It must be then asked whether the deficits that constitute clinical apraxia (however fractionated) relate to what we think of as being the skills underlying handedness in any normally accepted sense of this term. If they do not, then there really is no conflict between "handedness" being associated with one hemisphere and control of "praxis," in the sense of an overall ability to carry out purposeful movement, being vested in the opposite hemisphere (see Raymer et al., 1999).

PATHOLOGICAL LEFT-HANDEDNESS

A distinction between "natural" and "pathological" left-handers was drawn by Gordon (1921), who stated, "... there are certainly two distinct types of left-handedness: (1) those who are naturally left-handed .... (2) those who are naturally right-handed, but who have been driven to the use of left hand [sic] in some of their activities owing to some defect of the nervous or muscular systems" (p. 349).

It has long been claimed (but see Previc, 1996) that there is an elevated frequency of mixed- and left-handedness, and reduced frequency of strong right-handedness, in cases of severe epilepsy and "mental handicap" (see Harris & Carlson, 1988; Pipe, 1988, 1990; Mandal et al., 1998). An increased frequency of mixed- or left-handedness has also been claimed in a large number of developmental disorders (for review, see Geschwind & Galaburda, 1987; Bishop, 1990b).

An explanation for the higher incidence of non-right-handedness in certain clinical populations was proposed by Satz (1972) and developed by Soper and Satz (1984). The model is based on the assumption that in a proportion of cases of pre- or perinatal unilateral lesions, the damage will be such as to cause a shift in control of the preferred hand from one hemisphere to the other. If lesions of the left and right cerebral hemispheres are equiprobable, then the fact that most people are destined to become right-handers will mean that more individuals will have their handedness shifted from right to left than from left to right. This will disproportionately increase the number of individuals manifesting left-handedness in the population of brain-damaged individuals. The outcome is a higher frequency of left-handedness among the brain-damaged population relative to the population at large.

The effects of early cerebral injury may be asymmetric. Hiscock et al. (1989) compared children with left or right hemiplegia on tests of hand preference, and strength and skill, as well as length of hand and foot. The mean length of the hand (and foot) was smaller on the side opposite the presumed lesion, but hand preference scores did not distinguish the two hemiplegic groups. In terms of skill asymmetry, however, the left hemiplegic group were more asymmetrical than the right hemiplegic group, as would be expected if most individuals are destined by birth (rather than by training) to become right-handed. This result therefore suggests that "manual specialization is determined early in life and cannot be reversed completely even by a combination of lateralized brain pathology and unilateral practice with the originally nondominant hand" (p. 184).

While the pathological left-handedness (PLH) model (for review, see Harris & Carlson, 1988) accounts for a raised incidence of sinistrality among people with brain damage, it does not explain left-handedness among the neurologically undamaged population without further assumptions being made. One is that very early subtle cerebral insult or anomaly sufficient to cause a "shift" in handedness may occur at a given stage of brain development, yet not be serious enough to produce any noticeable neurological impairment. Bishop (1984) argued that in such cases one would expect to see particularly poor performance of the nonpreferred hand compared with the preferred hand. She confirmed her prediction (see also Williams et al., 1992) of a raised incidence of left-handers in a group of normal schoolchildren showing this pattern of hand skill. In a later publication (Bishop, 1990b) she calculated that in the normal population approximately 1 case in 20 of left-handedness is due to pathological causes.

Alan A. Beaton

The notion of PLH was rejected by McManus (1983) except for the theoretically trivial case in which a severely hemiplegic person can not use one limb. Peters (1990a) also raised doubts, pointing out that "within the context of left-handedness it is not entirely clear [what] is meant by pathology ... if there are no overt neurological problems, why should one talk of a case of pathological left-handedness?" (p. 173).

Related to the PLH model is the view that in the absence of other signs of pathology, left-handedness (or non-right-handedness) arises from complications associated with birth stress, such as hypoxia. The origins of this idea, which in recent times has been promoted most energetically by Bakan and his colleagues (Bakan, 1990; see also Coren & Searleman, 1990; Coren, 1995), can be found in the Bible (Bakan, 1990). One problem with this hypothesis in its simplest form (see Schwartz, 1990; Previc, 1996 for reviews) is that it is unrealistic to suppose that a significant proportion of the population would be right-handed (making humans the only all-right-handed species) if it were not for a significant degree of birth stress (which nonetheless leaves them without conspicuous impairment). A second difficulty is that there have been many failures to find any significant association even in fairly large samples (McManus, 1981; Nachson & Denno, 1987; Schwartz, 1990; Dellatolas et al., 1991) between handedness and birth complications as recorded at the time of birth or between handedness and factors, such as birth order, presumed to be associated with birth stress.

Searleman et al. (1989) carried out a meta-analysis and found little or no support for the hypothesis that birth order was related to handedness, but did find a weak though statistically significant association between birth stress and non-right-handedness. In a subsequent article (Coren & Searleman, 1990) it was concluded that "Although the size of the effect was quite small for any individual birth stressor, ... when birth stressors are considered collectively, there is some validity to the hypothesis that birth stress is correlated with deviations from right-handedness" (p. 18). Schwartz (1988), however, found large discrepancies between hospital records and mothers' reports of the events surrounding the birth of their offspring which raises some doubt as to the reliability of one or both kinds of report, at least in some circumstances or in some institutions.

Adverse prenatal as well as perinatal factors surrounding birth may be seen (Bakan, 1990) as comprising a "continuum of reproductive casuality." Coren and Porac (1980) reported an effect of maternal age on offspring handedness, but this was not replicated by Ashton (1982). The latter found a significant association between self-reported pregnancy risks (specifically, very quick labor and premature birth) and left-handedness in daughters but not in sons. Subsequently, Coren (1990) reported that frequency of left-handedness (definition not given) in college students increased as a function of maternal age at parturition. Bakan (1991) reported that the student offspring of mothers who were said to have smoked during pregnancy were as a group less biased toward use of the right hand, and reported more pregnancy and birth complications, than students whose mothers were said not to have smoked in pregnancy.

McKeever et al. (1995) concluded that about 29% of female left-handers "may owe their sinistrality to factors associated with high risk parity and maternal ages over 32." However, since birth complications were unrelated to handedness of offspring, it was speculated that "age-related hormonal changes or uterine condition changes could be involved" (p. 553).

Doubts have been raised about the reliability of subjects' reports of their own birth stress. Focusing on the mothers' recall rather than the reports of the offspring, Ellis and Peckham (1991) reported that mothers of left-handers recalled significantly greater stress throughout pregnancy than did the mothers of mixed- or right-handers. It was suggested that this was compatible with the view that "stress" hormones secreted by the mother during pregnancy can affect the cortical functioning of the offspring.

Even if the birth stress hypothesis in its strongest form does not command a great deal of support, it may be that factors associated with certain kinds of births—those which are very early or premature (less than about 34 weeks gestation) and are associated with very low birth weight (less than 1000 gms)—do lead to an increase in left- or mixed-handedness (e.g. Ross et al., 1987; O'Callaghan et al., 1993; Powls et al., 1996) despite some negative reports (Ashton, 1982; Tan & Nettleton, 1980). Certainly MRI scans at age 14–15 years have revealed a high incidence of brain abnormalities among preterm as compared with full-term children (Stewart et al., 1999).

In a large-scale prospective investigation of perinatal birth "stressors" (such as low birth weight, multiple births, forceps delivery, or resuscitation of the infant) Williams et al. (1992) found that infants who had been resuscitated or were one of twins or triplets were significantly more likely to be left-handed (as assessed by drawing hand) at age 5 years than were infants who had not experienced such perinatal stress. There was, however, no significant association between low or extremely low birth weight and subsequent sinistrality in this study.

In the study by Ross et al. (1987) parental handedness was assessed; it was apparent that there was no difference in the distribution of right-, left-, and mixed-handedness between the parents of full-term and of premature, extremely low birth weight infants. Thus there is no reason from this study to believe that non-right-handed parents are more likely to produce premature and low birth weight infants. It should be noted, however, that Ross et al. did not distinguish between the handedness of mothers and fathers. Coren (1995) reported that mothers (aged 17–27 years, so as to reduce the potential effect of maternal age) who were non-right-handed were more likely to have birth-stressed children than were right-handed mothers. A similar pattern was not found for fathers. Coren suggested that having had a difficult birth is passed on from a mother, through her own "internal conditions," to a daughter.

If the pathology model can explain some instances of left-handedness, which it assuredly can, it would require turning the model on its head to attempt to explain the (numerically much larger) phenomenon of right-handedness. It is thus not a serious candidate as an explanation of the major feature of human laterality, right-handedness.

WITELSON'S THEORY

Witelson (1985) reported in a postmortem study that the posterior region of the corpus callosum was larger in nonconsistent right-handers than in consistent right-handers (although this has often been referred to by others as showing a difference between left- and right-handers). She subsequently confirmed (Witelson, 1989) that the isthmus was larger in male but not female nonconsistent right-handers. In males, isthmal area correlated significantly with a measure of handedness (Witelson & Goldsmith, 1991). As a result of such findings, Witelson and Nowakowski (1991) proposed what might be called a callosal theory of handedness. They wrote:

The hypothesis elaborated here is that one determinant of hand preference and the pattern of functional asymmetries in the adult is the amount of naturally occurring loss of callosal axons which occurs during late fetal and early postnatal periods. . . .

. . . In the case of handedness, the specific hypothesis is that lateralization changes towards right-handedness with increases in axon loss over time. (p. 328)

Witelson and Nowakowski (1991) suggest that axon loss might contribute to the anatomical basis of hand preference in one of two ways. Either axon loss could operate on a symmetric brain in an asymmetric fashion, or axon loss could operate (symmetrically or asymmetrically) on an already asymmetric brain. The first possibility, operating on a symmetric brain, was thought unlikely because indications of perisylvian neuroanatomic asymmetry have been reported as early as the first trimester of pregnancy (Chi et al., 1977). Because callosal area was not found by Witelson (1989) to be related to handedness in females, Witelson and Nowakowski suggested that "loss of callosal axons may not be a factor in lateralization in women, at least in relation to hand preference" (p. 329).

Witelson (1991) expanded her arguments to include a role for androgenic hormones (a group of hormones to which testosterone belongs; for the sake of simplicity, Witelson used the specific hormone testosterone to apply to the entire group). There is, in fact, evidence from animal research that hormones play some role in determining a sex difference in callosal size (see Fitch & Dennenberg, 1998 for review). Witelson wrote: "I hypothesize that in men, lower levels of testosterone lead to less axon elimination, a larger callosal isthmus and associated temporo-parietal structures, greater left handedness (less consistent-right-hand preference) and greater bihemispheric representation of cognitive skills (less functional asymmetry), and that these same factors are not similarly operative in the development of the female brain" (pp. 142–143).

Witelson's theory, it will be noted, attributes higher rates of left-handedness in men to relatively low levels of fetal testosterone, whereas the same effect was attributed by Geschwind, Behan, and Galaburda (see above) to high levels of testosterone. Although Witelson argued that the larger corpus callosum in men is not due to postnatal factors (Witelson, 1991, p. 142), a possible role for experience in the size of the callosum is suggested by findings that the anterior callosum is enlarged in musicians who began to play their instruments before the age of 7 years (Schlaug et al., 1995) in comparison with those who began after this age.

Since publication of Witelson's original reports, many other post-mortem and in vivo studies have investigated differences in relation to callosal size as a function of handedness. The literature on handedness and sex differences in relation to callosal size is controversial (for reviews, see Driesen & Raz, 1995; Beaton, 1997; Bishop & Wahlsten, 1997). Driesen and Raz (1995) carried out a meta-analysis which showed that so-called left-handers had on average (for seven studies) larger total callosal areas than right-handers. The measurement of handedness, however, has often been inadequate or idiosyncratic (see Beaton, 1997). Given the striking individual variation in callosal size (Bleier et al., 1986), large subject samples are required to adequately assess morphological characteristics of the callosum in relation to other variables. Nonetheless, it is of interest in the context of Liepmann's model of left hemisphere motor dominance that some attention has centered on putative handedness differences in callosal morphology. It is possible to infer from Witelson's hypothesis how variation in callosal size might relate to skill differences between the hands. However, it is difficult not to be skeptical regarding the implication of the hypothesis that handedness is determined by different factors in males and in females, given the similarity in the handedness distributions for the two sexes.

PREVIC'S THEORY

Previc (1991) has argued that the emergence of one hand as the more skilled is a consequence of the specialization of the left lower limb for anti-gravity extension (i.e., for postural support). This is itself related, in Previc's view, to greater strength of vestibulospinal reflexes on the left, which in turn is due to an otolithic asymmetry leading to a dopaminergic asymmetry in the basal ganglia (see Glick et al., 1982; Kooistra & Heilman, 1988). The otolithic asymmetry leading to stronger vestibulospinal reflexes on the left side is attributed by Previc to asymmetry in orientation of the fetus in the womb relative to the mother's midline. He maintains that, in evolutionary terms, the adoption of an upright posture and method of locomotion led to asymmetry in the position of the fetus, and hence to unequal vestibular stimulation. Levinson (1990), too, has suggested that handedness and cerebral dominance might relate to vestibular asymmetry.

Schaeffer (1928) reported that blindfolded subjects walk, swim and steer a car in a consistently biased direction toward one side or the other, with no difference between three left- and three right-handers in directional turning bias during blindfolded walking. However, Bracha et al. (1987) reported a bias in turning during everyday activity. The direction of bias was related to participants' "dominant side." Furthermore, in a preliminary study in my laboratory that investigated directional turning preference in a cycling task, we found a difference between left- and right-handers. It may be, then, that handedness and turning biases are related through dopaminergic asymmetry, and that handedness is in part determined by some asymmetry in neurotransmitter substance. Previc (1991) argues that "The greater dopaminergic content of the left basal ganglia presumably underlies the predominance of rightward turning, rightward postural deviations, and, ultimately, right-handedness in humans" (p. 314). However, the theory (see also Previc, 1996) is insufficiently specified at the present time to address most of the features of handedness outlined earlier in this chapter.

STRUCTURAL ASPECTS OF HANDEDNESS

For a complete account of handedness, theories such as those outlined above need to be underpinned by some plausible account of the mechanisms presumed to give rise to the relevant effects. Such mechanisms may involve structural as well as functional attributes. Indeed, the belief that "cerebral dominance is based in most instances on asymmetries of structure" (Geschwind & Galaburda, 1985, p. 428) is implicit in many accounts of handedness. More recent reports of hemispheric neuroanatomical asymmetry (White et al., 1994, but see White et al., 1997a, b; Amunts et al., 1996, 1997, 2000) in brain regions representing the hand have been regarded as showing that handedness has a neurobiological basis, and are discussed elsewhere in this volume.

Asymmetries in thresholds of motor evoked potentials in response to transcranial magnetic stimulation (TMS) have been correlated with both hand preference scores (Triggs et al., 1994) and left-right manual performance differences (Triggs et al., 1997; see also Li et al., 1996). This implies that handedness is related to localized asymmetry in some aspect of neural functioning. The implication is strengthened by demonstrations (in studies using different techniques) of reversed patterns of hemispheric asymmetry of activation in left-handers compared with right-handers (Li et al., 1996; Volkmann et al., 1998; Taniguchi et al., 1998) while they perform simple unimanual tasks with the preferred hand.

A question arises, however, as to whether regional anatomic or neurophysiological asymmetry between the hemispheres derives purely from extensive experience of unilateral hand use or whether an initial asymmetry itself determines, at least in part, the side of hand dominance. The fact that neuroanatomical asymmetry has been observed in a group of children (Amunts et al., 1997) does not answer this question, since we do not know whether it was present before hand preference was established in individual cases. There is considerable evidence that the extent of cortex representing the fingers can be expanded with practice (see, e.g., Elbert et al., 1995; Wang et al., 1995) but it is equally possible that a person develops strong hand preference as a result of a preexisting asymmetry in sensorimotor representation.

Furthermore, there is evidence that the volume of the right hand is greater than that of the left hand (Purves et al., 1994), and the surface area also might be expected to differ. Certainly in my own laboratory we have found the breadth of the right hand to be slightly greater than that of the left. Such size differences might be related to a difference in muscle mass and/or bone size (see Steele, 2000) brought about by differential hand use, and might be expected to have cortical correlates. Conceivably, the neuroanatomic and neurophysiological findings are a reflection of this. In this context it is of interest that complexity of dendritic organization in the presumed hand region of the cortex has been related to differences in finger dexterity and hand function characteristic of a person's working life (Scheibel et al., 1990).

Whatever the explanation of the structural and functional asymmetries reported, I am extremely doubtful that the neurobiological underpinnings of handedness will be found only in the cortex, and particularly only in the primary motor area. Current theories in neuropsychology are moving away from the idea of circumscribed brain centers serving distinct psychological functions and toward a more dynamic conception of cognitive and motor activity mediated by cerebral circuits involving the integrated action of different brain regions. In addition to the primary motor cortex, areas of the brain involved in movement planning and execution include the premotor area, supplementary motor area, and anterior cingulate area (see Roland & Zilles,

1996 for review). These areas are connected with each other and with subcortical regions and the spinal cord. At the very least the supplementary motor area is likely to be involved in handedness (see Jäncke et al., 2000) and possibly even in spinal mechanisms (see Melsbach et al., 1996). It is also conceivable that the somatosensory cortex is involved through sensory feedback mechanisms (see Okuda et al., 1995; Mima et al., 1999). Given the crucial involvement of the cerebellum and other subcortical structures in motor control, it seems to me almost certain that these, too, are functionally related to handedness (see also Peters, 1995; McManus & Cornish, 1997). In fact, a recent PET study showed that asymmetric activation of the nigrostriatal system is related to performance asymmetry between the hands (Fuente-Fernández et al., 2000).

A difference in the relative volume of the left and right cerebellar hemispheres in relation to handedness was reported by Snyder et al. (1995), but the functional correlates, if any, remain obscure. In a functional imaging study Jäncke et al. (1999) reported that when volunteers made unimanual responses, cerebellar activation varied according to whether the preferred or nonpreferred hand was used, being greater for the nonpreferred hand. The precise significance of the pattern of activation recorded is not known because the motor functions of the cerebellum are still a subject of debate (compare reviews by Thach et al., 1992 and by Stein & Glickstein, 1992). Conceivably, the greater activation associated with the nonpreferred than the preferred hand reflects greater difficulty in performing the experimental task.

In a classic paper on the effects of cerebellar damage Holmes (1917) wrote:

'The majority of the abnormalities of movement ... refer to those in which the larger and more proximal group of muscles are concerned, but similar disturbances can be observed in the finer and more elaborate actions of the hand'.... When a man with a right-sided cerebellar lesion was given a pair of scissors he had, in the first place, difficulty in grasping them correctly, then failed to direct them properly and was unable to move the blades regularly and appropriately when he attempted to cut a piece of paper with them. (p. 490).

This description bears a remarkable resemblance to the performance of my own left hand and suggests that the cerebellum, along with the basal ganglia (for reviews, see Bhatia & Marsden, 1994; Brooks, 1995), is involved in the kinds of skilled activity for which individuals show a decided unimanual preference. Certain actions become automatic with practice, a process to which the cerebellum is thought to make a major contribution, and yet require very fine adjustments of the hand and fingers. In threading a needle, for example, or in drawing or painting a picture, steadiness of the hand is required; in spreading jam, shaving, or cutting the top off an egg, one must exert an appropriate degree of force; in playing a musical instrument, the fingers must move at just the right velocity. Such parameters may be computed by the globus pallidus (Hoover & Strick, 1993; see Brooks, 1995 for dissenting view).

The implicit view that handedness resides, so to speak, in the primary motor area of the cortex probably owes something to demonstrations in the split-brain monkey (Brinkman & Kuypers, 1972, 1973) and human (Gazzaniga et al., 1967) that the distal musculature of the upper limb is represented exclusively in the contralateral motor cortex. However, Lawrence and Kuypers (1968) showed that though relatively independent finger movements by rhesus monkeys were abolished by bilateral interruption of the pyramidal tracts, the animals were able "to reach accurately with either hand to pick up morsels of food by closure of all fingers in concert" (p. 9) only three weeks after the operation. Nor did pyramidectomy abolish the so-called precision or pincer grip in which an object is held between the thumb and one finger. This suggests that the subcorticospinal pathways can support accurate movements of the hand and some movements of the fingers with a fair degree of dexterity.

Although handedness may not relate exclusively to the cortex, there is little doubt that direction and degrees of handedness are more closely related to the functioning of the hemisphere contralateral than ipsilateral to the preferred hand. This raises the possibility that handedness is intimately connected to functional and possibly structural aspects of the pyramidal tract. About 75–90% of pyramidal tract fibers cross at the medulla oblongata to form the crossed lateral corticospinal tract. It has been reported that in human fetal and neonatal material the spinal cord is asymmetrical in the majority of cases by virtue of the fact that a greater number of corticospinal fibers from the bulbar pyramids cross from left to right, and at a higher level, than in the reverse direction (Yakovlev & Rakic, 1966; Yakovlev & Lecours, 1967; see also Kertesz & Geschwind, 1971). Thus more fibers descend on the right side of the cord (Nathan et al., 1990). The proportion of cases in which fibers from the left hemisphere crossed at a higher level than those from the right was 87% in a sample of 100 neonate brains examined by Yakovlev and Rakic (1966), and 73% in the 158 adult specimens examined by Kertesz and Geschwind (1971). This side of the cord was larger in 40 of the 53 asymmetric cords (from a total of 74) examined by Nathan et al. (1990). However, no relation between handedness and pyramidal crossing was observed in the study by Kertesz and Geschwind (1971). It is also worth noting that in a review of the human pyramidal tract Davidoff (1990) concludes that "corticospinal fibers alone may not be sufficient to produce ... fine movements; a number of indirect cortico-fugal pathways must also function to produce voluntary movement" (p. 337).

SOME CONCLUDING SPECULATIONS

Depite the common tendency to think of the hands as being controlled exclusively from the contralateral hemisphere, for many tasks, perhaps even all, this is almost certainly an oversimplification, since most movements of the hands will be accompanied by movements of the arms that are recognized to be controlled bilaterally. In point of fact, the term "handedness" may be something of a misnomer, since a preference for one upper limb can be seen not only in tasks involving primarily the fingers or wrist of one hand, as in writing, but also in tasks such as throwing or catching (Newman, 1934; Watson & Kimura, 1989) which involve the upper arm(s) and body. Kimura and Davidson (1975) showed that on a tapping task superiority of the right arm and shoulder (see also Todor et al., 1982; Peters & Pang, 1992) was as marked as for the hands (which would not be expected if handedness were linked to control only of the distal musculature). Even actions that are referred to as manual reaction time tasks often involve an arm movement to take the hand from an initial starting position to a target.

Not only are movements of the upper arm controlled bilaterally, but recent findings from different methodologies, including EEG (Urbano et al., 1996), PET (Shibasaki et al., 1993), MRI (Kim et al., 1993; Boecker et al., 1994; Li et al., 1996), and TMS (Wasserman et al., 1994), suggest that in humans cortical control of even single finger movements is not exclusively contralateral, particularly for more cognitively complex or demanding tasks (Sadato et al., 1996), and may give rise to quite widespread areas of brain activation (e.g., Deiber et al., 1991). The implication is surely that behaviors associated with skilled actions of the preferred hand are mediated by brain circuits which involve both cerebral hemispheres rather than being confined to one.

It has long been considered likely that ipsilateral motor pathways contribute to the degree of functional recovery which is seen after unilateral brain damage (Gooddy & McKissock, 1951; R. D. Jones et al., 1989; Wasserman et al., 1994). If they do, why should they not relate to degree of hand skill in the intact brain? Poor ipsilateral control of the nonpreferred hand relative to the preferred hand might help to explain its inferiority in skilled performance. However, research with commissurotomized patients (Gazzaniga et al., 1967; Zaidel & Sperry, 1977; Trope et al., 1987) suggests that control of the right hand by the right hemisphere is not as good as ipsilateral control of the left hand. Chen et al. (1997) conclude from a review of relevant literature, and from their own research using TMS, that ipsilateral mortor cortex is "involved in the control of fine finger movements, with the left hemisphere playing a greater role than the right hemisphere" (p. 286). On the face of it, this observation does not accord well with the fact that (in dextral subjects) degree of right-handedness is determined by variation in skill of the left hand.

Neuroimaging (Kawashima et al., 1993; Dassonville et al., 1997) and MEG (magnetoencephalography) studies (Volkmann et al., 1998) indicate that during unilateral movements, the left hemisphere-left hand system in right-handers (the opposite might hold for left-handers—see data of Li et al., 1996) is activated to a greater degree than the right hemisphere-right hand system. Together with the findings referred to above, this implies that ipsilateral pathways might be subject to inhibition, possibly through callosal mechanisms. In a review of split-brain work, Zaidel and Sperry (1977) concluded that "... it would appear that volitional motor control of the ipsilateral hand, in either hemisphere, normally involves regulation not only through direct ipsilateral pathways but also through callosal fibres to the contralateral motor centres of the opposite hemisphere" (p. 201).

That the callosum may inhibit communication between the two cerebral hemispheres has been proposed by a number of authors (see Cook, 1984; Hoptman & Davidson, 1994; Chiarello & Maxfield, 1996) although callosally mediated interhemispheric effects may also be excitatory (e.g., Meyer et al., 1995). Since it appears from animal research that the cortical representations of the digits themselves are only sparsely connected through the callosum (Jenny, 1979; Rouiller et al., 1994), it is probable that interhemispheric excitation or inhibition occurs between areas other than the primary motor cortices.

Congenital absence of the corpus callosum is associated in at least some cases with impaired control of the fingers (Reynolds & Jeeves, 1977; Meerwaldt, 1983). Might the callosum not participate (see Geffen et al., 1994) in a complex interplay between contralateral and ipsilateral motor pathways? It may not be irrelevant that there is a statistical association between the side of hand and eye dominance (see McManus et al., 1999; Porac, 1997; Annett, 1999b, 2000). Both forms of laterality may share a common mechanism (but see Papousek & Schulter, 1999), since the hand and the eye are in each case linked to crossed and uncrossed pathways. Ocular dominance (in one sense of the word, at least) would seem to require a mechanism of inhibition; why not, then, handedness?

Research with rats (Rosen et al., 1989) and humans (Aboitiz et al., 1992) suggests that the number of fibers (of a particular diameter) present in a given callosal region is inversely related to the degree of left-right asymmetry in associated cortical regions. Annett (1992b) has drawn attention to certain parallels between relative hand skill and asymmetry of the planum temporale. If performance differences between the hands do indeed relate in some way to anatomic brain asymmetry (see Steinmetz et al., 1991), and hence to callosal connectivity, then it is to be expected that the corpus callosum and hand preference are functionally related.

Experiments on intermanual transfer of training (Hicks, 1974; Byrd et al., 1986; Parlow & Kinsbourne, 1989) have suggested that transcallosal effects from one hemisphere to the other may in some cases be asymmetric (Marzi et al., 1991; Bisiacchi et al., 1994; Hoptman & Davidson, 1994). Certainly there are indications in the literature that interhemispheric transfer effects may differ between left- and right-handers (e.g., Potter & Graves, 1988; Gorynia & Egenter, 2000). Mirror writing, which might also reflect a callosal mechanism, has been reported in some studies to be more efficient in left- than in right-handers (Tankle & Heilman, 1983; Tucha et al., 2000). I suggested some time ago (Beaton, 1985) that attentional factors might be involved in the concordance between different manifestations of lateral dominance. More recently my collaborators and I (Beaton et al., 2000) have proposed that age-related changes in certain aspects of lateralized behavior may be linked to attentional or resource-allocating functions of the corpus callosum (see Arguin et al., 2000). Perhaps we should consider more carefully the possible influence of callosal function on the expression of handedness itself.

REFERENCES

Aboitiz, F., Scheibel, A. B., Fisher, R. S., & Zaidel, E. (1992). Fiber composition of the human corpus callosum. *Brain Research, 598*, 143–153.

Amunts, K., Jäncke, L., Mohlberg, H., Steinmetz, H., & Zilles, K. (2000). Interhemispheric asymmetry of the human motor cortex related to handedness and gender. *Neuropsychologia, 38*, 304–312.

Amunts, K., Schlaug, G., Schleicher, A., Steinmetz, H., Dabringhaus, A., Roland, P. E., & Zilles, K. (1996). Asymmetry in the human motor cortex and handedness. *Neuroimage, 4*, 216–222.

Amunts, K., Schmidt-Passos, F., Schleicher, A., & Zilles, K. (1997). Postnatal development of interhemispheric asymmetry in the cytoarchitecture of human area 4. *Anatomy and Embryology, 196*, 393–402.

Annett, M. (1970). A classification of hand preference by association analysis. *British Journal of Psychology, 61*, 303–321.

Annett, M. (1975). Hand preference and the laterality of cerebral speech. *Cortex, 11*, 305–328.

Annett, M. (1976). A co-ordination of hand preference and skill replicated. *British Journal of Psychology, 67*, 587–592.

Annett, M. (1979). Family handedness in three generations predicted by the right shift theory. *Annals of Human Genetics, 42*, 479–491

Annett, M. (1983). Hand preference and skill in 115 children of two left-handed parents. *British Journal of Psychology, 74*, 17–32.

Annett, M. (1985). *Left, right, hand, brain: The right shift theory.* Hove, U.K.: Lawrence Erlbaum Associates.

Annett, M. (1988). Comments on Lindesay: Laterality shift in homosexual men. *Neuropsychologia, 26*, 341–343.

Annett, M. (1991). Predicting from the right shift theory. *Behavioral and Brain Sciences, 14*, 338–341.

Annett, M. (1992a). Five tests of hand skill, *Cortex, 28*, 583–600.

Annett, M. (1992b). Parallels between asymmetries of planum temporale and of hand skill. *Neuropsychologia, 30*, 951–962.

Annett, M. (1994). Handedness as a continuous variable with dextral shift: Sex, generation, and family handedness in subgroups of left- and right-handers. *Behavior Genetics, 24*, 51–63.

Annett, M. (1995a). The right shift theory of a genetic balanced polymorphism for cerebral dominance and cognitive processing. *Cahiers de Psychologie Cognitive/Current Psychology of Cognition, 14,* 1–53.

Annett, M. (1995b). The fertility of the right shift theory. *Cahiers de Psychologie Cognitive/Current Psychology of Cognition, 14,* 623–650.

Annett, M. (1996). In defence of the right shift theory. *Perceptual and Motor Skills, 82,* 115–137.

Annett, M. (1999a). Left-handedness as a function of sex, maternal versus paternal inheritance, and report bias. *Behavior Genetics, 29,* 103–114.

Annett, M. (1999b). Eye dominance in families predicted by the right shift theory. *Laterality, 4,* 167–172.

Annett, M. (2000). Predicting combinations of left and right asymmetries. *Cortex, 36,* 485–505.

Annett, M., & Alexander, M. P. (1996). Atypical cerebral dominance: Predictions and tests of the right shift theory. *Neuropsychologia, 34,* 1215–1227.

Annett, M., & Kilshaw, D. (1983). Right and left hand skill—II. Estimating the parameters of the distribution of L-R differences in males and females. *British Journal of Psychology, 74,* 269–281.

Archibald, Y. M. (1987). Persisting apraxia in two left-handed, aphasic patients with right-hemisphere lesions. *Brain and Cognition, 6,* 412–428.

Arguin, M., Lassonde, M., Quattrini, A., Del Pesce, M., Foschi, N., & Papo, I. (2000). Divided visuo-spatial attention systems with total and anterior callosotomy. *Neuropsychologia, 38,* 283–291.

Ashton, G. C. (1982). Handedness: An alternative hypothesis. *Behavior Genetics, 12,* 125–147.

Bakan, P. (1990). Nonright-handedness and the continuum of reproductive casualty. In S. Coren (Ed.), *Left-handedness behavioural implications and anomalies* (pp. 33–76). North-Holland: Elsevier Science Publishers.

Bakan, P. (1991). Handedness and maternal smoking during pregnancy. *International Journal of Neuroscience, 56,* 161–168.

Barnsley, R. H., & Robinovitch, M. S. (1970). Handedness: Proficiency versus stated preference. *Perceptual and Motor Skills, 30,* 343–362.

Beaton, A. A. (1985). *Left side, right side: A review of laterality research.* London: Batsford; New Haven, CT: Yale University Press.

Beaton, A. A. (1995). Hands, brains and lateral thinking: An overview of the right shift theory. *Cahiers de Psychologie Cognitive/Current Psychology of Cognition, 14,* 481–495.

Beaton, A. A. (1997). The relation of planum temporale asymmetry and morphology of the corpus callosum to handedness, gender, and dyslexia: A review of the evidence. *Brain and Language, 60,* 255–322.

Beaton, A. A., Hugdahl, K., & Ray, P. (2000). Lateral asymmetries and interhemispheric transfer in aging: A review and some new data. In M. K. Mandal, M. B. Bulman-Fleming, & G. Tiwari (Eds.), *Side bias: A neuropsychological perspective* (pp. 101–152). Dordrecht, Netherlands: Kluwer Academic Publishers.

Beaton, A. A., & Moseley, L. G. (1984). Anxiety and the measurement of handedness. *British Journal of Psychology, 75*, 275–278.

Beaton, A. A., Williams, L., & Moseley, L. G. (1984). Handedness and hand injuries. *Journal of Hand Surgery: British and European Version, 19B*, 158–161.

Bell, J., & Gabbard, C. (2000). Foot preference changes through adulthood. *Laterality, 5*, 63–68.

Benton, A. L., Meyers, R., & Polder, G. J. (1962). Some aspects of handedness. *Psychiatrica et Neurologica, 144*, 321–337.

Bhatia, K. P., & Marsden, C. D. (1994). The behavioural and motor consequences of focal lesions of the basal ganglia in man. *Brain, 117*, 859–876.

Bishop, D. V. M. (1984). Using non-preferred hand skill to investigate pathological left-handedness in an unselected population. *Developmental Medicine and Child Neurology, 26*, 214–226.

Bishop, D. V. M. (1989). Does hand proficiency determine hand preference? *British Journal of Psychology, 80*, 191–199.

Bishop, D. V. M. (1990a). On the futility of using familial sinistrality to subclassify handedness groups. *Cortex, 26*, 153–155.

Bishop, D. V. M. (1990b). *Handedness and developmental disorder*. Oxford: Blackwell.

Bishop, K. M., & Wahlsten, D. (1997). Sex differences in the human corpus callosum: Myth or reality? *Science and Behavioural Reviews, 21*, 581–601.

Bisiacchi, P., Marzi, C. A., Nicoletti, R., Carena, G., Mucignat, C., & Tomaiuolo, F. (1994). Left-right asymmetry of callosal transfer in normal human subjects. *Behavioural Brain Research, 64*, 173–178.

Bleier, R., Houston, L., & Byne, W. (1986). Can the corpus callosum predict gender, age, handedness or cognitive differences? *Trends in Neurosciences, 9*, 391–394.

Boecker, H., Kleinschmidt, A., Requardt, M., Hänicke, W., Merboldt, K. D., & Frahm, J. (1994). Functional cooperativity of human cortical motor areas during self-paced simple finger movements: A high-resolution MRI study. *Brain, 117*, 1231–1239.

Bol, P., Scheirs, J., & Spanjaard, L. (1996). Meningitis and the evolution of right-handedness. *Cortex, 33*, 1–23.

Bracha, H. S., Seitz, D. J., Otemaa, J., & Glick, S. D. (1987). Rotational movement (circling) in normal humans: Sex difference and relationship to hand, foot and eye preference. *Brain Research, 411*, 231–235.

Brackenridge, C. J. (1981). Secular variation in handedness over ninety years. *Neuropsychologia, 19*, 459–462.

Brinkman, J., & Kuypers, H. G. J. M. (1972). Split-brain monkeys: Cerebral control of ipsilateral and contralateral arm, hand, and finger movements. *Science, 176,* 536–539.

Brinkman, J., & Kuypers, H. G. J. M. (1973). Cerebral control of contralateral and ipsilateral arm, hand and finger movements in the split-brain rhesus monkey. *Brain, 96,* 653–674.

Brooks, D. J. (1995). The role of basal ganglia in motor control: Contributions from PET. *Journal of the Neurological Sciences, 128,* 1–13.

Bryden, M. P. (1977). Measuring handedness with questionnaires. *Neuropsychologia, 15,* 617–624.

Bryden, M. P., McManus, I. C., & Bulman-Fleming, M. B. (1994a). Evaluating the empirical support for the Geschwind-Behan-Galaburda model of cerebral lateralization. *Brain and Cognition, 26,* 103–167.

Bryden, M. P., McManus, I. C., & Bulman-Fleming, M. B. (1994b). GBG, BMB, R & L, X & Y . . . Reply to commentaries. *Brain and Cognition, 26,* 312–326.

Bryden, M. P., Roy, E. A., McManus, I. C., & Bulman-Fleming, M. B. (1997). On the genetics and measurement of human handedness. *Laterality, 2,* 317–336.

Bryden, M. P., Singh, M., Steenhuis, R. E., & Clarkson, K. L. (1994). A behavioural measure of hand preference as opposed to hand skill. *Neuropsychologia, 32,* 991–999.

Bryden, M. P., & Steenhuis, R. E. (1991). Issues in the assessment of handedness. In F. L. Kitterle (Ed.), *Cerebral laterality: Theory and research* (pp. 35–51). Hillsdale, NJ: Lawrence Erlbaum Associates.

Buchanan, A. (1862). Predominance of right hand over left. *Transactions of the Philosophical Society of Glasgow, 5,* 142–167.

Byrd, R., Gibson, M., & Gleason, M. H. (1986). Bilateral transfer across ages 7 to 17 years. *Perceptual and Motor Skills, 62,* 87–90.

Calvert, G. A., & Bishop, D. V. M. (1998). Quantifying hand preference using a behavioural continuum. *Laterality, 3,* 255–268.

Carlier, M., Dumont, A. M., Beau, J., & Michel, F. (1993). Hand performance of French children on a finger-tapping test in relation to handedness, sex, and age. *Perceptual and Motor Skills, 6,* 931–940.

Carter-Saltzman, L. (1980). Biological and sociocultural effects on handedness: Comparison between biological and adoptive families. *Science, 209,* 1263–1265.

Chamberlain, H. D. (1928). The inheritance of left-handedness. *Journal of Heredity, 19,* 557–559.

Chang, K. S. F., Hsu, F. K., Chan, S. T., & Chan, Y. B. (1960). Scrotal asymmetry and handedness. *Journal of Anatomy, 94,* 543–548.

Chau, N., Remy, E., Pétry, D., Huguenin, P., Bourgkard, E., & André, J. M. (1998). Asymmetry correction equations for hand volume, grip and pinch strengths in healthy working people. *European Journal of Epidemiology, 14,* 71–77.

Chen, R., Cohen, L. G., & Hallett, M. (1997). Role of the ipsilateral motor cortex in voluntary movement. *Canadian Journal of Neurological Sciences, 24,* 284–291.

Chi, J. G., Dooling, E. C., & Gilles, F. H. (1977). Left-right asymmetries of the temporal speech areas of the human fetus. *Archives of Neurology, 34,* 346–348.

Chiarello, C., & Maxfield, L. (1996). Varieties of interhemispheric inhibition, or how to keep a good hemisphere down. *Brain and Cognition, 30,* 81–108.

Collins, R. L. (1985). On the inheritance of direction and degree of asymmetry. In S. D. Glick (Ed.), *Cerebral lateralization in nonhuman species* (pp. 41–71). New York: Academic Press.

Connolly, K. J., & Bishop, D. V. M. (1992). The measurement of handedness: A cross-cultural comparison of samples from England and Papua New Guinea. *Neuropsychologia, 30,* 13–26.

Cook, N. D. (1984). Homotopic callosal inhibition. *Brain and Language, 23,* 116–125.

Corballis, M. C. (1997). The genetics and evolution of handedness. *Psychological Review, 104,* 714–727.

Corballis, M. C., Lee, K., McManus, I. C., & Crow, T. J. (1996). Location of the handedness gene on the X and Y chromosomes. *American Journal of Medical Genetics (Neuropsychiatric Genetics), 67,* 50–52.

Coren, S. (1990). Left-handedness in offspring as a function of maternal age at parturition. *New England Journal of Medicine, 322,* 1673.

Coren, S. (1995). Family patterns in handedness: Evidence for indirect inheritance mediated by birth stress. *Behavior Genetics, 25,* 517–524.

Coren, S., & Porac, C. (1980). Birth factors and laterality: The effects of birth order, parental age and birth stress on four indices of lateral preference. *Behavior Genetics, 10,* 123–138.

Coren, S., & Searleman, A. (1990). Birth stress and left-handedness: The rare trait marker model. In S. Coren (Ed.), *Behavioral implications and anomalies* (pp. 3–32). North Holland: Elsevier Science Publishers.

Crow, T. J. (1995). A Darwinian approach to the origins of psychosis. *British Journal of Psychiatry, 167,* 12–25.

Crow, T. J. (1998). Sexual selection, timing and the descent of man: A theory of the genetic origins of language. *Cahiers de Psychologie Cognitive/Current Psychology of Cognition, 17,* 1079–1114.

Crow, T. J., Crow, L. R., Done, T. J., & Leask, S. J. (1998). Relative hand skill predicts academic ability: Global deficits at the point of hemispheric indecision. *Neuropsychologia, 36,* 1275–1282.

Curt, F., De Agostini, M., Maccario, J., & Dellatolas, G. (1995). Parental hand preference and manual functional asymmetry in preschool children. *Behavior Genetics, 25,* 525–535.

Curt, F., Maccario, J., & Dellatolas, G. (1992). Distributions of hand preference and hand skill asymmetry in preschool children: Theoretical implications. *Neuropsychologia, 30,* 27–34.

Curt, F., Mesbah, M., Lellouch, J., & Dellatolas, G. (1997). Handedness scale: How many and which items? *Laterality, 2,* 137–154.

Dassonville, P., Zhu, X., Urgubil, K., Kim, S., & Ashe, J. (1997). Functional activation in motor cortex reflects the direction and the degree of handedness. *Proceedings of the National Academy of Sciences, USA, 94,* 14015–14018.

Davidoff, R. A. (1990). The pyramidal tract. *Neurology, 40,* 332–339.

Davis, A., & Annett, M. (1994). Handedness asymmetries as a function of twinning, age and sex. *Cortex, 30,* 105–111.

De Agostini, M., Khamis, A. H., Ahui, A. M., & Dellatolas, G. (1997). Environmental influences in hand preference: An African point of view. *Brain and Cognition, 35,* 151–167.

Deiber, M. P., Passingham, R. E., Colebatch, J. G., Friston, K. J., Nixon, P. D., & Frackowiak, R. S. J. (1991). Cortical areas and the selection of movement: A study with positron emission tomography. *Experimental Brain Research, 84,* 393–402.

Dellatolas, G., & Curt, F. (1995). The distribution of cerebral dominance in the general population and its cognitive implications need further study. *Cahiers de Psychologie Cognitive/Current Psychology of Cognition, 14,* 537–542.

Dellatolas, G., Moreau, T., Jallon, P., & Lellouch, J. (1993). Upper limb injuries and handedness plasticity. *British Journal of Psychology, 84,* 201–205.

Dellatolas, G., Tubert, P., Castresana, A., Mesbah, M., Giallonardo, T., Lazaratou, H., & Lellouch, J. (1991). Age and cohort effects in adult handedness. *Neuropsychologia, 29,* 225–261.

De Renzi, E., Motti, F., & Nichelli, P. (1980). Imitating gestures: A quantitative approach to ideomotor apraxia. *Archives of Neurology, 37,* 6–10.

Dodrill, C. B. (1979). Sex differences on the Halstead-Reitan neuropsychological battery and on other neuropsychological measures. *Journal of Clinical Psychology, 35,* 236–241.

Driesen, N. R., & Raz, N. (1995). The influence of sex, age, and handedness on corpus callosum morphology: A meta-analysis. *Psychobiology, 23,* 240–247.

Elbert, T., Pantev, C., Wienbruch, C., Rockstroh, B., & Taub, E. (1995). Increased cortical representation of the fingers of the left hand in string players. *Science, 270,* 305–307.

Elliott, D., & Chua, R. (1996). Manual asymmetries in goal directed movements. In D. Elliott & E. Roy (Eds.), *Manual asymmetries in motor performance* (pp. 143–158). Boca Raton, FL: CRC Press.

Ellis, L., & Peckham, W. (1991). Prenatal stress and handedness among offspring. *Pre- and Peri-Natal Psychology Journal, 6,* 135–144.

Falek, A. (1958). Handedness: A family study. *American Journal of Human Genetics, 11,* 52–62.

Fitch, R. H., & Denenberg, V. H. (1998). A role for ovarian hormones in sexual differentiation of the brain. *Behavioural and Brain Sciences, 21,* 311–352.

Fleishman, E. A., & Hempel, W. E. (1954). A factor analysis of dexterity tests. *Personnel Psychology, 7,* 15–32.

Foundas, A. L., Hong, K., Leonard, C. M., & Heilman, K. M. (1998). Hand preference and magnetic resonance imaging asymmetries of the central sulcus. *Neuropsychiatry, Neuropsychology and Behavioural Neurology, 11,* 65–71.

Fuente-Fernández, R. de la, Kishore, A., Calne, D. B., Ruth, T. J., & Stoess, A. J. (2000). Nigrostriatal dopamine system and motor lateralization. *Behavioural Brain Research, 112,* 63–68.

Galaburda, A. M., Corsiglia, J., Rosen, G. D., & Sherman, G. F. (1987). Planum temporale asymmetry: Reappraisal since Geschwind and Levitsky. *Neuropsychologia, 25,* 853–868.

Gangestad, S. W., & Yeo, R. A. (1994). Parental handedness and relative hand skills: A test of the developmental instability hypothesis. *Neuropsychology, 8,* 572–578.

Gangestad, S. W., Yeo, R. A., Shaw, P., Thoma, R., Daniel, W. F., & Korthank, A. (1996). Human leukocyte antigens and hand preference: Preliminary observations. *Neuropsychology, 10,* 423–428.

Gardner, R. A., & Broman, M. (1979). The Purdue pegboard: Normative data on 1334 school children. *Journal of Clinical Child Psychology,* (Fall), 56–162.

Gazzaniga, M. S., Bogen, J. E., & Sperry, R. W. (1967). Dyspraxia following division of the cerebral commissures. *Archives of Neurology, 16,* 606–612.

Geffen, G. M., Jones, D. J., & Geffen, L. B. (1994). Interhemispheric control of manual motor activity. *Behavioural Brain Research, 64,* 131–140.

Gersh, F., & Damasio, A. R. (1981). Praxis and writing of the left hand may be served by different callosal pathways. *Archives of Neurology, 38,* 634–636.

Geschwind, N., & Behan, P. (1982). Left-handedness: Association with immune disease, migraine, and developmental learning disorder. *Proceedings of the National Academy of Sciences, USA, 79,* 5097–5100.

Geschwind, N., & Galaburda, A. M. (1985). Cerebral lateralization. Biological mechanisms, associations, and pathology: 1. A hypothesis and program for research. *Archives of Neurology, 42,* 428–459.

Geschwind, N., & Galaburda, A. M. (1987). *Cerebral lateralization: Biological mechanisms, associations and pathology.* Cambridge, MA: MIT Press.

Geschwind, N., & Kaplan, E. (1962). A human cerebral deconnection syndrome. *Neurology, 12,* 675–685.

Geschwind, N., & Levitsky, W. (1968). Human brain: Left-right asymmetries in temporal speech region. *Science, 161,* 186–187.

Gilbert, A. N., & Wysocki, C. J. (1992). Hand preference and age in the United States. *Neuropsychologia, 30,* 601–608.

Glees, P., & Cole, J. (1952). Ipsilateral representation in the cerebral cortex: Its significance in relation to motor function. *The Lancet*, June 14, 1191–1192.

Glick, S. D., Ross, D. A., & Hough, L. B. (1982). Lateral asymmetry of neurotransmitters in human brain. *Brain Research, 234*, 53–63.

Goldenberg, G., Wimmer, A., Holzner, F., & Wessely, P. (1985). Apraxia of the left limbs in a case of callosal disconnection: The contribution of medial frontal lobe damage. *Cortex, 21*, 135–148.

Gooddy, W., & McKissock, W. (1951). The theory of cerebral localisation. *The Lancet*, March 3, 481–483.

Gordon, H. (1921). Left-handedness and mirror writing, especially among defective children. *Brain, 43*, 313–368.

Gorynia, I., & Egenter, D. (2000). Intermanual coordination in relation to handedness, familial sinistrality and lateral preferences. *Cortex, 36*, 1–18.

Grimshaw, G. M., Bryden, M. P., & Finegan, J.-A. K. (1995). Relations between prenatal testosterone and cerebral lateralization in children. *Neuropsychology, 9*, 68–79.

Guiard, Y., Diaz, G., & Beaubaton, D. (1983). Left-hand advantage in right-handers for spatial constant error. *Neuropsychologia, 21*, 111–115.

Habib, M., Touze, F., & Galaburda, A. M. (1990). Intrauterine factors in sinistrality: A review. In S. Coren (Ed.), *Left-handedness: Behavioural implications and anomalies* (pp. 99–128). North-Holland: Elsevier Science Publishers.

Harris, L. (1980). Left-handedness: Early theories, facts and fancies. In J. Herron (Ed.), *The neuropsychology of left-handedness* (pp. 3 –78). San Diego: Academic Press.

Harris, L. (1990). Cultural influences on handedness: Historical and contemporary theory and evidence. In S. Coren (Ed.), *Left handedness: Behavioural implications and anomalies* (pp. 195–258). Amsterdam: Elsevier Science Publishers.

Harris, L. J., & Carlson, D. F. (1988). Pathological left-handedness: An analysis of theories and evidence. In D. L. Molfese & S. J. Segalowitz (Eds.), *Brain lateralization in children: Developmental implications* (pp. 289–372). New York: Guildford Press.

Hatta, T., & Nakatsuka, Z. (1976). Note on hand preference of Japanese people. *Perceptual and Motor Skills, 42*, 530.

Healey, J. M., Liederman, J., & Geschwind, N. (1986). Handedness is not a unidimensional trait. *Cortex, 22*, 33–53.

Heilman, K. M., Coyle, J. M., Gonyea, E. F., & Geschwind, N. (1973). Apraxia and agraphia in a left hander. *Brain, 96*, 21–28.

Heilman, K. M., Gonyea, E. F., & Geschwind, N. (1973). Apraxia and agraphia in a right hander. *Cortex, 10*, 284–288.

Heilman, K. M., & Rothi, L. J. G. (1993). Apraxia. In K. M. Heilman & E. Valenstein (Eds.), *Clinical neuropsychology* (pp. 141–163). New York: Oxford University Press.

Helleday, J., Siwers, B., Ritzen, M., & Hugdahl, K. (1994). Normal lateralization for handedness and ear advantage in a verbal dichotic listening task in women with congenital adrenal hyperplasia (CAH). *Neuropsychologia, 32*, 875–880.

Helsen, W. F., Starkes, J. L., Elliott, D., & Buekers, M. J. (1998). Manual asymmetries and saccadic eye movements in right-handers during single and reciprocal aiming movements. *Cortex, 34*, 513–529.

Hepper, P. G., McCartney, G. R., & Shannon, E. A. (1998). Lateralised behaviour in first trimester human foetuses. *Neuropsychologia, 36*, 531–534.

Hepper, P. G., Shahidullah, S., & White, R. (1991). Handedness in the human fetus. *Neuropsychologia, 29*, 1107–1111.

Hildreth, G. (1950). The development and training of hand dominance: V. Training of handedness. *Journal of Genetic Psychology, 76*, 101–144.

Hiscock, C. K., Hiscock, M., Benjamins, D., & Hillman, S. (1989). Motor asymmetries in hemiplegic children: Implications for the normal and pathological development of handedness. *Developmental Neuropsychology, 5*, 169–186.

Hicks, R. E. (1974). Asymmetry of bilateral transfer. American Journal of Psychology, 87, 667–674.

Holmes, G. (1917). The symptoms of acute cerebellar injuries due to gunshot injuries. *Brain, 40*, 461–535.

Hoosain, R. (1990). Left handedness and handedness switch amongst the Chinese. *Cortex, 26*, 451–545.

Hoover, J. E., & Strick, P. L. (1993). Multiple output channels in the basal ganglia. *Science, 259*, 819–821.

Hoptman, M. J., & Davidson, R. J. (1994). How and why do the two cerebral hemispheres interact? *Psychological Bulletin, 116*, 195–219.

Hugdahl, K., Zaucha, K., Satz, P., Mitrushina, M., & Miller, E. (1996). Left-handedness and age: Comparing writing/drawing and other manual activities. *Laterality, 1*, 177–183.

Humphrey, M. E. (1951). Consistency of hand usage: A preliminary enquiry. *British Journal of Educational Psychology, 21*, 214–225.

Humphry, G. M. (1861). *The human foot and the human hand.* Cambridge: Macmillan.

Ingram, D. (1975). Motor asymmetries in young children. *Neuropsychologia, 13*, 95–102.

Inman, W. S. (1924). An enquiry into the origin of squint, left-handedness and stammer. *The Lancet*, August 2, 211–215.

Jänke, L., Peters, M., Himmelbach, M., Nösselt, T., Shah, J., & Steinmetz, H. (2000). fMRI study of bimanual coordination. *Neuropsychologia, 38*, 164–174.

Jäncke, L., Specht, K., Mirzazade, S., & Peters, M. (1999). The effect of finger-movement speed of the dominant and the subdominant hand on cerebellar activation: A functional magnetic resonance imaging study. *Neuroimage, 9*, 497–507.

Jenny, A. B. (1979). Commissural projections of the cortical hand motor area in monkeys. *Journal of Comparative Neurology, 188*, 137–146.

Jones, G. V., & Martin, M. (2000). A note on Corbalis (1997) and the genetics and evolution of handedness: Developing a unified distributional model from the sex-chromosomes gene hypothesis. *Psychological Review, 107*, 213–218.

Jones, R. D., Donaldson, I. M., & Parkin, P. P. (1989). Impairment and recovery of ipsilateral sensory-motor function following unilateral cerebral infarction. *Brain, 12*, 113–132.

Kauranen, K., & Vanharanta, H. (1996). Influences of ageing, gender and handedness on motor performance of upper and lower extremities. *Perceptual and Motor Skills, 82*, 515–525.

Kawashima, R., Yamada, K., Kinomura, S., Yamaguchi, T., Matsui, H., Yoshioka, S., & Fukuda, H. (1993). Regional cerebral blood flow changes of cortical motor areas and prefrontal areas in humans related to ipsilateral and contralateral hand movement. *Brain Research, 623*, 33–40.

Kertesz, A., & Geschwind, N. (1971). Patterns of pyramidal decussation and their relationship to handedness. *Archives of Neurology, 24*, 326–332.

Kilshaw, D., & Annett, M. (1983). Right- and left-hand skill. I: Effects of age, sex and hand preference showing superior skill in left-handers. *British Journal of Psychology, 74*, 253–268.

Kim, S.-G., Ashe, J., Hendrich, K., Ellermann, J. M., Merkle, H., Ugurbil, K., & Georgopoulos, A. P. (1993). Functional magnetic resonance imaging of motor cortex: Hemispheric asymmetry and handedness. *Science, 261*, 615–617.

Kimura, D. (1982). Left-hemisphere control of oral and brachial movements and their relation to communication. *Philosophical Transactions of the Royal Society of London, 298*, 135–149.

Kimura, D. (1993). *Neuromotor mechanisms in human communication.* Oxford Psychology Series, no. 20. Oxford: Oxford University Press.

Kimura, D., & Davidson, W. (1975). Right arm superiority for tapping with distal and proximal joints. *Journal of Human Movement Studies, 1*, 199–202.

Kimura, D., & Vanderwolf, C. H. (1970). The relation between hand preference and the performance of individual finger movements by left and right hands. *Brain, 93*, 769–774.

King, G. D., Hannay, H. J., Masek, B. J., & Burns, J. W. (1978). Effects of anxiety and sex on neuropsychological tests. *Journal of Consulting and Clinical Psychology, 46*, 375–376.

Klar, A. J. S. (1996). A single locus, RGHT, specifies preference for hand utilization in humans. *Cold Spring Harbor Symposia on Quantitative Biology, 61*, 59–65.

Koch, H. (1933). A study of the nature, measurement and determination of hand preference. *Genetic Psychology Monographs, 13*, 117–221.

Komai, T., & Fukuoka, G. (1934). A study on the frequency of left-handedness and left-footedness among Japanese school children. *Human Biology, 66*, 33–42.

Kooistra, C. A., & Heilman, K. M. (1988). Motor dominance and lateral asymmetry of the globus pallidus. *Neurology, 38,* 388–391.

Laland, K. N., Kumm, J., Van Horn, J. D., & Feldman, M. W. (1995). A gene-culture model of human handedness. *Behavior Genetics, 25,* 433–445.

Lalumière, M. L., Blanchard, R., & Zucker, K. J. (2000). Sexual orientation and handedness in men and women: A meta-analysis. *Psychological Bulletin, 126,* 575–592.

Lausberg, H., Göttert, R., Münßinger, U., Boegner, F., & Marx, P. (1999). Callosal disconnection syndrome in left-handed patient due to infarction of the total length of the corpus callosum. *Neuropsychologia, 37,* 253–265.

Lawrence, D. G., & Kuypers, H. G. J. M. (1968). The functional organization of the motor system in the monkey. 1. The effects of bilateral pyramidal lesions. *Brain, 91,* 1–14.

Leask, S. J., & Crow, T. J. (1997). How far does the brain lateralize?: An unbiased method for determining the optimum degree of hemispheric specialization. *Neuropsychologia, 35,* 1381–1387.

Levinson, H. N. (1990). Diagnostic value of cerebellar-vestibular tests detecting learning disabilities, dyslexia, and attention deficit disorder. *Perceptual and Motor Skills, 71,* 67–82.

Levy, J. (1976). A review of evidence for a genetic component in the determination of handedness. *Behavior Genetics, 6,* 429–453.

Levy, J., & Nagylaki, T. (1972). A model for the genetics of handedness. *Genetics, 72,* 117–128.

Levy, J., & Reid, M. (1976). Variations in writing posture and cerebral organization. *Science, 194,* 337–339.

Li, A., Yetkin, Z., Cox, R., & Haughton, V. M. (1996). Ipsilateral hemisphere activation during motor and sensory tasks. *American Journal of Neuroradiology, 17,* 651–655.

Liepmann, H., & Maas, O. (1907). Ein fall von linksseitiger agraphie und apraxie bei rechtsseitiger lähmung. *Zeitschrift für Psychologie und Neurologie, 10,* 214–227.

Macdonell, R. A. L., Shapiro, B. E., Chiappa, K. H., Helmers, S. L., Cros, D., Day, B. J., & Shahani, B. T. (1991). Hemispheric threshold differences for motor evoked potentials produced by magnetic coil stimulation. *Neurology, 41,* 1441–1444.

Mandal, M. K., Pandey, G., Das, C. T., & Bryden, M. P. (1998). Handedness in mental retardation. *Laterality, 3,* 221–225.

Marchant, L. F., McGrew, W. C., & Eibl-Eibesfeldt, I. (1995). Is human handedness universal? Ethological analyses from three traditional cultures. *Ethology, 101,* 239–258.

Marchetti, C., & Della Sala, S. (1997). On crossed apraxia. Description of a right-handed apraxic patient with right supplementary motor area damage. *Cortex, 33,* 341–354.

Marzi, C. A., Bisiacchi, P., & Nicoletti, R. (1991). Is interhemispheric transfer of visuomotor information asymmetric? Evidence from a meta-analysis. *Neuropsychologia, 29,* 1163–1177.

The Nature and Determinants of Handedness

McKeever, W. F. (2000). A new family handedness sample with findings consistent with X-linked transmission. *British Journal of Psychology, 91*, 21–39.

McKeever, W. F., Cerone, L. J., & Chase-Carmichael, C. (2000). Developmental instability and right shift theory hypotheses concerning correlate of familial sinistrality: Negative findings. *Laterality, 5*, 97–110.

McKeever, W. F., Cerone, L. J., Suter, P. J., & Wu, S. M. (2000). Family size, miscarriage proneness, and handedness: Tests of the hypothesis of the developmental instability theory of handedness. *Laterality, 5*, 111–120.

McKeever, W. F., Suter, P. J., & Rich, D. A. (1995). Maternal age and parity correlates of handedness: Gender, but no parental handedness modulation of effects. *Cortex, 31*, 543–553.

McKeever, W. F., & VanEys, P. P. (1989). Inverted handwriting posture in left handers is related to familial sinistrality incidence. *Cortex, 25*, 581–589.

McManus, I. C. (1981). Handedness and birth stress. *Psychological Medicine, 11*, 485–496.

McManus, I. C. (1983). Pathologic left-handedness: Does it exist? *Journal of Communication Disorders, 16*, 315–344.

McManus, I. C. (1985a). Right- and left-hand skill: Failure of the right shift model. *British Journal of Psychology, 76*, 1–16.

McManus, I. C. (1985b). Handedness, language dominance and aphasia: A genetic model. *Psychological Medicine, Monograph Supplement, 8*, 1–40.

McManus, I. C. (1991). The inheritance of left-handedness. In G. R. Bock & J. Marsh (Eds.), *CIBA Foundation symposium 162: Biological asymmetry and handedness* (pp. 251–267). Chichester, UK: Wiley.

McManus, I. C. (1995). Familial sinistrality: The utility of calculating exact genotype probabilities for individuals. *Cortex, 3*, 3–24.

McManus, I. C., & Bryden, M. P. (1991). Geschwind's theory of cerebral lateralization: Developing a formal, causal model. *Psychological Bulletin, 110*, 237–253.

McManus, I. C., & Bryden, M. P. (1992). The genetics of handedness, cerebral dominance and lateralization. In I. Rapin and S. Segalowitz (Eds.), *Handbook of neuropsychology: 10-developmental neuropsychology* (pp. 115–144). Amsterdam: Elsevier.

McManus, I. C., & Bryden, M. P. (1993). The neurobiology of handedness, language, and cerebral dominance. In M. F. Johnson (Ed.), *Brain development and cognition: A reader* (pp. 679–702). Oxford: Blackwell.

McManus, I. C., & Cornish, K. M. (1997). Fractionating handedness in mental retardation: What is the role of the cerebellum? *Laterality, 2*, 81–90.

McManus, I. C., Kemp, I. R., & Grant, J. (1986). Differences between fingers and hands in tapping ability: Dissociation between speed and regularity. *Cortex, 22*, 461–473.

McManus, I. C., Murray, B., Doyle, K., & Baron-Cohen, S. (1992). Handedness in childhood autism shows a dissociation of skill and preference. *Cortex, 28*, 373–381.

McManus, I. C., Porac, C., Bryden, M. P., & Boucher, R. (1999). Eye-dominance, writing hand, and throwing hand. *Laterality, 4,* 173–192.

McManus, I. C., Shergill, S., & Bryden, M. P. (1993). Annett's theory that individuals heterozygous for the right shift gene are intellectually advantaged: Theoretical and empirical problems. *British Journal of Psychology, 84,* 517–537.

Meerwaldt, J. D. (1983). Disturbances in spatial perception in a patient with agenesis of the corpus callosum. *Neuropsychologia, 21,* 161–165.

Melsbach, G., Wohlschläger, A., Spiess, M., & Güntürkün, O. (1996). Morphological asymmetries of motoneurons innervating upper extremities: Clues to the anatomical foundations of handedness? *International Journal of Neuroscience, 86,* 217–224.

Meyer, B. U., Roricht, S., von Einsiedel, G., Kruggel, F., & Weindl, A. (1995). Inhibitory and excitatory interhemispheric transfers between motor cortical areas in normal humans and patients with abnormalities of the corpus callosum. *Brain, 118,* 429–440.

Milner, B., & Kolb, B. (1985). Performance of complex arm movements and facial-movement sequences after cerebral commissurotomy. *Neuropsychologia, 23,* 791–799.

Mima, T., Sadato, N., Yazawa, S., Hanakawa, T., Fukuyama, H., Yonekura, Y., & Shibasaki, H. (1999). Brain structures related to active and passive finger movements in man. *Brain, 122,* 1989–1997.

Moffat, S. D., & Hampson, E. (1996). Salivary testosterone levels in left- and right-handed adults. *Neuropsychologia, 34,* 225–233.

Morgan, M. J., & Corballis, M. C. (1978). On the biological basis of human laterality II. The mechanisms of inheritance. *The Behavioral and Brain Sciences, 2,* 270–279.

Morgan, M. J., & McManus, I. C. (1988). The relationship between brainedness and handedness. In F. C. Rose, R. Whurr, & M. Wyke (Eds.), *Aphasia* (pp. 85–130). London: Whurr.

Nachshon, I., & Denno, D. (1987). Birth stress and lateral preferences. *Cortex, 23,* 45–58.

Nass, R., Baker, S., Speiser, P., Virdis, R., Balsamo, A., Cacciari, E., Loche, A., Dumic, M., & New, M. (1987). Hormones and handedness: Left-hand bias in female congenital adrenal hyperplasia patients. *Neurology, 37,* 711–715.

Nathan, P. W., Smith, M. C., & Deacon, P. (1990). The corticospinal tracts in man: course and location of fibres at different segmental levels. *Brain, 113,* 303–324.

Newman, H. H. (1934). Dermatoglyphics and the problem of handedness. *American Journal of Anatomy, 55,* 277–322.

O'Callaghan, M. J., Burn, Y. R., Mohay, H. A., Rogers, Y., & Tudehope, D. I. (1993). Handedness in extremely low birth weight infants. *Cortex, 29,* 629–637

O'Connor, J. T. (1890). Right-handedness. *Science,* Vol. XVI, 331–332.

Ogle, W. (1871). On dextral pre-eminence. *Transactions of the Royal Medical and Chirurgical Society of London, 54,* 297–301.

Okuda, B., Tanaka, H., Tomino, Y., Kawabata, K., Tachibana, H., & Sugita, M. (1995). The role of the left somatosensory cortex in human hand movement. *Experimental Brain Research, 106,* 493–498.

Oldfield, R. C. (1971). The assessment and analysis of handedness: The Edinburgh inventory. *Neuropsychologia, 9,* 87–113.

Palmer, A. R., & Strobeck, C. (1986). Fluctuating asymmetry: Measurement, analysis, patterns. *Annual Review of Ecological Systems, 17,* 391–421.

Palmer, R. E., & Corballis, M. C. (1996). Predicting reading ability from handedness measures. *British Journal of Psychology, 87,* 609–620.

Papousek, I., & Schulter, G. (1999). Quantitative assessment of five behavioural laterality measures: Distributions of scores and intercorrelations among right-handers. *Laterality, 4,* 345–362.

Parlow, S. E., & Kinsbourne, M. (1989). Asymmetrical transfer of training between hands. *Brain and Cognition, 11,* 98–113.

Parson, B. S. (1924). *Left handedness: A new interpretation.* New York: Macmillan.

Payne, M. A. (1987). Impact of cultural pressures on self-reports of actual and approved hand use. *Neuropsychologia, 25,* 247–258.

Perelle, I. B., Ehrman, L., & Manowitz , J. W. (1981). Human handedness: The influence of learning. *Perceptual and Motor Skills, 53,* 967–977.

Peters, M. (1990a). Phenotype in normal left-handers: An understanding of phenotype is the basis for understanding mechanism and inheritance of handedness. In S. Coren (Ed.), *Left handedness: Behavioral implications and anomalies* (pp. 167–192). Elsevier Science Publishers.

Peters, M. (1990b). Subclassification of non-pathological left-handers poses problems for theories of handedness. *Neuropsychologia, 28,* 279–289.

Peters, M. (1992). How sensitive are handedness prevalence figures to differences in questionnaire classification procedures? *Brain and Cognition, 18,* 208–215.

Peters, M. (1995). Handedness and its relation to other indices of cerebral lateralization. In R. J. Davidson & K. Hugdahl (Eds.), *Brain asymmetry* (pp. 183–214). Cambridge, MA: MIT Press.

Peters, M. (1998). Description and validation of a flexible and broadly usable handedness questionnaire. *Laterality, 3,* 77–96.

Peters, M., & Durding, B. M. (1978). Handedness measured by finger tapping: A continuous variable. *Canadian Journal of Psychology/Revue Canadienne de Psychologie, 32,* 257–261.

Peters, M., & Durding, B. (1979). Left-handers and right-handers compared on a motor task. *Journal of Motor Behavior, 11,* 103–111.

Peters, M., & Pang, J. (1992). Do "right-armed" lefthanders have different lateralization of motor control for the proximal and distal musculature? *Cortex, 28,* 391–399.

Pipe, M.-E. (1988). Atypical laterality and retardation. *Psychological Bulletin, 104,* 343–347.

Pipe, M.-E. (1990). Mental retardation and left-handedness: Evidence and theories. In S. Coren (Ed.), *Left-handedness: Behavioural implications and anomalies* (pp. 293–318). North-Holland: Elsevier Science Publishers.

Plante, E., Boliek, C., Binkiewicz, A., & Erly, W. K. (1996). Elevated androgen, brain development and language/learning disabilities in children with congenital adrenal hyperplasia. *Developmental Medicine and Child Neurology, 38,* 423–437.

Porac, C. (1995). Genetic vs. environmental contributions to human handedness: Insights gained from studying individuals with unilateral hand injuries. *Behavior Genetics, 25,* 447–455.

Porac, C. (1996). Hand and foot preference in young and older adults: A comment on Gabbard and Iteya. *Laterality, 1,* 207–213.

Porac, C. (1997). Eye preference patterns among left-handed adults. *Laterality, 2,* 305–316.

Porac, C., & Coren, S. (1981). *Lateral preferences and human behavior.* New York: Springer-Verlag.

Porac, C., Coren, S., & Searleman, A. (1986). Environmental factors in hand preference formation: Evidence from attempts to switch the preferred hand. *Behavior Genetics, 16,* 250–261.

Potter, S. M., & Graves, R. E. (1988). Is interhemispheric transfer related to handedness and gender? *Neuropsychologia, 26,* 319–325.

Powls, A., Botting, N., Cooke, R. W. I., & Marlow, N. (1996). Handedness in very-low-birthweight (VLBW) children at 12 years of age: Relation to perinatal and outcome variables. *Developmental Medicine and Child Neurology, 38,* 594–602.

Previc, F. H. (1991). A general theory concerning the prenatal origins of cerebral lateralization in humans. *Psychological Review, 98,* 299–334.

Previc, F. H. (1996). Nonright-handedness, central nervous system and related pathology, and its lateralization: A reformulation and synthesis. *Developmental Neuropsychology, 12,* 443–515.

Provins, K. A. (1997a). The specificity of motor skill and manual asymmetry: A review of the evidence and its implications. *Journal of Motor Behaviour, 29,* 183–192.

Provins, K. A. (1997b). Handedness and speech: A critical reappraisal of the role of genetic and environmental factors in the cerebral lateralization of function. *Psychological Review, 104,* 554–571.

Purves, D., White, L. E., & Andrews, T. J. (1994). Manual asymmetry and handedness (trophic interactions/somatic symmetry). *Proceedings of the National Academy of Sciences, USA, 91,* 5030–5032.

Pye-Smith, P. H. (1871). On left-handedness. *Guy's Hospital Reports, 16,* 141–146.

Rapcsack, S. Z., Rothi, L. J. G., & Heilman, K. M. (1987). Apraxia in a patient with atypical cerebral dominance. *Brain and Cognition, 6*, 450–463.

Raymer, A. M., Merians, A. S., Adair, J. C., Schwartz, R. L., Williamson, D. J. G., Rothi, L. J. G., Poizner, H., & Heilman, K. M. (1999). Crossed apraxia: Implications for handedness. *Cortex, 35*, 183–199.

Reynolds, D. M., & Jeeves, M. A. (1977). Further studies of tactile perception and motor coordination in agenesis of the corpus callosum. *Cortex, 13*, 257–272.

Riddoch, M. J., Humphreys, G. W., & Price, C. J. (1989). Routes to action: Evidence from apraxia. *Cognitive Neuropsychology, 6*, 437–454.

Rigal, R. A. (1992). Which handedness: Preference or performance? *Perceptual and Motor Skills, 75*, 851–866.

Risch, N., & Pringle, G. (1985). Segregation analysis of human hand preference. *Behavior Genetics, 15*, 385–400.

Roland, P. E., & Zilles, K. (1996). Functions and structures of the motor cortices in humans. *Current Opinion in Neurobiology, 6*, 773–781.

Rosen, G. D., Sherman, G. F., & Galaburda, A. M. (1989). Interhemispheric connections differ between symmetrical and asymmetrical regions. *Neuroscience, 33*, 525–533.

Ross, G., Lipper, E. G., & Auld, P. A. M. (1987). Hand preference of four-year-old children: Its relationship to premature birth and neurodevelopmental outcome. *Developmental Medicine and Child Neurology, 29*, 615–622.

Rothi, L. J. G., Ochipa, C., & Heilman, K. M. (1991). A cognitive neuropsychological model of limb praxis. *Cognitive Neuropsychology, 8*, 443–458.

Rouiller, E. M., Babalian, A., Kazennikov, O., Moret, V., Yu, X.-H., & Wiesendanger, M. (1994). Transcallosal connections of the distal forelimb representations of the primary and supplementary motor cortical areas in macaque monkeys. *Experimental Brain Research, 102*, 227–243.

Roy, E. A. (1996). Hand preference, manual asymmetries, and limb apraxia. In D. Elliot & E. A. Roy (Eds.), *Manual asymmetries in motor performance* (pp. 215–236). London: CRC Press.

Roy, E. A., & Elliott, D. (1989). Manual asymmetries in aimed movements. *Quarterly Journal of Experimental Psychology, 41A*, 501–516.

Sadato, N. V., Campbell, G., Ibáñez Deiber, M.-P., & Hallett, M. (1996). Complexity affects regional cerebral blood flow change during sequential finger movements. *Journal of Neuroscience, 16*, 2693–2700.

Sanders, G., Wright, H. V., & Ellis, C. (1989). Cerebral lateralization of language in deaf and hearing people. *Brain and Language, 36*, 555–579.

Satz, P. (1972). Pathological left-handedness: An explanatory model. *Cortex, 8*, 121–135.

Satz, P., & Soper, H. V. (1986). Left-handedness, dyslexia, and autoimmune disorder: A critique. *Journal of Clinical and Experimental Neuropsychology, 8*, 453–458.

Schachter, S. C. (1994). Handedness in women with intrauterine exposure to diethyl-stilbestrol. *Neuropsychologia, 32,* 619–623.

Schaeffer, A. A. (1928). Spiral movements in man. *Journal of Morphology, 45,* 293–398.

Scheibel, A., Conrad, T., Perdue, S., Tomiyasu, U., & Wechsler, A. (1990). A quantitative study of dendrite complexity in selected areas of the human cerebral cortex. *Brain and Cognition, 12,* 85–101.

Scheirs, J. G. M., & Vingerhoets, A. J. J. M. (1995). Handedness and other laterality indices in women prenatally exposed to DES. *Journal of Clinical and Experimental Neuropsychology, 17,* 725–730.

Schlaug, G., Jäncke, L., Huang, Y., Steiger, J., & Steinmetz, H. (1995). Increased corpus callosum size in musicians. *Neuropsychologia, 33,* 1047–1055.

Schmidt, S. L., Oliveira, R. M., Krahe, T. E., & Filgueiras, C. C. (2000). The effects of hand preference and gender on finger tapping performance asymmetry by the use of an in-frared light measurement device. *Neuropsychologia, 38,* 529–534.

Schwartz, M. (1988). Discrepancy between maternal report and hospital records. *Developmental Psychology, 4,* 303–304.

Schwartz, M. (1990). Left-handedness and prenatal complications. In S. Coren (Ed.), *Left-handedness: Behavioural implications and anomalies* (pp. 75–97). Amsterdam: Elsevier Science Publishers.

Searleman, A., Coren, S., & Porac, C. (1989). Relationship between birth order, birth stress, and lateral preferences: A critical review. *Psychological Bulletin, 105,* 397–408.

Shibasaki, H., Sadato, N., Lyshkow, H., Yonekura, Y., Honda, M., Nagamine, T., Suwa-zono, S., Magata, Y., Ikeda, A., Miyazaki, M., Fukuyama, H., Asato, R., & Konishi, J. (1993). Both primary motor cortex and supplementary motor area play an important role in complex finger movement. *Brain, 116,* 1387–1398.

Smith, G. E. (1927). *The evolution of man.* London: Oxford University Press.

Snyder, P. J. (2000). Evolutionary bases for cerebral localization of higher cognitive functions. *Brain and Language, 73,* 127–131.

Snyder, P. J., Bilder, R. M., Wu, H., Bogerts, B., & Lieberman, J. A. (1995). Cerebellar volume asymmetries are related to handedness: A quantitative MRI study. *Neuropsychologia, 33,* 407–419.

Soper, H. V., & Satz, P. (1984). Pathological left-handedness and ambiguous handedness: A new explanatory model. *Neuropsychologia, 22,* 511–515.

Speigler, B. J., & Yeni-Komishan, G. H. (1983). Incidence of left-handed writing in a college population with reference to family patterns of hand preference. *Neuropsychologia, 21,* 651–659.

Steele, J. (2000). Handedness in past human populations: Skeletal markers. *Laterality, 5,* 193–220.

Steenhuis, R. E., & Bryden, M. P. (1989). Different dimensions of hand preference that relate to skilled and unskilled activities. *Cortex*, *25*, 289–304.

Steenhuis, R. E., & Bryden, M. P. (1999). The relation betwen hand preference and hand performance: What you get depends upon what you measure. *Laterality*, *4*, 3–26.

Stein, J. F., & Glickstein, M. (1992). Role of the cerebellum in visual guidance of movement. *Physiological Reviews*, *72*, 967–1017.

Steinmetz, H., Volkmann, J., Jäncke, L., & Freund, H.-J. (1991). Anatomical left-right asymmetry of language-related temporal cortex is different in left- and right-handers. *Annals of Neurology*, *29*, 315–319.

Stewart, A. L., Rifkin, L., Amess, P. N., Kirkbride, V., Townsend, J. P., Miller, D. H., Lewis, S. W., Kingsley, D. P. E., Moseley, I. F., Foster, O., & Murray, R. M. (1999). Brain structure and neurocognitive and behavioural function in adolescents who were born very preterm. *The Lancet*, *353*, 1653–1657.

Sutton, P. R. (1963). Handedness and facial asymmetry: Lateral position of the nose in two racial groups. *Nature*, *198*, 909.

Tambs, K., Magnus, P., & Berg, K. (1987). Left-handedness in twin families: Support of an environmental hypothesis. *Perceptual and Motor Skills*, *64*, 155–170.

Tan, L. E., & Nettleton, N. C. (1980). Left handedness, birth order and birth stress. *Cortex*, *16*, 363–373.

Taniguchi, M., Yoshimine, T., Cheyne, D., Kato, A., Kihara, T., Ninomiya, H., Hirata, M., Hirabuki, N., Nakamura, H., & Hayakawa, T. (1998). Neuromagnetic fields preceding unilateral movements in dextrals and sinistrals. *NeuoroReport*, *9*, 1497–1502.

Tankle, R. S., & Heilman, K. M. (1983). Mirror writing in right-handers and in left-handers. *Brain and Language*, *19*, 115–123.

Tapley, S. M., & Bryden, M. P. (1985). A group test for the assessment of performance between the hands. *Neuropsychologia*, *23*, 515–519.

Thach, W. T., Goodkin, H. P., & Keating, J. G. (1992). The cerebellum and adaptive coordination of movement. *Annual Review of Neuroscience*, *15*, 403–442.

Todor, J. I., Kyprie, P. M., & Price, H. L. (1982). Lateral asymmetries in arm, wrist and finger movements. *Cortex*, *18*, 515–523.

Trankell, A. (1955). Aspects of genetics in psychology. *American Journal of Human Genetics*, *7*, 264–276.

Triggs, W. J., Calvanio, R., & Levine, M. (1997). Transcranial magnetic stimulation reveals a hemispheric asymmetry correlate of intermanual differences in motor performance. *Neuropsychologia*, *35*, 1355–1363.

Triggs, W. J., Calvanio, R., Levine, M., Heaton, R. K., & Heilman, K. M. (2000). Predicting hand preference with performance on motor tasks. *Cortex*, *36*, 679–689.

Triggs, W. J., Calvanio, R., Macdonell, R. A. L., Cros, D., & Chiappa, K. H. (1994). Physiological motor asymmetry in human handedness: Evidence from transcranial magnetic stimulation. *Brain Research, 636,* 270–276.

Trope, I., Fishman, B., Gur, R., Sussman, N., & Gur, R. (1987). Contralateral and ipsilateral control of fingers collowing callosotomy. *Neuropsychologia, 25,* 287–291.

Tucha, O., Aschenbrenner, S., & Lange, K. W. (2000). Mirror writing and handedness. *Brain and Language, 73,* 432–441.

Urbano, A., Babiloni, C., Onorati, P., & Babiloni, F. (1996). Human cortical activity related to unilateral movements. A high resolution EEG study. *NeuroReport, 8,* 203–206.

Velay, J.-L., & Benoit-Dubrocard, S. (1999). Hemispheric asymmetry and interhemispheric transfer in reaching programming. *Neuropsychologia, 37,* 895–903.

Volkmann, J., Schnitzler, A., Witte, O. W., & Freund, H.-J. (1998). Handedness and asymmetry of hand representation in human motor cortex. *Journal of Neurophysiology, 79,* 2149–2154.

Volpe, B. T., Sidtis, J. J., & Gazzaniga, M. S. (1981). Can left-handed writing posture predict cerebral language laterality? *Archives of Neurology, 38,* 637–638.

Wang, X., Merzenich, M. M., Sameshima, K., & Jenkins, W. M. (1995). Remodelling of hand representation in adult cortex determined by timing of tactile stimulation. *Nature, 378,* 71–75.

Wassermann, E. M., Pascual-Leone, A., & Hallet, M. (1994). Cortical motor representation of the ipsilateral hand and arm. *Experimental Brain Research, 100,* 121–132.

Watson, N. V., & Kimura, D. (1989). Right-hand superiority for throwing but not for intercepting. *Neuropsychologia, 27,* 1399–1414.

Weber, A. M., & Bradshaw, J. L. (1981). Levy and Reid's neurological model in relation to writing hand posture: An evaluation. *Psychological Bulletin, 90,* 74–88.

Wharton, H. T. (1884). Right-sidedness. *Nature, 29,* 477.

White, L. E., Andrews, T. J., Hulette, C., Richards, A., Groelle, M., Paydarfar, J., & Purves, D. (1997a). Structure of the human sensorimotor system. I: Morphology and cytoarchitecture of the central sulcus. *Cerebral Cortex, 7,* 18–30.

White, L. E., Andrews, T. J., Hulette, C., Richards, A., Groelle, M., Paydarfar, J., & Purves, D. (1997b). Structure of the human sensorimotor system. II: Lateral symmetry. *Cerebral Cortex, 7,* 31–47.

White, L. E., Lucas, G., Richards, A., & Purves, D. (1994). Cerebral asymmetry and handedness. *Nature, 368,* 197–198.

Wile, I. R. (1934). *Handedness: Right and left.* Boston: Lothrop, Lee and Shepard.

Williams, C. S., Buss, K. A., & Eskenazi, B. (1992). Infant resuscitation is associated with an increased risk of left-handedness. *American Journal of Epidemiology, 136,* 277–286.

Wilson, D. (1886). Palaeolithic dexterity. *Transactions of the Royal Society of Canada, 11,* 119–138.

Witelson, S. F. (1985). The brain connection: The corpus callosum is larger in left-handers. *Science, 229,* 665–668.

Witelson, S. F. (1989). Hand and sex differences in the isthmus and genu of the human corpus callosum: A postmortem morphological study. *Brain, 112,* 799–835.

Witelson, S. F. (1991). Neural sexual mosaicism: Sexual differentiation of the human temporo-parietal region for functional asymmetry. *Psychoneuroendocrinology, 16,* 131–153.

Witelson, S. F., & Goldsmith, C. H. (1991). The relationship of hand preference to anatomy of the corpus callosum in men. *Brain Research, 545,* 175–182.

Witelson, S. F., & Nowakowski, R. S. (1991). Left out axons make men right: A hypothesis for the origin of handedness and functional asymmetry. *Neuropsychologia, 29,* 327–333.

Yakovlev, P. I., & Lecours, A. R. (1967). The myelogenetic cycles of regional maturation of the brain. In A. Monkowski (Ed.), *Regional development of the brain in early life* (pp. 3–70). Oxford: Blackwell.

Yakovlev, P. I., & Rakic, P. (1966). Patterns of decussation of bulbar pyramids and distribution of pyramidal tracts on two sides of the spinal cord. *Transactions of the American Neurological Association, 91,* 366–367.

Yeo, R. A., & Gangestad, S. W. (1993). Developmental origins of variation in human hand preference. *Genetica, 89,* 281–296.

Yeo, R. A., Gangestad, S. W., & Daniel, W. F. (1993). Hand preference and developmental instability. *Psychobiology, 21,* 161–168.

Yeo, R. A., Gangestad, S. W., Thoma, R., Shaw, P., & Repa, K. (1997). Developmental instability and cerebral lateralization. *Neuropsychology, 11,* 552–561.

Zaidel, D., & Sperry, R. W. (1977). Some long term motor effects of cerebral commissurotomy in man. *Neuropsychologia, 15,* 193–204.

II Neuroimaging and Brain Stimulation Studies

5 Characterizing Functional Asymmetries with Brain Mapping

Karl J. Friston

This chapter deals with the experimental design and analysis of functional brain imaging studies, with a special emphasis on asymmetry and lateralization in functional brain architectures. It considers the neurobiological motivations for different designs and describes some of the standard approaches that have been developed to analyze data. Functional neuroimaging (positron emission tomography [PET] and functional magnetic resonance imaging [fMRI]) are generally used to make inferences about functional anatomy on the basis of evoked patterns of cortical activity. An important issue, in design and analysis, is the relationship between conceptual models of brain organization and neurophysiological responses, and how this relationship is realized in terms of the statistical models used to analyze neuroimaging data. This chapter begins by reviewing the distinction between functional specialization and integration, and how these principles serve as the motivation for common analytic approaches.

Statistical parametric mapping is used to identify functionally specialized brain regions. The alternative perspective, that provided by functional integration, requires a different set of (multivariate) approaches that examine the changes in activity in one region in relationship to another. Statistical parametric mapping is a voxel-based approach (a voxel is a volume element of the image), employing standard inferential statistics, to make comments about regionally specific responses to experimental factors at that voxel. The general ideas behind statistical parametric mapping are described, and illustrated with the different sorts of inferences that can be made with various designs and analytic perspectives on the data. A PET study of verbal fluency is used to show how laterality issues can be addressed at a number of levels, highlighting the crucial role of *hemisphere by condition interactions* in making inferences about lateralization. This chapter concludes by reviewing functional integration and effective connectivity, and extending the illustrative examples of previous sections to address asymmetries in intra- and interhemispheric coupling.

FUNCTIONAL SPECIALIZATION AND INTEGRATION

The brain appears to adhere to two fundamental principles of functional organization: *functional integration* and *functional specialization*, where the integration within and among specialized areas is mediated by effective connectivity. The distinction relates to that between "localizationism" and "(dis)connectionism" that dominated thinking about cortical function in the nineteenth century. Since the early anatomic theories of Gall, the identification of a particular brain region with a specific function has become a central theme in neuroscience. However, functional localization per se was not easy to demonstrate. For example, a meeting that took place in London on August 4, 1881, addressed the difficulties of attributing function to a cortical area, given the dependence of cerebral activity on underlying connections (Phillips et al., 1984). This meeting's title was "Localization of Function in the Cortex Cerebri." Goltz, although accepting the results of electrical stimulation in dog and monkey cortex, considered the excitation method to be inconclusive, in that the behaviors elicited might have originated in related pathways, or current could have spread to distant centers. In short, the excitation method could not be used to infer functional localization because localizationism discounted interactions, or functional integration, among different brain areas. It was proposed that lesion studies could supplement excitation experiments.

Ironically, it was observations on patients with brain lesions some years later (see Absher & Benson, 1993) that led to the concept of "disconnection syndromes" and the refutation of localizationism as a complete or sufficient explanation of cortical organization. Functional localization implies that a function can be localized in a cortical area, whereas specialization suggests that a cortical area is specialized for some aspects of perceptual or motor processing, where this specialization can be anatomically segregated within the cortex. The cortical infrastructure supporting a single function may then involve many specialized areas whose union is mediated by the functional integration among them. Functional specialization and integration are not exclusive; they are complementary. Functional specialization is meaningful only in the context of functional integration, and vice versa.

The functional role of any component (e.g., cortical area, subarea, neuronal population, or neuron) of the brain is largely defined by its connections. Certain patterns of cortical projections are so common that they could amount to rules of cortical connectivity. "These rules revolve around one, apparently, overriding strategy that the cerebral cortex uses—that of functional segregation" (Zeki, 1990).

Functional segregation demands that cells with common functional properties be grouped together. This architectural constraint in turn necessitates both convergence and divergence of cortical connections. Extrinsic connections, among cortical regions, are not continuous but occur in patches or clusters. This patchiness has, in some instances, a clear relationship to functional segregation. For example, the secondary visual area V2 has a distinctive cytochrome oxidase architecture, consisting of thick stripes, thin stripes, and interstripes. When recordings are made in V2, directionally selective (but not wavelength or color selective) cells are found exclusively in the thick stripes. Retrograde (i.e., backward) labeling of cells in V5 is limited to these thick stripes. All the available physiological evidence suggests that V5 is a functionally homogeneous area that is specialized for visual motion.

Evidence of this nature supports the notion that patchy connectivity is the anatomical infrastructure that underpins functional segregation and specialization. If it is the case that neurons in a given cortical area share a common responsiveness (by virtue of their extrinsic connectivity) to some sensorimotor or cognitive attribute, then this functional segregation is also an anatomical one. Challenging a subject with the appropriate sensorimotor attribute or cognitive process should lead to activity changes in, and only in, the area of interest. This is the model upon which the search for regionally specific effects with functional neuroimaging is based.

The analysis of functional neuroimaging data involves several steps that can be broadly divided into (1) spatial preprocessing, (2) estimating the parameters of a statistical model, and (3) making inferences about modeled effects, using the parameter estimates and their associated statistics. Figure 5.1 depicts the series of transformations that constitute the data analysis stream for a typical neuroimaging analysis. In this chapter we will focus on model estimation and inference, and

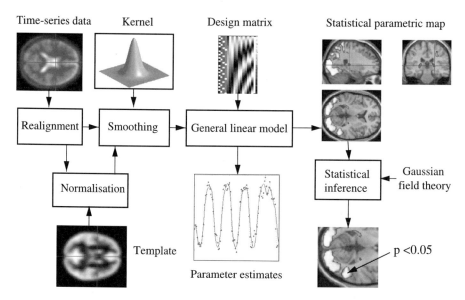

Time-series data   Kernel   Design matrix   Statistical parametric map

Realignment → Smoothing → General linear model →

Normalisation

Template

Parameter estimates

Statistical inference ← Gaussian field theory

p <0.05

Figure 5.1 This schematic depicts the transformations that start with the imaging time series and end with a statistical parametric map (SPM). SPMs can be thought of as X-rays of the significance of an effect. Voxel-based analyses require the data to be in the same anatomical space. This is achieved by first realigning the data to remove the effects of subject movement. After realignment the images are subject to nonlinear warping so that they match a template that already conforms to a standard anatomical space. After smoothing, the general linear model is employed to (1) estimate the parameters of the model and (2) derive the appropriate univariate test statistic at each and every voxel (see figure 5.2). The test statistics (usually T- or F-statistics) constitute the SPM. The final stage is to make statistical inferences on the basis of the SPM, using Gaussian field theory (see figure 5.3), and to characterize the responses observed, using the fitted responses or parameter estimates.

how questions about the lateralization of specialization and integration can be addressed.

Functional mapping studies are usually analyzed with some form of statistical parametric mapping. Statistical parametric mapping refers to the construction of statistical maps to test hypotheses about regionally specific effects (Friston et al., 1995). Statistical parametric maps (SPMs) are image processes with voxel values that are, under the null hypothesis, distributed according to a known probability density function (usually Student's T- or F-distributions). The success of statistical parametric mapping is largely due to the simplicity of the idea: that one analyzes each and every voxel, using any standard (univariate) statistical test. The resulting statistical parameters are assembled into an image, the SPM. SPMs are interpreted as spatially extended statistical processes by referring to the probabilistic behavior of Gaussian fields (Friston et al., 1995; Worsley et al., 1996). Gaussian fields model both the univariate probabilistic characteristics of an SPM and any spatial covariance structure. "Unlikely" excursions of the SPM are interpreted as regionally specific effects, attributable to the sensorimotor or cognitive process that has been manipulated experimentally. Statistical analysis corresponds to modeling the data in order to partition observed neurophysiological responses into components of interest, confounds, and error. Almost universally the models employed are examples of the general linear model (see figure 5.2).

The General Linear Model

The general linear model is an equation $\mathbf{Y} = \mathbf{X}\boldsymbol{\beta} + \boldsymbol{\varepsilon}$ that expresses the observed response variable $\mathbf{Y}$ in terms of a linear combination of explanatory variables $\mathbf{X}$ plus a well-behaved error term (Friston et al., 1995). The general linear model is variously known as "analysis of covariance" or "multiple regression analysis," and subsumes simpler variants, such as the "T-test" for a difference in means, to more elaborate linear convolution models such as finite impulse response (FIR) models. The matrix $\mathbf{X}$ that contains the explanatory variables (e.g., designed effects or confounds) is called the "design matrix." Each column of the design matrix corresponds to some effect one has built into the experiment or that may confound the results. These are variously referred to as explanatory variables, covariates, regressors or, in fMRI, stimulus functions.

The example in figure 5.2 relates to an fMRI study of visual stimulation under four conditions. The effects on the response variable are modeled in terms of functions of the presence of these conditions (i.e., boxcars smoothed with a hemodynamic response function, a function that models the delay and dispersion of neuronal response after it is transduced by the brain into a hemodynamic change). These condition-specific effects constitute the first four columns of the design matrix. There then follows a series of terms that are designed to remove or model low-frequency variations in signal due to artifacts such as aliased biorhythms. The final column is whole brain activity.

The relative contribution of each of these columns is assessed using least squares, and inferences about these contributions are made using

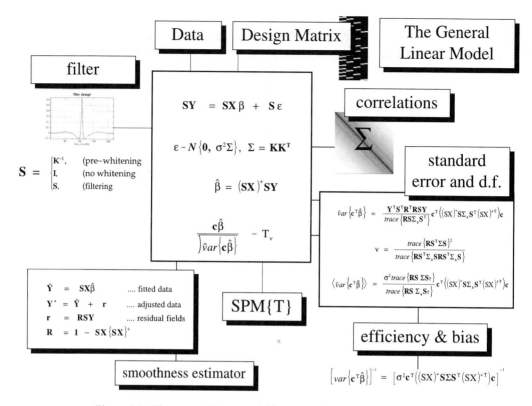

Figure 5.2 The general linear model is an equation expressing the response variable **Y** in terms of a linear combination of explanatory variables in a design matrix **X** and an error term with assumed or known autocorrelation **Σ**. In fMRI the data can be filtered with a convolution matrix **S**, leading to a general linear model that includes (intrinsic) serial correlations and applied (extrinsic) filtering. Different choices of **S** correspond to different filtering schemata (*upper left*). The parameter estimates obtain in a least squares sense, using the pseudoinverse (denoted by +) of the filtered design matrix. Generally an effect of interest is specified by a vector of contrast weights **c** that give a weighted sum or compound of parameter estimates **cβ̂**, referred to as a contrast. The T-statistic is simply this contrast divided by the estimated standard error. The ensuing T-statistic is distributed with **v** degrees of freedom. The equations for the estimated variance of the contrast estimate and the degrees of freedom associated with the error variance are provided in the *right-hand panel*. Efficiency is simply the inverse of the contrast estimate variance. Discrepancies between the actual and assumed intrinsic correlations (**Σ** and **Σ_a**, respectively) can result in systematic bias in the actual and estimated variance of the contrast. These expressions are useful when assessing the relative efficiency and robustness of a model. The parameter estimates can either be examined directly or used to compute the fitted responses (see *lower left panel*). Adjusted data are data from which estimated confounds have been removed. The residuals **r** are obtained from applying the residual-forming matrix **R** to the data. These residual fields are used to estimate the smoothness of the component fields of the SPM used in Gaussian field theory (see figure 5.3).

T- or F-statistics, depending upon whether one is looking at a particular linear combination or all of them together. The operational equations are shown in figure 5.2. In this figure's scheme the general linear model has been extended to incorporate intrinsic autocorrelations among the error terms and to allow for some specified filtering or smoothing of the data. These extensions are required for the analysis of fMRI time series, where the data can be correlated from scan to scan. For PET data one usually assumes the error terms are independent (see the legend of figure 5.2 for details).

These equations can be used to implement a vast range of statistical analyses. The issue is therefore not so much the mathematics but the formulation of a design matrix X appropriate to the study design and the inferences that are sought. The design matrix can contain both covariates and indicator variables. Each column of X has an associated unknown parameter. Some of these parameters will be of interest (e.g., the effect of a particular sensorimotor or cognitive condition or the regression coefficient of hemodynamic responses on reaction time). The remaining parameters will be of no interest, and pertain to nuisance or confounding effects (e.g., the effect of being a particular subject or the regression slope of voxel activity on global activity).

Inferences about the parameter estimates are made using their estimated variance. This allows one to test the null hypothesis that all the estimates are 0, using the F-statistic to give an SPM{F}, or that some particular linear combination (e.g., a subtraction) of the estimates is 0, using an SPM{T}. The T-statistic is obtained by dividing a contrast or compound (specified by contrast weights) of the ensuing parameter estimates by the standard error of that compound. The latter is estimated using the variance of the residuals about the least-squares fit. An example of contrast weights would be $[-1 \quad 1 \quad 0 \quad 0 \ldots]$ to compare the differential responses evoked by two conditions, as modeled by the first two condition-specific regressors in the design matrix. If several parameter estimates are potentially interesting (e.g., using polynomial expansions [Büchel et al., 1996] or basis functions of some parameter of interest), then the SPM{F} is employed.

Statistical Inference and the Theory of Gaussian Fields

Inferences using SPMs can be of two sorts, depending on whether one knows where to look in advance. With an anatomically constrained

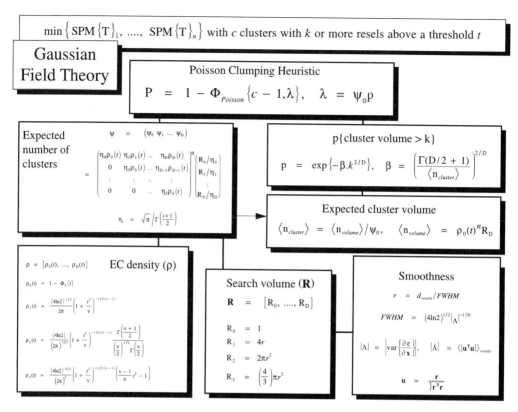

$$\min \left\{ \mathrm{SPM} \left\{ \mathrm{T} \right\}_1, \; ...., \; \mathrm{SPM} \left\{ \mathrm{T} \right\}_n \right\} \text{ with } c \text{ clusters with } k \text{ or more resels above a threshold } t$$

Gaussian Field Theory

Poisson Clumping Heuristic

$$P \;=\; 1 - \Phi_{Poisson} \left\{ c - 1, \lambda \right\}, \quad \lambda = \psi_0 p$$

Expected number of clusters

$$\psi \;=\; (\psi_0 \; \psi_1 \; ... \; \psi_D)$$

$$= \begin{pmatrix} \eta_0 \rho_0(t) & \eta_1 \rho_1(t) & ... & \eta_D \rho_D(t) \\ 0 & \eta_0 \rho_0(t) & ... & \eta_{D-1}\rho_{D-1}(t) \\ \vdots & \vdots & \ddots & \vdots \\ 0 & 0 & ... & \eta_0 \rho_0(t) \end{pmatrix}^n \begin{pmatrix} R_0/\eta_0 \\ R_1/\eta_1 \\ \vdots \\ R_D/\eta_D \end{pmatrix}$$

$$\eta_i \;=\; \sqrt{\pi} \Big/ \Gamma\!\left(\tfrac{i+1}{2} \right)$$

$p\{\text{cluster volume} > k\}$

$$p \;=\; \exp\left\{ -\beta . k^{2/D} \right\}, \quad \beta = \left(\frac{\Gamma(D/2 + 1)}{\langle n_{cluster} \rangle} \right)^{2/D}$$

Expected cluster volume

$$\langle n_{cluster} \rangle = \langle n_{volume} \rangle / \psi_0, \quad \langle n_{volume} \rangle = \rho_0(t)^n R_D$$

$$\rho = [\rho_0(t), \; ...., \; \rho_D(t)]$$

EC density (ρ)

$$\rho_0(t) = 1 - \Phi_T(t)$$

$$\rho_1(t) = \frac{(4\ln 2)^{1/2}}{2\pi}\left(1 + \frac{t^2}{v}\right)^{-1/2(v-1)}$$

$$\rho_2(t) = \frac{(4\ln 2)}{(2\pi)^{3/2}}\left(1 + \frac{t^2}{v}\right)^{-1/2(v-1)} \frac{\Gamma\!\left(\frac{v+1}{2}\right)}{\left(\frac{v}{2}\right)^{1/2}\Gamma\!\left(\frac{v}{2}\right)}$$

$$\rho_3(t) = \frac{(4\ln 2)^{3/2}}{(2\pi)^2}\left(1 + \frac{t^2}{v}\right)^{-1/2(v-1)}\left(\frac{v-1}{n}t^2 - 1\right)$$

Search volume (R)

$$R = [R_0, \; ...., \; R_D]$$

$$R_0 = 1$$

$$R_1 = 4r$$

$$R_2 = 2\pi r^2$$

$$R_3 = \left(\frac{4}{3}\right)\pi r^3$$

Smoothness

$$r = d_{voxels} / FWHM$$

$$FWHM = (4\ln 2)^{1/2}|\Lambda|^{-1/D}$$

$$|\Lambda| = \left| var\left\{ \frac{\partial \varepsilon}{\partial x} \right\} \right|, \quad |\hat{\Lambda}| = \langle |u^\mathrm{T} u| \rangle_{voxels}$$

$$u = \frac{r}{\sqrt{r^\mathrm{T} r}}$$

Figure 5.3 The theory of Gaussian fields. If one knows where to look beforehand, then inference can be based on the value of the statistic at the specified location in the SPM without correction. If, however, one does not have an anatomical constraint a priori, then an adjustment or correction for multiple dependent comparisons has to be made. These corrections are usually made using distributional approximations from the theory of Gaussian fields. This schematic deals with the most general case of n SPM{T}s whose voxels all survive a common threshold t (i.e., a conjunction). The central probability, upon which all voxel, cluster, or set-level inferences rest, is the probability P of getting c or more clusters with k or more resels (resolution elements) above this threshold. By assuming that clusters behave like a multidimensional point process (i.e., the Poisson clumping heuristic), P can be determined from the distribution of c—that is, assumed to be Poisson with an expectation that is the product of the expected number of clusters, of any size, and the probability that any cluster will be bigger than k resels. The latter probability is shown using a form for a single Z-variate field constrained by the expected number of resels per cluster ($\langle . \rangle$ denotes expectation or average). The expected number of resels per cluster is simply the total number of resels divided by the expected number of clusters. The expected number of clusters is estimated with the Euler characteristic (EC), effectively the number of blobs minus the number of holes. This estimate is in turn a function of the EC density for the statistic in question (with v degrees of freedom) and the

hypothesis about effects in a particular brain region, the uncorrected p-value associated with the height or extent of that region in the SPM can be used to test the hypothesis. With an anatomically open hypothesis (i.e., a null hypothesis that there is no effect anywhere in the brain) a correction for multiple dependent comparisons is necessary. The theory of Gaussian fields provides a way of computing this corrected p-value which takes into account the fact that neighboring voxels are not independent, by virtue of smoothness in the original data. Provided the data are sufficiently smooth, the correction based on Gaussian field theory is less severe (i.e., is more sensitive) than a Bonferroni correction for the number of voxels. Figure 5.3 provides an overview of the equations that underlie Gaussian field theory and its application to inference in SPMs. Interested readers are referred to the legend of figure 5.3. However, it is sufficient to note that there exists a mathematical framework which provides adjusted p-values that are corrected for the volume encompassed by the analysis.

EXPERIMENTAL DESIGN

In this section we will consider the different sorts of design that can be employed in neuroimaging studies and how these approaches can be harnessed to look at laterality in functional neuroimaging. We will review categorical, conjunction, parametric, and factorial approaches, and then reprise them to address lateralization using a PET study of verbal fluency.

Categorical Designs, Cognitive Subtraction, and Conjunctions

The tenet of cognitive subtraction is that the difference between two tasks can be formulated as a separable cognitive or sensorimotor component, and that the regionally specific differences in hemodynamic

resel counts. The EC density is the expected EC per unit of D-dimensional volume of the SPM, where the D-dimensional volume of the search space is given by the corresponding element in the vector of resel counts. The resel count can be thought of as a volume metric that has been normalized by the smoothness of the SPM's component fields expressed in terms of the full width at half maximum (FWHM). This is estimated from the determinant of the variance-covariance matrix of the first spatial derivatives of $\mathbf{u}$, the normalized residual fields $\mathbf{r}$. In this example, equations for a sphere of radius r are given. Φ denotes the cumulative distribution function for the subscripted statistic in question.

responses identify the corresponding functionally specialized area. Early applications of subtraction range from the functional anatomy of word processing (Petersen et al., 1989) to functional specialization in extrastriate cortex (Lueck et al., 1989). The latter studies involved presenting visual stimuli with and without some sensory attribute (e.g., color, motion, etc.). The areas highlighted by subtraction were identified with homologous areas in monkeys that showed selective electrophysiological responses to equivalent visual stimuli.

Cognitive conjunctions (Price & Friston, 1997) can be thought of as an extension of the subtraction technique, in the sense that conjunctions combine a series of subtractions. In subtraction we test a hypothesis pertaining to the activation in one task, relative to another. In conjunction analyses, several hypotheses are tested conjointly, asking whether all the activations, in a series of task pairs, are jointly significant. Conjunction analyses allow one to demonstrate this context-insensitive nature of regional responses. As will be shown later, this approach can be used to identify bilateral cortical responses, with enhanced sensitivity, by simply asking where activations are jointly significant in both hemispheres.

Parametric Designs

The premise behind parametric designs is that regional physiology will vary systematically with the degree of cognitive or sensorimotor processing or deficits thereof. Examples of this approach include the PET experiments of Grafton et al. (1992) that demonstrated significant correlations between hemodynamic responses and the performance of a visually guided motor tracking task. These relationships or "neurometric functions" may be linear or nonlinear. Using polynomial regression, in the context of the general linear model, one can identify nonlinear relationships between stimulus parameters (e.g., stimulus duration or presentation rate) and evoked responses. To do this, one usually uses an SPM{F} (see Büchel et al., 1996).

The example provided in figure 5.4 illustrates subtraction, conjunction, and parametric approaches to design and analysis. These data were obtained from an fMRI study of visual motion processing using radially moving dots. The stimuli were presented over a range of speeds, using isoluminant and isochromatic stimuli. To identify areas involved in visual motion, a stationary dots condition was subtracted from the moving dots conditions (see contrast weights, *upper right*). To ensure significant motion-sensitive responses, using both color and luminance cues, a conjunction of the equivalent subtractions was assessed under both viewing contexts (i.e., when using color and luminance cues). Areas V5 and V3a are seen in the ensuing SPM{T}. The responses in left V5, shown in the lower panel, speak to a compelling inverted U relationship between speed and evoked response that peaks at around 8 degrees/s. It is this sort of relationship that parametric designs try to characterize. Interestingly, the form of these speed-dependent responses was similar, using both sorts of motion cues, although luminance cues are seen to elicit a greater response. From the point of view of a factorial design, there is a main effect of cue (isoluminant vs. isochromatic), a main (nonlinear) effect of speed, but no speed by cue interaction.

Factorial Designs

At its simplest, an interaction represents a change in a change. Interactions are associated with factorial designs where two or more factors are combined in the same experiment. The effect of one factor, on the effect of the other, is assessed by the interaction term. Factorial designs have a wide range of applications (e.g., assessing physiological adaptation with time by condition interactions). Psychopharmacological activation studies are examples of factorial designs. In these studies, cognitively evoked responses are assessed before and after administration of a drug. The interaction term reflects the modulatory drug effect on the task-dependent activation. Factorial designs have an important role in the context of the logic of cognitive subtraction and additive factors by virtue of being able to test for interactions, or "context-sensitive activations" (i.e., to demonstrate the fallacy of "pure insertion." (See Friston, Price, et al., 1996). These interaction effects can sometimes be interpreted as (1) the integration of the two or more (cognitive) processes or (2) the modulation of one process by another.

Clearly, from the point of view of lateralization, every neuroimaging experiment can be construed as a factorial design in which the same experiment is replicated in the right and left hemispheres. Significant asymmetry or lateralization reduces, in this context, to hemisphere by task, or condition, interactions. We will pursue this and related issues in the next section.

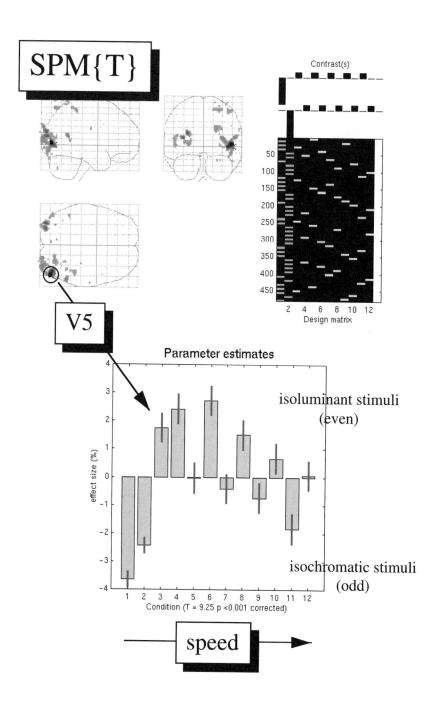

LATERALIZATION IN A PET STUDY OF VERBAL FLUENCY

In this section we will use the above perspectives to look at lateralization issues in a single PET data set. These data have been used in many previous communications to illustrate some of the basic principles of data analysis, and they serve the same purpose here. These data came from a PET study of paced FAS orthographic verbal fluency in which five subjects were asked to produce words beginning with a heard letter (word generation) or simply repeat the letter (word shadowing). Each subject was scanned 12 times, alternating between word generation and word shadowing. The order of the conditions was reversed for each successive subject. The crucial differences between the two tasks comprise the intrinsic generation of a word representation and the mnemonic processes required to keep track of the words already produced. By virtue of the fact that the orthographic fluency task was paced, the sensorimotor components of the tasks were matched.

A Categorical Perspective

The simplest analysis, for this design, is a subtractive one in which we compare the fluency against the shadowing conditions. The resulting activations can be associated with the cognitive components that discriminate between the two tasks, namely, the intrinsic generation of representations and working memory processes that monitor words already produced. This comparison is effected with the contrast $[-1 \quad 1 \quad 0]$, where the shadowing condition-specific effects are mod-

Figure 5.4 (*Top right*) This is an image representation of the design matrix. The contrasts are the vectors of contrast weights defining the linear compounds of parameters tested. The contrasts are displayed over the column of the design matrix that corresponds to the effects in question. The design matrix here includes condition-specific effects (boxcars convolved with a hemodynamic response function). Odd columns correspond to stimuli shown under isochromatic conditions, and even columns model responses to isoluminant stimuli. The first two columns are for stationary stimuli, and the remaining columns are for conditions of increasing speed. The final column is a constant term. (*Top left*) SPM{T} is a maximum-intensity projection of the SPM{T} conforming to the standard anatomical space of Talairach and Tournoux (1988). The T-values here are the minimum T-values from both contrasts, thresholded at $p = .001$ uncorrected. The most significant conjunction is seen in left V5. (*Bottom*) Plot of the condition-specific parameter estimates for this voxel. The T-value was 9.25 ($p < .001$ corrected; see figure 5.3).

eled in the first column of the design matrix, and the fluency effects in the second. The results of this analysis are shown in figure 5.5. The SPM here has been thresholded at $p = .05$ corrected (corresponding to a T-value of 5.00), and shows three cortical activation and three cerebellar effects. The cortical activations were expressed in the region of the anterior cingulate, Broca's area (BA 44), and the dorsomedial thalamus. The table provides (from left to right) (1) the number of clusters and the probability of getting this number or more by chance; (2) the number of voxels in each cluster and the probability of getting this number or more by chance (corrected for the search volume and for each cluster considered alone); (3) the T-values of voxel maxima in each cluster and the equivalent Z-score with the associated p-values (corrected and uncorrected), and finally (4) the location, in mm, according to the atlas of Talairach and Tournoux (1988). There is clear anecdotal evidence of left lateralization here with contralateral effects in the cerebellum. However, before we look at these more rigorously, what about symmetrical or bilateral effects?

A Conjunction Perspective

Suppose one wanted to identify cortical regions that showed a significant bilateral activation in this paradigm. A significant bilateral effect is effectively a conjunction of significant activations in the right and left hemispheres that can be tested using a conjunction analysis. To enable this analysis, the data and design matrix are augmented to include the original data flipped across the midline. Effectively we are treating voxels in homologous parts of the two hemispheres as the same voxel examined in the context of belonging first to the right hemisphere and then to the left. The resulting design matrix, shown in figure 5.6, demonstrates how the activation effects are modeled separately for the right and left hemispheres. The conjunction of the two contrasts, shown above the design matrix, finds areas that are jointly significant in both contrasts. The ensuing SPM{T} was thresholded at $p = .05$ corrected. This corrected threshold corresponds to the situation where $n = 2$ in figure 5.3 (i.e., the case where the SPM comprises the minimum of two component SPMs, in this case activation on the right and on the left). If either of the two component SPMs falls below threshold, the voxel is not shown. Surviving voxels therefore represent areas that show true bilateral effects.

Karl J. Friston

Fluency activations

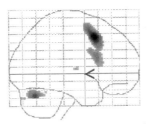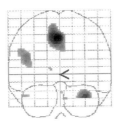

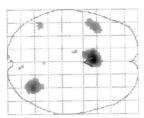

SPM{T}

Statistics: *volume summary (p–values corrected for entire volume)*

set–level		cluster–level			voxel–level				x,y,z (mm)
p	c	$p_{corrected}$	k_E	$p_{uncorrected}$	$p_{corrected}$	T	$(Z_{\equiv})$	$p_{uncorrected}$	
0.000	8	0.000	833	0.000	0.000	9.32	(7.75)	0.000	-2 14 46
					0.000	7.06	(6.27)	0.000	-10 4 58
		0.000	241	0.000	0.000	7.63	(6.67)	0.000	32 -66 -28
		0.000	267	0.000	0.000	6.51	(5.87)	0.000	-42 16 22
					0.002	5.85	(5.36)	0.000	-50 8 28
					0.010	5.47	(5.06)	0.000	-40 22 14
		0.004	14	0.076	0.007	5.56	(5.13)	0.000	-48 -56 -28
		0.032	1	0.642	0.014	5.37	(4.98)	0.000	8 -84 -32
		0.017	4	0.328	0.014	5.36	(4.98)	0.000	-12 -12 6
		0.032	1	0.642	0.022	5.23	(4.87)	0.000	6 -80 -32
		0.032	1	0.642	0.038	5.08	(4.74)	0.000	2 -52 -24

Figure 5.5 Subtractive analysis of the verbal fluency data set. (*Top*) SPM{T} testing for the differences between intrinsic and extrinsic word generation. This SPM has been thresholded at $p = .05$ corrected. This SPM is shown in the same format as in figure 5.4. (*Bottom*) Tabular display of the results in terms of sets of clusters, clusters of voxels, and voxels. Z_E denotes the Z-score equivalent of the corresponding T-statistic.

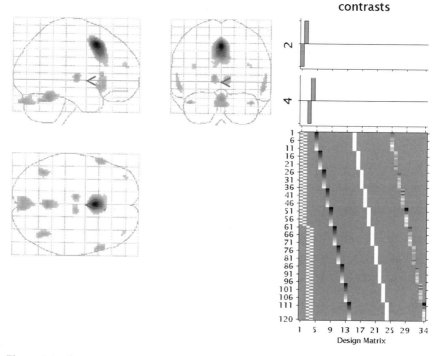

Figure 5.6 Conjunction analysis of bilateral effects. (*Right*) Design matrix used in this analysis. Here the explanatory variables have been augmented to accommodate the flipped images. In addition to condition-specific effects, for the two hemispheres, in the first four columns, subject-specific time and global effects have been included as nuisance variables. The contrast weight vectors are shown above the design matrix. (*Left*) SPM{T} testing for the conjunction, thresholded at $p = .05$ corrected.

Note that there are some areas which were not revealed by the simple subtraction or simple main effect analysis in figure 5.5. This is because conjunction analyses are generally more sensitive. This enhanced sensitivity results from mutual constraints on the search in one component SPM that is provided by the other. The ensuing adjustment of the *p*-values is therefore ameliorated, allowing the threshold to be lowered while maintaining the same specificity at a corrected level. Bilateral effects in the dorsomedial thalami are now clearly evident, with the emergence of bilateral effects in the inferior frontal gyri and anterior middle frontal gyri. Note, however, that Broca's area and the left dorsolateral prefrontal cortex (DLPFC) do not show bilateral activation.

The use of conjunction analysis of bilateral effects has already been exploited in the context of voxel-based morphometry (VBM). VBM uses SPMs to assess, not functional differences among scans, but structural or morphometric differences in gray matter density. The detection of bilateral effects is particularly important in children, where neuropsychological impairment is more likely to be associated with bilateral brain damage. This is thought to reflect the fact that hemispheric specialization increases during neurodevelopment, rendering unilateral damage in children less disruptive (Salmond et al., 2000).

A Factorial Perspective

In the previous subsection we looked for bilateral effects. Here we address lateralized responses in terms of hemisphere by condition interactions. Using the augmented model above, we can now test formally for more activation in one hemisphere, relative to the other, using a contrast that tests explicitly for this differential activation (i.e., the interaction). The contrast weights [1 −1 −1 1] test for activations that are significantly greater in the left hemisphere than they are in the right. The results of this analysis, shown in figure 5.7, demonstrate that, in relation to the right hemisphere, the left prefrontal activations are more extensive than revealed by the simple subtraction analysis. The DLPFC effect now extends into the middle frontal gyrus and BA 46. There are also some left-sided parietal responses of smaller anatomical extent (but still very significant). Taken together with the subtraction analysis, this suggests that the homologous right DLPFC deactivates during fluency. Examining the parameter estimates shows this to be the case (see the lower panel of figure 5.7). Indeed, the homologous right region shows an effect that is nearly as large as the left, but in the opposite direction. The interpretation of this may be related to interactions between the right and left hemispheres, and speaks to the importance of functional integration among specialized regions. This is the subject of the last section.

EFFECTIVE CONNECTIVITY AND FUNCTIONAL INTEGRATION

There is a necessary relationship between approaches to characterizing functional integration and multivariate analyses because the latter are necessary to model interactions among brain regions. Multivariate

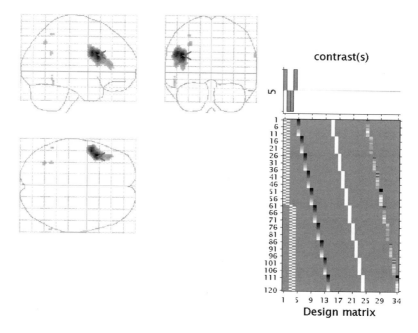

contrast(s)

Design matrix

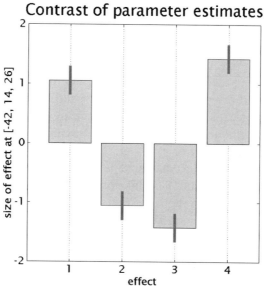

Figure 5.7 Interaction analysis testing for lateralized effects. (*Top*) Design matrix and SPM{T}, as in figure 5.6. (*Bottom*) Condition and hemisphere-specific parameter estimates for a voxel in the DLPFC. The first two estimates are for the right hemisphere, and the second pair are for the left. The lines represent the standard error of these estimates.

approaches can be divided into those which are inferential and those which are data-led or exploratory. Most are based on the singular value or eigen decomposition of the between-voxel covariances in a neuroimaging time series.

Eigenimage Analysis and Related Approaches

Friston et al. (1993) introduced voxel-based PCA of neuroimaging time series to characterize distributed brain systems implicated in sensorimotor, perceptual, or cognitive processes. These distributed systems are identified with principal components or eigenimages that correspond to spatial modes of coherent brain activity. This approach represents one of the simplest multivariate characterizations of functional neuroimaging time series and falls into the class of exploratory analyses. Principal component or eigenimage analysis generally uses singular value decomposition (SVD) to identify a set of orthogonal spatial modes that capture the greatest amount of variance, expressed over time. As such, the ensuing modes embody the most prominent aspects of the variance-covariance structure of a given time series. Noting that the covariances among brain regions is equivalent to functional connectivity (see below) renders eigenimage analysis particularly interesting because it was among the first ways of addressing functional integration (i.e., connectivity) in the human brain.

Subsequently eigenimage analysis has been elaborated in a number of ways. Notable among these are canonical variate analysis and multidimensional scaling (Friston, Poline, et al., 1996). Canonical variate analysis (CVA) was introduced in the context of ManCova (multivariate analysis of covariance), and uses the generalized eigenvector solution to maximize the variance that can be explained by some explanatory variables relative to error. CVA can be thought of as an extension of eigenimage analysis that refers explicitly to some explanatory variables and allows for statistical inference.

Functional and Effective Connectivity

Imaging neuroscience has firmly established functional specialization as a principle of brain organization in man. The functional integration of specialized areas has proven more difficult to assess. Functional integration is usually inferred on the basis of correlations among measurements of neuronal activity. Functional connectivity has been defined as *correlations between remote neurophysiological events*. However, correlations can arise in a variety of ways. For example, in multiunit electrode recordings they can result from stimulus-locked transients evoked by a common input or reflect stimulus-induced oscillations mediated by synaptic connections (Gerstein & Perkel, 1969).

Integration within a distributed system is usually better understood in terms of *effective connectivity*. Effective connectivity refers explicitly to *the influence that one neural system exerts over another*, at either a synaptic (i.e., synaptic efficacy) or a population level. It has been proposed that "the [electrophysiological] notion of effective connectivity should be understood as the experiment- and time-dependent, simplest possible circuit diagram that would replicate the observed timing relationships between the recorded neurons" (Aertsen & Preissl, 1991). This speaks to two important points: (1) Effective connectivity is dynamic and activity- and time-dependent, and (2) it depends upon a model of the interactions. The models used in functional neuroimaging can be classified as (1) those based on regression models (see next section) or (2) structural equation modeling (i.e., path analysis) (McIntosh et al., 1994).

Linear models of effective connectivity assume that the multiple inputs to a region are linearly separable and fixed. This precludes any contextual change in connectivity induced by experimental factors or, indeed, activity in other regions. We will consider two important examples of nonlinear effects and how they are modeled: (1) activity-dependent modulation of pathways in the visual system, and (2) how coupling with a reference region changes in one experimental context relative to another.

Characterizing Nonlinear Coupling Among Brain Areas

Linear models preclude activity-dependent connections that are expressed in one sensorimotor or cognitive context and not in another. The resolution of this problem lies in adopting nonlinear models that include interactions among inputs. These interactions can be construed as a context- or activity-dependent modulation of the influence that one region exerts over another, where that context is instantiated by activity in further brain regions exerting modulatory effects. From the point of view of regression models, modulatory effects can be modeled with nonlinear input-output models, in particular a Volterra series formulation. (This formulation can be thought of as a polynomial regression on the activity of areas providing inputs, both now and in the recent past.) Because the kernels are high-order, they embody interactions over time and among inputs. The influence of one region j on another region i can therefore be divided into two components: (1) the direct influence of j on i, irrespective of the activities elsewhere, and (2) an activity-dependent component that represents an interaction with inputs from the remaining regions.

The example provided in figure 5.8 addresses the modulation of visual cortical responses by attentional mechanisms and the mediating

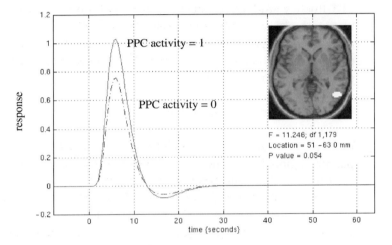

Figure 5.8 Characterization of effects of V2 inputs on V5 and the modulation of these effects by posterior parietal cortex (PPC), using simulated inputs at different levels of PPC activity. The broken line represents estimates of V5 responses when PPC activity = 0 according to a second-order Volterra model with inputs based on the activity in V2, PPC, and the pulvinar (all normalized to 0 mean and unit standard deviation). The simulated input from V2 corresponded to a square wave of 500 ms duration convolved with a hemodynamic response function. The solid curve represents the same response when PPC activity is 1. It is evident that V2 has an activating effect on V5 and that PPC increases the responsiveness of V5 to these inputs. The insert shows all the voxels in V5 that evidenced a modulatory effect ($p < .05$ uncorrected). These voxels were identified by thresholding the SPM{F} testing for the contribution of second-order effects involving V2 and PPC while treating all other components as confounds. Results for one subject are shown. Subjects were studied with fMRI under identical stimulus conditions (visual motion subtended by radially moving dots) while manipulating the attentional component of the task (detection of velocity changes).

role of activity- or context-sensitive changes in effective connectivity. Figure 5.8 shows a characterization of this modulatory effect in terms of the increase in V5 (a motion-sensitive area) responses, to a simulated V2 (early visual area) input, when posterior parietal activity is 0 (broken line) and when it is high (solid line). This sort of result suggests that parietal activity may be a sufficient explanation for attentional modulation of visually evoked extrastriate responses.

The dynamic or context-sensitive aspects of coupling among brain areas has an important implication for assessing effective connectivity: It implies that the more interesting questions are framed in terms of *changes* in effective connectivity. In the final subsection we return to the PET fluency study, used in the previous section, and ask whether any inference can be made about *asymmetries in coupling*, as opposed to regional responses in any one region. This question can be addressed using a simple analysis of changes in coupling, referred to as psychophysiological interactions.

Psychophysiological Interactions

In an analysis of psychophysiological interactions, one is trying to explain a regionally specific response in terms of an interaction between the presence of a sensorimotor or cognitive process and activity in another part of the brain (Friston et al., 1997). This approach is interesting from two points of view. First, the explanatory variables used to predict activity in any brain region (i.e., the response variable) comprise a standard predictor variable based on the experimental design (in this instance, which hemisphere the data came from) and a response variable from another part of the brain. The second reason that this analysis is interesting is that it employs techniques usually used to make inferences about functional specialization to infer something about integration. The statistical model employed for testing for psychophysiological interactions is a simple regression model of effective connectivity that embodies nonlinear (second-order or modulatory) effects. As such, this class of model speaks directly to functional integration of a contextual sort.

Consider the functional integration between prefrontal and temporal cortices. Is the ipsilateral coupling between the DLPFC and temporoparietal systems greater in the left hemisphere than in the right? Is the left-to-right interhemispheric coupling greater than the right-to-left? These questions can be addressed using the regression slopes of activity in remote brain regions, on DLFPC activity, as a measure of effective connectivity between the candidate region and the DLPFC. Asymmetries in coupling correspond to a right-left difference in the regression slope. This difference is simply an interaction, and can be tested for in exactly the same way as in the previous section. However, here the explanatory variables pertaining to the conditions are replaced by activity measures in the DLPFC. These activities are usually taken to be the first local eigenvariate around the voxel of interest (a regional mean, weighted in accordance with the local covariance structure).

The lower panel of figure 5.9 shows the locale and activity over (60×2) scans for the DLFPC voxel identified in figure 5.7. These activities were entered as explanatory variables into a design matrix, as shown in figure 5.9 (upper right panel), modeling effects separately for the flipped and nonflipped data. The regions showing a significant decrease in regression slope (i.e., negative coupling) in the left hemisphere, relative to the right, are shown in the SPM{T} (upper left panel). These results suggest that, relative to the right DLPFC, the left DLPFC expresses a significantly greater intrahemispheric and interhemispheric coupling with both the ipsilateral and contralateral temporoparietal regions. A significant intrahemispheric coupling asymmetry is demonstrated with the medial prefrontal cortex. Another asymmetric coupling involves the posterior basotemporal region, often associated with naming, and in this case is interhemispheric. Note that this analysis will highlight increased negative coupling and decreased positive coupling, depending on whether the coupling itself is positive or negative. Most of the regions shown in this SPM deactivated during the shadowing condition and are therefore negative.

In short, these augmented negative couplings reflect the fact that as activity in the prefrontal regions increases, the temporoparietal regions decreases. This coupling is significantly more pronounced in the left hemisphere than in the right, and involves both intra- and interhemispheric influences of the DLPFC. Note that there are no regions implicated by the SPM in the right DLPFC. This is because the left-to-right coupling is exactly the same as the right-to-left coupling.

CONCLUSION

In summary, some form of statistical parametric mapping can identify functionally specialized brain areas. The nature of the specialization

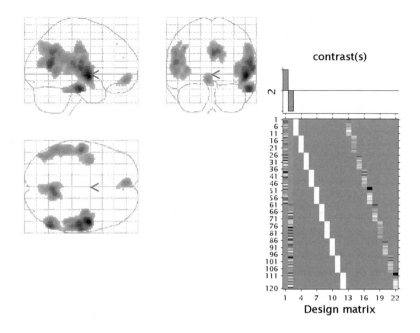

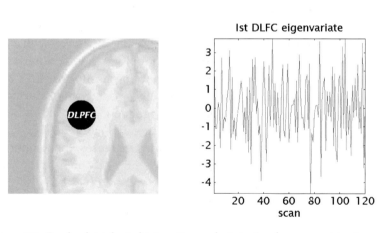

Figure 5.9 Psychophysiological interaction analysis testing for asymmetries in coupling with the DLPFC. (*Upper panels*) Design matrix and SPM{T}, as in figures 5.6 and 5.7. (*Lower panels*) Position of the DLPFC region selected (*left*), and the activity over all scans (*right*), in terms of the first eigenvariate of the voxels within a 4 mm sphere of the selected DLPFC voxel.

and the interactions between various cognitive or sensorimotor factors in engendering a brain response can be established using simple subtraction, parametric, or multifactorial designs. A factorial approach to the data is especially relevant in the context of laterality issues because the hemisphere from which the data came can be treated as an experimental factor. This enables the application of conjunction analyses to test for bilateral effects and the use of interactions to test for lateralization of functionally specific responses.

Functional integration is usually assessed using some form of multivariate analysis, framed in terms of effective connectivity. Recent advances in modeling effective connectivity emphasize nonlinear interactions among inputs to an area in "causing" its response. A simple variant of these (psychophysiological interactions), is easily applicable to most brain imaging studies and can be used to address asymmetry in the coupling among brain regions within and between the hemispheres. The examples provided in this chapter serve to show what is possible with modern imaging techniques and standard analytic procedures, and speak to the usefulness of neuroimaging in characterizing the asymmetry of functional brain architectures.

ACKNOWLEDGMENT

The Wellcome Trust supported this work.

REFERENCES

Absher, J. R., & Benson, D. F. (1993). Disconnection syndromes: An overview of Geschwind's contributions. *Neurology, 43*, 862–867.

Aertsen, A., & Preissl, H. (1991). Dynamics of activity and connectivity in physiological neuronal networks. In H. G. Schuster (Ed.), *Non linear dynamics and neuronal networks* (pp. 281–302). New York: VCH Publishers.

Büchel, C., Wise, R. J. S., Mummery, C. J., Poline, J.-B., & Friston, K. J. (1996). Nonlinear regression in parametric activation studies. *NeuroImage, 4*, 60–66.

Friston, K. J., Frith, C., Liddle, P., & Frackowiak, R. S. J. (1993). Functional connectivity: The principal component analysis of large data sets. *Journal of Cerebral Blood Flow and Metabolism, 13*, 5–14.

Friston, K. J., Holmes, A. P., Worsley, K. J., Poline, J.-B., Frith, C. D., & Frackowiak, R. S. J. (1995). Statistical parametric maps in functional imaging: A general linear approach. *Human Brain Mapping, 2*, 189–210.

Friston, K. J., Poline, J.-B., Holmes, A. P., Frith, C. D., & Frackowiak, R. S. J. (1996). A multivariate analysis of PET activation studies. *Human Brain Mapping, 4*, 140–151.

Friston, K. J., Price, C. J., Fletcher, P., Moore, C., Frackowiak, R. S. J., & Dolan, R. J. (1996). The trouble with cognitive subtraction. *NeuroImage, 4*, 97–104.

Friston, K. J., Büchel, C., Fink, G. R., Morris, J., Rolls, E., & Dolan, R. J. (1997). Psychophysiological and modulatory interactions in neuroimaging. *NeuroImage, 6*, 218–229.

Gerstein, G. L., & Perkel, D. H. (1969). Simultaneously recorded trains of action potentials: Analysis and functional interpretation. *Science, 164*, 828–830.

Grafton, S., Mazziotta, J., Presty, S., Friston, K. J., Frackowiak, R. S. J., & Phelps, M. (1992). Functional anatomy of human procedural learning determined with regional cerebral blood flow and PET. *Journal of Neuroscience, 12*, 2542–2548.

Lueck, C. J., Zeki, S., Friston, K. J., Deiber, M. P., Cope, N. O., Cunningham, V. J., Lammertsma, A. A., Kennard, C., & Frackowiak, R. S. J. (1989). The colour centre in the cerebral cortex of man. *Nature, 340*, 386–389.

McIntosh, A. R., & Gonzalez-Lima, F. (1994). Structural equation modelling and its application to network analysis in functional brain imaging. *Human Brain Mapping, 2*, 2–22.

Petersen, S. E., Fox, P. T., Posner, M. I., Mintun, M., & Raichle, M. E. (1989). Positron emission tomographic studies of the processing of single words. *Journal of Cognitive Neuroscience, 1*, 153–170.

Phillips, C. G., Zeki, S., & Barlow, H. B. (1984). Localisation of function in the cerebral cortex: Past, present and future. *Brain, 107*, 327–361.

Price, C. J., & Friston, K. J. (1997). Cognitive conjunction: A new approach to brain activation experiments. *NeuroImage, 5*, 261–270.

Salmond, C., Ashburner, J., Vargha-Khadhem, F., Gadian, D., & Friston, K. J. (2000). Detecting bilateral abnormalities with voxel-based morphometry. *Human Brain Mapping, 11*, 223–232.

Talairach, P., & Tournoux, J. (1988). *A stereotactic coplanar atlas of the human brain.* Stuttgart: Thieme.

Worsley, K. J., Marrett, S., Neelin, P., Vandal, A. C., Friston, K. J., & Evans, A. C. (1996). A unified statistical approach for determining significant signals in images of cerebral activation. *Human Brain Mapping, 4*, 58–73.

Zeki, S. (1990). The motion pathways of the visual cortex. In C. Blakemore (Ed.), *Vision: Coding and efficiency* (pp. 321–345). Cambridge: Cambridge University Press.

6 Anatomical Brain Asymmetries and Their Relevance for Functional Asymmetries

Lutz Jäncke and Helmuth Steinmetz

Anatomical brain asymmetries (or morphological brain asymmetries) are macroscopic and microscopic structural (cyto-, myelo-, glio-, or angioarchitectonic) differences between both brain hemispheres. Such right-left differences are often designated as asymmetries or lateralizations. Macroanatomical right-left differences can be found for the volume of both hemispheres, for the volume of specific brain areas, for the gyrification pattern, and for the form and length of certain sulci. With regard to the microscopic level, the number, volume, or density of neurons and glial cells, as well as the intra- and interhemispheric wiring, also can contribute to morphological interhemispheric differences. Morphological brain asymmetries were first described around the turn of the twentieth century. These first reports concerned right-left asymmetries on the lateral surface of the brain in the perisylvian region, including the sylvian fissure (Eberstaller, 1884; Cunningham, 1892). These initial studies noted right-left differences in the length and angulation of the sylvian fissure, with the left being longer and running more horizontal than the right.

In addition to this external asymmetry, it was also noted by Pfeifer (1920, 1936) and by von Economo and Horn (1930) that within the sylvian fissure, the transverse gyri (Heschl gyri) and the extent of cortical surface (planum temporale) posterior to the Heschl gyrus showed marked variation in gross morphology, with the left often being larger. Pfeifer also found that there were mostly two Heschl gyri on the right hemisphere, but only one on the right (Pfeifer's rule). In spite of these observations (and some early speculations about their possible functional implications made by Flechsig [1908] and von Economo & Horn [1930]), no hypothesis of the possible relationship of neuroanatomical variation to functional asymmetry could reasonably be made or tested by the early neuroanatomists (von Bonin, 1962).

Following the seminal work of Geschwind and Levitsky (1968), who first measured the exposed planum temporale in a large number of specimens, the hypothesis of an association between these morphological asymmetries and functional asymmetries became the topic of much consideration. With the advent of magnetic resonance imaging (MRI) techniques, the examination of anatomical asymmetries as well as of anatomical markers of interhemispheric connectivity has increased substantially. MRI techniques now provide the opportunities to obtain anatomical measures and to relate these measures to functional measures of lateralized psychological processes. Applying these new techniques further, neuroanatomical asymmetries have been observed, including asymmetries of the hippocampus, the central sulcus, the cerebellum, and the size of motoneurons in the spinal cord. In the following we will review the current status of research by focusing on those anatomical asymmetries which have revealed reliable morphological right-left differences associated with functional asymmetries.

PERISYLVIAN ANATOMICAL ASYMMETRIES

Sylvian Fissure

The lateral or sylvian fissure (SF) is the most prominent fissure of the primate brain hemisphere. Unlike sulci, the SF is not formed by an infolding of the cortex, but results from an uneven growth of the outer cortex leading to the opercularization of inner (insular) structures. Unique to the human brain is the extensive degree of opercularization of frontal, parietal, and temporal brain regions, which form the banks of the SF. This anatomical feature allows for great morphological variation among hemispheres, both between and within subjects. SF variability was noted early on and became the subject of several studies. Qualitative and quantitative analysis of the variability of this region have been performed by Eberstaller (1884, 1890), Cunningham (1892), Rubens et al. (1976), Steinmetz, Fürst, et al. (1990), Witelson and Kigar (1992), and Ide et al. (1996, 1999). These studies have largely agreed in dividing the SF into a main horizontal segment (with an anterior and posterior portion, ASF and PSF) and four additional rami (anterior ascending ramus, anterior horizontal ramus, posterior ascending ramus,

Lutz Jäncke and Helmuth Steinmetz

posterior descending ramus; abbreviated AAR, AHR, PAR, PDR, respectively; figure 6.1).

According to the length of the posterior horizontal SF or the size of the PAR and PDR, at least two subtypes of SF can be distinguished: (1) one that is more common on the left hemisphere and is characterized by a long horizontal part of the SF, and (2) a second type that is more common on the right hemisphere and typically is characterized by a relatively small posterior horizontal part of the SF. In some studies the ascending ramus was frequently absent on the left hemisphere (Steinmetz, Rademacher, et al., 1990) or the left ascending ramus was directed more upward and forward (instead of upward and backward) (Ide et al., 1996). In addition, the horizontal part of the sylvian fissure is much more strongly angulated upward on the right hemisphere and is more horizontally located on the left hemisphere. Most interestingly, when the two hemispheres of each subject are matched, no correspondence is observed between the fissurization pattern of one hemisphere and the other, indicating that fissurization develops independently in each hemisphere (figure 6.1).

Older studies suggest that this apparent morphological asymmetry might already exist in the fetal brain. For instance, Cunningham (1892), who examined six fetal brains between the ages of 7.5 and 8.5 months, reported that the mean SF length was greater and the upward slope was less on the left side than on the right side, the same pattern he observed in the adult brain. LeMay and Culebras (1972) reported that examination of the external surfaces of ten fetal brains revealed that in each case the end of the SF was higher on the right than on the left side in relation to the dorsoventral axis of the brain. This asymmetry was observed in a fetal brain as young as the 16th gestational week. Thus, these findings may support the assumption that this morphological asymmetry is perhaps genetically determined. Recent studies in monkeys (Cheverud et al., 1990) and in monozygotic human twins have reported important findings seeming to corroborate a possible genetic origin for the fissurization pattern of primary fissures (Lohmann et al., 1999). There are, however, also findings challenging this view (Steinmetz et al., 1995). In this context, findings by Yeni Komshian and Benson (1976) and Gannon et al. (1998), who examined the shape of the sylvian fissure or the planum temporale size in nonhuman primates, are most interesting. Both reported human-like asymmetries for chimpanzees that were not found in phylogenetic older primates (Yeni

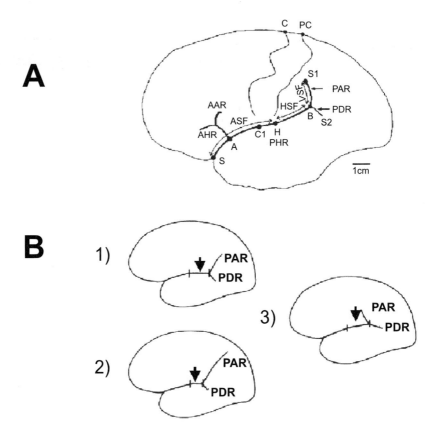

Figure 6.1 (*A*) Tracing of one hemisphere showing the general morphology of the sylvian fissure (SF) and associated landmarks. S, anterior end of the SF; A, point at which the anterior ascending ramus (AAR) and anterior horizontal ramus (AHR) join the SF; H, point at which the transverse sulcus of Heschl on the supratemporal plane meets or can be extended to the lateral edge of the SF; B: point of bifurcation of the posterior end of the main horizontal branch of the SF; C, central sulcus; PC, precentral sulcus; C1, point where the central sulcus meets or is extended to meet the SF; S1, end of the posterior ascending ramus; S2, end of the posterior descending ramus; ASF, anterior part of the SF, located between S and H; HSF, horizontal part of the SF located between H and B; PAR, posterior ascending ramus of the SF located between B and S1; PDR, posterior descending ramus of the SF located between B and S2. (Adapted from Witelson & Kigar, 1992.) (*B*) Three common types of SF morphology. (*1*) and (*2*) show pattern where the ascending branch of the posterior SF (PAR) is longer than the descending (PDR). In (*1*) the horizontal part of the SF (HSF) is relatively long (typical for left hemispheres), while in (*2*) the brain has a relatively small HSF (typical for right hemispheres). In (*3*) the ascending ramus of the posterior SF (PAR) is distorted and directed forward. (Partly adapted from Ide et al., 1996.)

Komshian & Benson, 1976). Thus, the latter authors concluded that this phylogenetic evolution of a left-larger-than-right SF asymmetry in the higher primates might be related to the phylogeny of functional lateralization.

Until now, only two papers directly relating SF measures to measures of functional lateralization have been published. Witelson and Kigar (1992) examined the brains of 67 cancer patients who had consented to neuropsychological testing before death. They found that men having consistent right-hand preference had longer horizontal segments in both hemispheres compared to men not having such preference. Hellige et al. (1998) reported that the length of the right hemisphere SF negatively correlates with the error rate for detecting briefly presented consonant-vowel-consonant trigrams to the left or right visual half-field. Thus, these findings obtained in relatively small samples do not support the idea that SF asymmetries are directly related to functional lateralizations.

In addition to the hemispheric differences for the posterior parts of the SF, there seem to be hemispheric differences for the anterior branches of the SF as well. For example, Ide et al. (1999) pointed out that on the right hemisphere either the anterior horizontal or the anterior ascending ramus dominates in size. Thus, mainly only one principal ramus dominates on the right hemisphere. On the left hemisphere, however, both anterior rami typically are equally well developed and of the same size. A less common pattern, which Ide et al. labeled the Y-shaped pattern, was characterized by a common stem for both anterior rami. This pattern is evenly distributed in both hemispheres. This fissurization pattern may relate to some of the few findings reporting hemispheric asymmetries with respect to the volume measures of what is thought to be Broca's area. Ide et al. suggest that the degree of cortical folding is larger in the anterior perisylvian region by virtue of the expansion of areas 44 and 45.

Studies designed to measure gross anatomical asymmetries in Broca's area revealed partly contradictory results. Several studies, using different kinds of measurements, examined the hemispheric and sex-related differences of the anterior speech areas, such as the pars opercularis and pars triangularis of the inferior frontal gyrus. An earlier study by Wada et al. (1975) measured the external surface of the pars triangularis and found this area to be slightly larger in the right hemisphere. Using a more adequate total surface method, Albanese et al. (1989) later found the opposite. More recently, Foundas et al. (1996) measured the volume of the pars triangularis on MRI scans of subjects who had undergone an intracarotid sodium amytal test to establish the side of speech lateralization. They found that 10 out of 11 right-handed subjects had a larger left pars triangularis, a finding that was consistent with each subject's side of speech lateralization.

Complementary to these findings, Leonard (1997) reported that verbal fluency correlates with the asymmetry of the pars triangularis in subjects with above-average intelligence. However, two recent studies challenged these findings. In one study 108 normal adult brains were analyzed by means of magnetic resonance imaging (Tomaiuolo et al., 1999). These authors noted a considerable variability in the shape and location of the pars opercularis across brains and between hemispheres. There was also no significant difference between sex and side of asymmetry of the pars opercularis. Finally, a study by Amunts et al. (1999) on 10 postmortem brains suggested a trend toward left-larger-than-right asymmetry for area 44 but not for area 45. It is interesting to note that in this study, the borders of areas 44 and 45 did not coincide with gross sulcal landmarks, thereby bringing into question macroscopic volumetric approaches at least for this brain area.

Planum Temporale and Planum Parietale

Anatomical Definition The brain region that has attracted by far the most attention with respect to cerebral asymmetry is the planum temporale (PT). The PT is a roughly triangular structure on the supratemporal plane within the sylvian fissure. The precise anatomical definition of the PT has been the subject of some debate (Westbury et al., 1999). However, the most widely used definition accords with Pfeifer's (Pfeifer, 1920) and von Economo and Horn's (1930) first delineations of the PT, a definition that was later adopted by Steinmetz, Fürst, et al. (1990). According to this definition, the anterior border of the PT is defined by Heschl's sulcus, which is the sulcus behind the first (most anterior) transverse gyrus of Heschl. Using this definition of the anterior border, any additional transverse gyrus is included in the PT. The posterior border of the PT is much more a matter of dispute than the anterior border, the main problem being whether to include or exclude the posterior rami of the sylvian fissure. Most current research has

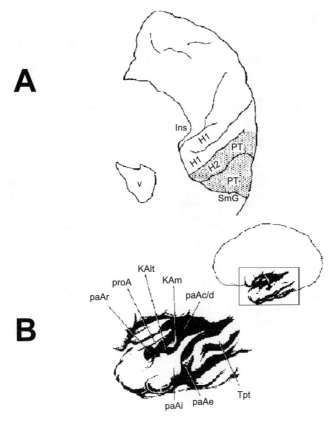

Figure 6.2 (*A*) Tracing of a horizontal slice through the planum temporale. Ins, insula; H1, H2, first and second Heschl gyri; PT, planum temporale; SmG, supramarginal gyrus; V, ventricle. (*B*) Cytoarchitectonic areas on the superior temporal plane. KAm and KAlt, primary auditory koniocortex; pa: parakoniocortex; Tpt, coniocortex from the typ Tpt.

adopted definitions that exclude at least the posterior ascending ramus. This definition also allows separation of the PT from the planum parietale (PP), which is formed by the cortex covering the posterior bank of the posterior ascending ramus of the sylvian fissure (figures 6.2 and 6.3; see also plate 1).

The cytoarchitecture of the perisylvian region is complex, and its intersubject variation has not been intensively studied in humans. The few studies that have been published revealed the following main findings pertaining to the PT and the PP. First, two studies found left-larger-than-right asymmetries for nonprimary cytoarchitectonic areas

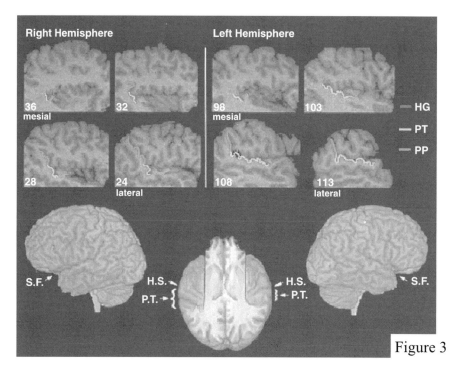

Figure 6.3 Example of delineated anatomical regions on the superior temporal plane of a representative brain. Tracing line in red indicates Heschl's gyrus (HG); in yellow, the planum temporale (PT); and in green, the planum parietale (PP). Reconstructed brain in the lower row indicates the position of Hesch's sulcus (H.S.) and the PT. (Courtesy of Gottfried Schlaug.) See plate 1 for color version.

covering the PT (area TB of von Economo and Horn (1930) and area Tpt of Galaburda and Sanides (1980) and Galaburda et al. (1978). Other researchers exerted more caution in interpreting their findings because of problems defining the exact borders of higher-order auditory cortices in this area (Braak, 1978). Thus, further studies using quantitative cytoarchitectonics are needed. Second, asymmetries have been described for neuronal packing density (Seldon, 1982) and neuronal microcircuitry of higher-order cortex covering the posterolateral PT (Galuske et al., 2000). Both studies suggested a more complex degree of organization on the left. Third, so far, no cytoarchitectonic asymmetries have been found for the areas covering the inferior parietal lobule (Schulze, 1962).

Structural-Functional Correlations Although adopting different definitions, the vast majority of anatomical studies have revealed prominent leftward PT asymmetries in terms of length, area, or volume measures. Following the work of Geschwind and Levitsky (1968), who first measured PT length in a large number of specimens, several other studies examined PT asymmetry with respect to both lateral length and surface area. Most of these studies have been reviewed in detail (Steinmetz, 1996; Shapleske et al., 1999). In summary, they revealed a left-larger-than-right asymmetry of the PT in approximately 70–80% of unselected adult and infant brains studied in vivo or postmortem. Quantitative analysis of PT asymmetry with respect to either PT area or PT length revealed smaller right PT areas or length measures ranging from 55 to 80% of the right PT measure related to the left PT. On average, the size of the right PT expressed as a percentage of left PT ($PT_{R\%L}$) is 76.6% for the area measurements and 65.4% for the length measurements. In contrast to the PT, which is situated on the superior temporal gyrus, the PP belongs to the inferior parietal lobe. This area is usually lateralized to the right, and has also been linked to functional lateralization (Jäncke et al., 1994).

Because the left PT (1) coincides with the core of Wernicke's speech area, (2) functional neuroimaging consistently shows an involvement of the left PT in phonological and phonetic processing (Fiez et al., 1996; Tzourio et al., 1998; Buchanan et al., 2000), and (3) the PT is anatomically larger on the left, it has been suggested that PT asymmetry may be part of the anatomical foundation of speech lateralization. However, residual ambiguity exists regarding the true functional significance of PT asymmetry. One strategy to confirm this supposed structure-function relationship is to correlate indices of functional lateralization directly and within individuals with PT asymmetry. This has been done in only a few studies. One set of investigations related PT asymmetries to handedness measures because these measures are easy to obtain and are related to other functional asymmetries, including language and spatial abilities (Steinmetz et al., 1991; Jäncke, Schlaug, et al., 1994; Habib et al., 1995; Steinmetz et al., 1995; Foundas et al., 1995).

In summary, these studies showed reduced leftward (but not inverted) PT asymmetry in normal left-handers compared to right-handers. A representative finding of PT asymmetry with respect to handedness is shown in figure 6.4, which summarizes our own data

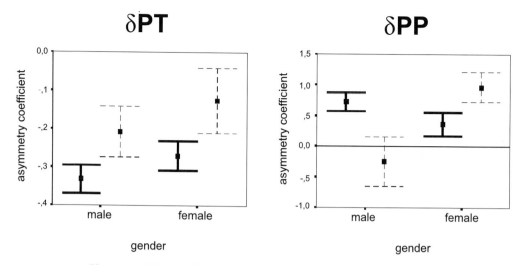

Figure 6.4 Mean coefficients of anatomic asymmetry (δ) of the planum temporale (δPT) and the planum parietale (δPP) broken down for handedness (RH: bold lines, LH: dotted lines) and gender groups (total n = 141). Negative δPT or δPP values (y-axis) indicate leftward, and positive values rightward, asymmetry. Error bars indicate standard errors of mean.

based on the largest sample of healthy young volunteers published until now (N = 250; Jäncke, Schlaug, et al., 1994). A further interesting finding of this and similar studies is that there is no gender difference in terms of absolute PT size and PT asymmetry, thus opposing the assumption that women might have smaller PT asymmetries (Kulynych et al., 1994).

Since handedness is only imperfectly related to functional lateralization of cognitive functions (like verbal or spatial processing), it is necessary to relate PT asymmetry to other indices of functional lateralization. In one study of this kind it was found that language lateralization followed the direction of PT asymmetry in a small sample of presurgical patients also undergoing the intracarotid test (Foundas et al., 1994). Two further studies have related anatomical PT asymmetry to measures of auditory lateralization. Jäncke and Steinmetz (1993) administered a number of dichotic listening tasks to a sample of left- and right-handed subjects and obtained PT measurements from MRI. They found no relationship between direction or degree of dichotic ear advantage and quantitative measurements of PT asymmetry. However, they also found that ear advantage scores from the different dichotic

Lutz Jäncke and Helmuth Steinmetz

tests were only poorly related to each other, forcing them to conclude that these dichotic tests were unreliable to infer auditory lateralization. In addition, the subjects were randomly selected right- and left-handers; the vast majority showed either a right ear advantage or no ear advantage on dichotic testing. There was no subject with a reversed ear advantage (left ear advantage).

A more recent study by Moffat et al. (1998) circumvented the problems of the aforementioned study by examining a sample of young adult left-handed males who were tested with the fused dichotic words test (FDWT). This dichotic test has been shown to be a valid noninvasive instrument for classifying individuals according to their speech lateralization. For example, Zatorre (1989) administered this test to a sample of left- and right-handed patients who also underwent sodium amytal testing. He found that 36 out of 38 patients (95%) with known exclusive left or right hemisphere representation of speech were correctly classified on the basis of the direction of their ear advantage score on the FWDT. On the basis of this test, Moffat et al. identified left-handers with left- or right-hemisphere speech lateralization. Their results demonstrate a strong leftward PT asymmetry among left-handed subjects with left hemisphere speech representation (N = 9), but no consistent PT asymmetry among left-handed subjects with right hemisphere speech representation (N = 7).

Provided that the FWDT is a valid noninvasive test for predicting speech lateralization, this study does not support the view that PT asymmetry per se is the anatomical substrate for auditory speech lateralization. Instead, it might be that the absolute size of PT is more important with regard to functional aspects. Consistent with this hypothesis, Tzourio et al. (1998) found significant positive correlations between the left PT surface size and the amount of cerebral blood flow increase in this area as measured with positron emission tomography during story listening. These results may indicate that the size of the left PT is the relevant anatomical landmark for language dominance or for superior performance in language-related tasks.

This contention is also supported by a study on two groups of professional musicians, one with and one without absolute pitch (Schlaug et al., 1995). Interestingly, the absolute pitch musicians turned out to have extraordinarily large left PT areas, while the right PT was about in the same size range as found for normal controls (figure 6.5). Absolute pitch is a rare ability enabling the performer to verbally designate a tone without a reference tone. It is presumed that this ability is depen-

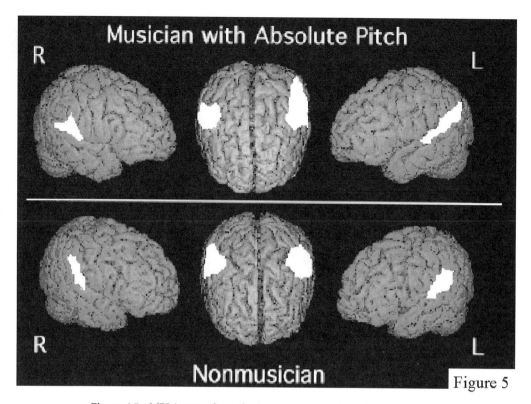

Figure 6.5 MRI images from the brain of a musician with perfect pitch (*top*) and the brain of a nonmusician (*bottom*). In the musician, the left planum temporale (white clusters) is larger. (Courtesy of Gottfried Schlaug.)

dent on additional verbal functions enabling these musicians to categorize tones, an ability that is unusual for human tone perception since it is usually performed in a continuously and noncategorical manner. It is thought that this additional function is implemented early in life by increasing the neural network (thus increasing the volume of gray and white matter). Most of the absolute pitch musicians started their musical training before the age of seven, thus supporting the idea that the additional implementation of cortical volume within the PT region follows some kind of external stimulation. A general genetic determination of PT asymmetry or exaggerated PT asymmetry in professional musicians is unlikely from the present point of view because there is virtually no concordance with regard to direction or degree of PT asymmetry within normal monozygotic twins (Steinmetz et al., 1995).

Lutz Jäncke and Helmuth Steinmetz

It remains to be shown whether the PP may be another structural marker of human brain laterality measurable in vivo. Anatomically, the PP is part of the inferior parietal lobule. Depending on the individually variable posterior extension of the sylvian fissure, the PP is covered mostly by the cytoarchitectonic area 40 or, in some hemispheres, area 39 of Brodmann (1909). It is tempting to speculate that rightward PP asymmetry may be related to right parietal specialization for aspects of nonverbal higher-order cognition. Thus, the inferior parietal lobule has been considered to be a nodal point of a network subserving directed attention or spatial working memory, functions that are lateralized to the right hemisphere. A further interesting finding of our own studies is that the direction of PP asymmetry is basically unrelated to PT asymmetry (Jäncke, Schlaug, et al., 1994). This fits with recent morphological studies examining the shape and size of various parts of the sylvian fissure (Ide et al., 1999). These findings are also altogether in concordance with neuropsychological data from lesion studies suggesting that the lateralizations of linguistic and spatial abilities are more or less statistically independent (Bryden et al., 1983).

PT Asymmetries in Clinical Populations   Meanwhile, there are numerous reports on temporal lobe abnormalities in schizophrenics, persons suffering from dyslexia, and children with other developmental language disorders (for a summary see Shapleske et al., 1999; see also Chapter 18 in this volume). With respect to schizophrenia, there have been reports of reduced left temporal lobe volume, reduced left superior temporal lobe volume, or larger left posterior sylvian fissures in schizophrenics compared to controls. Investigations of PT size or asymmetry in schizophrenics compared with controls have yielded mixed results. In summary, these studies revealed no difference in PT asymmetry, reversed PT asymmetry (right > left), a reduction of the normal left-larger-than-right PT asymmetry, or a normal left-larger-than-right PT asymmetry, with a slightly increased left PT in schizophrenics. Because all these studies differ in sample size, anatomical definitions, and inclusion criteria for the patients (e.g., family history), it is currently difficult to draw firm conclusions.

Similar objections might hold for anatomical studies performed with subjects suffering from developmental dyslexia or developmental language disorders. While older studies revealed symmetrical PTs in postmortem brains of dyslexics (Galaburda, 1993), more recent MRI studies have reported either reversed PT asymmetries, no PT asymmetries, or exaggerated leftward PT asymmetry (summarized in Shapleske et al., 1999; and Beaton, 1997).[1] As in the studies of schizophrenics, numerous methodological problems in these studies relate to (1) differences in the assessment and operationalized diagnostic criteria used to accurately document the presence and severity of the clinical disorder, (2) the exclusion of other learning disabilities, and (3) the anatomical definitions of the PT.

Conclusion

The distinct asymmetric fissurization pattern of the sylvian fissure is likely to result from differences in the relative growth of specific cortical regions, which in turn may be directly or indirectly related to divergent modes of cortical processing. There are clear left-right differences in terms of shape and size of different SF measures. Whether these asymmetries are directly or indirectly related to functional asymmetries (e.g., language lateralization) is still a matter of dispute. A particular promising perisylvian substructure is the PT, for which several authors have shown that the left PT is usually larger than the right. In addition, it is the only anatomical structure that has been shown to vary considerably with measures of functional lateralizations (e.g., handedness and partial auditory lateralization). This relationship is, however, far from perfect, perhaps for several reasons. First, there is currently no widely accepted consensus about the exact anatomical borders of the PT, mainly because of the lack of correspondence between anatomical landmarks and cytoarchitectonic borders (for instance, the cytoarchitectonic area Tpt did not correspond to the anatomically defined PT in the cases studied by Galaburda and Sanides [1980], and it is likely that the cytoarchitectonic borders vary within brains or between brains). Second, the prevalence of leftward PT asymmetry in right-handers, or even in unselected samples, is far below the >95% frequency of left hemisphere language dominance in clinical populations. (However, it should be noted that the latter figure concerns the lateralization of speech production, whereas auditory speech perception is less asymmetrically organised; the auditory-related PT is more likely to subserve perceptive functions). Third, functional asymmetries vary due to attentional or learning factors, and thus add variability to studies trying to elucidate structure-function relationships.

Lutz Jäncke and Helmuth Steinmetz

In addition, one may also be skeptical about the "bigger is better" hypotheses underlying such "neophrenological" studies. However, there are precedents for larger regions that subserve more complex functioning. For example, in the primary sensory areas, the macular region in vision has a greater area of representation than do the peripheral fields; in somatesthesia the hand is represented by a larger region than the trunk; and the right posterior hippocampus has recently been reported to enlarge as a result of its intensive use (Maguire et al., 2000). At a speculative level, such larger regions may allow for advantages in neural circuitry. Whether an increase in volume is due to an increase in the number of neurons or to an increase of connectivity has to be shown in future studies. Currently there is evidence supporting both assumptions.

Although the presumably embryonic mechanisms leading to perisylvian asymmetries are currently unknown, there is some evidence that these asymmetries are largely nongenetic in origin. Since PT asymmetries appear in utero and are unlikely to change after birth (Preis et al., 1998), early-acting epigenetic factors may play an important role in the development of PT asymmetry. Among such factors could be fetal position, cytoplasmic and maturational left-right gradients, fetal testosterone, chance, or early use-dependent growth, to mention just a few.

ASYMMETRY OF THE PRIMARY MOTOR CORTEX

A further candidate structure that may be related to functional lateralization is the hand motor area (see also Chapter 4 in this volume). Surprisingly few studies have focussed on anatomical asymmetries directly related to handedness. Older theories dating from the 19th and the beginning of the 20th centuries proposed that nonneuronal asymmetries of, for instance, blood supply to the extremities, or arm length or bone weight, were genetically fixed and would determine handedness (Hyrtl, 1882; Theile, 1884; Haase & Dehner, 1893). The study of possible anatomical correlates or underpinnings of handedness was reopened by a study published by Purves et al. (1994). These authors demonstrated that right-handed individuals have larger right hands than left hands. Based on what is known about trophic interactions between neurons and targets, such findings would seem to predict that the relevant parts of the sensorimotor system are correspondingly asymmetrical. This assumption was partly substantiated by the finding that there was a leftward asymmetry in central sulcus depth in the region of the functional hand representation of postmortem brains with unknown handedness (White et al., 1994) (but see also the opposite findings of the same group (White et al., 1997a, 1997b).

Using MRI, Amunts et al. (1996, 2000) measured the intrasulcal length of the precentral gyrus—that is, the depth of the central sulcus (CS)—as an estimate of the size of the hand motor area. This measure was obtained from the horizontal slices of linearly normalized brains. The intrasulcal length of the posterior contour of the precentral gyrus was measured as an indicator of the size of the primary motor cortex (i.e., Brodmann's area 4 in the hand representation area in a dorsoventral sequence of 35 horizontal sections). The sections extended from Talairach coordinates $z = 69$ to $z = 35$, thus including the functional hand representation.

In summary, these MRI studies revealed four results. First, right-handed males showed a clear leftward asymmetry of the CS depth for the superior horizontal slices from $z = 70$ to about $z = 50$, while left-handed males showed a rightward asymmetry. Second, right-handed professional keyboard players who had received intensive bimanual training from early childhood were more symmetrical both in hand skill tests and in the sulcal depths. Third, the absolute length of the CS was related to the age of commencement of musical training, such that those musicians who had started early in life with musical training revealed the largest CS on both sides. Fourth, the asymmetry of the CS depth varied according to handedness only in men; for women there was no interhemispheric asymmetry, not even among consistent-right-handed women (figure 6.6).

These findings suggest that the anatomical asymmetry in the depth of the CS may depend on an interaction of handedness and gender, and also on the amount or duration of hand skill training. These findings fit well with data from a recent MEG study analyzing dipoles during simple hand and finger movements (Volkmann et al., 1998). The authors found a larger volume of dipole sources in the primary motor cortex of the preferred hand than the nonpreferred hand in both right- and left-handers. Further studies provide evidence that handedness may have anatomical correlates not only in the asymmetry of the primary hand motor cortex but also in the spinal cord (Melsbach et al., 1996). There is also evidence for an asymmetric volume of the anterior and posterior cerebellum correlating with handedness (Snyder et al., 1995).

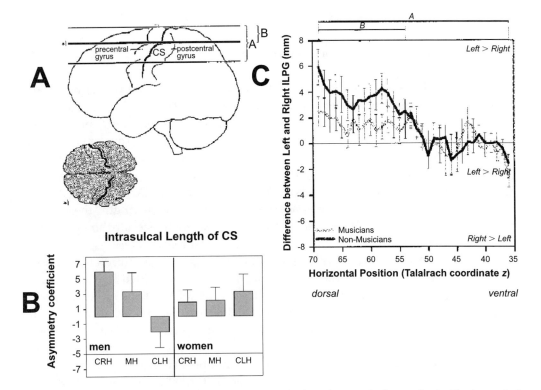

Figure 6.6 (*A*) Schematic diagram of the lateral view of a human brain. The intrasulcal length of the posterior bank of the precentral gyrus was analyzed in 35 horizontal slices (Talairach region from z = 69 to z = 35 mm). The intrasulcal length of both hemispheres is shown as a thick black line on a model horizontal section with Talairach coordinates z = 54 mm. CS, central sulcus. (*B*) Mean asymmetry coefficients (AC ± SE) for depth of central sulcus (CS). Mean ACs were calculated for the entire sequence of horizontal sections (from z = 69 to z = 35), and then averaged within each group. Differences in the three groups of handedness were influenced by gender. In males, the mean AC decreases linearly from CRH over MH to CLH. (*C*) Differences between left and right intrasulcal length (mean ± SEM) in 30 right-handed controls and 21 right-handed professional musicians. Musicians showed significantly lower degrees of asymmetry than controls. The most pronounced difference between musicians and controls were found between Talairach coordinates z = 69 and z = 54.

THE CORPUS CALLOSUM

Anatomy of the Corpus Callosum

A further anatomical structure that is likely to play a role in functional lateralization is the corpus callosum (CC). The CC is a massive tract containing roughly $200-350 \times 10^6$ fibers connecting both hemispheres. Interestingly, across this tract only 2% of cortical neurons of both hemispheres are interconnected. A commonly used method to subdivide the midsagittal section of the CC into macroscopic subregions is the partition proposed by Witelson (1989), in which the CC is arbitrarily divided into three regions according to the maximal length: the anterior third (genu), the mid third (truncus), and the posterior third. The posterior third is further divided into the splenium (posterior fifth) and the adjacently located isthmus (region between the mid third and the splenium). In some studies, the mid third is also divided into an anterior and a posterior part (figure 6.7). The anterior third is a rather large and bulbous region containing fibers connecting the prefrontal cortices. The mid third is a slender region containing projections from the motor, somatosensory, and auditory cortices. It is presumed that the anterior part of the mid third contains mostly fibers connecting the motor and sensory cortices and that the posterior third should contain fibers connecting the auditory cortices. The isthmus and the splenium are believed to contain fibers connecting superior temporal, parietal, and occipital areas.

Although this method of subdividing the CC is widely used for the purpose of morphometry, it is not without problems, because it is biased by local variability in callosal shape. This issue is particularly critical because gender differences in the shape of the CC have been reported (De Lacoste-Utamsing & Holloway, 1982; Allen et al., 1991). An efficient alternative method to delineate CC subareas has been proposed by Denenberg et al. (1991). The basic principle is to divide the midsagittal CC area into 99 percentile widths along a curved longitudinal axis drawn through the middle of the CC (figure 6.7). Subjecting these width measures to factor analysis revealed at least seven covarying clusters of widths according to which CC subdivisions can be obtained. More recent approaches work with CC area measurements that are normalized into a stereotaxic space. One possibility is to outline the three-dimensional shape of the CC of stereologically normal-

Lutz Jäncke and Helmuth Steinmetz

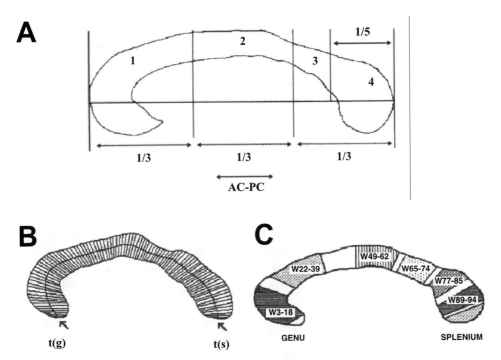

Figure 6.7 (*A*) Drawing illustrating the definition of five midsagittal CC subareas. 1, genu of the CC; 2, truncus; 3, isthmus; 4, splenium; AC-PC: reference line connecting the anterior and posterior commissures. (*B*) Tracing of a human CC showing the 99 widths and the central axis. Placement of the terminal points, t(g) and t(s), is based on the minimum sum-widths criterion. (Adapted from Denenberg et al., 1991.) (*C*) Seven subregions derived from a factor analysis in Denenberg et al. (1991).

ized brains and to subject these volumes to further statistical analyses (Narr et al., 2000) (figure 6.8).

A further recently applied method requires two steps. First, the brains are linearly normalized. Then each individual's CC size is measured in comparison to a reference template. This measurement is accomplished by elastically adapting the template to the shape of each individual CC. The resulting shrinkage or expansion of the template is quantified at each point by a deformation function, a collection of coefficients measuring how much the template has to be contorted around each point to move into spatial registration with each individual's CC (Davatzikos & Resnick, 1998). Between-group differences or correlations with other variables (i.e., performance measures) with respect to

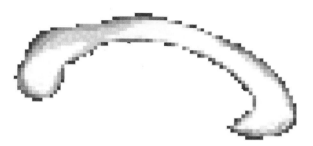

Figure 6.8 Example of an averaged CC area (across 20 subjects) obtained from stereotaxic normalized brain volumes. Black voxels indicate high variability measures and white voxels indicate less variability.

these deformation functions can then be statistically tested independently of a priori anatomical definitions.

Very few studies have delineated the fiber types or fiber numbers in the human CC. The most recent and most carefully done study has been published by Aboitiz et al. (Aboitiz, Scheibel, Fisher, et al., 1992). Employing light microscopic techniques in 20 postmortem brains, they discovered that the callosal fibers ranged from 0.4 to 15 mm in diameter, allowing for estimated interhemispheric transmission times between 1 ms and 30 ms. The most common fiber diameter was between 0.6 and 1 mm. Interestingly, there were regional differences in terms of the proportions and densities of fibers of distinct diameter. Fast-conducting, large-diameter fibers (>3 mm) were more concentrated in the posterior mid third and the splenium, which may correspond to the representation of primary and secondary sensorimotor areas, particularly auditory and somatosensory (posterior mid third) and visual (splenium). On the other hand, callosal subregions likely to connect higher-order association areas are mainly composed of small-diameter, slower-conducting fibers.

This is of interest because callosal fibers connecting primary and secondary areas are relatively few, and are restricted to representations near the sensory or motor midline, while in higher-order areas callosal neurons can be found more homogeneously (Innocenti, 1986). In primary and secondary visual, as well as somatosensory, cortices, fast-conducting large callosal fibers probably serve the fusion of the two hemirepresentations in both hemispheres, while in auditory areas they may represent an additional stage of fast bilateral interaction in the au-

Lutz Jäncke and Helmuth Steinmetz

ditory pathway that serves auditory space perception. It is important to note that Aboitiz et al. identified these fibers with light microscopy. However, there are also many very small unmyelinated fibers that are undetectable with this method. Their number has often been underestimated. For example, Innocenti (1986) reports that when a count of callosal fibers in the cat was made with the electron microscope, the total number of callosal fibers was five times that reported on the basis of light microscopy. These results suggest that in humans, half or more of all callosal fibers are unmyelinated. Such fiber types seem not to be well suited for a fast interchange of information between sensory and motor areas, particularly when such information must serve to guide movement. However, they may be suited for the guidance of global and relatively slow attentional processes, and their enormous numbers are commensurate with the demands of such processes.

Structural-Functional Correlations

Because of the obvious role of the CC in interhemispheric integration, morphometric research has focused on potential links between the size of the CC or its subregions and behavioral laterality effects. One hypothesis is that because the CC mainly connects homotopic cortices in the left and right hemisphere, its size may be inversely related to the degree of behavioral and anatomical left-right asymmetry (Ringo et al., 1994). This hypothesis is supported by Rosen et al. (1989, 1990), who found a negative correlation between the density of callosal terminations and volumetric asymmetries in the somatomotor cortex (Rosen et al., 1989). This association indicated that greater density of callosal terminations is associated with a more symmetric structure between hemispheres.

Research into the effect of handedness—the most pronounced marker of behavioral asymmetry—on callosal morphology has only partly supported these anatomical findings. Witelson (1985, 1989; Witelson & Goldsmith, 1991), in a series of postmortem studies, found that the CC of non-consistent-right-handed men tended to be thicker than that of consistent-right-handed men. Some in vivo MRI studies have supported Witelson's postmortem findings. There is, however, little agreement about the region of the callosum responsible for this effect. One MRI study favored the anterior body (Habib et al., 1991), and others, the isthmus (Clarke & Zaidel, 1994; Moffat et al., 1998). Still other MRI studies have failed to find an effect of handedness on the size of the CC or of any specific callosal region (Kertesz et al., 1987; O'Kusky et al., 1988; Reinarz et al., 1988; Steinmetz et al., 1992; Hines et al., 1992; Jäncke et al., 1997), or have found complex hand x gender interactions upon various CC subareas (Cowell et al., 1993).

A further set of studies measured auditory or visual behavioral asymmetry measures and related them to CC morphology measures. Significant negative correlations between CC size and behavioral asymmetry indices were found for free-recall verbal dichotic listening tests in two studies (O'Kusky et al., 1988; Hines et al., 1992). Two further studies found negative correlations between CC size and the magnitude of the right-ear advantage in the dichotic listening tests (Clarke et al., 1993; Yazgan et al., 1995). However, no such correlations have been found by others using verbal dichotic listening or visual half-field tests (Kertesz et al., 1986; Clarke et al., 1993; Clarke & Zaidel, 1994; Jäncke & Steinmetz, 1994; Hellige et al., 1998).

Researchers have also been concerned with potential links between the size of the CC and the level of behavioral performance, either overall or when stimuli are presented directly to only one hemisphere. For example, Jäncke & Steinmetz (1994) found that mean reaction time in a dichotic consonant-vowel monitoring task decreased as the area of the CC increased. That is, a larger CC was associated with better overall performance. More recently, Davatzikos and Resnick (1998), applying a new method for quantifying CC morphology in a large sample of 114 individuals, revealed that the bulbosity of the CC correlated with cognitive performance (card rotations, figural memory, verbal memory, Boston naming, and letter fluency) in women, indicating that larger callosal size was associated with better performance.

However, this was not always the case. For example, Robichon and Habib (1998) found the midsagittal area of the CC to be larger in a group of dyslexic adults than in a group of age-matched controls. Furthermore, within the dyslexic group, various phonological impairments became more severe as the size of certain callosal regions increased. In addition, Clarke et al. (1993; Clark & Zaidel, 1994) found significant negative correlations of the right-ear scores in a dichotic listening task with the total CC area, with the area of the anterior third of the CC, and with the area of the anterior midbody. There were no significant correlations between any CC area and the left-ear scores. For their male participants alone, the correlations of the right-ear score with the area of the isthmus and with the area of the splenium also were significantly negative. Clarke et al. suggest that, for the task they used, a larger CC leads to an increase in functional inhibition from the nonspecialized hemisphere to the specialized hemisphere—as if a larger CC permits more erroneous, interference-causing cross talk from the nonspecialized to the specialized hemisphere. Contrary to intuitions that an increase in callosal communication would enhance performance, it may be that for some strongly lateralized domains like phonetic processing, increased communication via a larger CC can be detrimental to the performance of at least one hemisphere.

Although the relation between behavioral asymmetry measures and CC morphology remains a matter of dispute, there is strong evidence that anatomical perisylvian asymmetry and CC morphology are related to one other. Aboitiz, Scheibel, & Zaidel (1992) investigated the relation between callosal connectivity and perisylvian anatomical asymmetry. They measured the asymmetry of sylvian fissure length between Heschl's gyrus and the end of the posterior ascending branch. An inverse relationship was found between the magnitude of this asymmetry and the size and the axon number of the isthmus. This relation was stronger for males than for females. Their finding receives some support from a recent in vivo morphometric study reporting a significant negative correlation between an absolute value of hemispheric asymmetry and the size of the CC in males but not in females (Dorion et al., 2000). However, it is necessary to point out that the authors used two sagittal brain area measures for estimating brain size (De Lacoste et al., 1990). Together, these findings suggest that increasing perisylvian asymmetry or general brain asymmetry (and hence increasing hemispheric specialization) is associated with a sex-dependent decrease in interhemispheric communication.

Interestingly, a recent primate study also revealed a negative correlation between brain asymmetry measures or handedness and CC size, suggesting that the evolution of hemispheric asymmetry may have been accompanied by a progressive reduction of interhemispheric connectivity (Hopkins & Marino, 2000).

Gender Differences or Brain Size Effects?

It is still a matter of dispute whether there are gender differences in the size or shape of various components of the CC. This research has a tradition dating back to the work of Bean (1906) and Mall (1909), who analyzed postmortem brains. Although these researchers did not find convincing evidence for strong gender differences with respect to the size or shape of the CC, this debate was revived by de Lacoste and Holloway (De Lacoste-Utamsing & Holloway, 1982; De Lacoste & Holloway, 1986), who suggested—on the basis of relatively few postmortem brains—that females have a larger splenium than males. This finding was taken as supporting evidence that females have a stronger interhemispheric connectivity, reflecting their more bilateral processing of various psychological functions compared to men. These first findings have received some support in later research, but a recent carefully performed meta-analytic review of the relevant literature clearly suggests that there is no significant gender difference in terms of size or shape of the CC or its subregions (Bishop & Wahlsten, 1997).

Our own studies on a large sample of healthy adults and children, applying in vivo morphometry, also revealed no gender difference for CC size measures (absolute or normalized to total CC size) (Jäncke et al., 1997, 1999). An important finding of this study, however, was that although the cross-sectional area of the CC increases with forebrain volume, this increase is less than proportional to forebrain volume. Related to this less-than-proportional increase of the CC with increasing forebrain size is the finding that CC ratios (CC area is related to forebrain volume) correlated negatively with forebrain volume. The allometric equations ($\log CC = a + b^* \log[\text{forebrain volume}]$) suggest that the relationship between CC and forebrain volume follows the geometrical rule that a cross-sectional area of a three-dimensional object is scaled nonisometrically to the volume of this object (figure 6.9).

A further step of our analysis involved the between-gender comparison for small and large brains. This analysis revealed that small brains, irrespective of gender, had relatively larger CC areas than large brains. Therefore, we conclude that forebrain volume is the main factor determining CC size. Since women have on average approximately 10–15% smaller brains, gender differences in CC size might mostly or exclusively be explained by brain size differences. Based on present anatomical knowledge, a functional interpretation of this inverse relationship between forebrain size and relative callosal size must remain speculative. Let us assume that the packing densities and branching patterns of callosal neurons and axons do not depend on brain size. In this case our

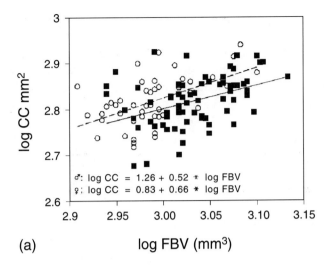

(a)

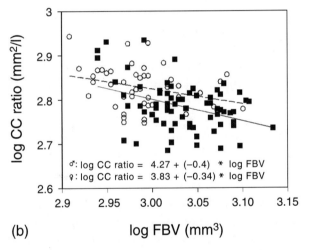

(b)

Figure 6.9 (*a*) Total corpus callosum (CC in log mm²) and forebrain volume (FBV in log l); (*b*) total corpus callosum ratio (CC/FBV in log mm²/l) and forebrain volume (FBV in log l). (Data taken from Jäncke et al., 1997.) Unfilled circles represent women; filled squares, men. Regression slopes for women are dashed.

Anatomical Brain Asymmetries

study would indicate that the degree of interhemispheric connectedness decreases with increasing human brain size. This would concur with theoretical predictions made by Ringo and coworkers (Ringo, 1991; Ringo et al., 1994). They argued that as brain size is scaled up, there must be a fall in interhemispheric connectivity, due to the increasing time constraints of transcallosal conduction delay. Consequently, functionally related neuronal elements would cluster in one hemisphere, so that increasing brain size would be the driving force in the phylogeny of hemispheric specialization. With regard to callosal connectivity, the present morphometric data can provide empirical support for this conjecture.

Developmental Aspects

Theories to explain interhemispheric differences in CC morphology include naturally occurring regressive events, such as death of neurons and elimination of axon collaterals (Cowan et al., 1984; LaMantia & Rakic, 1990). However, this axonal elimination is thought to occur prior to most environmental influences. On the other hand, it has been proposed that functional maturation of the CC extends into late childhood and adolescence, and coincides with the termination of its myelination cycle. According to Rakic and Yakovlev (1968) and Yakovlev and Lecours (1967), the CC is one of the latest fiber tracts in the central nervous system to be myelinated. Furthermore, in vivo imaging has revealed that increases of callosal size can be seen at least up to the middle of the third decade, with a maximum during the first decade of human life (Allen et al., 1991; Cowell et al., 1992; Pujol et al., 1993). The presumed progression in maturation of the CC may thus correspond to the continuing changes in cortical synaptic density that occur throughout childhood (Huttenlocher, 1979; Kinney et al., 1988).

In animal studies of postnatal development of the CC, the number of callosal axons in neonates exceeds that of young adults, suggesting that normal development involves the remodeling of axonal projections between the two hemispheres with a subsequent elimination of callosal axons. However, the reduction in the number of callosal axons, which reflects the selective elimination of axon collaterals or callosal neurons during early development, can be manipulated experimentally by altering sensory or motor experience during early development (Innocenti & Frost, 1979; Berrebi et al., 1988). Other studies of humans and nonhumans have suggested a considerable degree of callosal plasticity during brain development until adulthood (Zilles, 1992; Pujol et al., 1993). In addition, several recent studies have revealed significant correlations between posterior and mid regions of the CC with age even when forebrain volume was controlled for (Giedd et al., 1996).

Taken together, these results suggest an anterior-to-posterior maturation gradient with continued maturation of posterior CC regions even in adulthood. It is likely that this maturation gradient is somehow linked to a similar maturation gradient of higher association areas since a large portion of callosal fibers emanate from these (Pandya & Seltzer, 1986). Thus, during the development of the CC, factors such as intense training could play an important role in the determination of callosal fiber composition and size. This, then, would fit well within a concept of callosal plasticity as an adaptive structural-functional process following changes in stimulation intensity. A finding that is compatible with the concept of such an adaptive structural-functional process has been published by Schlaug et al. (1995). These authors found that the anterior CC was significantly larger in highly professional musicians than in well-matched controls. This difference was due to a much larger anterior CC in the subgroup of musicians who had begun musical training before the age of seven. This larger CC was taken as evidence for a more efficient interhemispheric communication between the frontal cortices containing the motor areas subserving and supporting bimanual coordination, which is essential for skillful playing of an instrument.

Conclusion

Taken together, there are still only equivocal and controversial findings regarding the relation between CC morphology and functional measures. This may be due to some methodological but also theoretical reasons. First, the measurement of functional asymmetries is often confounded by the operation of cognitive intermediates such as attention or memory. Behavioral asymmetry tests may not be reliable measures of functional lateralization because attention or memory may influence the performance on these tests substantially.

Second, slight differences in test design may evoke strong differences in behavioral asymmetry. For example, processing of the test material presented to the left or right hemisphere might follow either the "direct access" or the "callosal transfer" model, depending on the nature of the task. According to the "callosal transfer" model, only the dominant hemisphere processes the relevant information, so that laterality effects are expected to reflect callosal transfer from the nondominant to the dominant hemisphere. In contrast, the "direct access" model has suggested that the nondominant hemisphere is also capable of processing this information, but less efficiently than the contralateral one. It has been shown that "easy" material presented to the subdominant hemisphere is processed according to the "direct access" model, while more complex material requires some kind of callosal transfer in order to tie in the specialized hemisphere in the processing of the material (Karnath et al., 1991). Thus, it may be possible that complex behavioral asymmetry tests may more strongly rely on callosal transfer processes, while easier material is processed according to the "direct access" model without any participation of the CC.

Third, a further problem relates to the handedness measurement. Although many researchers argue that handedness can be inferred by asking for writing hand preference, this matter is much more complicated, as has been demonstrated in a wealth of studies (for a summary see also Peters, 1995, 1998). A result of this complicated status is that there is currently no consensus for classifying right- or left-handers. Some researchers have used the Annett classification scheme, while others prefer the continuous preference measures or the self-classification of the writing hand. Regardless of which method is used for handedness classification, each method imposes its own problems, causing considerable variability and hampering between-study comparisons.

Fourth, another problem for morphometric studies of the CC is the unsolved question whether CC area measures are indeed valid indices of the number of callosal fibers. The aforementioned study by Aboitiz et al. (1992a) demonstrated that CC subarea sizes are positively related only to the number of small-diameter (slow-conducting) callosal fibers, but not to the number of large-diameter (fast-conducting) axons. Thus, only performance measures of psychological functions utilizing collosal transfer via these smaller fibers might correlate with sagittal CC area size. The large-caliber fibers of more than 3 mm diameter most likely serve to cement together the cortical regions subserving the two half-fields of vision, to improve auditory sound localization, or to enhance bimanual coordination. These fibers, however, are so few and variable in density that they may fail to show a relation with callosal size. The small-diameter fibers delineated by Aboitiz et al. allow for interhemispheric transfer times in the range of 15 to 30 ms, which are reasonable transfer times for cognitive functions as estimated by dichotic monitoring experiments (Jäncke et al., 1994).

As mentioned above, the number of callosal fibers in humans has been estimated only by light microscope until now, but there is reasonable evidence that the CC contains at least two to five times more unmyelinated fibers, which can be measured only with electron microscopy. Given the likely fact that more than half of all CC fibers are small and unmyelinated, one might assume that CC size is more strongly related to the number of these fibers. Since the estimated interhemispheric transfer time for these very small fibers is about 300 ms, it is plausible to argue that these fibers are unsuited for the fast interchange of information. However, they may be well suited for the guidance of global and relatively slow attentional processes. Thus, it is possible that CC size is more strongly related to attentional processes mediating between both hemispheres. Unfortunately, there is no study of a possible relationship between attentional switching processes and CC size.

Fifth, an unsolved problem relates to the methods used to delineate CC area or volume. The method that has been most used may be too imprecise, and any comparable subdivision probably is also influenced by the shape or bending of the CC. For example, a strongly curved CC may have a smaller isthmus and a less curved CC may have a larger isthmus (applying the method outlined in figure 6.6). A possible solution for this problem might be to work with linearly normalized brains and to subject the white matter volumes including the CC on a voxel-wise basis to further statistical analysis. However, these methods are not free from methodological problems. It is, for example, unknown whether the shape of the CC is somehow related to brain size. If that is the case, a linear normalization of brains of different sizes will not correct for this influence.

An important future question will be whether there is a relationship between brain size, established behavioral (e.g., language lateralization), and structural asymmetries (e.g., planum temporale and planum parietale asymmetry; Steinmetz et al., 1991). If there is a relation between brain size and asymmetry, larger brains should demonstrate stronger anatomical and functional asymmetries. This then may provide clues for the phylogeny of hemispheric dominance in the higher primates (Ringo, 1991; Ringo et al., 1994).

FURTHER ANATOMICAL ASYMMETRIES

Several studies have demonstrated or suggested brain anatomical asymmetries in areas different from those described in the previous chapters. These asymmetries include those of left versus right hemispheric volume and hemispheric shape, as well as between-hemisphere differences in smaller target structures like the hippocampus. A relatively old and easy-to-measure overall brain asymmetry in humans and nonhumans is the petalia pattern. Petalias are the frontal and parieto-occipital protrusions of the skull and underlying hemisphere. In humans and nonhuman primates, petalia asymmetries have largely been examined using endocasts, CT scans, X-rays, and, recently, MRI scans. The most common petalia asymmetry found in humans is a left parieto-occipital versus right frontal bias. That is, the posterior left hemisphere and skull protrude further outward than the posterior right hemisphere and skull, while the opposite pattern is found for the anterior hemisphere and skull (LeMay & Culebras, 1972; LeMay, 1976, 1977, 1981, 1992; LeMay & Kido, 1978; Kertesz et al., 1986; Zilles et al., 1996). Interestingly, it was demonstrated recently that the great apes exhibit a right frontal and left occipital directional asymmetry in cerebral width (a classical measure of petalia), while there was no significant directional asymmetry in either the Old or New World monkeys (Hopkins & Marino, 2000).

The functional significance of these findings remains unclear. There is, however, some evidence that this petalia pattern is somehow related to functional asymmetries. For example, in left-handed humans the typical petalia pattern seems to be reduced (LeMay et al., 1972). In addition, the great apes, which show typical petalia patterns, are more right-handed compared to the other taxonomic ape families not showing the typical petalia pattern, at least for some measures of hand preference, such as bipedal reaching and coordinated bimanual actions. Thus, at one level of analysis, functional differences in asymmetry appear to map onto neuroanatomical differences, but this conclusion assumes that differences among species in the direction of hand preference are indeed real rather than an artifact of certain testing circumstances or situations (McGrew & Marchant, 1997). However, whether

Lutz Jäncke and Helmuth Steinmetz

these petalia asymmetries are indeed related to functional asymmetries in humans and nonhuman primates has to be evaluated in future studies applying more sophisticated methods similar to those used by Zilles and coworkers (Semendeferi et al., 1998; Zilles et al., 2001).

A further anatomical asymmetry related to function has been reported by Willerman et al. (1992). They estimated the size of both hemispheres in 39 college students and correlated these anatomical measures with prorated WAIS-R IQ scores (verbal IQ minus performance IQ). In men, they found that a relatively larger left hemisphere predicted better verbal than nonverbal scores, whereas in women a larger left hemisphere predicted relatively better nonverbal than verbal scores. These results were taken as evidence for a gender-specific brain organization underlying gender-specific psychological functions. The rationale behind this interpretation is that the left hemisphere houses language functions, and the right, nonverbal functions. Besides the fact that this is a very coarse dichotomy, this study also had some methodological problems, including small sample size and the morphometric method used to estimate brain size differences. The small sample size (n = 39) is susceptible to false positive errors, and thus requires further crossvalidation by independent studies, and the morphometric method used for measuring brain size differences is not precise enough from the current point of knowledge. These authors calculated the number of voxels from four sagittal MRI slices of each hemisphere and used these measurements to predict the volume of each hemisphere. However, De Lacoste et al. (1990) have demonstrated that such measures are unreliable for estimating total brain size. Because of these objections, we would like not to draw too firm conclusions from these data, although we have to admit that this is an interesting approach to studying interindividual differences in brain organization.

A more recent and spectacular finding has been provided by Maguire et al. (2000), who obtained structural MRIs of the brains of licensed London taxi drivers known to possess extensive navigation experience. Applying conventional in vivo morphometrical methods (delineating regions of interest) and newly developed voxel-based morphometry methods, the authors found that the volume of the posterior hippocampi were significantly larger relative to those of control subjects. A more anterior hippocampal region was larger in control subjects than in taxi drivers. These anatomical data correspond to animal and human studies demonstrating that the posterior hippocampus is involved in spatial learning as well as in the generation of spatial maps. Most interestingly, right hippocampal volume correlated with the amount of time spent as a taxi driver (positively in the posterior, and negatively in the anterior, hippocampus). These data suggest that changes in hippocampal gray matter on the right are acquired, introducing the possibility of local plasticity in the structure of the healthy adult human brain as a function of increasing exposure to an environmental stimulus.

BRAIN SIZE AND COGNITIVE ABILITIES

Since the 1970s there has been a resurgence in the study of simple mental and biological processes underlying general intelligence (g). This approach derives from ideas proposed over 100 years ago by Sir Francis Galton. The view that intelligence is largely heritable and driven by differences in the speed of simple mental processes, themselves ultimately based on brain physiology, has drawn fresh evidence from the genetic work conducted by Bouchard (1998; Bouchard et al., 1990). The hypothesis that brain size has some influence on intellectual function is an old one, and it initially took the questionable premise that one could infer brain size from head circumference. Nevertheless, the mean correlation between head size and measured IQ from more than 30 studies was positive, although small (r = 0.2) (Jensen, 1994). The emergence of MR techniques enables a more conclusive statement to be made regarding the size of the relationship between brain size and IQ.

Several papers have indicated a sizable relation between brain size, as determined by MRI, and IQ (mean r = 0.4). Each of these studies has problems posed by method and interpretation or by the findings themselves. We will not go into deeper discussions of each of these studies here, but we will emphasize at least some critical points that are important to consider. First, it must be kept in mind that neural systems, by definition, have evolved to interact with the environment, and the very significant expansion of brain size after birth, driven by growth of synapses and cortical interconnections, is interactive with environmental input. Thus, nutritional and environmental conditions that foster good development of intelligence can be expected to foster good physical brain development as well. Thus, family background, socioeconomic status, cross-assortative mating, and cultural influences potentially affect both brain anatomy and behavior in the same direction independently, which could result in noncausal associations between brain size and cognitive ability. If one controls for such influences, correlations between brain size and cognitive abilities disappear completely (Schoenemann et al., 2000).

Second, there is a wealth of quantitative features of the brain that are related to brain size, including the number of cortical neurons, average cortical thickness, average neuron density, extent of axodendritic arborization, neuron/glia ratios, and various neurochemical measures. Which of these features influence cognitive ability is unknown. Also, brain size is a crude anatomical measure. As discussed in the previous chapters, there is substantial anatomical variation in individual brain regions that are not directly related to brain size. Thus it may be that a larger volume in a particular region is compensated by a smaller volume in another region. A further possibility may be that there are volumetric differences in small brain areas which are too small to influence overall brain weight (e.g., hippocampus). Taken together, individual differences in brain size (within species) are usually unrelated to fundamental structural and functional differences, except during early development or in the case of brain damage.

However, while further comparisons of individual brain size and cognitive ability do not appear to be promising, the question of differences in brain anatomy between genders still requires more attention. Sex hormones may well influence brain growth, development, and left-right asymmetry. Thus, in a recent in vivo MRI study of 80 healthy men and women, Gur and colleagues (1999) found that women have a higher percentage of gray matter, whereas men have a higher percentage of white matter and of cerebrospinal fluid. In addition, the percentage of gray matter was higher in the left hemisphere. Although this may eventually turn out to be one of many unconfirmed studies in the field of brain morphometry, the underlying question clearly deserves further study.

FUTURE RESEARCH

Great progress has been made in disentangling possible structure-function relationships. This progress was possible because of the tremendous technical developments introduced by computer scientists and neuroanatomists. These developments are a vivid example of interdisciplinary research in the cognitive neurosciences. Because this field is constantly expanding, one can expect further high potential findings in the near future. A very important innovation is the possibility to analyze greater sample sizes of brains within a reasonable time, thus preventing the false positive findings very often published in earlier neuroanatomical studies of this kind.

NOTE

1. Two recent population-based studies applying refined morphometric measures of the PT and the PP indicate only subtle morphological abnormalities in the left perisylvian brain region for dyslexic children (Hugdahl et al., 1998; Heiervang et al., 2000).

REFERENCES

Aboitiz, F., Scheibel, A. B., Fisher, R. S., & Zaidel, E. (1992). Fiber composition of the human corpus callosum. *Brain Research, 598*, 143–153.

Aboitiz, F., Scheibel, A. B., & Zaidel, E. (1992). Morphometry of the sylvian fissure and the corpus callosum, with emphasis on sex differences. *Brain, 115*, 1521–1541.

Albanese, E., Merlo, A., Albanese, A., & Gomez, E. (1989). Anterior speech region. Asymmetry and weight-surface correlation. *Archives of Neurology, 46*, 307–310. (See comments.)

Allen, L. S., Richey, M., Chai, Y., & Gorski, R. (1991). Sex differences in the cerebral cortex and the corpus callosum of the living human being. *Journal of Neuroscience, 11*, 933–942.

Amunts, K., Jäncke, L., Mohlberg, H., Steinmetz, H., & Zilles, K. (2000). Interhemispheric asymmetry of the human motor cortex related to handedness and gender. *Neuropsychologia, 38*, 304–312.

Amunts, K., Schlaug, G., Schleicher, A., Steinmetz, H., Dabringhaus, A., Roland, P. E., & Zilles, K. (1996). Asymmetry in the human motor cortex and handedness. *Neuroimage, 4*(3, pt. 1), 216–222.

Amunts, K., Schleicher, A., Burgel, U., Mohlberg, H., Uylings, H. B., & Zilles, K. (1999). Broca's region revisited: Cytoarchitecture and intersubject variability. *Journal of Comparative Neurology, 412*, 319–341.

Bean, R. B. (1906). Some racial peculiarities of the negro brain. *American Journal of Anatomy, 5*, 353–432.

Beaton, A. A. (1997). The relation of planum temporale asymmetry and morphology of the corpus callosum to handedness, gender, and dyslexia: A review of the evidence. *Brain and Language, 60*, 255–322.

Berrebi, A. S., Fitch, R., Ralphe, D., Denenberg, J., Friedrich, V., & Denenberg, V. H. (1988). Corpus callosum: Region-specific effects of sex, early experience and age. *Brain Research, 438*, 216–224.

Bishop, K. M., & Wahlsten, D. (1997). Sex differences in the human corpus callosum: Myth or reality? *Neuroscience and Biobehavioral Reviews, 21,* 581–601.

Bouchard, T. J., Jr. (1998). Genetic and environmental influences on adult intelligence and special mental abilities. *Human Biology, 70,* 257–279.

Bouchard, T. J., Jr., Lykken, D. T., McGue, M., Segal, N. L., & Tellegen, A. (1990). Sources of human psychological differences: The Minnesota Study of Twins Reared Apart. *Science, 250,* 223–228.

Braak, H. (1978). On magnopyramidal temporal fields in the human brain—probable morphological counterparts of Wernicke's sensory speech region. *Anatomy and Embryology.* (Berlin), *152,* 141–169.

Brodmann, K. (1909). *Vergleichende Lokalisationslehre der Grosshirnrinde.* Leipzig: Barth.

Bryden, M. P., Hecaen, H., & DeAgostini, M. (1983). Patterns of cerebral organization. *Brain and Language, 20,* 249–262.

Buchanan, T. W., Lutz, K., Mirzazade, S., Specht, K., Shah, N. J., Zilles, K., & Jäncke, L. (2000). Recognition of emotional prosody and verbal components of spoken language: An fMRI study. *Cognitive Brain Research, 9,* 227–238.

Cheverud, J. M., Falk, D., Vannier, M., Konigsberg, L., Helmkamp, R. C., & Hildebolt, C. (1990). Heritability of brain size and surface features in rhesus macaques (*Macaca mulatta*). *Journal of Heredity, 81,* 51–57.

Clarke, J. M., Lufkin, R. B., & Zaidel, E. (1993). Corpus callosum morphometry and dichotic listening performance: Individual differences in functional interhemispheric inhibition? *Neuropsychologia, 31,* 547–557.

Clarke, J. M., & Zaidel, E. (1994). Anatomical-behavioral relationships: Corpus callosum morphometry and hemispheric specialization. *Behavioral Brain Research, 64,* 185–202.

Cowan, W. M., Fawcett, J. W., O'Leary, D. D., & Stanfield, B. B. (1984). Regressive events in neurogenesis. *Science, 225,* 1258–1265.

Cowell, P. E., Allen, L. S., Zalatimo, N. S., & Denenberg, V. (1992). A developmental study of sex and age interactions in the human corpus callosum. *Developmental Brain Research, 66,* 187–192.

Cowell, P. E., Kertesz, A., & Denenberg, V. H. (1993). Multiple dimensions of handedness and the human corpus callosum. *Neurology, 43,* 2353–2357.

Cunningham, D. J. (1892). Contribution to the surface anatomy of the cerebral hemispheres. *The Academy House,* 77–160.

Davatzikos, C., & Resnick, S. M. (1998). Sex differences in anatomic measures of interhemispheric connectivity: Correlations with cognition in women but not men. *Cerebral Cortex, 8,* 635–640.

De Lacoste, M. C., Adesanya, T., & Woodward, D. J. (1990). Measures of gender differences in human brain and their relationship to brain weight. *Biological Psychiatry, 28,* 931–942.

De Lacoste, M. C., & Holloway, R. L. (1986). Sex differences in the fetal human corpus callosum. *Human Neurobiology, 5,* 93–96.

De Lacoste-Utamsing, M. C., & Holloway, R. L. (1982). Sexual dimorphism in the human corpus callosum. *Science, 216,* 1431–1432.

Denenberg, V. H., Cowell, P. E., Fitch, R., Kertesz, A., & Kenner, G. II. (1991). Corpus callosum: Multiple parameter measurements in rodents and humans. *Physiology and Behavior, 49,* 433–437.

Dorion, A. A., Chantome, M., Hasboun, D., Zouaoui, A., Marsault, C., Capron, C., & Duyme, M. (2000). Hemispheric asymmetry and corpus callosum morphometry: A magnetic resonance imaging study. *Neuroscience Research, 36,* 9–13.

Eberstaller, O. (1884). Zur oberflächenanatomie der grosshirn-hemisphären. Vorläufige mitteilung: Das untere scheitelläppchen. *Wiener Medizinische Blätter, 21,* 644–646.

Eberstaller, O. (1890). *Das stirnhirn. Ein beitrag zur anatomie der oberfläche des grosshirns.* Vienna: Urban & Schwarzenberg.

Economo, C. von, & Horn, L. (1930). Über Windungsrelief, Maße und Rindenarchitektonik der Supratemporalfläche, ihre individuellen und ihre Seitenunterschiede. *Zeitschrift für Neurologie und Psychiatrie, 130,* 678–757.

Fiez, J. A., Raichle, M. E., Balota, D. A., Tallal, P., & Petersen, S. E. (1996). PET activation of posterior temporal regions during auditory word presentation and verb generation. *Cerebral Cortex, 6,* 1–10.

Flechsig, P. (1908). Bemerkungen über die hörsphäre des menschlichen gehirns. *Zentralblatt, 27,* 61–67.

Foundas, A. L., Leonard, C. M., Gilmore, R., Fennell, E., & Heilman, K. M. (1994). Planum temporale asymmetry and language dominance. *Neuropsychologia, 32,* 1225–1231.

Foundas, A. L., Leonard, C. M., Gilmore, R. L., Fennell, E. B., & Heilman, K. M. (1996). Pars triangularis asymmetry and language dominance. *Proceedings of the National Academy of Sciences, USA, 93,* 719–722.

Foundas, A. L., Leonard, C. M., & Heilman, K. M. (1995). Morphologic cerebral asymmetries and handedness. The pars triangularis and planum temporale. *Archives of Neurology, 52,* 501–508.

Galaburda, A. M. (1993). Neurology of developmental dyslexia. *Current Opinion in Neurobiology, 3,* 237–242.

Galaburda, A. M., & Sanides, F. (1980). Cytoarchitectonic organization of the human auditory cortex. *Journal of Comparative Neurology, 190,* 597–610.

Galaburda, A. M., Sanides, F., & Geschwind, N. (1978). Human brain: Cytoarchitectonic left-right asymmetries in the temporal speech region. *Archives of Neurology, 35,* 812–817.

Galuske, R. A., Schlote, W., Bratzke, H., & Singer, W. (2000). Interhemispheric asymmetries of the modular structure in human temporal cortex. *Science, 289,* 1946–1949. (See comments.)

Gannon, P. J., Holloway, R. L., Broadfield, D. C., & Braun, A. R. (1998). Asymmetry of chimpanzee planum temporale: Humanlike pattern of Wernicke's brain language area homolog. *Science, 279,* 220–222.

Geschwind, N., & Levitsky, W. (1968). Human brain: Left-right asymmetries in temporal speech region. *Science, 161,* 186–187.

Giedd, J. N., Rumsey, J. M., Castellanos, F. X., Rajapakse, J. C., Kaysen, D., Vaituzis, A. C., Vauss, Y. C., Hamburger, S. D., & Rapoport, J. L. (1996). A quantitative MRI study of the corpus callosum in children and adolescents. *Develeopmental Brain Research, 91,* 274–280.

Gur, R. C., Turetsky, B. I., Matsui, M., Yan, M., Bilker, W., Hughett, P., & Gur, R. E. (1999). Sex differences in brain gray and white matter in healthy young adults: Correlations with cognitive performance. *Journal of Neuroscience, 19,* 4065–4072.

Haase, C., & Dehner, P. (1893). Unsere Truppen in körperlicher Beziehung. *Archiv für Anatomie und Entwicklungsgeschichte,* 249–256.

Habib, M., Gayraud, D., Oliva, A., Regis, J., Salamon, G., & Khalil, R. (1991). Effects of handedness and sex on the morphology of the corpus callosum: A study with brain magnetic resonance imaging. *Brain and Cognition, 16,* 41–61.

Habib, M., Robichon, F., Levrier, O., Khalil, R., & Salamon, G. (1995). Diverging asymmetries of temporo-parietal cortical areas: A reappraisal of Geschwind/Galaburda theory. *Brain and Language, 48,* 238–258.

Heiervang, E., Hugdahl, K., Steinmetz, H., Inge, S. A., Stevenson, J., Lund, A., Ersland, L., & Lundervold, A. (2000). Planum temporale, planum parietale and dichotic listening in dyslexia. *Neuropsychologia, 38,* 1704–1713.

Hellige, J. B., Taylor, K. B., Lesmes, L., & Peterson, S. (1998). Relationships between brain morphology and behavioral measures of hemispheric asymmetry and interhemispheric interaction. *Brain and Cognition, 36,* 158–192.

Hines, M., Chiu, L., McAdams, L. A., Bentler, P. M., & Lipcamon, J. (1992). Cognition and the corpus callosum: Verbal fluency, visuospatial ability, and language lateralization related to midsaggital surface areas of callosal subregions. *Behavioral Neuroscience, 106,* 3–14.

Hopkins, W. D., & Marino, L. (2000). Asymmetries in cerebral width in nonhuman primate brains as revealed by magnetic resonance imaging (MRI). *Neuropsychologia, 38,* 493–499.

Hugdahl, K., Heiervang, E., Nordby, H., Smievoll, A. I., Steinmetz, H., Stevenson, J., & Lund, A. (1998). Central auditory processing, MRI morphometry and brain laterality: Applications to dyslexia. *Scandinavian Audiology Supplementum, 49,* 26–34. (In process citation.)

Huttenlocher, P. R. (1979). Synaptic density in human frontal cortex—Developmental changes and effects of aging. *Brain Research, 163,* 195–205.

Hyrtl, J. (1882). *Lehrbuch der Anatomie des Menschen, mit Rücksicht auf physiologische Begründung und praktische Anwendung.* Vienna.

Ide, A., Dolezal, C., Fernandez, M., Labbe, E., Mandujano, R., Montes, S., Segura, P., Verschae, G., Yarmuch, P., & Aboitiz, F. (1999). Hemispheric differences in variability of fissural patterns in parasylvian and cingulate regions of human brains. *Journal of Comparatvive Neurology, 410,* 235–242.

Ide, A., Rodriguez, E., Zaidel, E., & Aboitiz, F. (1996). Bifurcation patterns in the human sylvian fissure: Hemispheric and sex differences. *Cerebral Cortex, 6,* 717–725.

Innocenti, G. M. (1986). What is so special about callosal connections. In F. Lepore, M. Ptito, & H. H. Jasper (Eds.), *Two hemispheres—one brain. Functions of the corpus callosum* (pp. 75–82). New York: Alan R. Liss.

Innocenti, G. M., & Frost, D. O. (1979). Abnormal visual experience stabilizes juvenile patterns of interhemispheric connections. *Nature, 280,* 231–234.

Jäncke, L., Preis, S., & Steinmetz, H. (1999). The relation between forebrain volume and midsagittal size of the corpus callosum in children. *NeuroReport, 10,* 2981–2985.

Jäncke, L., Schlaug, G., Huang, Y., & Steinmetz, H. (1994). Asymmetry of the planum parietale. *NeuroReport, 5,* 1161–1163.

Jäncke, L., Staiger, J. F., Schlaug, G., Huang, Y., & Steinmetz, H. (1997). The relationship between corpus callosum size and forebrain volume. *Cerebral Cortex, 7,* 48–56.

Jäncke, L., & Steinmetz, H. (1993). Auditory lateralization and planum temporale asymmetry. *NeuroReport, 5,* 169–172.

Jäncke, L., & Steinmetz, H. (1994). Interhemispheric transfer time and corpus callosum size. *NeuroReport, 5,* 2385–2388.

Jensen, A. R. (1994). Psychometric g related to differences in head size. *Personality and Individual Differences, 17,* 597–606.

Karnath, H. O., Schumacher, M., & Wallesch, C. W. (1991). Limitations of interhemispheric extracallosal transfer of visual information in callosal agenesis. *Cortex, 27,* 345–350.

Kertesz, A., Black, S. E., Polk, M., & Howell, J. (1986). Cerebral asymmetries on magnetic resonance imaging. *Cortex, 22,* 117–127.

Kertesz, A., Polk, M., Howell, J., & Black, S. E. (1987). Cerebral dominance, sex, and callosal size in MRI. *Neurology, 37,* 1385–1388.

Kinney, H. C., Brody, B. A., Kloman, A. S., & Gilles, F. H. (1988). Sequence of central nervous system myelination in human infancy. II. Patterns of myelination in autopsied infants. *Journal of Neuropathology and Experimental Neurology, 47,* 217–234.

Kulynych, J. J., Vladar, K., Jones, D. W., & Weinberger, D. R. (1994). Gender differences in the normal lateralization of the supratemporal cortex: MRI surface-rendering morphometry of Heschl's gyrus and the planum temporale. *Cerebral Cortex, 4,* 107–118.

LaMantia, A., & Rakic, P. (1990). Axon overproduction and elimination in the corpus callosum of the developing rhesus monkey. *Journal of Neuroscience, 10,* 2156–2175.

LeMay, M. (1976). Morphological cerebral asymmetries of modern man, fossil man, and nonhuman primate. *Annals of the New York Academy of Sciences, 280,* 349–366.

LeMay, M. (1977). Asymmetries of the skull and handedness. *Journal of the Neurological Sciences, 32,* 243–253.

LeMay, M. (1981). Are there radiological changes in the brains of individuals with dyslexia. *Bulletin of the Orton Society, 31,* 135–141.

LeMay, M. (1992). Left-right dissymmetry, handedness. *American Journal of Neuroradiology, 13,* 493–504.

LeMay, M., & Culebras, A. (1972). A human brain: Morphological differences in the hemispheres demonstrable by carotid angiography. *New England Journal of Medicine, 287,* 168–170.

LeMay, M., & Kido, D. K. (1978). Asymmetries of the cerebral hemispheres on computed tomograms. *Journal of Computer Assisted Tomography, 2,* 471–476.

Leonard, C. M. (1997). Language and the prefrontal cortex. In N. A. Krasnegor, G. Reid Lyon, & P. S. Goldman-Rakic (Eds.), *Development of the prefrontal cortex. Evolution, neurobiology, and behavior* (pp. 141–166). Baltimore: Paul Brookes.

Lohmann, G., von Cramon, D. Y., & Steinmetz, H. (1999). Sulcal variability of twins. *Cerebral Cortex, 9,* 754–763.

Maguire, E. A., Gadian, D. G., Johnsrude, I. S., Good, C. D., Ashburner, J., Frackowiak, R. S., & Frith, C. D. (2000). Navigation-related structural change in the hippocampi of taxi drivers. *Proceedings of the National Acadamy of Sciences, USA, 97,* 4398–4403.

Mall, F. P. (1909). On several anatomical characters of the human brain, said to vary according to race and sex, with especial reference to the weight of the frontal lobe. *American Journal of Anatomy, 9,* 1–32.

McGrew, W. C., & Marchant, L. F. (1997). On the other hand: Current issues in and meta-analyses of the behavioral laterality of hand function in nonhuman primates. *Yearbook of Physical Anthrophology, 40,* 201–232.

Melsbach, G., Wohlschlager, A., Spiess, M., & Güntürkün, O. (1996). Morphological asymmetries of motoneurons innervating upper extremities: Clues to the anatomical foundations of handedness? *International Journal of Neuroscience, 86,* 217–224.

Moffat, S. D., Hampson, E., & Lee, D. H. (1998). Morphology of the planum temporale and corpus callosum in left handers with evidence of left and right hemisphere speech representation. *Brain, 121*(pt. 12), 2369–2379.

Narr, K. L., Thompson, P. M., Sharma, T., Moussai, J., Cannestra, A. F., & Toga, A. W. (2000). Mapping morphology of the corpus callosum in schizophrenia. *Cerebral Cortex, 10,* 40–49.

O'Kusky, J., Strauss, E., & Kosaka, B. (1988). The corpus callosum is larger with right hemisphere cerebral speech dominance. *Annals of Neurology, 24,* 379–383.

Pandya, D. N., & Seltzer, B. (1986). The topography of commissural fibers. In F. Lepore, M. Ptito, & H. H. Jasper (Eds.), *Two hemispheres—one brain. Functions of the corpus callosum* (pp. 47–73). New York: Alan R. Liss.

Peters, M. (1995). Handedness and its relation to other indices of cerebral lateralization. In R. J. Davidson & K. Hugdahl (Eds.), *Brain asymmetry* (pp. 183–214). Cambridge, MA: MIT Press.

Peters, M. (1998). Description and validation of a flexible and broadly usable hand preference questionnaire. *Laterality, 3,* 77–96.

Pfeifer, R. A. (1920). Myelogenetisch-anatomische untersuchungen über das kortikale ende der hörleitung. *Leipzig,* 54.

Pfeifer, R. A. (1936). Pathologie der hörstrahlung und der corticalen hörsphäre. In O. Bumke & O. Förster (Eds.), *Handbuch der neurologie.* Berlin: Springer-Verlag.

Preis, S., Jäncke, L., Schittler, P., Huang, Y., & Steinmetz, H. (1998). Normal intrasylvian anatomical asymmetry in children with developmental language disorder. *Neuropsychologia, 36,* 849–855.

Pujol, J., Vendrell, P., Junque, C., Marti Vilata, J. L., & Capdevila, A. (1993). When does human brain development end? Evidence of corpus callosum growth up to adulthood. *Annals of Neurology, 34,* 71–75.

Purves, D., White, L. E., & Andrews, T. J. (1994). Manual asymmetry and handedness. *Proceedings of the National Academy of Sciences, USA, 91,* 5030–5032.

Rakic, P., & Yakovlev, P. I. (1968). Development of the corpus callosum and cavum septi in man. *Journal of Comparative Neurology, 132,* 45–72.

Reinarz, S. J., Coffman, C. E., Smoker, W. R., & Godersky, J. C. (1988). MR imaging of the corpus callosum: Normal and pathologic findings and correlation with CT. *American Journal of Roentgenology, 151,* 791–798.

Ringo, J. L. (1991). Neuronal interconnection as a function of brain size. *Brain, Behavior and Evolution, 38,* 1–6.

Ringo, J. L., Doty, R. W., Demeter, S., & Simard, P. Y. (1994). Time is of the essence: A conjecture that hemispheric specialization arises from interhemispheric conduction delay. *Cerebral Cortex, 4,* 331–343.

Robichon, F., & Habib, M. (1998). Abnormal callosal morphology in male adult dyslexics: Relationships to handedness and phonological abilities. *Brain and Language, 62,* 127–146.

Rosen, G. D., Sherman, G. F., Emsbo, K., Mehler, C., & Galaburda, A. M. (1990). The midsagittal area of the corpus callosum and total neocortical volume differ in three inbred strains of mice. *Experimental Neurology, 107,* 271–276.

Rosen, G. D., Sherman, G. F., & Galaburda, A. M. (1989). Interhemispheric connections differ between symmetrical and asymmetrical brain regions. *Neuroscience, 33,* 525–533.

Rubens, A. B., Mahowald, M. W., & Hutton, J. T. (1976). Asymmetry of the lateral (sylvian) fissures in man. *Neurology, 26,* 620–624.

Schlaug, G., Jäncke, L., Huang, Y., Staiger, J. F., & Steinmetz, H. (1995). Increased corpus callosum size in musicians. *Neuropsychologia, 33*, 1047–1055.

Schlaug, G., Jäncke, L., Huang, Y., & Steinmetz, H. (1995). In vivo evidence of structural brain asymmetry in musicians. *Science, 267*, 699–701. (See comments.)

Schoenemann, P. T., Budinger, T. F., Sarich, V. M., & Wang, W. S. (2000). Brain size does not predict general cognitive ability within families. *Proceedings of the National Academy of Sciences, USA, 97*, 4932–4937.

Schulze, H. A. F. (1962). Quantitative untersuchungen zur frage der individuellen variationen und der hemisphärendifferenzen der corticalen areale des unteren parietalläppchens. *Journal für Hirnforschung, 4*, 486–517.

Seldon, H. L. (1982). Structure of human auditory cortex. III. Statistical analysis of dendritic trees. *Brain Research, 249*, 211–221.

Semendeferi, K., Armstrong, E., Schleicher, A., Zilles, K., & Van Hoesen, G. W. (1998). Limbic frontal cortex in hominids: A comparative study of area 13. *American Journal of Physical Anthropology, 106*, 129–155.

Shapleske, J., Rossell, S. L., Woodruff, P. W., & David, A. S. (1999). The planum temporale: A systematic, quantitative review of its structural, functional and clinical significance. *Brain Research Review, 29*, 26–49.

Snyder, P. J., Bilder, R. M., Wu, H., Bogerts, B., & Lieberman, J. A. (1995). Cerebellar volume asymmetries are related to handedness: A quantitative MRI study. *Neuropsychologia, 33*, 407–419.

Steinmetz, H. (1996). Structure, function, and cerebral asymmetry: In vivo morphometry of the planum temporale. *Neuroscience and Biobehavioral Reviews, 20*, 587–591.

Steinmetz, H., Fürst, G., & Freund, H. J. (1990). Variation of perisylvian and calcarine anatomical landmarks within stereotaxic proportional coordinates. *American Journal of Neuroradiology, 11*, 1123–1130.

Steinmetz, H., Herzog, A., Schlaug, G., Huang, Y., & Jäncke, L. (1995). Brain (a)symmetry in monozygotic twins. *Cerebral Cortex, 5*, 296–300.

Steinmetz, H., Jäncke, L., Kleinschmidt, A., Schlaug, G., Volkmann, J., & Huang, Y. (1992). Sex but no hand difference in the isthmus of the corpus callosum. *Neurology, 42*, 749–752. (See comments.)

Steinmetz, H., Rademacher, J., Jäncke, L., Huang, Y.X., Thron, A., & Zilles, K. (1990). Total surface of temporoparietal intrasylvian cortex: Diverging left-right asymmetries. *Brain and Language, 39*, 357–372.

Steinmetz, H., Volkmann, J., Jäncke, L., & Freund, H. J. (1991). Anatomical left-right asymmetry of language-related temporal cortex is different in left- and right-handers. *Annals of Neurology, 29*, 315–319.

Theile, F. W. (1884). *Gewichtsbestimmung zur Entwicklung des Muskelsystems und des Skeletts beim Menschen. Durch eine biographische notiz eingeleitet von W. His.* Halle: Engelmann.

Tomaiuolo, F., MacDonald, J. D., Caramanos, Z., Posner, G., Chiavaras, M., Evans, A. C., & Petrides, M. (1999). Morphology, morphometry and probability mapping of the pars opercularis of the inferior frontal gyrus: An in vivo MRI analysis. *European Journal of Neuroscience, 11,* 3033–3046.

Tzourio, N., Nkanga-Ngila, B., & Mazoyer, B. (1998). Left planum temporale surface correlates with functional dominance during story listening. *NeuroReport, 9,* 829–833.

Volkmann, J., Schnitzler, A., Witte, O. W., & Freund, H. (1998). Handedness and asymmetry of hand representation in human motor cortex. *Journal of Neurophysiology, 79,* 2149–2154.

von Bonin, G. (1962). Anatomical asymmetries of the cerebral hemispheres. In V. B. Mountcastle (Ed.), *Interhemispheric relations and cerebral dominance* (pp. 1–6). Baltimore: Johns Hopkins University Press.

Wada, J. A., Clarke, R., & Hamm, A. (1975). Cerebral hemispheric asymmetry in humans. Cortical speech zones in 100 adult and 100 infant brains. *Archives of Neurology, 32,* 239–246.

Westbury, C. F., Zatorre, R. J., & Evans, A. C. (1999). Quantifying variability in the planum temporale: A probability map. *Cerebral Cortex, 9,* 392–405.

White, L. E., Andrews, T. J., Hulette, C., Richards, A., Groelle, M., Paydarfar, D., & Purves, D. (1997a). Structure of the sensorimotor system. I: Morphology and cytoarchitecture of the central sulcus. *Cerebral Cortex, 7,* 18–30.

White, L. E., Andrews, T. J., Hulette, C., Richards, A., Groelle, M., Paydarfar, D., & Purves, D. (1997b). Structure of the sensorimotor system. II: Lateral symmetry. *Cerebral Cortex, 7,* 31–47.

White, L. E., Lucas, G., Richards, A., & Purves, D. (1994). Cerebral asymmetry and handedness. *Nature, 368,* 197–198. (Letter.)

Willerman, L., Schultz, R., Rutledge, J. N., & Bigler, E. D. (1992). Hemispheric size asymmetry predicts relative verbal and nonverbal intelligence differently in the sexes: An MRI study of structure-function relations. *Intelligence, 16,* 315–328.

Witelson, S. F. (1985). The brain connection: The corpus callosum is larger in left-handers. *Science, 229,* 665–668.

Witelson, S. F. (1989). Hand and sex differences in the isthmus and genu of the human corpus callosum. A postmortem morphological study. *Brain, 112*(pt. 3), 799–835.

Witelson, S. F., & Goldsmith, C. H. (1991). The relationship of hand preference to anatomy of the corpus callosum in men. *Brain Research, 545,* 175–182.

Witelson, S. F., & Kigar, D. L. (1992). Sylvian fissure morphology and asymmetry in men and women: Bilateral differences in relation to handedness in men. *Journal of Comparative Neurology, 323,* 326–340.

Yakovlev, P. I., & Lecours, A. R. (1967). The myelogenetic cycles of regional maturation of the brain. In A. Minkowsky (Ed.), *Regional development of the brain in early life* (pp. 3–70). Oxford: Blackwell.

Yazgan, M. Y., Wexler, B. E., Kinsbourne, M., Peterson, B., & Leckman, J. F. (1995). Functional significance of individual variations in callosal area. *Neuropsychologia, 33,* 769–779.

Yeni Komshian, G. H., & Benson, D. A. (1976). Anatomical study of cerebral asymmetry in the temporal lobe of humans, chimpanzees, and rhesus monkeys. *Science, 192,* 387–389.

Zatorre, R. J. (1989). Perceptual asymmetry on the dichotic fused words test and cerebral speech lateralization determined by the carotid sodium amytal test. *Neuropsychologia, 27,* 1207–1219.

Zilles, K. (1992). Neuronal plasticity as an adaptive property of the central nervous system. *Anatomischer Anzeiger, 174,* 383–391.

Zilles, K., Dabringhaus, A., Geyer, S., Amunts, K., Qu, M., Schleicher, A., Gilissen, E., Schlaug, G., & Steinmetz, H. (1996). Structural asymmetries in the human forebrain and the forebrain of non-human primates and rats. *Neuroscience and Biobehavioral Review, 20,* 593–605.

Zilles, K., Kawashima, R., Dabringhaus, A., Fukuda, H., & Schormann, T. (2001). Hemispheric shape of European and Japanese brains: 3-D MRI analysis of intersubject variability, ethnical, and gender differences. *Neuroimage, 13,* 262–271.

7 Transcranial Magnetic Stimulation Studies of Asymmetry of Cognitive Functions in the Brain

Alvaro Pascual-Leone and Vincent Walsh

In the past decades, neuroimaging techniques such as computerized tomography (CT), magnetic resonance imaging (MRI), positron emission tomography (PET), magnetoencephalography (MEG), and electroencephalography (EEG) have shaped the way in which we model behavior. Anatomical neuroimaging techniques have produced ever more detailed descriptions of the extent of lesions produced by brain injury. Functional neuroimaging methods have revealed associations between various behaviors and patterns of activity in cortical and subcortical structures. Functional MRI and PET can inform us about the *location* of a brain activity associated with a function, and event-related potentials (ERPs) using EEG or MEG can provide information about the *timing* of a brain activation during a task. Careful design of neuroimaging experiments may allow us to conclude with reasonable certainty that the correlation of brain activity with behavior is likely to be due to a causal connection (i.e., that the brain activity produces the behavior).

Nevertheless, imaging alone can never provide proof of that assertion. Transcranial magnetic stimulation (TMS) is the only noninvasive technique available that allows us to *interfere* actively with brain function, and thus investigate the relationship between focal cortical activity and behavior, trace the timing at which a cortical region contributes to a given task, and map the functional connectivity between brain regions (Pascual-Leone, Bartres-Faz, et al., 1999; Pascual-Leone & Walsh, 2001; Walsh & Rushworth, 1999; Walsh & Cowey, 2000).

TMS is based on Faraday's principles of electromagnetic induction. A pulse of current flowing through a coil of wire generates a brief magnetic field pulse that will induce a secondary current in any nearby conductor. The rate of change of the magnetic field determines the magnitude of the current induced. When the stimulating coil is discharged over a subject's head, the generated magnetic field passes through the subject's scalp and skull without attenuation (decaying only by the square of the distance), and induces a current in the subject's brain that can stimulate the neural tissue. TMS can be applied in single pulses, pairs of stimuli of the same or different intensity to the same or different brain regions, or a series of pulses at rates of up to 50 Hz (repetitive TMS or rTMS). Single-pulse TMS appears to be safe, but rTMS can cause undesirable side effects, including seizures even in healthy subjects. In either case, appropriate precautions and safety and ethical guidelines should be followed (Wasserman, 1998).

Single-pulse TMS can be used to probe the level of excitability of a cortical region by varying the intensity of the stimuli and establishing the threshold for evoking a given response. This application is particularly obvious when TMS is delivered to the motor cortex and is used to induce twitches of contralateral limb muscles that can be recorded using electromyographic techniques as motor evoked potentials (figure 7.1; Rothwell, 1997). However, the same methodology can be employed by applying TMS to the somatosensory cortex and recording the induction of paresthesias (Amassian et al., 1991), or to the occipital cortex and recording the subject's perception of phosphenes, brief flashes of light evoked by depolarization of visual cortical neurons (Marg and Rudiak, 1994; Stewart et al., 2001).

Paired-pulse TMS can be used in much the same manner to provide greater insight into corticocortical excitability (Kujirai et al., 1993; Pascual-Leone et al., 1998). Typically, two stimuli are delivered to the same brain area, a subthreshold (conditioning) stimulus and thereafter a suprathreshold (test) stimulus. Depending on the interval between the two stimuli, the response to the test stimulus is differentially modulated by the preceding conditioning stimulus, which provides insight into inhibitory or excitatory corticocortical connections (figure 7.1). These effects appear to depend on the cortical region and to be influenced by the task being tested (Oliveri et al., 2000).

Trains of rTMS (at appropriate intensity and frequency of stimulation) can be used to transiently disrupt the function of a given cortical target, thus creating a temporary "virtual brain lesion" (Pascual-Leone, Bartres-Faz, et al., 1999; Pascual-Leone & Walsh, 2001; Walsh & Rushworth, 1999; Walsh & Cowey, 2000). In this type of application, rTMS is

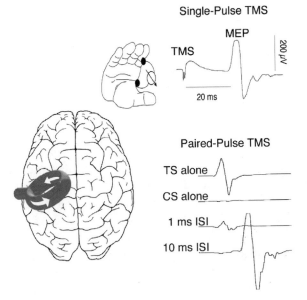

Single-Pulse TMS

MEP

TMS

200 μV

20 ms

Paired-Pulse TMS

TS alone

CS alone

1 ms ISI

10 ms ISI

Figure 7.1 Schematic representation of TMS application to the motor cortex to induce motor-evoked potentials (MEPs) in contralateral hand muscles. MEPs to single-pulse stimulation and to paired-pulse stimulation are presented. Note the lack of response to the conditioning stimulus (CS), which is set at subthreshold intensity. When CS precedes the test stimulus (TS) by 1 ms, the MEP is markedly smaller (compared to the response to TS alone). Conversely, there is facilitation of the response to TS preceded by CS at an interstimulus interval (ISI) of 10 ms. See text for details.

a useful first step, helping to address the question of whether a given brain region is functionally relevant for a given behavior, and inviting subsequent studies to analyze the timing of this causal contribution. In such studies, single stimuli are applied, thus disrupting activity for only some tens of milliseconds and providing information on *when* activity contributes essentially to task performance (the "chronometry" of cognition).

In this fashion, single-pulse TMS applied to the motor cortex can investigate the timing of the engagement of the motor cortex in the execution of motor programs (Day et al., 1989); applied to the somatosensory cortex, it can provide insight into the time course of tactile perception (Cohen et al., 1991); and applied to the occipital cortex, it can explore the chronometry of detection and perception of visual stimuli (Amassian et al., 1989). In a similar kind of application, paired-pulse

TMS can be applied to two different brain regions at different times in order to investigate the chronometric interaction between them during a given task. This has recently been illustrated in a study on the role of feedback connections between visual areas MT+/V5 (motion area) and V1 (primary visual cortex) in visual awareness (Pascual-Leone and Walsh, 2001).

Our knowledge about the precise mechanisms of action of TMS is still limited, despite studies in animal models and in neurosurgical patients. For example, we still know little about the spatial resolution of TMS or the depth of stimulation in the brain, and we cannot say which neural elements are likely to be most sensitive to TMS in a particular area of brain or during a given task. Nevertheless, despite these limitations, TMS promises to reshape the way we investigate brain-behavior relations. The majority of TMS experiments in cognitive neuroscience rely on the fact that a TMS stimulus applied to any given brain area will disrupt the neural processing which is going on at the time. If that processing was contributing essentially to the performance of a given task, we can expect to observe deterioration in performance. We will then be able to conclude that there was a functional connection between activity in the stimulated brain area and the assessed behavior. At this level of resolution (cognitive, rather than spatial or temporal), we can trust the technique and need not know precisely which elements in the brain were activated by the stimulus.

TMS IN STUDIES OF BRAIN ASYMMETRY

Fundamentally, three different types of studies can be conducted with TMS to investigate the asymmetry of cognitive functions in the brain. In all its forms of application, TMS can be used as single-pulse, paired-pulse, or repetitive stimulation. In addition, TMS can be applied on-line (i.e., during the performance of a given task) or off-line (prior to a task, in order to influence performance, or before and after a task, in order to evaluate the effect that the given task might have on cortical excitability or TMS effects) (figure 7.2).

First, TMS can be used as a probe to demonstrate interhemispheric asymmetric representations. The studies of Triggs et al. (1994, 1997, 1999) examining the motor cortical output maps to the preferred and nonpreferred hands are good examples of this type of application, and are discussed below. Speech arrest studies might represent the same

Alvaro Pascual-Leone and Vincent Walsh

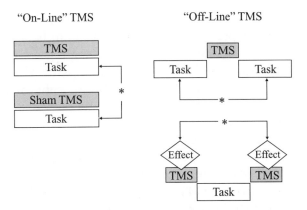

"On-Line" TMS   "Off-Line" TMS

Figure 7.2 Schematic representation of the different paradigms of TMS application in the study of cognitive functions: on-line TMS and off-line TMS are represented. See text for details.

type of application, but in this case the subject is asked to perform a task and the brain is hence not at rest, but rather is engaged in a specific task, while being probed. Therefore, we might consider this as an instance in which TMS is used to probe the lateralized effects of tasks. The subject is engaged in a task that might preferentially activate one hemisphere over the other. TMS is then used to demonstrate such asymmetric activation. The studies of modulation of the right and left motor cortical outputs during reading (Tokimura et al., 1996) or mood induction (Tormos et al., 1997) are fine examples of this type of application. Finally, TMS can be used to demonstrate the neurobiological basis of cognitive functions that are lateralized. Studies on speech and language, memory, or attention are suitable examples for this form of TMS application that will be discussed in greater detail in this chapter.

There have been a number of studies on mood effects of TMS that could also be used to exemplify applications of TMS in the study of lateralized neural functions and that deserve mention. In normal subjects, rTMS to the left hemisphere appears to induce transient sadness and anxiety, while the same stimulation applied to the right prefrontal cortex can lead to increased happiness and energy (Pascual-Leone, Catala et al., 1996; George et al., 1996). These effects of rTMS on mood have been extended to patients with depression, where rTMS might in fact have a therapeutic potential, though results are still unclear and quite debated (George & Bellmaker, 2000; Reid et al., 1998;

Sackeim, 2000). Nevertheless, it is interesting to note that in the application of TMS in depression, there also appears to be a lateralization of effects, such that an antidepressant effect might be evoked by high-frequency stimulation of the left (but not the right) dorsolateral prefrontal cortex (George ct al., 1997; Pascual-Leone, Rubio, et al., 1996), or by low-frequency stimulation of the right (but not the left) dorsolateral prefrontal cortex (Klein et al., 1999).

Given the differential effects of rTMS on motor cortical excitability depending on stimulation frequency (Maeda et al., 2000; Pascual-Leone, Valls-Sole et al., 1994), it seems reasonable to suspect that similar differences are present when rTMS is applied to the dorsolateral prefrontal cortex, and that the differential results of low- and high-frequency rTMS of the right and of the left side on depressive symptoms reveal bihemispheric asymmetries in the control of mood and affect.

TMS AS A PROBE OF ASYMMETRIC REPRESENTATION IN THE BRAIN: HANDEDNESS

The studies on the asymmetry of cortical motor representation depending on hand preference are a good illustration of the application of TMS in the study of asymmetries in the brain. Mcdonell et al. (1991) observed hemispheric asymmetry in the threshold for induction of motor evoked potentials (MEPs) in a group of 19 right-handed subjects. The threshold for eliciting MEPs in the right hand was significantly lower than the threshold for eliciting MEPs in the left hand. These findings were subsequently confirmed and extended by Triggs et al. (1994) in a study on 60 subjects. In right-handers, the MEP threshold for the left hand was lower than the one for the right hand, while in left-handers the reverse asymmetry was demonstrated (Triggs et al., 1994). The hemispheric asymmetry in MEP thresholds correlated with hand differences in finger tapping and pegboard dexterity measures (Triggs et al., 1997). It should be noted that other TMS studies have failed to find similar results (Cicinelli et al., 1997; Wilson et al., 1993), and it seems clear that very careful attention to methodological questions is critical. More recently, using detailed TMS mapping techniques with a focal, 8-shaped coil, Triggs et al. (1999) were able to show that the cortical output maps for the abductor pollicis brevis (APB) and the first dorsal interosseous (FDI) muscles of the preferred hand were larger than those of the nonpreferred hand (figure 7.3).

Alvaro Pascual-Leone and Vincent Walsh

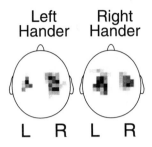

Left   Right
Hander   Hander

L   R   L   R

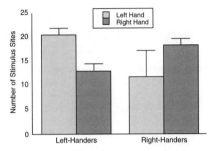

Figure 7.3 The top two figures illustrate representative examples of motor cortical output maps to the right and left first dorsal interosseous muscles (FDI) in a left-handed and a right-handed subject. Note the larger output maps for the muscle of the preferred hand in both instances. The lower bar histogram displays the average results of all subjects studied. The sizes of the motor output maps are quantified by the number of scalp locations over which TMS led to induction of motor evoked potentials in the contralateral FDI. Note the greater number of scalp positions for the maps of the preferred hands, in both right- and left-handed subjects. (Modified from Triggs et al., 1997, with permission.)

These findings are consistent with those obtained by Nudo et al. (1992), using intracortical microstimulation to investigate the motor representations in squirrel monkeys. In these animals, the cortical motor representations contralateral to the hand that the animals preferred for performing tasks which required independent finger control were both larger and more complex than the corresponding representation contralateral to the nonpreferred hand. However, demonstrating that handedness is associated with asymmetry in the motor cortical output maps of the preferred and the nonpreferred hands (in animals or humans) does not differentiate whether such asymmetry reflects differential use of the two hands or whether it is evidence of a biological predisposition for preferential hand use.

There is no doubt that motor output maps as determined by TMS are markedly altered by training and experience (Cohen et al., 1998; Pascual-Leone, Tarazona et al., 1999). Indeed, the impact of use can be very rapid and dramatic, as demonstrated by the study of motor cortical outputs to the preferred reading finger in Braille readers. In these subjects the cortical output maps can be shown to change significantly following a day at work (reading Braille for 4–6 hours) or after a weekend without Braille reading (Pascual-Leone et al., 1995). Studies of motor cortical outputs during development ought to be most informative in this regard, because they would allow the demonstration of possible motor cortical output asymmetries prior to the development of clear hand preference, and follow the establishment of asymmetries with use. TMS can indeed be used for such serial studies on the development of cortical output maps and corticospinal projections (Heinen et al., 1998; Müller et al., 1992; Nezu et al., 1997), so that in the future it might inform on this issue.

TMS TO PROBE THE LATERALIZED EFFECTS OF TASKS: EFFECTS OF READING AND MOOD INDUCTION

Following an observation by Schaafsma (1988), Tokimura et al. (1996) investigated the enhancement of motor responses from hand muscles during speech. They recorded compound motor action potentials from relaxed FDI muscles of both hands while subjects performed a variety of speech output tasks. Spontaneous speech increased the size of the MEPs bilaterally, and reading aloud increased only MEPs evoked by TMS to the dominant hemisphere. For ten normal right-handed subjects, this facilitation by reading aloud was uniformly larger in the right hand, appeared reliably on consecutive days, and was independent of the language used. For three normal left-handed subjects, two had increases only in the left hand, and one had bilateral facilitation. The authors hypothesized that reading aloud may increase excitability of the motor hand area in the dominant hemisphere, and that this procedure might represent a simpler and safer alternative to rTMS for assessment of cerebral dominance.

Using essentially the same methodology and study design, Tormos et al. (1997) asked whether a similar facilitatory effect of the corticospinal projection can be induced by mentally evoking different emotionally charged thoughts, and whether this facilitatory effect shows a lateralization. A lateralization of such a facilitatory effect can be hypothesized since neuroimaging and lesion studies show lateralized contributions of left and right prefrontal cortex to mood. Right-handed subjects (n = 14) sat comfortably in a room with dimmed light. The head was held in a constant position by means of a specially designed device with a chin and a forehead rest. The same device held two magnetic stimulation coils in position, one over the right hemisphere and one over the left. Stimuli were delivered pseudo randomly through the right or the left stimulation coil. Electromyography (EMG) was recorded from the right and left FDI muscles. Stimulation intensity was chosen so that at rest, peak-to-peak amplitude of the MEPs ranged from 0.5 to 1.5 mV. Stimulation was delivered as single bipolar pulses with interstimulus intervals of at least 10 s.

In each subject 120 trials were recorded in 4 blocks of 30 trials. Each trial consisted of an instruction for the subject and the application of a single TMS stimulus to either the right or the left hemisphere. Throughout the study the subjects were instructed to maintain the FDI relaxed. Continuous EMG monitoring with visual and auditory feedback was used to assure FDI relaxation. Three instructions were possible, and were intermixed randomly: (1) add mentally in steps of 3, starting with a given number; (2) try to evoke feelings of sadness by thinking back to a time when you felt particularly blue; (3) try to evoke feelings of happiness by thinking back to a time when you felt particularly elated. These instructions were presented in standardized form, using a neutral voice recording on an audiotape. Magnetic stimuli were applied 5 to 10 s following the instructions. This interval was varied randomly. Each block consisted of 10 trials of each instruction, 5 with right-sided and 5 with left-sided TMS. The order of the trials in each block was random, and counterbalanced across blocks and subjects.

All subjects felt able to follow the instructions without difficulty and all tolerated the procedure without side effects. The MEPs evoked by right and left hemispheric stimulation during mental counting were of comparable amplitude, while the MEPs evoked from the left hemisphere (right FDI recording) were larger during thinking of sad thoughts and markedly suppressed during thinking happy thoughts (figure 7.4). Thinking sad thoughts led to a significant lateralized effect on MEP amplitude, with MEPs evoked from the left hemisphere being facilitated. Conversely, there was the inverse effect for thinking happy thoughts. This led to a facilitation of MEPs evoked from the right hemisphere, but

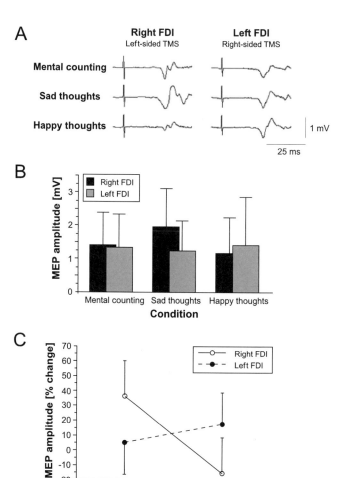

Figure 7.4 (*A*) Representative examples of the motor evoked potentials (MEP) induced by left or right hemispheric transcranial magnetic stimulation (TMS) in right and left first dorsal interosseous muscle (FDI), respectively. (*B*) Bar histograms of the MEP amplitude (mean and standard deviation in all 14 subjects) evoked by TMS in right or left FDI during the three different conditions. (*C*) Line graph of the MEP amplitude (mean and standard deviation in all 14 subjects), expressed as percentage change from the control condition (mental counting), depending on self-induced emotion. (Modified from Tormos et al., 1997, with permission.)

Alvaro Pascual-Leone and Vincent Walsh

a reduction in the amplitude of the MEPs evoked from the left. In two subjects an additional experiment was conducted to evaluate the relative contributions of spinal and cortical mechanisms to the described phenomena. H-reflexes on the right or left flexor muscles in the forearm (FCR) did not show any significant modulation with either thinking sad or happy thoughts. Nevertheless, the cortical TMS-evoked MEPs showed prominent modulation in both subjects, depending on the affective content of the thoughts.

Therefore, Tormos et al.'s (1997) results show a differential, lateralized effect of self-induced sad and happy thoughts on corticospinal excitability. The left hemispheric corticospinal projection shows an increase in corticospinal excitability when the subjects evoke sad thoughts, while there is a reduction in excitability during happy thoughts. Conversely, the right hemispheric corticospinal projection shows the opposite modulation by sad and happy thoughts. The experiment with H-reflexes supports the notion that this modulation of corticospinal excitability takes place at supraspinal, presumably cortical, level. Overall, the modulation of left hemispheric corticospinal excitability by self-induced emotions was much greater. Certainly, the method use for mood induction in this study is rather loose and poorly controlled. Further, better behaviorally controlled studies are desirable. However, the findings illustrate the potential of TMS to reveal asymmetric effects of tasks on cortical and corticospinal excitability.

PROBING THE NEURAL CIRCUITRY OF LATERALIZED FUNCTIONS: SPEECH AND LANGUAGE

One of the most dramatic effects of TMS is the induction of speech arrest, and this represents a clear example of the use of rTMS to demonstrate asymmetric representations in the human brain. Several investigators have reported that rTMS over left frontal cortex can cause subjects to cease speaking or to stutter or repeat segments of words. Pascual-Leone et al. (1991) were the first to induce speech arrest (25 Hz rTMS with a round coil) in a population of epileptic subjects awaiting surgery. The TMS determination of the dominant hemisphere in all six subjects matched that obtained in the Wada test.

The Wada test, named for its inventor, Dr. Jun Wada, is extensively used in preoperative evaluation for neurosurgical interventions near language areas. Wada testing involves placing an angiography catheter in the internal carotid artery and injecting sodium amobarbital in order to anesthetize the corresponding arterial territories of one hemisphere for several minutes. During this time the examiner can assess the language and memory capabilities of the other hemisphere. The Wada test is hampered by significant risks and potential pitfalls. Risks associated with the placement of the angiography catheter result in approximately 4% morbidity. Technical problems include normal and pathological variations in the branches and territories perfused by the internal carotid artery, overflow of drug into other vascular territories, and unpredictable interindividual variations in the effects of the same dose.

Interpretation of the results is complicated by the limited time available for testing, and by simultaneous behavioral changes (including hemiparesis, mood changes, and somnolence). Furthermore, repeat testing is very difficult. Therefore, replacement of the invasive Wada test with a noninvasive, safe procedure would indeed be most welcome. The results of TMS studies in this respect have been variable, largely because of the different hardware and criteria for speech arrest adopted by different groups, and at this point, there is not sufficient evidence to support such a claim.

The induction of speech arrest by TMS was replicated, again in epileptic patients, by Jennum et al. (1994; 30 Hz rTMS), who also found a strong concordance with the results of the Wada test. In studies that may require hundreds of trials, 25 and 30 Hz are too high frequencies, given current safety guidelines (Wasserman, 1996); a later study by Epstein, Lah et al. (1996) identified 4–8 Hz as the optimum range of rTMS frequency for induction of speech arrest in normal subjects. They were also able to distinguish between speech arrest associated with frontal cortex stimulation and absent effects of TMS on facial muscles, and speech arrest associated with loss of control of the facial muscles.

Three recent studies (Epstein et al., 1999; Bartres-Faz et al., 1999; Stewart et al., 2001) also obtained speech arrest lateralized to the left hemisphere with frontal stimulation. Epstein et al. suggest that their effects are due to motor cortex stimulation, but this is difficult to reconcile with the left unilateral dominance of the effects and also with the results of the other two studies that provide independent anatomical and physiological evidence of a dissociation between frontal stimulation and pure motor effects. Bartres-Faz's and Stewart's studies locate

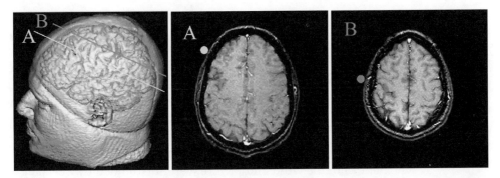

Figure 7.5 The results in a representative subject are presented. The 3-D reconstruction of the subject's head MRI (*left*) demonstrates the sites of TMS application and the level of the axial slices of fMRI displayed in the other two panels. The middle figure illustrates the statistically significant fMRI BOLD changes observed during the performance of the verbal fluency task, and marks on the scalp show the location of the TMS coil for induction of speech arrest. Note that speech arrest is induced by TMS over brain regions that are activated during the verbal fluency task. The figure at right shows the most representative slice of fMRI BOLD activity corresponding to a motor task consisting of opening and closing the right hand, which is shown to be directly under the TMS scalp position that evokes hand movements (but does not lead to speech arrest). Note that the changes corresponding to the motor areas appear more posterior than those responsible for the word generation task. The latter include the areas targeted by rTMS during speech arrest. (Modified from Bartres-Faz et al., 1998, with permission.) See plate 2 for color version.

the critical site of stimulation over the middle frontal gyrus, dorsal to the inferior frontal gyrus and what is usually referred to as Broca's area (figure 7.5; plate 2). These findings are in agreement with lesion data, electrical stimulation mapping, and PET studies, all of which have shown several areas, including the middle temporal gyrus, to be important in speech production.

Speech arrest can be obtained from direct electrical stimulation of so many brain regions that it clearly will be very difficult to try to pin down a single area with TMS. On the other hand, TMS can be used to produce language-related dissociations that address theoretical questions. This area is wide open for new approaches using TMS: Human lesions that produce language deficits typically are large; animal lesions of course cannot address the question of language. In such studies, TMS can be applied at intensity levels too low to induce arrest but sufficient to incur reaction time costs in verbal tasks. Indeed, Pascual-Leone et al. (1991) noted that counting errors and paraphasias could be induced by rTMS to the same sites that led to speech arrest, but at lower stimulation intensities. Flitman et al. (1998) applied rTMS over frontal and parietal lobes while subjects judged whether a word was congruent with a simultaneously presented picture. Subjects were slower to verify the congruency when TMS was applied to the frontal site of the dominant hemisphere. However, it is not clear whether they were impaired on any particular cognitive aspect of this task or performance was affected by TMS simply because the load on the language system was greater than in the control condition that required stating whether or not the word and picture were surrounded by a rectangular frame.

Stewart et al. (2001) have begun to probe parts of the language system by taking the prediction that BA37 has a role in phonological retrieval and object naming. Repetitive pulse TMS was applied over the posterior region of BA37 of the left and right hemispheres and over the vertex. Repetitive TMS had significant effects on picture naming but no effect on word reading, nonword reading, or color naming. Thus, with respect to object encoding and naming, the posterior region of BA37 would seem to be critical for recognition.

Picture naming was also examined by Töpper et al. (1998), who applied single-pulse TMS over Wernicke's area and motor cortex. Somewhat paradoxically, TMS over Wernicke's area 500–1000 msecs prior to picture presentation resulted in faster reaction times than control trials. The effect was specific to task and area, and the authors concluded that TMS "is able to facilitate lexical processes due to a general preactivation of language-related neuronal networks when delivered over Wernicke's area." While these effects are intriguing, they raise several questions about why TMS would have facilitatory effects within a system.

Paradoxical lesion effects, such as disruption of a given area resulting in disinhibition of another, remote site, need to be considered alongside generalized arousal within the language system. More than in any other kind of result, it is important that the apparently facilitatory effects of TMS are grounded in theoretical frameworks and that the mechanisms proposed in one modality are applicable to others. Further studies of these effects are clearly necessary.

Shapiro et al. (2001) used TMS to study grammatical distinctions in the frontal cortex and demonstrated the role of the left frontal cortex in representation of verbs as a grammatical class. Selective deficits in producing verbs relative to nouns in speech are well documented in neuropsychology and have been associated with left-hemisphere frontal cortical lesions resulting from a variety of causes. This functional-anatomical link, though problematic, has led some researchers to propose that verb retrieval is mediated by left frontal or frontostriatal circuits that also subserve motor planning.

Previous attempts to verify the neural substrates of verb retrieval with data from unimpaired speakers have been inconclusive. Though electrophysiological studies have shown increased left-lateralized anterior positivity when verbs are produced (compared to nouns), functional neuroimaging either has failed to reveal differences in patterns of activation between nouns and verbs or has shown that verb generation recruits a patchwork of areas in the left hemisphere (see Shapiro et al., 2001 for discussion). It is not obvious from these data whether frontal circuits are necessarily and specifically engaged in verb production.

Shapiro et al. (2001) used rTMS to target a portion of prefrontal cortex along the midfrontal gyrus anterior and superior to Broca's area while subjects performed a linguistic task involving regular nouns or verbs. Eight right-handed native speakers of English aged 20 to 29 years (mean = 21.6 years) participated in the study. The experiment was divided into four blocks, each of which consisted of two sets of 80 trials separated by an interval of 300 pulses of rTMS at 1 Hz and 110% of the motor threshold intensity, applied with a focal 8-shaped coil. A 10-minute rest period followed each block to allow the effects of rTMS to wash out. The first two blocks were control blocks in which the TMS coil was positioned to produce a sensation similar to real stimulation, but no cortical interference.

In each trial the subject was presented with a stimulus word (either a noun or a verb) for 250 ms, followed for another 250 ms by a symbolic cue indicating the morphological form in which the word was to be produced aloud—singular or plural for nouns (e.g., *song*, *songs*), third-person singular or plural for verbs (e.g., *sings*, *sing*). Plural and singular stimulus words were paired randomly with cues so that the required manipulation (if any) for each stimulus was unpredictable. It is important to note that given the task design, the manipulations were phonologically identical for nouns and verbs, involving addition and subtraction of the morpheme (s). Nouns and verbs were presented in alternate blocks in an order that varied by subject.

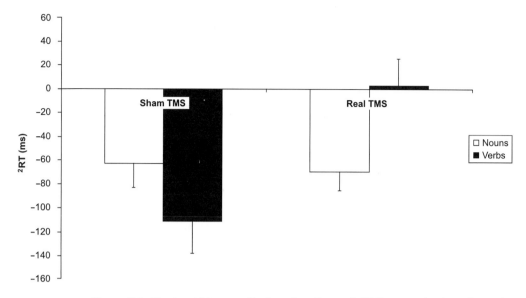

Figure 7.6 The bar histogram displays the effects of rTMS on production of pseudo words used as nouns and verbs (see text for details). As with real words, statistically equivalent decreases in average response latency were observed after sham stimulation for both nouns and verbs. However, real rTMS to the left, but not to the right, frontal cortex led to a decrease in average response time for nouns (due to practice effect) following the rTMS, but no such decrease for verbs. Therefore, the results demonstrate a critical role of left prefrontal cortex in processing verbs, since disruption of function in this area prevented the expected practice-induced decrease in response times. (Modified from Shapiro et al., 2001, with permission.)

Figure 7.6 summarizes the results. Following sham stimulation, average response latencies decreased markedly from baseline for both nouns and verbs. The magnitude of this decrease did not differ significantly between word classes when compared for individual subjects, and there was no interaction between time and grammatical class. When real stimulation was applied, the results were strikingly different. There was again a decrease in average response time for nouns, identical to the decrease in the sham condition. However, average response time for verbs *increased* following rTMS, a change that was both qualitatively and quantitatively different from that seen after sham stimulation, and that suggests verb production had been specifically hindered.

Alvaro Pascual-Leone and Vincent Walsh

Word production is a multistage process with separate components involved in the computation of a word's meaning, grammatical function, and sound structure; nouns and verbs may differ prototypically in any or all of these dimensions. The results of Shapiro et al. (2001) demonstrate for the first time that neural circuits in the left frontal cortex adjacent to Broca's area are critical at some stage in the spoken production of verbs by unimpaired individuals, and illustrate the potential of TMS in studies of linguistic processing and asymmetry of language.

PROBING THE NEURAL CIRCUITRY OF LATERALIZED FUNCTIONS: VERBAL MEMORY

Language-related memory function has been studied by Grafman et al. (1994). Subjects received rTMS at 20 Hz, 120% of motor threshold for 500 msecs over one of several cortical sites while they were presented with a list of words. Focal TMS was applied, using a specially designed water-cooled coil, to right or left temporo-occipital, temporoparietal, midtemporal, and dorsolateral frontal regions. Recall of the words was then tested. Selective deficits in recall were produced only by rTMS over left midtemporal or either left or right dorsolateral frontal stimulation when the stimulation was applied either at the onset or with a delay of 250 ms after onset of the visual word display. The authors concluded that this impairment represented a failure of retrieval from long-term memory and speculated that the regional effects of rTMS on recall might be due to disruptive effects on lateralized cortical semantic consolidation processes temporally, and on bihemispheric, contextual consolidation processes frontally.

Düzel et al. (1996) used single-pulse TMS to evaluate verbal working memory in epilepsy patients. They found subtle, focal effects on the digit span test: only with left hemisphere stimulation and only in patients with left temporal origin of seizures. The total number of digit span errors was unchanged; but the number of recency errors decreased significantly with left temporal stimulation, and increased significantly with TMS over the vertex. Düzel et al. relate these results to a specialized verbal subsystem, the phonological loop, that may involve the supramarginal gyrus and posterior temporal lobe. They speculate that left temporal lobe epilepsy may represent a preexisting lesion of this physiological system whose effects were compounded by those of

TMS. This study illustrates, in regard to the application of TMS to the study of asymmetry of cortical functions, the intriguing suggestion of an interaction between the laterality of the underlying pathology, the asymmetry of hemispheric activation for a given task, and the effects of TMS.

Mottaghy et al. (2000) investigated the effect of repetitive TMS (rTMS) over the left or right dorsolateral prefrontal cortex on the performance in a two-back verbal working memory task and correlated these behavioral effects with the changes induced in regional cerebral blood flow (rCBF) in the involved neuronal network. Stimulation of the midline frontal cortex served as a reference condition because this brain region is thought not to play a critical role in working memory.

Subjects saw 20 letters (A–D five times each, in a randomized order) and were instructed to press one of two buttons with the index or ring finger of the right hand to indicate whether each presented letter was the same (ring finger) or not the same (index finger) as the letter presented two earlier in the sequence. In the control task (0-back condition) they had to press the left button each time an X was presented and the right button each time a Y was presented. Repetitive TMS was applied while the subjects performed the task in the PET scanner. Stimulation was delivered with a figure-eight coil centered over F3, F4, or Fz of the international 10–20 system for stimulation of the left dorsolateral prefrontal cortex, right dorsolateral prefrontal cortex, or midline frontal cortex, respectively. Precise anatomical information about the brain area stimulated in each subject was obtained by a three-dimensional reconstructed brain MRI in which vitamin A capsules were taped onto the stimulated scalp locations (F4, F3, and Fz). Subjects received a single train of rTMS at 4 Hz and 110% of the individual motor threshold intensity during the two-back or the reference condition that was started with the bolus injection of ^{15}O-butanol and stopped after 30 seconds.

rTMS to right or left dorsolateral prefrontal cortex significantly impaired performance in the working memory task, whereas rTMS to the midline frontal cortex did not interfere with the performance (figure 7.7; plate 3). Performance on the control task was not affected by rTMS to any of the target areas. Therefore, no asymmetry of the TMS effects was detected at the behavioral level. However, the PET data revealed a rather different picture. During the task, bilateral dorsolateral prefrontal cortex (Brodmann area [BA] 9/46), premotor areas (BA6), the anterior cingulate (BA24/32), bilateral inferior parietal areas (BA39/40), the precuneus (BA7), and the cerebellum were activated. Comparison of the

Alvaro Pascual-Leone and Vincent Walsh

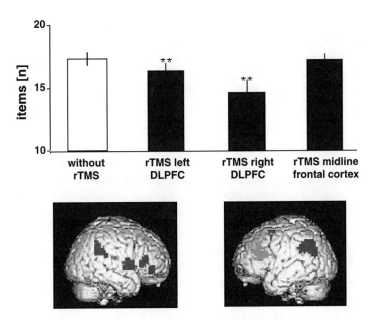

Figure 7.7 The bar histogram displays the number of correct items (n = 20) in the task, depending on stimulation condition. The first bar represents the performance in the two-back working-memory task without rTMS; the second, with rTMS over the left dorsolateral prefrontal cortex; the third, with rTMS over the right dorsolateral prefrontal cortex; and the fourth, with rTMS over the midline prefrontal cortex. ** = $p < .01$ (paired t-test). The bottom part of the figure shows the spatial distribution of rCBF changes. Specifically, the deactivations induced by rTMS of the left (green) and the right (blue) dorsolateral prefrontal cortex are shown as an overlay on a 3-D surface-rendered anatomical MR ($p < .01$; $k = 20$) to illustrate the differences in TMS-induced changes in brain activity despite similar behavioral effects. (Modified from Mottaghy et al., 2000, with permission.) See plate 3 for color version.

conditions with and without rTMS over the left or the right prefrontal cortex revealed that rTMS reduced activity in the targeted brain region but also changed the activation of the distributed network.

In spite of the seemingly similar behavioral consequences, rTMS-induced deactivations in the distributed, bihemispheric network were different for right and left prefrontal stimulation (figure 7.7). rTMS to the left dorsolateral prefrontal cortex (F3) led to significant reductions in rCBF in the left prefrontal cortex. rTMS to the right dorsolateral prefrontal cortex (F4) significantly decreased activity in right prefrontal, but also in bilateral parietal areas (BA7/40) and the left prefrontal cortex. Stimulation of the midline frontal cortex did not lead to a significant rCBF change in the involved network of brain regions.

This study combining rTMS and PET exemplifies a novel approach to demonstrating relations between brain activity and behavior. Mottaghy et al. (2000) demonstrate with PET that rTMS to the prefrontal cortex modulates the cortical neural circuitry subserving working memory by changing the activation patterns of the involved, distributed neuronal network. The transient disruption of either right or left dorsolateral prefrontal cortex results in a significant deterioration in the performance of the memory task, emphasizing the crucial role of normal bilateral prefrontal cortex activity for working memory. However, despite the similar behavioral consequences, the changes in activation of elements of a distributed network are different for right and left dorsolateral prefrontal cortex stimulation.

It is important to realize, as Lomber and Payne (1999) have argued regarding experiments with cooling probes, that transient disruption of a given cortical region tells us mostly about the capacity of the rest of the brain to adjust (react/adapt) to it. Hence, "functional connectivity experiments" combining TMS with functional imaging might in fact reveal the capacity of the brain to rapidly adjust to the disruption of a given area in the attempt to maintain behavior. In this case, neuroimaging studies associated with TMS during a task illustrate bihemispheric asymmetry that the behavioral measures themselves fail to capture.

Paus et al. (1997, 1998, 1999) were the first to introduce TMS combined with functional neuroimaging as a method to map neural connections in the living human brain. TMS is used to directly stimulate a selected cortical area while simultaneously measuring changes in brain activity, indexed by CBF, with PET. Ilmoniemi et al. (1997) used a similar approach in combining TMS with quantitative EEG. To date, these studies, except the one by Mottaghy et al. (2000), discussed above, have not addressed questions of bihemispheric asymmetry. Nevertheless, the combination of TMS with neuroimaging provides a novel tool to probe hemispheric differences in brain connectivity.

PROBING THE NEURAL CIRCUITRY OF LATERALIZED FUNCTIONS: ATTENTION

A different application of TMS that has illustrated bihemispheric asymmetry consists of studies on neglect and attention, an area in which much neurological literature would support a notion of functional laterality with the right parietal lobe playing a critical role. The ability to focus attention is normally taken for granted. The existence of special attentional mechanisms often becomes apparent only when they fail. Patients with unilateral lesions in regions of the parietal and premotor cortex frequently show (hemi)neglect with reduced spatial attention to sensory stimulation in the contralateral hemispace. Human spatial attention appears to be remarkably lateralized, since left hemineglect, caused by damage to the right hemisphere, is much more frequently encountered and more severe than right hemineglect. These deficits are more apparent during bilateral stimulation with the patient demonstrating extinction to double simultaneous stimulation.

Modeling neurological patients by transient disruption of focal brain areas with TMS allows the study of brain-behavior relationships avoiding the whim and limitations of natural lesions (Pascual-Leone, Bartres-Faz, et al., 1999). Replicating the effects seen in patients is a good starting point for a TMS study, but it may also be a good end point. Replication is rarely exact, and the differences between real and the virtual patients can be important. In the first demonstration of attentional effects with rTMS, stimulation was applied at 25 Hz to the occipital, parietal, or temporal cortices (Pascual-Leone, Gomez-Tortosa, et al., 1994). The aim was to study visual extinction to double simultaneous stimulation. Patients showing extinction can detect and identify targets that are presented singly in one visual field, but fail to detect the left-sided stimulus when right- and left-sided stimuli are presented at the same time. Repetitive TMS of the right parietal cortex duly reproduced visual extinction of left visual field stimuli when two targets were presented. But left parietal stimulation produced the phenomenon with equal facility. The difference between the real and virtual patients can be accounted for by invoking plastic reorganization following brain damage.

A study by Oliveri, Rossini et al. (1999) elegantly illustrates the potential of TMS in providing chronometric information to the causal role of a given cortical region for a behavior, and expands these findings on TMS in the study of bihemispheric asymmetry in attention and neglect. Oliveri et al. used TMS in a tactile stimulus detection task to demonstrate that the right, but not the left, parietal cortex is critical for detection not only of contralateral but also of ipsilateral stimuli. They found that bimanual discrimination is more readily disrupted than unimanual tasks, but only during right (not left) parietal TMS. Most important, they showed that the contribution of the right parietal cortex takes place 40 ms after the tactile stimuli are applied, suggesting involvement of late cortical events.

Olivieri, Rossini et al. (1999) then applied TMS to patients with right hemispheric lesions. When stimuli were applied simultaneously to both hands, patients often failed to detect the stimulus on the left side. Stimulation (at intensities 10% higher than used in normal subjects) of left frontal, but not parietal, cortex significantly reduced the rate of extinction. Therefore, as in the animal model (Lomber and Payne, 1996), transient disruption of the healthy hemisphere restores spatial attention and improves neglect. These results support the notion of an interhemispheric competition (possibly asymmetrical) of cortical or subcortical structures to explain spatial attention.

This notion of interhemispheric competition in guiding attention was directly put to the test by Hilgetag et al. (2001), using an off-line rTMS paradigm. They found ipsilateral enhancement of visual attention, compared to normal performance (figure 7.8), produced by rTMS of the parietal cortex at stimulation parameters known to reduce cortical excitability. Healthy, right-handed volunteers received rTMS (1 Hz, 10 mins) over right or left parietal cortex (at P3 or P4 EEG coordinate point, respectively). This type of stimulation is expected to transiently disrupt cortical function by inducing a depression of excitability that outlasts the duration of the rTMS train itself (Chen et al., 1997; Maeda et al., 2000).

Subsequently, subjects' attention to ipsilateral visual targets improved significantly while contralateral attention diminished. In addition, correct detection of bilateral stimuli decreased significantly, coupled with an increase in erroneous responses for ipsilateral unilateral targets. Application of the same rTMS paradigm to motor cortex and sham magnetic stimulation indicated that the effect was specific for stimulation of parietal cortex. These results underline the potential of focal brain dysfunction to produce behavioral improvement and provide experimental support for models of visuospatial attention based on the interhemispheric competition of cortical components in a large-scale attentional network.

CONCLUSIONS

Transcranial magnetic stimulation, applied as single pulses, paired-pulses, or trains of repetitive stimulation, provides a unique oppor-

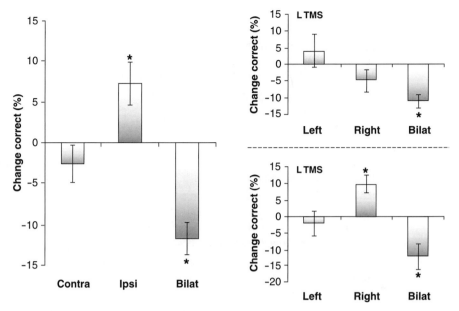

Figure 7.8 Changes in correct stimulus detection after parietal rTMS. The diagrams are based on changes in the number of correctly detected stimuli (relative to the total number of presented stimuli), averaged for both stimulus sizes and all subjects. (*a*) The pooled data show a significant increase in performance ipsilateral to the parietal rTMS location (increase in relative percentage, 7.3%; SEM, 2.6%) and a trend to decreased contralateral performance (reduction by 2.5%; SEM, 2.3%). In addition, detection of bilateral stimuli decreased significantly (−11.7%; SEM, 2.0%). These trends are also apparent after separating data for (*b*) left parietal TMS and (*c*) right parietal rTMS. Significant trends (as determined by z-tests) are marked by asterisks. (Modified from Hilgetag et al., 2001, with permission.)

tunity to study causal relationships between focal brain function and behavior. Using TMS, we can model patients by creating "virtual lesions" and study the chronometry of the functional contribution of a given brain area to a behavior. We can also combine TMS with functional imaging methods, and hence can study functional brain connectivity at rest or during task performance. All these possibilities can be implemented in the study of brain asymmetry. Using TMS on-line (during task performance), or off-line (before a task, and comparing performance before and after the task), it is possible to demonstrate interhemispheric asymmetric representations, probe the potentially lateralized effects of tasks, and explore the neurobiological basis of cognitive functions that are lateralized.

REFERENCES

Amassian, V. E., Cracco, R. Q., Maccabee, P. J., Cracco, J. B., Rudell, A. P., & Eberle, L. (1989). Suppression of visual perception by magnetic coil stimulation of human occipital cortex. *Electroencephalography and Clinical Neurophysiology, 74,* 458–462.

Amassian, V. E., Somasundaram, M., Rothwell, J. C., Britton, T., Cracco, J. B., Cracco, R. Q., Maccabee, P. J., & Day, B. L. (1991). Paraesthesias are elicited by single pulse, magnetic coil stimulation of motor cortex in susceptible humans. *Brain, 114,* 2505–2520.

Bartres-Faz, D., Pujol, J., Deus, J., Tormos, J. M., Keenan, J., & Pascual-Leone, A. (1999). Identification of brain areas from which TMS induces speech arrest in normal subjects. *Neuroimage, 9,* S1051.

Chen, R., Classen, J., Gerloff, C., Celnik, P., Wassermann, E. M., Hallett, M., & Cohen, L. G. (1997). Depression of motor cortex excitability by low-frequency transcranial magnetic stimulation. *Neurology, 48,* 1398–1403.

Cicinelli, P., Traversa, R., Bassi, A., Scivoletto, G., & Rossini, P. M. (1997). Interhemispheric differences of hand muscle representation in human motor cortex. *Muscle and Nerve, 20,* 535–542.

Cohen, L. G., Bandinelli, S., Sato, S., Kufta, C., & Hallett, M. (1991). Attenuation in detection of somatosensory stimuli by transcranial magnetic stimulation. *Electroencephalography and Clinical Neurophysiology, 81*(5), 366–376.

Cohen, L. G., Ziemann, U., Chen, R., Classen, J., Hallett, M., Gerloff, C., et al. (1998). Studies of neuroplasticity with transcranial magnetic stimulation. *Journal of Clinical Neurophysiology, 15,* 305–324.

Day, B. L., Rothwell, J. C., Thompson, P. D., Maertens de Noordhout, A., Nakashima, K., Shannon, K., & Marsden, C. D. (1989). Delay in the execution of voluntary movement by electrical or magnetic brain stimulation in intact man. Evidence for the storage of motor programs in the brain. *Brain, 112,* 649–663.

Düzel, E., Hufnagel, A., Helmstaedter, C., & Elger, C. (1996). Verbal working memory components can be selectively influenced by transcranial magnetic stimulation in patients with left temporal lobe epilepsy. *Neuropsychologia, 34,* 775–783.

Epstein, C. M., Lah, J. K., Meador, K., Weissman, J. D., Gaitan, L. E., & Dihenia, B. (1996). Optimum stimulus parameters for lateralized suppression of speech with magnetic brain stimulation. *Neurology, 47,* 1590–1593.

Epstein, C. M., Meador, K. J., Loring, D. W., Wright, R. J., Weissman, J. D., Sheppard, S., et al. (1999). Localization and characterization of speech arrest during transcranial magnetic stimulation. *Clinical Neurophysiology, 110,* 1073–1079.

Epstein, C. M., Meador, K., Weissman, J. D., Puhalovich, F., Lah, J. K., Gaitan, L. E., Sheppard, S., & Davey, K. R. (1996). Localization of speech arrest with transcranial magnetic brain stimulation. *Journal of Clinical Neurophysiology, 13,* 387–390.

Flitman, S. S., Grafman, J., Wassermann, E. M., Cooper, V., O'Grady, J., Pascual-Leone, A., & Hallett, M. (1998). Linguistic processing during repetitive transcranial magnetic stimulation. *Neurology, 50*, 175–181.

George, M. S., & Bellmaker, R. H. (2000). *Transcranial magnetic stimulation in neuropsychiatry.* Washington D.C.: American Psychiatric Association Press.

George, M. S., Wassermann, E. M., Kimbrell, T. A., Little, J. T., Williams, W. E., Danielson, A. L., et al. (1997). Mood improvement following daily left prefrontal repetitive transcranial magnetic stimulation in patients with depression: A placebo-controlled crossover trial. *American Journal of Psychiatry, 154*, 1752–1756.

George, M. S., Wassermann, E. M., Williams, W. A., Steppel, J., Pascual-Leone, A., Basser, P., et al. (1996). Changes in mood and hormone levels after rapid-rate transcranial magnetic stimulation (rTMS) of the prefrontal cortex. *Journal of Neuropsychiatry and Clinical Neurosciences, 8*, 172–180.

Grafman, J., Pascual-Leone, A., Alway, D., Nichelli, P., Gomez-Tortosa, E., & Hallett, M. (1994). Induction of a recall deficit by rapid-rate transcranial magnetic stimulation. *NeuroReport, 5*, 1157–1160.

Heinen, F., Fietzek, U. M., Berweck, S., Hufschmidt, A., Deuschl, G., & Korinthenberg, R. (1998). Fast corticospinal system and motor performance in children: Conduction precedes skill. *Pediatric Neurology, 19*, 217–221.

Hilgetag, C. C., Theoret, H., & Pascual-Leone, A. (2001). Enhanced visual spatial attention ipsilateral to rTMS-induced "virtual lesions" of human parietal cortex. Is the speech arrest induced by repetitive transcranial magnetic stimulation due to disruption of the motor cortex? *Nature Neuroscience, 4*, 953–957.

Ilmoniemi, R. J., Virtanen, J., Ruohonen, J., Karhu, J., Aronen, H. J., Naatanen, R., et al. (1997). Neuronal responses to magnetic stimulation reveal cortical reactivity and connectivity. *NeuroReport, 8*, 3537–3540.

Jennum, P., Friberg, L., Fuglsang-Frederiksen, A., & Dam, M. (1994). Speech localization using repetitive transcranial magnetic stimulation. *Neurology, 44*, 269–273.

Klein, E., Kreinin, I., Chistyakov, A., Koren, D., Mecz, L., Marmur, S., et al. (1999). Therapeutic efficacy of right prefrontal slow repetitive transcranial magnetic stimulation in major depression: A double-blind controlled study. *Archives of General Psychiatry, 56*, 315–320.

Kujirai, T., Caramia, M. D., Rothwell, J. C., Day, B. L., Thompson, B. D., & Ferbert, A. (1993). Cortico-cortical inhibition in human motor cortex. *Journal of Physiology* (London), *471*, 501–520.

Lomber, S. G., & Payne, B. R. (1996). Removal of 2 halves restores the whole—reversal of visual hemineglect during bilateral cortical or collicular inactivation in the cat. *Visual Neuroscience, 13*, 1143–1156.

Lomber, S. G., & Payne, B. R. (1999). Assessment of neural function with reversible deactivation methods. *Journal of Neuroscience Methods, 86*, 105–108.

Macdonell, R. A. L., Shapiro, B. E., Chiappa, K. H., Helmers, S. L., Cross, D., Day, B. J., et al. (1991). Hemispheric threshold differences for motor evoked potentials produced by transcranial magnetic cortical stimulation. *Neurology, 41,* 1441–1444.

Maeda, F., Keenan, J. P., Tormos, J. M., Topka, H., & Pascual-Leone, A. (2000). Modulation of corticospinal excitability by repetitive transcranial magnetic stimulation. *Clinical Neurophysiology, 111,* 800–805.

Marg, E., & Rudiak, D. (1994). Phosphenes induced by magnetic stimulation over the occipital brain: Description and probable site of stimulation. *Optometry and Vision Science, 71,* 301–311.

Mottaghy, F. M., Krause, B. J., Kemna, L. J., Töpper. R., Tellmann, L., Beu, M., Pascual-Leone, A., & Müller-Gärtner, H. W. (2000). Modulation of the neural circuitry subserving verbal working memory by repetitive transcranial magnetic stimulation. *Neuroscience Letters, 280,* 167–170.

Müller, K., Homberg, V., Aulich, A., & Lenard, H. G. (1992). Magnetoelectrical stimulation of motor cortex in children with motor disturbances. *Electroencephalography and Clinical Neurophysiology, 85,* 86–94.

Nezu, A., Kimura, S., Uehara, S., Kobayashi, T., Tanaka, M., & Saito, K. (1997). Magnetic stimulation of motor cortex in children: Maturity of corticospinal pathway and problem of clinical application. *Brain and Development, 19,* 176–180.

Nudo, R. J., Jenkins, W. M., Merzenich, M. M., Prejean, T., & Grenda, R. (1992). Neurophysiological correlates of hand preference in primary motor cortex of adult squirrel monkeys. *Journal of Neuroscience, 12,* 2918–2949.

Oliveri, M., Caltagirone, C., Filippi, M. M., Traversa, R., Cicinelli, P., Pasqualetti, P., & Rossini, P. M. (2000). Paired transcranial magnetic stimulation protocols reveal a pattern of inhibition and facilitation in the human parietal cortex. *Journal of Physiology, 529,* 461–468.

Oliveri, M., Rossini, P. M., Pasqualetti, P., Traversa, R., Cicinelli, P., Palmieri, M. G., et al. (1999). Interhemispheric asymmetries in the perception of unimanual and bimanual cutaneous stimuli. A study using transcranial magnetic stimulation. *Brain, 122,* 1721–1729.

Oliveri, M., Rossini, P. M., Traversa, R., Cicinelli, P., Filippi, M. M., Pasqualetti, P., et al. (1999). Left frontal transcranial magnetic stimulation reduces contralesional extinction in patients with unilateral right brain damage. *Brain, 122,* 1731–1739.

Pascual-Leone, A., Bartres-Faz, D., & Keenan, J. P. (1999). Transcranial magnetic stimulation: Studying the brain-behaviour relationship by induction of "virtual lesions." *Philosophical Transcripts of the Royal Society of London, Biological Sciences, 354,* 1229–1238.

Pascual-Leone, A., Catalá, M. D., & Pascual-Leone Pascual, A. (1996). Lateralized effect of rapid-rate transcranial magnetic stimulation of the prefrontal cortex on mood. *Neurology, 46,* 499–502.

Pascual-Leone, A., Gates, J. R., & Dhuna, A. (1991). Induction of speech arrest and counting errors with rapid-rate transcranial magnetic stimulation. *Neurology, 41,* 697–702.

Pascual-Leone, A., Gomez-Tortosa, E., Grafman, J., Alway, D., Nichelli, P., & Hallett, M. (1994). Induction of visual extinction by rapid-rate transcranial magnetic stimulation of parietal lobe. *Neurology, 44,* 494–498.

Pascual-Leone, A., Rubio, B., Pallardo, F., & Catalá, M. D. (1996). Rapid-rate transcranial magnetic stimulation of left dorsolateral prefrontal cortex in drug-resistant depression. *Lancet, 348,* 233–237.

Pascual-Leone, A., Tarazona, F., Keenan, J. P., Tormos, J. M., Hamilton, R., & Catalá, M. D. (1999). Transcranial magnetic stimulation and neuroplasticity. *Neuropsychologia, 37,* 207–217.

Pascual-Leone, A., Tormos, J. M., Keenan, J., Tarazona, F., Canete, C., & Catalá, M. D. (1998). Study and modulation of human cortical excitability with transcranial magnetic stimulation. *Journal of Clinical Neurophysiology, 15*(4), 333–343.

Pascual-Leone, A., Valls-Sole, J., Wassermann, E. M., & Hallett, M. (1994). Responses to rapid-rate transcranial magnetic stimulation of the human motor cortex. *Brain, 117,* 847–858.

Pascual-Leone, A., & Walsh, V. (2001). Fast backprojections from the motion area to the primary visual area necessary for visual awareness. *Science, 292,* 510–512.

Pascual-Leone, A., Walsh, V., & Rothwell, J. (2000). Transcranial magnetic stimulation in cognitive neuroscience—virtual lesion, chronometry, and functional connectivity. *Current Opinion in Neurobiology, 10,* 232–237.

Pascual-Leone, A., Wassermann, E. M., Sadato, N., & Hallett, M. (1995). The role of reading activity on the modulation of motor cortical outputs to the reading hand in Braille readers. *Annals of Neurology, 38,* 910–915.

Paus, T. (1999). Imaging the brain before, during, and after transcranial magnetic stimulation. *Neuropsychologia, 37,* 219–224.

Paus, T., Jech, R., Thompson, C. J., Comeau, R., Peters, T., & Evans, A. C. (1997). Transcranial magnetic stimulation during positron emission tomography: A new method for studying connectivity of the human cerebral cortex. *Journal of Neuroscience, 17,* 3178–3184.

Paus, T., Jech, R., Thompson, C. J., Comeau, R., Peters, T., & Evans, A. C. (1998). Dose-dependent reduction of cerebral blood flow during rapid-rate transcranial magnetic stimulation of the human sensorimotor cortex. *Journal of Neurophysiology, 79,* 1102–1107.

Paus, T., & Wolforth, M. (1998). Transcranial magnetic stimulation during PET: Reaching and verifying the target site. *Human Brain Mapping, 6,* 399–402.

Reid, P. D., Shajahan, P. M., Glabus, M. F., & Ebmeier, K. P. (1998). Transcranial magnetic stimulation in depression. *British Journal of Psychiatry, 173,* 449–452.

Rothwell, J. C. (1997). Techniques and mechanisms of action of transcranial stimulation of the human motor cortex. *Journal of Neuroscience Methods, 74*(2), 113–122.

Sackeim, H. A. (2000). Repetitive transcranial magnetic stimulation: What are the next steps? *Biological Psychiatry, 48,* 959–961.

Schaafsma, A. (1988). Changes in excitability demonstrated by electrical stimulation of the motor cortex in man. *Journal of Physiology* (London), *412*, (abstract).

Shapiro, K., Pascual-Leone, A., Mottaghy, F. M., Gangitano, M., & Caramazza, A. (2001). Grammatical distinctions in the left frontal cortex. *Journal of Cognitive Neuroscience, 13*, 713–720.

Stewart, L. M., Walsh, V., & Rothwell, J. C. (2001). Motor and phosphene thresholds: A TMS correlation study. *Neurospychologia, 39*, 114–119.

Tokimura, H., Tokimura, Y., Oliviero, A., Asakura, T., & Rothwell, J. C. (1996). Speech-induced changes in corticospinal excitability. *Annals of Neurology, 40*, 628–634.

Töpper, R., Mottaghy, F. M., Brugmann, M., Noth, J., & Huber, W. (1998). Facilitation of picture naming by focal transcranial magnetic stimulation of Wernicke's area. *Experimental Brain Research, 121*, 371–378.

Tormos, J. M., Cañete, C., Tarazona, F., Catalá, M. D., Pascual-Leone Pascual, A., & Pascual-Leone, A. (1997). Lateralized effects of self-induced sadness and happiness on corticospinal excitability. *Neurology, 49*, 487–491.

Triggs, W. J., Calvanio, R., & Levine, M. (1997). Transcranial magnetic stimulation reveals a hemispheric asymmetry correlate of intermanual differences in motor performance. *Neuropsychologia, 35*, 1355–1363.

Triggs, W. J., Calvanio, R., Macdonell, R. A., Cros, D., & Chiappa, K. H. (1994). Physiological motor asymmetry in human handedness: Evidence from transcranial magnetic stimulation. *Brain Research, 636*, 270–276.

Triggs, W. J., Subramanium, B., & Rossi, F. (1999). Hand preference and transcranial magnetic stimulation asymmetry of cortical motor representation. *Brain Research, 835*, 324–329.

Walsh, V., & Cowey, A. (2000). Transcranial magnetic stimulation and cognitive neuroscience. *Nature Reviews, 1*, 73–79.

Walsh V., & Rushworth, M. (1999). A primer of magnetic stimulation as a tool for neuropsychology. *Neuropsychologia, 37*, 125–135.

Wassermann, E. M. (1998). Risk and safety of repetitive transcranial magnetic stimulation: Report and suggested guidelines from the International Workshop on the Safety of Repetitive Transcranial Magnetic Stimulation, June 5–7, 1996. *Electroencephalography and Clinical Neurophysiology, 108*, 1–16.

Wilson, S. A., Thickbroom, G. W., & Mastaglia, F. L. (1993). Transcranial magnetic stimulation mapping of the motor cortex in normal subjects. The representation of two intrinsic hand muscles. *Journal of the Neurological Sciences, 118*, 134–144.

III   Visual Laterality

8 Interaction between the Hemispheres and Its Implications for the Processing Capacity of the Brain

Marie T. Banich

This chapter presents an overview of current knowledge regarding interaction between the cerebral hemispheres. Its main theme is that interaction between the hemispheres is not simply a mechanism whereby the hemispheres keep "in sync" by sharing information between them. Rather, interaction between the hemispheres has a somewhat unexpected emergent property—that of modulating the attentional capacity of the brain. I cite evidence supporting this proposal from studies of split-brain patients in whom the cortical commissures have been severed, from studies of individuals in whom transmission of information between the hemispheres is disrupted, and from neurologically intact individuals. In order to put this work into perspective, the chapter first provides an overview of the channels by which information is transferred between the hemispheres. The next section of the chapter emphasizes a series of studies performed in our laboratory that demonstrate how communication between the hemispheres can have the emergent property of modulating the brain's information-processing capacity and its attentional functioning. The last section of the chapter discusses the implications of such findings for understanding different aspects of brain function and for expanding our conceptions of the underlying problems in various neuropsychological disorders.

CHANNELS OF INTERCHANGE BETWEEN THE CEREBRAL HEMISPHERES

Classic work by Sperry and colleagues performed during the 1960s and 1970s with monkeys and humans revealed that the cortical commissures are critical for the transfer of information between the hemispheres (see, e.g., Trevarthen, 1990). This fact was most dramatically demonstrated in split-brain patients, who are unable to compare most types of information when they are presented to different hemispheres. Since that time, our knowledge about the nature of interaction between the hemispheres has become increasingly refined.

Rather than conceptualizing interaction between the hemispheres as a unitary phenomenon, as was done initially, it has become apparent that communication between the hemispheres occurs via a series of "channels" that are utilized in a temporally cacophonous manner. This symphony of heterogeneous signals is carried over distinct channels, both over the 200 to 800 million nerve fibers that compose the corpus callosum and over subcortical commissures. There are major and minor routes of communication between the hemispheres in terms of the information carried, the fidelity of the information sent, and the speed at which information is transmitted. These channels have both relative autonomy and some functional specialization.

The notion of a channel will be discussed in three senses. The first sense of a channel is an anatomical one. There are several commissures that connect the cerebral hemispheres, and each commissure can be considered a channel. The corpus callosum is the largest channel, but there are others as well, such as the anterior commissure and the hippocampal commissure. The second sense of a channel is a route of information transfer that is dedicated to carrying a specific type of information. For example, visual information appears to be carried over certain regions of the callosum, whereas auditory information is transferred over others. Finally, one can also think of a channel in a temporal sense. Myelinated fibers can be thought of as fast channels and unmyelinated fibers as slow ones. These channels are usually separable, although not necessarily totally independent.

Anatomical Channels

When discussing interhemispheric processing, it is generally assumed that one is talking about callosal interaction, but this need not always be the case. Although the callosum is indeed the largest fiber tract connecting the two hemispheres, there are other fiber tracts that have a similar function (see Clarke & Zaidel, 1989 for an example of how these different routes may be identified). Hence cortical and subcortical channels will be distinguished in the discussion below.

Marie T. Banich

Cortical vs. Subcortical Channels

One way to determine exactly what type of information can be relayed by the corpus callosum is to determine whether a task can be performed by split-brain patients, in whom the cortical but not the subcortical commissures have been severed for the relief of epilepsy. If split-brain patients cannot integrate a particular type of information across the hemispheres, it is inferred that transfer of that type of information must be critically dependent on cortical commissures. In contrast, when information can be integrated across the hemispheres by these patients, it is assumed to occur via a subcortical route. The list of researchers who have used this logic is long (e.g., Cronin-Golumb, 1986; Johnson, 1984; Myers & Sperry, 1985; Trevarthen & Sperry, 1973). Converging evidence for the critical role of the callosum in information transfer is provided by examining integration of information across the hemispheres in acallosal patients in whom the callosum never formed (e.g., Jeeves, 1979).

Although researchers initially thought that little or no information presented to opposite hemispheres could be integrated by split-brain patients, subsequent studies suggested that certain types of information can indeed be integrated in the absence of cortical commissures. A series of studies by Sergent (e.g., 1990) is instructive in this regard. She demonstrated that although split-brain patients could not determine if items on either side of visual midline were identical, they could nonetheless make simple binary decisions about whether those same items belonged to similar categories (e.g., whether the digits had equal value or not). Evidence suggests that other commissures, such as the anterior commissure, may be capable of supporting transfer of such information. For example, Brown and colleagues (Brown et al., 1999) found that simple, overlearned, and easily encoded stimuli (such as letters) can be transferred between the hemispheres by the anterior commissure, especially when the set of possible items and responses is limited. From these results, it appears that the cortical commissures are critical for the transfer of higher-order information between the cerebral hemispheres.

It is not entirely clear, however, precisely what defines the nature of "higher-order" information that is transferred by the callosum. In the absence of the cortical commissures, abstract information about a particular digit, such as whether it is odd or even, can be transferred. And abstract categorical attributes of a face, such as whether a person is old or young, male or female, white or black, and other semantic information, such as person "not being nice" or "not being an American," can be communicated from the right hemisphere to the left. Information that cannot be transferred when the cortical commissures are severed or lacking is that which uniquely identifies an item, such as the exact value of a digit or the identity associated with a specific person's face.

Not only does transfer of information about an item's identity rely critically on the corpus callosum, but transfer of detailed information about spatial position appears to do so as well. Without a callosum, spatial localization of items across the midline is, at least in the visual modality, crude at best. Some ability to grossly localize information has been found in cases of cross comparisons of large moving objects in the periphery (Trevarthen & Sperry, 1973) (which presumably rely on integration of information at the level of the superior colliculus), decisions about relative position (e.g., above and below) (Sergent, 1991), and comparisons when a frame provides multiple cues (Holtzman, 1984).

There are two broad classes of information that can be integrated without the cerebral commissures: emotional information and aspects of spatial attention. Information about emotional tenor can be communicated via subcortical commissures. For example, Sperry et al. (1979) report that the emotional tone induced by information projected exclusively to the right hemisphere of a split-brain patient can be interpreted to a sufficient degree by the left hemisphere to influence its oral production. For example, when an array of pictures containing three strangers and her son was presented to the right hemisphere of split-brain patient N.G., her left hemisphere received enough information to enable her to point to her son and verbally report that she felt good about him.

At least certain aspects of directing attention remain unified after commissurotomy. This work has been reviewed by Gazzaniga (1987), so only highlights will be presented here. For example, responses by split-brain patients to a target in one visual field (and hence projected to a single hemisphere) are speeded when a cue has been previously presented in the opposite visual field in the analogous location (e.g., Holtzman et al., 1981). A control condition indicated that the information being integrated was attentional in nature and not spatial. Split-brain patients are unable to decide if two items, one on each side of midline, appeared in analogous locations in the visual fields, indicating that the cueing effect could not be due to integration of spatial locations across the hemispheres.

It should be noted that not all aspects of visuospatial attention are unified in split-brain patients. Although attention to a specific location in space can be integrated between the hemispheres, attentional search for a target in a complex visual array is not. Luck et al. (1994) found that visual search rates of split-brain patients were actually faster than those of neurologically intact subjects. Intact individuals had an identical search rate regardless of whether all the items were presented in one visual field (unilateral condition) or dispersed across both visual fields (bilateral condition). Although the split-brain patients had a search rate similar to neurologically intact individuals for unilateral trials, their search rate for the bilateral condition was twice as fast. Hence, the split-brain patients could search each half of space for a target independently and in parallel, whereas neurologically intact individuals could not. Confirmatory evidence that each of the disconnected hemispheres is able to control visuospatial attention independently has been provided by Arguin et al. (2000).

The work reviewed in this section of the chapter suggests that the cortical commissures are an interhemispheric "channel" critical for transferring information that precisely defines an item's attributes and for the specific localization of information in space. The next section will examine in more detail the ways in which the cortical commissures are organized to convey such information.

Information-Specific Channels Within the Callosum

Within the callosum there are various channels that are differentiated by the specific types of information they carry. This specificity is most obvious with regard to the segregation of signals in different sensory modalities, and appears to result from the topography of callosal connections. In general, fibers traversing the most anterior part of the callosum, the genu, connect prefrontal areas. The region of the callosum directly posterior to the genu connects the posterior superior frontal areas, followed by regions of the callosum that connect motor cortex and then, more posteriorly, somatosensory cortex. The caudal part of the body of the callosum connects more posterior regions, especially the temporo-parieto-occipital junction. The splenium also connects portions of the temporo-parieto-occipital junction, as well as dorsal parietal and occipital regions.

Neuroanatomical studies performed on rhesus monkeys (see Pandya & Seltzer, 1986 for a review) suggest that, in general, fibers from a given cortical region tend to occupy a specific place in the callosum and that little overlap exists between fibers from different brain regions. Confirmatory evidence in humans comes from studies of patients with partial callosal sections (e.g., Geffen, 1980) as well as individuals who have tumors in specific regions of the callosum (e.g., Geschwind & Kaplan, 1962), and studies of callosal degeneration after ischemic infarction (e.g., DeLacoste et al., 1985). A recently devised technique, diffusion tensor imaging, which shows the major directional axis along which white matter fibers are aligned, suggests that this segregation of fibers within the callosum can be highly specific. For example, within the splenium, fibers linking parietal regions are adjacent but just anterior to those connecting occipital regions (Conturo et al., 1999).

The anatomical organization of callosal connectivity has an important implication, namely, that different types of information are sent over different sections of the callosum. Behavioral research on individuals with an intact callosum does indeed suggest that interhemispheric channels can be separable. For example, behavioral dissociations suggest that visual and motor channels of information transfer may be distinct. In a series of studies A. D. Milner and colleagues (A. D. Milner & Lines, 1982; Rugg et al., 1984) examined interhemispheric transfer by comparing two conditions: one in which the hemisphere receiving a visual stimulus also controls the motor response (uncrossed condition), and one in which the visual signal is initially directed to one hemisphere, but the response is made by the other hemisphere (crossed condition). The difference between these two conditions (i.e., the crossed-uncrossed difference) is often taken as an estimate of the time needed for interhemispheric transfer (see Marzi, 1999 for a discussion of this technique, which is known as the Poffenberger paradigm).

When the dependent measure was vocal reaction time, the advantage observed for the uncrossed condition increased as the intensity of the stimulus decreased. From this finding it was inferred that the signal being transferred was sensory in nature because it varied with the intensity, a sensory characteristic of the stimulus. In contrast, when a manual rather than a vocal response was required, the uncrossed advantage did not vary with stimulus intensity, consistent with findings of other researchers (Berlucchi et al., 1971; Clarke & Zaidel, 1989), and suggesting the relay of a motor command.

A subsequent study in which estimates of interhemispheric transfer time were derived from EEG measures (Rugg et al., 1984) suggested that these signals were likely to be relayed by different regions of the callosum. Estimates of transfer time obtained at occipital lobe leads varied with signal intensity, whereas those obtained at central leads (i.e., over motor regions) did not. Further indicating that the visual and motor channels are indeed distinct, the estimate of interhemispheric transfer time calculated from verbal responses of a subject are uncorrelated with estimates calculated from manual responses in that same subject (St. John et al., 1987). Although there is evidence for distinct sensory channels, this segregation may not be absolute. For example, although it is generally assumed that fibers carrying somatosensory information are anterior to those carrying auditory information, there is some evidence of intermixing (Risse et al., 1989).

More recent studies have suggested that callosal channels can be specific not only with regard to modality, but also with regard to item attributes or representations within a given modality. For example, in one case study, a 14-year-old boy presented with letters in the left visual field (LVF) was unable to report them verbally or to write them with his right hand. This evidence suggests that information about letters received by the right hemisphere could not be transferred to the left. In contrast, he could identify forms or colors presented in the LVF, indicating that transfer of this material was possible. An MRI indicated a callosal lesion located in the ventroposterior end of the splenium, implicating this portion of the callosum as critical for transferring letter information (Suzuki et al., 1998). A converse case was reported by Funnell et al. (2000). In their patient, V.P., spared callosal fibers in the rostral and splenial end of the callosum allowed for transfer of word information, although information about color, shape, and size could not be transferred. Hence, these two case studies suggest that certain portions of the callosum may be specialized for transfer of very specific types of information even within a modality, in these cases within the visual modality.

The work described above provides evidence for a conceptualization of the callosum as consisting of separate channels that may have a fair degree of autonomy. The implication is that the callosum should not be thought of as a unitary system for information transfer, but rather may be better conceived of as a collection of systems with the ability to act independently.

Temporal Channels

Another way to conceptualize callosal channels is as an entity in time rather than in space. One can consider a temporal channel as a transfer of information that occurs within a particular temporal window or time frame. Variations in the degree of myelination of callosal fibers provides a potential anatomical substrate for temporal channels because increased myelination is associated with decreased transmission time. Relay of information by well myelinated as compared to unmyelinated fibers could form the basis of slow versus fast temporal channels. In fact, evidence derived from visual evoked potentials suggests that interhemispheric transfer of visual information occurs at four different ranges of speed: 4–8 Hz, 8–15 Hz, 15–20 Hz, and 20–32 Hz. Such time ranges are consistent with anatomical variations in the size of callosal fibers (Nalçaci et al., 1999).

Conceptually, one could argue that temporal channels are also likely to exist due to the time course of information processing. For example, when performing a complex task, it is likely that the transfer of motor commands to produce a final output is preceded, to some degree, by transfer of information between association areas, which in turn may be preceded by transfer between sensory regions. In fact, this temporal sequencing of transfer may be related to the degree of myelinization of callosal fibers. In both monkeys and humans, large myelinated callosal axons predominate in portions of the callosum connecting sensory areas relative to regions of the callosum connecting association areas (Lamantia & Rakic, 1990; Aboitiz et al., 1992).

Another way in which a temporal channel could be formed is by a series of neurons that are firing in phase. Conceptually, such phasic firing could occur even if the fibers were located in a spatially discontinuous manner and might not have similar degrees of myelination. Empirical evidence derived from electrophysiological recordings in cats suggests the existence of a substrate for such channels. Under certain conditions, such as when an object spans visual midline, regions in opposite hemispheres fire synchronously, a phenomenon that is eliminated by callosal deconnection (Engel et al., 1991). These findings suggest that the callosum can be critical in forming such phase-locked neuronal assemblies.

One interesting development with regard to the temporal dynamics of callosal relay is that transfer time between the hemispheres may not be symmetric. The meta-analysis of studies utilizing behavioral measures of the crossed-uncrossed difference to estimate interhemispheric transfer time suggested that transfer time from the right hemisphere to the left is faster than from the left to the right (Marzi et al., 1991). This

Marie T. Banich

conclusion was supported by a meta-analysis on ERP data (Brown et al., 1994), and has been found empirically to be uninfluenced by whether a task yields a left hemisphere or right hemisphere advantage (Larson & Brown, 1997).

The reason for such an asymmetry is not clear. One proposal is that this asymmetry in transfer time may be related to differences in attentional processing between the hemispheres—more specifically, the fact that the right hemisphere can direct attention to both the right and the left sides of space, whereas the left hemisphere has a much stronger bias to the contralateral side of space. If there is a delay in sending information from the left hemisphere (and hence right visual field [RVF]) to the right hemisphere, it may allow for better processing of LVF information by the right hemisphere (Larson & Brown, 1997).

Some researchers, although not conceptualizing the callosum as consisting of temporal channels, have suggested that the timing of callosal transfer may have important implications for information processing. Davidson et al. (1990) note that even in free vision, callosal transfer from one hemisphere to the other provides a source of redundant information that is useful in information processing. However, they have hypothesized that such redundant information may be useful only if it arrives within a narrow time window; otherwise its effect may be to disrupt the flow of information and hinder processing by causing interference. As this short review indicates, there is not much research that has attempted to address the issue of temporal channels associated interhemispheric transfer. Nonetheless, there are both theoretical considerations and experimental findings that suggest further exploration of this concept is likely to be fruitful.

EMERGENT PROPERTIES OF INTERHEMISPHERIC INTERACTION

Having reviewed the neuroanatomical and neurophysiological bases for communication transfer between the hemispheres, in this section of the chapter we turn our attention to the functional effects of interhemispheric communication. Clearly, one of its functions is to bind together processing performed by each hemisphere, such as integrating the sensory half-worlds in modalities such as the visual one, and coordinating asynchronous bimanual motor control (e.g., Preilowski, 1990). Yet, the major finding to come out of our laboratory since the mid-1980s is that interhemispheric interaction is much more than just a mechanism by which one hemisphere "photocopies" experiences and feelings for its partner. Rather, interhemispheric interaction has important emergent functions—functions that cannot be derived from the simple sum of its parts. Specifically, as is reviewed below, it serves to modulate the brain's computational capacity and its attentional functioning. Before we turn to a discussion of this body of work, however, we will first discuss some concrete evidence of the way in which interhemispheric processing has emergent properties.

We have garnered evidence for the emergent properties of inter-hemispheric communication by demonstrating that the nature of processing when both hemispheres are involved cannot be predicted by the processing performed by each hemisphere individually. We obtained such evidence in a paradigm that compared processing when information is directed unilaterally to a single hemisphere against that which occurs when both hemispheres receive some information. In our studies two words were either presented only in one visual field (RVF, LVF) or one word was presented in each visual field (bilateral visual field—BVF). The critical finding was that a manipulation of the font and case of the words did not affect performance across conditions for LVF or RVF trials. Nonetheless, this same manipulation did influence the pattern of performance across conditions on BVF trials (Banich & Karol, 1992).

If the whole is simply the sum of the parts, such a pattern of results should never have been observed. If communication between the hemispheres was completely constrained by processing within each hemisphere, then the lack of an effect of the font/case manipulation on unilateral trials would have predicted no effect of the font/case manipulation on BVF trials. These results make clear that processing of the hemispheres in relative isolation cannot be used to predict the effects of communication between the two hemispheres. Rather, interaction between the hemispheres can have effects on processing that are emergent, above and beyond those brought about by a single hemisphere.

Tenets of Our Model

If interaction between the hemispheres can have emergent properties, then how might these properties influence information processing? Our research has indicated that interaction between the hemispheres is particularly useful when tasks are attentionally and/or computationally

Marie T. Banich

demanding. Before we detail the support for this proposition, we first provide an outline of our model that explains the manner in which interhemispheric communication influences the processing capacity of the brain.

We posit that three major factors influence callosal interactions, and that these factors determine whether performance is superior when the critical information is restricted to a single hemisphere (within-hemisphere processing) or divided between them (across-hemisphere processing). These factors are (a) the degree to which the processing resources of a single hemisphere are taxed by the computational complexity of the task (b) the degree to which a communication overhead is imposed by callosal transfer, and (c) whether the informational complexity of the stimulus to be transferred exceeds the channel capacity of the callosum (or of the noncallosal commissures) of a given individual (see Banich & Brown, 2000 for a longer discussion).

When tasks are computationally simple, it is advantageous to have information processed by a single hemisphere. In this case, the processing resources of one hemisphere are ample for the task and interaction between the hemispheres imposes a communication overhead. The net result is an advantage for within-hemisphere processing. However, when task complexity increases to the point that the resources of a single hemisphere are overly taxed, another process comes into play. Under such conditions, it becomes advantageous to divide processing across the hemispheres so that more computational power can be brought to bear. Because both hemispheres can process almost all tasks to some degree (although in different manners), a division of processing is possible. Because the hemispheres are somewhat autonomous processors (e.g., Friedman & Polson, 1981), an interhemispheric division of processing provides extra computational power. This additional computational power more than offsets the overhead involved in callosal communication that is required for reintegration of information, leading to an advantage for across-hemisphere processing.

Channel capacity of the callosum influences whether a division of processing (and subsequent reintegration) is possible. In adults, the channel capacity of the callosum allows for transfer of most all types of information. However, under certain situations a limited channel capacity of the callosum may preclude an across-hemisphere advantage. For example, younger children cannot perform certain visuomotor tasks requiring integration between the hemispheres, nor can individuals with callosal agenesis, in whom the corpus callosum is missing (e.g., Chicoine et al., 2000).

A Role for Interhemispheric Interaction in Handling Computational Complexity

A large number of studies in our laboratory have indicated that interaction between the hemispheres becomes more helpful to performance as the computational complexity of a task increases. It should be noted that although all these studies indicate a shift with increasing computational demands toward greater utility for across-hemisphere relative to within-hemisphere processing, the size of the shift depends on the relative difference in complexity between the two tasks. If the difference in processing demands across the two tasks is large, a switch from a significant within- to a significant across-hemisphere advantage is observed. If the difference in complexity between the two tasks is smaller, a variety of patterns may be observed: There may be a significant reduction in the within-hemisphere advantage, there may be a shift to no difference between within- and across-hemisphere processing, or a slight across-hemisephre advantage may be observed. What is consistent across these studies, however, is a significant reduction in the size of the within-hemisphere advantage with increasing complexity. Here we briefly review some of these findings.

In one of our first studies, we manipulated computational complexity of the task by varying the number of computations required for a decision (Banich & Belger, 1990). In our relatively simple task, participants decided if a target letter was physically identical to either of two probes (e.g., A A). In the more demanding task, participants decided if a target letter had the same name as either of two probes (e.g., A a). Whereas the former task can be performed solely on the basis of physical characteristics of the stimulus, the latter task is more complex because it requires that the items be identified physically and, in addition, that a name be attached to the physical form.

In the paradigm we typically employ, the target item is located below fixation and somewhat laterally displaced in one visual field, while the two probes are presented above fixation and are more laterally displaced, one in each visual field. Individuals decide whether the bottom item "matches" one of the top items on a prespecified dimension. To assess the effect of interhemispheric interaction, we vary whether the target and matching probe are located in the same visual field (within-hemisphere trials) or in opposite visual fields (across-hemisphere trials). On across-hemisphere trials, interhemispheric interaction is critical because a correct decision cannot be made without comparing items presented to opposite hemispheres. In contrast, no such interaction is necessary to reach a correct decision on within-hemisphere trials. Half of the trials contain a match and half do not (figure 8.1).

For the physical identity task, responses were faster and more accurate when matching items were directed to only one hemisphere (within-hemisphere trials), compared to different hemispheres (across-hemisphere trials). However, the opposite was true for the name identity task: across-hemisphere trials were processed more quickly and accurately.

After this initial demonstration of the utility of interhemispheric interaction under conditions of high computational demands, we went on to demonstrate that this effect was not specific to the stimuli employed (i.e., letters), since it is also obtained when digits are used. We also demonstrated that an across-hemisphere advantage can be obtained for other complex decision processes. For example, an across-hemisphere advantage was observed for all of the following tasks: a summation task in which individuals determine whether the value of the target and probe equals or exceeds 10, an ordinal task in which individuals decide if the target is smaller in value than either probe (Banich & Belger, 1990), and a task in which individuals determine whether two letters in particular spatial positions are the second and third letters of a word they have just heard (Banich et al., 1990).

In all these experiments difficulty was manipulated by varying the complexity of decision while holding the nature of the input (e.g., digits) constant. Therefore, we set out to determine whether across-hemisphere processing would also prove to be advantageous if computational complexity was manipulated in some other manner. One of the first ways we did so was to vary the number of probe items. We created five-item analogues of our physical identity and name identity tasks with two probe items, rather than one, positioned in each visual field (Belger & Banich, 1992, 1998). Increasing the number of probe items heightens the computational requirements by extending the number of items to be recognized and compared before a decision can be reached. If across-hemisphere processing is particularly ad-

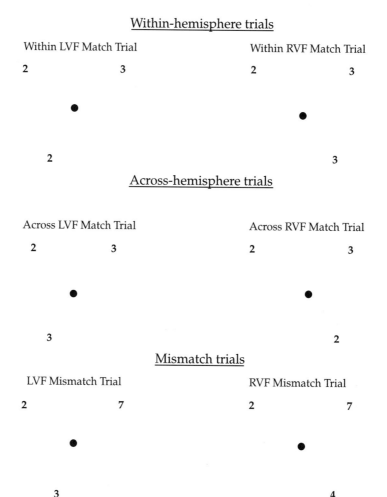

Figure 8.1 Sample trials for the physical identity task.

vantageous under conditions of high computational complexity, then across-hemisphere processing should be more advantageous for five-item, compared to three-item, tasks. This experiment also allowed us to examine whether the effects of computational complexity imposed by the decision process (physical identity vs. name identity) were separable from those imposed by the number of items to be identified and compared to the target (three- vs. five-item).

The results of these studies indicated that there is indeed an effect of complexity imposed by the number of items to be identified and compared to the target. Furthermore, this effect was separable from complexity imposed by increasing the number of steps required to reach a decision. Whereas a within-hemisphere advantage was observed for the three-item physical identity task, the five-item physical identity task yielded a modest across-hemisphere advantage. A larger across-hemisphere advantage was observed for the five-item name identity task, indicating a separable effect of the number of items to be identified and the number of steps required to reach a decision. Hence, this series of experiments indicated that the advantage afforded by across-hemisphere processing occurs across different types of stimuli, different types of decisions, and different manipulations of complexity

The Advantage Afforded by Interhemispheric Interaction Generalizes Across Modalities and Input Parameters

Having provided the basic evidence for the proposition that interhemispheric interaction is an effective method for dealing with computational complexity, we wished to further examine the robustness and generality of these effects. One nagging question was whether the effects were limited to the visual modality, since all of our experiments had been performed in that modality. Such an issue was of concern, because as we discussed above, there appear to be separate callosal channels for different types of sensory information. Hence, there existed the possibility that interaction between the hemispheres aids task complexity, but only for visual information. To determine whether across-hemisphere processing would also aid performance under computationally complex conditions in different sensory modalities, we devised tasks in the auditory and tactile domain that were as analogous as possible to those we had used in the visual modality (Passarotti et al., 2002).

In the auditory domain, we created dichotic tasks that were analogous to the physical identity and ordinal tasks previously employed in the visual modality (Banich & Belger, 1990). In our auditory task, individuals heard a dichotically presented pair of items consisting of a target digit and a foil (an animal name). The dichotic procedure was used to ensure that the target digit was processed primarily by the contralateral hemisphere (B. Milner et al., 1968). Following an interstimulus interval (ISI) (100 milliseconds for one group of participants and 250 for another), a pair of probe digits was presented dichotically. In the physical identity task, individuals decided whether either of the two probe digits was identical to the target digit presented earlier. In the ordinal task, they decided if either of the probe digits was larger in value than the target. To examine the effects of interhemispheric processing, we varied whether the target and matching probe item were presented to the same ear (within-hemisphere trials) or to opposite ears (across-hemisphere trials) (figure 8.2).

Consistent with results in the visual modality, within-hemisphere processing was less advantageous for the ordinal decision task, which

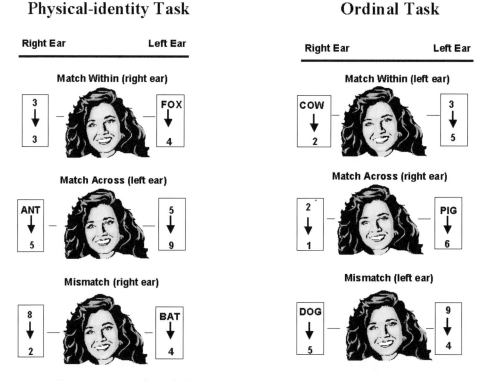

Figure 8.2 Example trials for the auditory versions of the physical identity and ordinal tasks. Individuals heard a target digit simultaneously with a foil (an animal name), presented to ensure dichotic presentation. Following an ISI of either 100 or 250 ms (represented by the arrows), a pair of digits was presented. Trials are labeled according to the ear receiving the target.

is more complex, than for the less complex physical identity task. Hence, the relationship between the utility of interhemispheric processing and computational complexity is not limited to the visual modality.

At the same time this study also provided important data to support the idea that computational complexity is the critical variable in producing an across-hemisphere advantage. All our prior work rested upon the assumption that the two tasks were processed identically except that the more computationally complex task involves at least one additional step in processing (the assumption of "pure insertion"). For example, the ordinal task involves the additional step of extracting a digit's value above and beyond the perceptual analysis and identification of items required in the physical identity task. However, this assumption might not be valid. For example, perceptual analysis may need to be more detailed or rigorous for a physical identity task than an ordinal decision task.

Manipulating the time constraints imposed on processing, as operationalized in this experiment by varying the ISI between the target item and the probes, provides a method of varying computational demands *without* varying the number or nature of the steps involved in reaching a decision. A shorter as compared to longer ISI (100 vs. 250 ms) between the two pairs of dichotic stimuli provides less time to process the target before presentation of the subsequent probes, resulting in greater computational demands for the 100 ms than 250 ms ISI condition. We predicted, therefore, that the within-hemisphere advantage would be lessened for the 100 ms as compared to the 250 ms ISI condition, especially for ordinal decision task, since more processing of the target is required (i.e., its value must be extracted). As expected, within-hemisphere processing was less advantageous for the 100 ms than the 250 ms ISI condition for the more demanding ordinal decision task.

A second experiment illustrated that the benefits of interhemispheric interaction for complex conditions extend to the tactile modality as well. In this study, we compared processing for a shape categorization task to a physical identity task. Individuals felt each side of a target shape (squares, circles, triangles, and rectangles) with the index finger of one hand. Then they felt each side of two probe shapes, one following the other. The fifth finger of one hand felt the first probe, and the fifth finger of the opposite hand felt the second probe. The effect of interhemispheric processing was examined by comparing those trials

Physical Identity Task

Category Identity Task

Match Within (left hand)

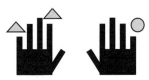

Match Within (right hand)

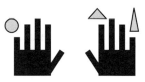

Match Across (right hand)

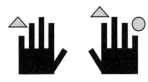

Match Across (left hand)

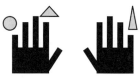

Mismatch (left hand)

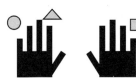

Mismatch (right hand)

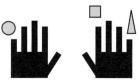

Figure 8.3 Example trials for the tactile physical- and category-identity tasks. On each trial, the individual sequentially explored each side of a target stimulus presented to the index finger. Next, each side of one probe was explored, followed by exploration of each side of another probe. Probes were presented to the fifth finger of each hand. Trials are labeled according to the hand receiving the target.

on which the target and matching probe were felt by fingers on the same hand (within-hemisphere trials) as compared to when they were felt by finger on opposite hands (across-hemisphere trials) (see figure 8.3 for example of some trials).

Because of the serial exploration of the items' contours in our task, the category task is less computationally complex than the physical identity task. In the category task, individuals only have to determine if items have the same number of sides positioned at the same angles. In contrast, the physical identity task requires an additional step—that of also determining if the sides of the items are the same length. Once again, we found that the within-hemisphere advantage was reduced for the more complex task, the physical identity task. Hence, the results of our studies in the auditory and tactile modalities indicate that the advantages afforded by interhemispheric processing are not limited to the auditory modality.

We have also investigated whether a particular aspect of our design, the uneven distribution of inputs across the hemispheres, might drive the across-hemisphere advantage either in part or totally. In our visual paradigm, one hemisphere receives one more input than the other (e.g., two items vs. one; three items vs. two). The rationale for designing the displays this way was to ensure that the number of inputs was equivalent on within- and across-hemisphere trials. This design feature ensured that the across-hemisphere advantage could be specifically attributed to a division of processing across the hemispheres, and ruled out the possibility that it merely resulted from a division of inputs between the hemispheres. In many paradigms, a hemisphere receives two inputs on within-hemisphere trials, but only one item on across-hemisphere trials. In such cases, it is not clear whether the across-hemisphere advantage derives from a division of inputs or a more central division of processing. Our paradigm ensures when across-hemisphere advantage is observed, it can be attributed to a central division of processing (see Banich & Shenker, 1994 for a longer discussion of this issue).

To rule out the possibility that our effects were totally driven by an unequal distribution of inputs, we compared the effects of inter-hemispheric processing for two types of displays, one with an uneven distribution of inputs across the hemispheres (our standard three-item arrays) and one with an even distribution (a four-item array containing two potential targets and two probes) (Weissman et al., 2000). Across-hemisphere processing was more advantageous for the name identity task than for the physical identity task for both the three- and four-item displays, confirming that the across-hemisphere advantage is not critically dependent on the inputs to the hemispheres being unequal. Yet, we found that the equality or inequality of the distribution of inputs did have an effect. Over both tasks, interhemispheric processing was more advantageous for the three-item displays than the four-item displays, suggesting that an uneven distribution of processing enhances the utility of interhemispheric processing. We propose that this effect occurs because a division of processing will be particularly useful when one hemisphere is relatively unburdened compared to the other: It can complete its processing and then be able to assist its partner.

Testing Our Model's Assumptions Regarding the Source of the Across-Hemisphere Advantage

Having shown that across-hemisphere processing is particularly helpful under computationally demanding conditions, the next step in our research program was to examine the validity of the mechanism that we had proposed for such an effect. In the first study, we specifically examined the assumption that the ability to divide processing across the hemispheres is critical in producing the across-hemisphere advantage. If this assumption is correct, then the across-hemisphere advantage should be *absent* for a computationally complex task that cannot be divided between the hemispheres. To put this idea to a test, we examined the effect of interhemispheric interaction on a rhyme task, since the critical aspect of the task, phonetic discrimination, can be performed *only* by the left hemisphere in right-handed individuals (Rayman & Zaidel, 1991). We designed our rhyme task to be comparable in computational demands and input characteristics to our other more complex tasks: Individuals viewed a vertically presented three-letter word (e.g., SEA) and decided if it rhymed with either of two probe letters (e.g., D, H), one presented in each visual field.

Despite the fact that the rhyme task was as computationally demanding as other tasks yielding an across-hemisphere advantage, a significant across-hemisphere advantage was not observed (Belger, 1993; Belger & Banich, 1998). This finding was even more compelling because the same participants who failed to exhibit an across-hemisphere advantage on the rhyme task did in fact exhibit an across-hemisphere advantage for other computationally complex tasks (e.g., name identity tasks). Hence, this study provided support for our assertion that interhemispheric interaction increases the processing capacity of the brain by allowing for a dispersal of processing load across the hemispheres.

In another study, we examined the assumption that computational complexity, rather than some general index of task difficulty, is critically related to the utility of across-hemisphere processing. If it is, then a manipulation that increases the response time to a task but does not increase the computational steps involved should not alter the utility of interhemispheric interaction. To evaluate this idea, we varied the perceptual discriminability of the stimuli utilized in the name identity and physical identity tasks, presenting items in a condition of either high contrast or low contrast. This was effective in manipulating the general difficulty of the task; reaction times to low-contrast stimuli were significantly elongated (40 ms) relative to high-contrast stimuli. Critically important, however, the relative advantage of interhemispheric processing did not vary between the two contrast conditions for either task (Weissman & Banich, 2000, experiment 2). This finding is consistent with our interpretation that the advantage afforded by across-hemisphere processing is linked to computational demands, not just to any manipulation that may make a task more difficult.

Finally, in what is probably one of the most important issues to address, we examined whether an across-hemisphere division processing is indeed how the brain handles complexity under everyday conditions. From one perspective, our experimental paradigm could be considered very artificial. In the across-hemisphere trials of our paradigm, we *force* the hemispheres to communicate to perform a task. Although across-hemisphere processing is indeed useful to task performance under the complex conditions in our experiments, it might be the case that the brain rarely, if ever, invokes such a strategy to meet computational demands. If so, all of the results described above would be of much less interest.

To investigate this critical issue, we created "indeterminate trials" that could be performed in one of two ways: by invoking within-hemisphere processing or by invoking across-hemisphere processing (Weissman & Banich, 2000). Our strategy was to determine whether performance on these indeterminate trials mimicked performance on within-hemisphere or on across-hemisphere trials. This strategy is reminiscent of that utilized by Hellige and colleagues (e.g., Hellige et al., 1988, 1989), who determined how processing occurs on BVF trials by comparing performance to unilteral RVF and unilateral LVF trials. We predicted that for low computational demands, processing on indeterminate trials would resemble that of within-hemisphere trials, whereas for high computational demands, they would resemble that of across-hemisphere trials.

In two experiments, we compared performance on "indeterminate" midline trials for the three-item physical identity and name identity tasks against performance on within- and across-hemisphere trials. On midline trials, the target item was positioned on midline, making the target's identity available to either hemisphere. Hence, the response could be generated either by a within-hemisphere comparison or by an across-hemisphere comparison. In the first experiment, responses to midline trials for the physical identity task were as fast and as accurate as within-field trials, and significantly different from across-field trials. In a second experiment, responses to midline trials for the name identity task were as fast and as accurate as across-field trials, but significantly different from within-field trials. Hence, these data suggest that under the lighter computational load imposed by the physical identity task, within-hemisphere processing is invoked on indeterminate trials, but under the heavier computational load imposed by the name identity task, across-hemisphere processing is utilized.

In a final experiment, we investigated this same issue utilizing a different paradigm that avoided the acuity differences between the central target on midline trials and laterally displaced target on within- and across-hemisphere trials. The display was a five-item array consisting of a lateralized target and four lateralized probes, two in each visual field. The target and probe items could be letters, digits or symbols, and the individual's task was to decide if the target and any of the probes came from the same category. To vary the computational demands imposed by the task, the temporal processing requirements of the task were manipulated. In the most demanding condition, all five items were presented simultaneously for 100 ms. In the condition with intermediate demands, the partially overlapping presentation condition, the four probes appeared for 50 ms, followed by all five items for 50 ms, followed by the target alone for 50 ms. In the least demanding condition, the sequential presentation condition, the four probes appeared for 100 ms, followed by the target for 100 ms. Notice that in all conditions, each item appears for a total of 100 ms. However, the processing load is more distributed over time in the sequential condition than in the partially overlapping condition, which in turn has a greater distribution over time than does the simultaneous condition.

To examine the effect of interhemispheric processing we once again compared performance on within-hemisphere and across-hemisphere trials against an "indeterminate" trial type. On within-field trials the target and two matching probes appeared in the same visual field (VF), whereas on across-field trials, the target appeared in one visual field and the two matching probes appeared in the other. Our "indeterminate" trials were divided trials, in that one matching probe was pre-

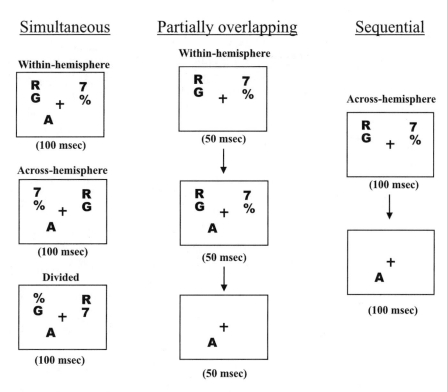

Figure 8.4 Example trials for the simultaneous, partially overlapping, and sequential conditions. In all conditions, each item is viewed for 100 ms.

sented in the same visual field as the target, and the other probe was presented in the opposite visual field. Hence, a match could be made either by detecting the matching probe in the same VF or by detecting the matching probe in the opposite VF (figure 8.4).

Consistent with our expectations regarding the complexity of our different conditions, overall reaction time (RT) increased from the sequential to partially overlapping condition and even more so to the simultaneous condition. Of critical importance, the increases in RT between conditions paralleled each other for the across- and divided conditions, both of which differed significantly from that for within-hemisphere trials. This result provides converging evidence that when either across- or within-hemisphere processing is possible, across-hemisphere processing underlies the performance of computationally complex tasks.

These studies provide strong evidence that the hemispheres dynamically couple and decouple their processing as a function of task complexity. When task demands are relatively simple, the hemispheres decouple their processing and work independently; when task demands are more complex, the hemispheres unite by invoking across-hemisphere processing. Hence, interhemispheric interaction provides a flexible and adaptable system for meeting the computational demands imposed upon the brain.

A Division of Processing Across the Hemispheres Can Modulate Attentional Control

The findings discussed above have implications that extend beyond cerebral asymmetry to the cognitive neuroscience of attentional control. Attentional mechanisms provide a means for dealing with the brain's capacity limitation, by providing a means for selecting material that is task-relevant across different stages of information processing: perceptual, central, and response-related. Our results suggest that dividing processing across the hemispheres can increase the overall processing capacity of the brain, suggesting that the dynamic coupling and decoupling of the hemispheres helps to modulate the allocation of attentional resources.

Given that we had observed a relationship between one aspect of attentional control (i.e., resource allocation) and interaction between the hemispheres, we decided to examine whether interhemispheric interaction might influence other aspects of attentional control, such as selective attention. This line of research utilized a variety of standard paradigms in which attention must be selectively directed to one aspect of a stimulus or a display while other information is ignored.

As a first step, we examined whether interaction between the hemispheres can modulate the degree of interference between global and local aspects of a hierarchical figure, so named because it consists of a global form composed of local elements. To assess the effects of attentional selection, processing of inconsistent hierarchical figures is compared to that of consistent figures. Consistent figures contain local elements that are identical to the global form (e.g., a large square composed of smaller squares), whereas inconsistent figures are composed of local elements that differ from the global form (e.g., a large square composed of smaller triangles). The individual's task is to identify the

Marie T. Banich

item based on its form at a specific level (e.g., the global level). This identification requires more attention for inconsistent than consistent stimuli because competing information from the unattended level must be filtered out. Reflecting these increased attentional demands, it takes longer to correctly respond to inconsistent as compared to consistent stimuli.

We specifically wished to examine the relationship between interhemispheric interaction and global/local interference because there was a claim about this relationship that was quite at odds with the results of our prior research. It had been suggested that global/local interference was actually *generated* by interhemispheric interaction that occurs when global information processed by the right hemisphere is intermixed with local information processed by the left hemisphere (e.g., Robertson et al., 1993; Polster & Rapcsak, 1994). In contrast, our prior research suggested that interaction between the hemispheres aids performance under attentionally demanding conditions, which would imply that interaction between the hemispheres should reduce (rather than produce) interference between global and local information.

To distinguish these two possibilities, we utilized our usual three-item arrays and had individuals decide if the target item matched one of the probes at a specific level (e.g., the local level) (Weissman & Banich, 1999). To manipulate attentional demands, we compared the effect of interhemispheric interaction for consistent items in which the matching items were identical at both the attended and unattended level against inconsistent items in which the items matched at the attended level (e.g., global) but not at the unattended level (e.g., the local).

The results indicated that global/local interference (the difference in RT between inconsistent trials and consistent trials) was significantly reduced on across- as compared to within-hemisphere trials regardless of whether stimuli were verbal or nonverbal. For hierarchical geometric forms (e.g., a square composed of triangles), the interference effect was 137 ms on within-hemisphere trials, but only 87 ms on across-hemisphere trials. Similarly, for hierarchical letters (e.g., an A composed of Os) the interference effect was 100 ms on within-hemisphere trials, but only 61 ms on across-hemisphere trials. Consistent with our prior work, these results suggest that interaction between the hemispheres aids attentional control, in this case by reducing interference.

We then became interested in better defining the locus of this effect. In our paradigm, inconsistent items can engender interference in multiple ways. First, they engender perceptual interference because the form of the items at the global and local levels is distinct. Second, they engender response interference because the relationship between items at the unattended level (which is inconsistent) leads to a different decision ("mismatch") than the relationship between the items at the attended level ("match").

To examine the degree to which perceptual aspects of attentional selection influenced our results, we compared the reduction in interference on across-hemisphere trials for two types of geometric hierarchical stimuli that vary in their perceptual characteristics. One set of hierarchical stimuli was composed of few local elements, whereas the other was composed of many local elements. When hierarchical figures are composed of few (as compared to many) elements, it hard to perceptually disembed the global and local levels (Kimchi & Palmer, 1985). The two levels tend to be integral dimensions, meaning that form at one level tends to influence the way in which form at the other level is perceived. In contrast, for many-element stimuli, the global and local levels are more separable, in that form at one level does not influence the perception of form at the other level. If interaction between the hemispheres aids attentional selection at the perceptual level, then it should reduce interference more for few-element than for many-element items, since the demands on attentional selection are greater for few- than for many-element arrays. Consistent with this prediction, interference was reduced more on across-hemisphere trials for few-element patterns (65 ms) than for many-element patterns (31 ms).

To demonstrate that our results generalized to other aspects of selective attention, we utilized a different paradigm, one in which individuals had to pay attention to the form of items while ignoring their color. While viewing our typical three-item arrays, individuals determined whether a target form was identical to either of two probe forms (e.g., squares, rectangles, triangles, ovals). The relationship between the color of the two items could either be concordant with their relationship in form (e.g., same form/same color) or discordant (e.g., same form/different color). The latter condition is more demanding attentionally because the relationship between the color of the two items needs to be ignored to reach the correct decision about their relationship in form. Not surprisingly, interhemispheric interaction was more helpful in the more attentionally demanding condition than in the less attentionally demanding condition (Banich & Passarotti, submitted). This study indicates that the relationship between interhemispheric interaction and attentional demands generalizes across aspects of selective attention—whether based on the spatial grain of items (i.e., the global vs. the local level) or two different attributes at the same spatial grain (i.e., color and form).

In our final study to examine the effects of interhemispheric interaction and attentional selection, we utilized a paradigm that varied in two significant ways from our prior studies. In this task, the to-be-ignored information was contained in an item separate from the task-relevant information, and an explicit comparison of information across the hemispheres was *not* required to perform the task. In this study we utilized a lateralized Stroop paradigm in which individuals were shown a colored box and a word, which were either positioned in the same visual field or in opposite visual fields (Shenker & Banich, submitted). As in the typical Stroop paradigm, individuals were asked to identify the colored item while ignoring the identity of the word. Such a task is attentionally demanding because word reading is relatively more automatic than color naming. Hence, attention must be directed away from the word and toward the color box.

Attentional demands were varied by manipulating the identity of the word: being either congruent, neutral, or incongruent with regard to the color of the box. Attentional demands are smallest when the word is congruent (e.g., "red" displayed along with a red box), because the word provides information that is redundant with the color information; intermediate on neutral trials (e.g., "lot" displayed along with a red box), because the word contains no task-relevant (i.e., color) information; and greatest in the incongruent condition (e.g., "red" displayed along with a blue box), because the word's identity must be ignored to correctly identify the box's color. The effect of interaction between the hemispheres was determined by comparing the degree to which the word influenced performance when it was positioned in the visual field opposite the box (across-hemisphere trials), as opposed to the same visual field (within-hemisphere trials). Although an explicit comparison of information is not required on across-hemisphere trials, the only way in which the word can influence performance on across-hemisphere trials is via callosal relay.

In addition to varying the attentional demands based on the identity of the word, we also manipulated attentional demands by varying the rate at which congruent trials appeared relative to other trials (constituting 17%, 40%, or 67% of all trials). As the congruency rate increases, individuals devote more attention to the word since probabilistically it is more likely to provide redundant information for identifying the color. This increased attention to the word increases facilitation by congruent words, but also increases the cost of interference on incongruent trials because the words are now a more potent source of interference.

The division of the word and color box across the hemispheres (as compared to being directed to the same hemisphere) modulated attentional demands with regard to both word type and congruency rate. The advantage for across-hemisphere as compared to within-hemisphere trials was greater on incongruent trials, which were the most attentionally demanding, as compared to neutral and congruent trials. Furthermore, with increasing congruency rate, across-hemisphere processing became more advantageous on incongruent trials (which entailed increasing attentional demands) and less advantageous on congruent trials (which entailed decreasing attentional demands).

These results are also important because they demonstrate that the attentional modulation afforded by interhemispheric interaction cannot be attributed to general callosal suppression of the relay/receipt of task-irrelevant information, in this case the word. If that were the case, the identity of the word should have little effect on performance. Rather, our results indicate that the advantage derived from dividing the word and color box across the hemispheres was *specifically* driven by the word's identity and the degree to which attention had to be engaged to ignore its identity to correctly identify the box's color. Likewise, the across-hemisphere advantage was also modulated by the variations in attentional demands imposed across different congruency rates. Hence, this study is consistent with other work in our laboratory indicating that interaction between the hemispheres varies dynamically with attentional demands.

Interhemispheric Interaction Across the Life Span

Having examined issues of interhemispheric interaction mainly with participants who were young adults, we were interested in the degree to which the effects we observed hold across the life span. Research performed by oursevles and others suggests that interhemispheric interaction may be particularly useful during those stages of life in which the resources of a single hemisphere are likely to be diminished.

We specifically examined whether a division of processing across the hemispheres aids performance under computationally complex conditions during childhood, as has been found in adults. Much evidence indicates that the functional connectivity of the hemispheres increases during childhood (e.g., Quinn & Geffen, 1986; Liederman et al., 1986) and that speed of callosal transmission decreases with age (e.g., Salamy, 1978; Hagelthorn et al., 2000). Hence we were interested in the ways in which these maturational changes might influence the role of interhemispheric interaction in information processing.

Conceptually, there are a number of distinct possibilities. One possibility is that the effect of interhemispheric interaction on performance changes very little with age. The critical factor influencing the utility of interhemispheric interaction during childhood may be the ability to divide processing across the hemispheres and then to reintegrate or cross-compare the results of such processing. Because children can integrate almost all information across the hemispheres (unlike split-brain patients), they may show a similar pattern to adults. From this perspective, the longer time needed by children than adults to transfer information across the callosum would be relatively insignificant. Another possibility is that decreases in callosal transfer time with age may reduce the cost or overhead associated with interhemispheric communication. If this were the case, one would expect the relative advantage of across-hemisphere processing to increase with age. A final possibility is that interhemispheric processing may be more advantageous for younger than for older children. Because younger children do not have the processing capacity of older children, they may need to rely more on across-hemisphere processing as a means to cope with increased computational demands.

To disentangle these possibilities, we examined the performance of school-age children (aged 6–14) on the physical identity task and name identity task for letters (Banich et al., 2000). In children, as in adults, across-hemisphere processing was more advantageous for the computationally more complex name identity task than for the less complex physical identity task. However, variations with age were also apparent—the younger the child, the larger the within-hemisphere advantage on the physical identity task, and the larger the across-hemisphere advantage on the name identity task. This finding suggests that the lessened capacity of a single hemisphere in younger children leads interaction between the hemispheres to especially beneficial when tasks are complex.

In an interesting parallel, Reuter-Lorenz and colleagues have reported analogous results in older adults (Reuter-Lorenz et al., 1999; Reuter-Lorenz & Stanczak, 2000). They examined the size of the across-hemisphere advantage in younger and older adults at three levels of task complexity by using the three-item physical identity, five-item physical identity, and five-item name identity tasks of Belger and Banich (1992, 1998). The older adults exhibited an across-hemisphere advantage for the tasks that were of intermediate and high complexity (five-item physical identity task, five-item name identity task), whereas the younger adults exhibited a significant across-hemisphere advantage only for the highest level of task complexity. In sum, across-hemisphere processing was useful to older adults at a lower level of task complexity than observed in younger adults. These findings, as well as our own with children, suggest that populations particularly challenged by computational complexity may invoke across-hemisphere processing as a mechanism to cope with increased computational demands.

INSIGHTS INTO BRAIN FUNCTION DERIVED FROM INTERHEMISPHERIC INTERACTION

Our increased knowledge of the emergent functions of interhemispheric interaction can shed light on numerous other phenomena and concepts in cognitive neuroscience and neuropsychology. These range from the results of neuroimaging studies to our understanding of deficits in neurological syndromes such as multiple sclerosis.

The idea that the brain deals with computational complexity by recruiting resources from both hemispheres is receiving confirmation from brain imaging studies. One interesting trend across numerous neuroimaging studies is that as computational complexity increases, activation that was restricted to a single hemisphere appears to spread across both. A prototypical example is provided in a study by Raye et al. (2000) in which they examined patterns of brain activation for two levels of memory demand. In the easier condition, individuals performed a forced-choice recognition task in which they decided which of a pair of items had been previously viewed. In the more difficult condition, individuals performed a successive recognition task in which they decided on each trial whether the presented item was old or new. Successive recognition is more difficult than forced-choice because the decision process cannot be aided by comparison with a foil (Macmillan & Creelman, 1991). Two types of stimuli were used: words, which should rely more on left-hemisphere mechanisms, and textures, which should rely more on right-hemisphere mechanisms.

In the forced-choice condition, activation was mainly unilateral and consistent with lateralization of function for each type of stimulus— there was greater activity in left prefrontal areas for words than for textures, whereas there was greater activity in the right prefrontal areas for textures than for words. Of most importance, however, was that for both tasks, activation was observed in *both* hemispheres in the more difficult successive condition. As the authors note, this is consistent with the idea that demanding conditions lead to a division of processing across the hemispheres, allowing for greater recruitment of neural resources to meet the increased computational demands (Banich, 1998).

An appreciation of the emergent properties of interhemispheric interaction may help to shed light on the pattern of difficulties observed in certain neurological syndromes. According to our model, a disruption of interaction between the hemispheres should lead to attentional problems. This expectation is supported by numerous studies in a variety of clinical populations. Probably the strongest evidence exists for multiple sclerosis (MS), a demyelinating disease that preferentially affects the corpus callosum and other periventricular white matter tracts (e.g., Barnard & Triggs, 1974; Simon et al., 1986). Individuals with MS exhibit disruptions in interhemispheric communication (e.g., Jacobson et al., 1983; Pelletier et al., 1993). Of greatest importance for the present purposes, the degree of callosal atrophy as measured by MRI is a better predictor of the ability to sustain attention (as assessed by multiple measures) than is the total amount of brain demyelination (Rao et al., 1989).

Another syndrome characterized by atypical morphology of the corpus callosum is schizophrenia. This atypical morphology cannot be explained by general brain atrophy (e.g., Woodruff et al., 1993) and has the functional consequence of disrupted interhemispheric interaction (e.g., David, 1993; Scarrone et al., 1993; Mohr et al., 2000). Concomitantly, schizophrenics have documented attentional disruptions in a variety of domains (e.g., Dawson et al., 1993; Cullum et al., 1993).

These disruptions distinguish individuals with schizophrenia from other individuals with psychopathology, such as those with affective disorders (e.g., Goldberg et al., 1993), and in some cases may precede psychotic symptomatology (e.g., Schreiber et al., 1992). To date, the linkage between interhemispheric processing and attentional abilities in schizophrenia has been investigated in only a handful of studies (Bellini et al., 1991; David, 1993).

Another disorder characterized by damage to the corpus callosum, both in adults (Levin et al., 1989; Vuilleumier & Assal, 1995) and in children (Benavidez et al., 1999), is closed head injury. Deficits in selective attention and divided attention are quite common in this disorder (Zoccolotti et al., 2000). Callosal atrophy is also present in Alzheimer's disease (Janowsky et al., 1996), but the degree to which such atrophy can predict attentional disorders remains to be seen.

At present, it is not clear for many of these disorders whether there is a direct linkage between disruptions in interhemispheric processing and attentional processing. Furthermore, attentional processes cover a broad domain of abilities. These include the ability to attend selectively to specific sensory information, such as spatial location or an item attribute (form, color), the ability to select particular representations to be placed in working memory, the ability to select specific responses, the ability to prioritize the performance of one task over the other, and the ability to remain vigilant. Future research will need to more carefully examine exactly which aspects of attentional function are linked to interhemispheric processing in these different neuropsychological syndromes.

Certain paradigms developed in our laboratory might fruitfully be applied to examine the degree to which degradation in interhemispheric interaction is linked to clinical symptomatology. For example, our auditory paradigm might be particularly useful in detecting early deficits in multiple sclerosis because it provides a means to examine computational complexity with regard to decision processes and temporal constraints. MS is characterized by an increase in speed of conduction of information between the hemispheres due to decreased myelination. Our auditory paradigm provides a means for examining how interaction between the hemispheres is affected by increasing load with regard to temporal constraints, as manipulated by the ISI between the dichotic pairs, separately from the influence of complexity of the decision processing, as manipulated in the physical identity vs. ordinal decision tasks. The ISI manipulation might be especially sensitive to detecting the first signs of compromised functioning due to degradation in callosal relay.

Ideally, the results from our auditory paradigm would with integrated with anatomical MR data demarcating the lesion load in specific regions of the callosum, electrophysiological measures providing an estimate of interhemispheric transfer time, and measures of the degree to which attentional functioning is compromised under nonlateralized conditions. Such a data set would provide a means for more definitely determining the degree to which hemispheric decoupling is linked to the attentional deficits observed in MS.

Our methods might also prove useful with other populations because they allow for an examination not only of within- versus across-hemisphere processing but also of lateralized effects. Many of our paradigms are designed so that the critical target stimulus is presented to only one hemisphere. Hence, performance on trials on which the target is directed to the left hemisphere can be compared to those on which the target is directed to the right hemisphere. This characteristic might be particularly useful in examining schizophrenia because this syndrome has been linked both to disruptions in left-hemisphere processing (e.g., Crow, 1997) and to left-hemisphere overactivation (e.g., Gur, 1978; Ferman et al., 1999). With our paradigms, lateralized effects could be examined, as well as their interrelationship, if any, to deficits in callosal functioning. A possible outcome of utilizing such paradigms might be a better understanding of subtypes of schizophrenic symptomatology, because different symptoms might be associated with abnormal left-hemisphere function, abnormal callosal function, or both.

ISSUES FOR THE FUTURE

Compared to our knowledge about lateralization of function, information about interhemispheric interaction is scant. There remains, therefore, a broad research agenda that needs to be addressed. As discussed above, increased understanding of interhemispheric interaction is likely to have important implications in a number of arenas. It may help to explain changes in cognitive processing across the life span, provide a framework for interpreting some of the results within the exploding domain of brain imaging research, and aid in providing a framework for understanding attentional deficits observed in various neurological syndromes. This section of the chapter will examine some of the issues that will require further examination and that also seem, at present, amenable to analysis.

One outstanding empirical issue is the degree to which callosal anatomy is related to its function. To date, this endeavor has been hampered somewhat by both methodological and theoretical limitations. Our knowledge of the functional anatomy of the corpus callosum is very coarse (e.g., knowing what functions can be ascribed to the posterior third of the callosum), and is derived mainly from patients who have circumscribed callosal lesions (e.g., Michel et al., 1996) or partial section of the corpus callosum (Risse et al., 1989). Furthermore, our knowledge of callosal connections in the human brain is derived mainly from postmortem samples (DeLacoste et al., 1985). Hence, most studies have examined the size of a section of the callosum and attempted to correlate that with some behavioral measure (e.g., Hines et al., 1992; Hellige et al., 1998) or some characteristics of a clinical syndrome (Downhill et al., 2000). Yet we do not really know what size of the callosum is indexing; it could vary from the degree of myelination of fibers, to the number of fibers, to the number of glia.

Recent development in imaging techniques may help to provide a means for providing a clearer understanding of the relationship between callosal morphology and function. The use of diffusion tensor imaging, which provides specific information on the organization of white matter fiber tracts, holds great promise for helping to delineate the integrity and pattern of connectivity of callosal fibers more carefully (e.g., Foong et al., 2000). If this method can be coupled with functional imaging techniques, such as fMRI, it might be able to provide a much more refined picture of the functional effects of specific callosal channels. Such functional data will also need to be linked to a behavioral paradigm that clearly isolates a cognitive operation which is related to callosal functioning. For example, one might want to examine whether there are separable callosal channels for the transfer of information about color and of form. Functional imaging techniques could be used to isolate the color- and form-specific processing regions. Callosal connections could be deduced using diffusion tensor imaging, and the functional connectivity could be deduced by juxtaposing activation for an across-hemisphere condition to a within-hemisphere condition during tasks that require processing of each of these visual attributes (i.e., color, form).

Marie T. Banich

Another promising area of research will be to investigate the degree to which disruptions in interhemispheric processing occur in particular disease states. It will be useful to demonstrate not only that a disruption in interhemispheric processing accompanies the disease state, but also that the disruption is in some way important or specific. There are numerous possible ways in which interhemispheric interaction could be linked to particular syndromes.

First, disrupted interhemispheric interaction could actually cause the syndrome. So, for example, it might be that dyslexia actually results from poor interhemispheric integration of the graphic forms of letters, preferentially processed by the right hemisphere, and phonological information about those letters, preferentially processed by the left.

Second, it might be that disrupted interhemispheric integration is just one manifestation of a larger and more ubiquitous deficit in neural processing. For example, some authors have suggested that schizophrenia is a disease typified by massive neural disorganization. In such a case, disrupted interhemispheric processing may be but one of many manifestations of neural disorganization without *causing* the cognitive and emotional dysfunction observed in schizophrenia.

Third, poor interhemispheric integration could be a specific marker for a syndrome but have no causative relationship. For example, it might be that attention deficit disorder causes poor interhemispheric processing, but that the disruption in interhemispheric processing is not the cause of the disorder—even if one could improve interhemispheric processing, the attention deficit disorder would remain.

Finally, the correlation between callosal function and some syndrome may be mediated by some other variables whose identity remains obscure. For example, acallosal individuals often have other anomalies, such as low intelligence. The developmental malformation that leads to the co-occurrence of callosal agenesis and low intelligence remains unknown. Understanding the manner in which interhemispheric interaction is related to various clinical disorders will be of paramount importance.

ACKNOWLEDGMENTS

I would like to thank all of my Ph.D. students who in the course of doing the research described in this chapter became my most invaluable colleagues: Aysenil Belger, Alessandra Passarotti, Joel Shenker, and Daniel Weissman. They have made pursuing this research more intellectually stimulating and more enjoyable than I could have ever imagined.

REFERENCES

Aboitiz, F., Scheibel, A. B., Fisher, R. S., & Zaidel, E. (1992). Individual differences in brain asymmetries and fiber composition in the human corpus callosum. *Brain Research, 598,* 154–161.

Arguin, M., Lassonde, M., Quattrini, A., Del Pesce, M., Foschi, N., & Papo, I. (2000). Divided visuo-spatial attention systems with total and anterior callosotomy. *Neuropsychologia, 38,* 283–291.

Banich, M. T. (1998). The missing link: The role of interhemispheric interaction in attentional processing. *Brain and Cognition, 36,* 128–157.

Banich, M. T., & Belger, A. (1990). Interhemispheric interaction: How do the hemispheres divide and conquer a task? *Cortex, 26,* 77–94.

Banich, M. T., & Brown, W. S. (2000). A life-span perspective on interaction between the cerebral hemispheres. *Developmental Neuropsychology, 18,* 1–10.

Banich, M. T., Goering, S., Stolar, N., & Belger, A. (1990). Interhemispheric processing in left- and right-handers. *International Journal of Neuroscience, 54,* 197–208.

Banich, M. T., & Karol, D. L. (1992). The sum of the parts does not equal the whole: Evidence from bihemispheric processing. *Journal of Experimental Psychology: Human Perception and Performance, 18,* 763–784.

Banich, M. T., & Passarotti, A. (submitted). Interhemispheric interaction aids task performance under conditions of selective attention. *Neuropsychology*

Banich, M. T., Passarotti, A. M., & Janes, D. (2000). Interhemispheric interaction during childhood: I. Neurologically intact children. *Developmental Neuropsychology, 18,* 33–51.

Banich, M. T., & Shenker, J. I. (1994). Investigations of interhemispheric processing: Methodological considerations. *Neuropsychology, 8*(2), 263–277.

Barnard, R. O., & Triggs, M. (1974). Corpus callosum in multiple sclerosis. *Journal of Neurology, Neurosurgery & Psychiatry, 37,* 1259–1264.

Belger, A. (1993). Influences of hemispheric specialization and interaction on task performance. Ph.D. dissertation, University of Illinois.

Belger, A., & Banich, M. T. (1992). Interhemispheric interaction affected by computational complexity. *Neuropsychologia, 30,* 923–931.

Belger, A., & Banich, M. T. (1998). Costs and benefits of integrating information between the cerebral hemispheres: A computational perspective. *Neuropsychology, 12,* 380–398.

Bellini, L., Abbruzzese, M., Gambini, O., Rossi, A., Stratta, P., & Scarone, S. (1991). Frontal and callosal neuropsychological performances in schizophrenia: Further evidence of possible attention and mnesic dysfunctions. *Schizophrenia Research, 5*(2), 115–121.

Benavidez, D. A., Fletcher, J. M., Hannay, H. J., Bland, S. T., Caudle, S. E., Mendelsohn, D. B., Yeakley, J., Brunder, D. G., Harward, H., Song, J., Perachio, N. A., Bruce, D., Scheibel, R. S., Lilly, M. A., Verger-Maestre, K., & Levin, H. S. (1999). Corpus callosum damage and interhemispheric transfer of information following closed head injury in children. *Cortex, 35*(3), 315–336.

Berlucchi, G., Heron, W., Hyman, R., Rizzolatti, G., & Umilta, C. (1971). Simple reaction times of ipsilateral and contralateral hand to lateralized visual stimuli. *Brain, 94*, 419–430.

Brown, W. S., Jeeves, M. A., Dietrich, R., & Burnison, D. S. (1999). Bilateral field advantage and evoked potential interhemispheric transmission in commissurotomy and callosal agenesis. *Neuropsychologia, 37*, 1165–1180.

Brown, W. S., Larson, E. B., & Jeeves, M. (1994). Directional asymmetries in interhemispheric transmission time: Evidence from visual evoked potentials. *Neuropsychologia, 32*, 439–448.

Chicoine, A. J., Proteau, L., & Lassonde, M. (2000). Absence of interhemispheric transfer of unilateral visuomotor learning in young children and individuals with agenesis of the corpus callosum. *Developmental Neuropsychology, 18*, 73–94.

Clarke, J. M., & Zaidel, E. (1989). Simple reaction times to lateralized light flashes: Varieties of interhemispheric communication routes. *Brain, 112*, 849–870.

Conturo, T. E., Lori, N. F., Cull, T. S., Akbudak, E., Snyder, A. Z., Shimony, J. S., McKinstry, R. C., Burton, H., & Raichle, M. E. (1999). Tracking neuronal fiber pathways in the living human brain. *Proceedings of the National Academy of Sciences, USA, 96*, 10422–10427.

Cronin-Golumb, A. (1986). Subcortical transfer of cognitive information in subjects with complete forebrain commissurotomy. *Cortex, 22*, 499–519.

Crow, T. J. (1997). Schizophrenia as a failure of hemispheric dominance for language. *Trends in Neurosciences, 20*, 339–343.

Cullum, C., Harris, J., Waldo, M., Smernoff, E., Madison, A., Nagamoto, H., Griffith, J., Adler, L., & Freedman, R. (1993). Neurophysiological and neuropsychological evidence for attentional dysfunction in schizophrenia. *Schizophrenia Research, 10*, 131–141.

David, A. S. (1993). Callosal transfer in schizophrenia: Too much or too little? *Journal of Abnormal Psychology, 102*, 573–579.

Davidson, R. J., Leslie, S. C., & Saron, C. (1990). Reaction time measures of interhemispheric transfer time in reading disabled and normal children. *Neuropsychologia, 28*, 471–485.

Dawson, M. E., Hazlett, E. A., Filion, D. L., Nuechterlein, K. H., & Schell, A. M. (1993). Attention and schizophrenia: Impaired modulation of the startle reflex. *Journal of Abnormal Psychology, 102*, 633–641.

DeLacoste, M. C., Kirkpatrick, J. B., & Ross, E. D. (1985). Topography of the human corpus callosum. *Journal of Neuropathology and Experimental Neurology, 44*, 578–591.

Downhill, J. E., Jr., Buchsbaum, M. S., Wei, T., Spiegel-Cohen, J., Hazlett, E. A., Haznedar, M. M., Silverman, J., & Siever, L. J. (2000). Shape and size of the corpus callosum in schizophrenia and schizotypal personality disorder. *Schizophrenia Research, 42*, 193–208.

Engel, A. K., Konig, P., Kreuter, A. K., & Singer, W. (1991). Interhemispheric synchronization of oscillatory neuronal responses in cat visual cortex. *Science, 252*, 1177–1179.

Ferman, T. J., Primeau, M., Delis, D., & Jampala, C. V. (1999). Global-local processing in schizophrenia: Hemispheric asymmetry and symptom-specific interference. *Journal of the International Neuropsychological Society, 5*, 442–451.

Foong, J., Maier, M., Clark, C. A., Barker, G. J., Miller, D. H., & Ron, M. A. (2000). Neuropathological abnormalities of the corpus callosum in schizophrenia: A diffusion tensor imaging study. *Journal of Neurology, Neurosurgery, & Psychiatry, 68*, 242–244.

Friedman, A., & Polson, M. C. (1981). The hemispheres as independent resource systems: Limited-capacity processing and cerebral specialization. *Journal of Experimental Psychology: Human Perception and Performance, 7*, 1031–1058.

Funnell, M. G., Corballis, P. M., & Gazzaniga, M. S. (2000). Insights into the functional specificity of the human corpus callosum. *Brain, 123*, 920–926.

Gazzaniga, M. S. (1987). Perceptual and attentional processes following callosal section in humans. *Neuropsychologia, 25*, 119–133.

Geffen, F. (1980). Phonological fusion after partial section of the corpus callosum. *Neuropsychologia, 18*, 613–620.

Geschwind, N., & Kaplan, E. (1962). A human cerebral disconnection syndrome. *Neurology, 12*, 675–685.

Goldberg, T. E., Gold, J. M., Greenberg, R., Griffin, S., Schulz, S. C., Pickar, D., Kleinman, J. E., & Weinberger, D. R. (1993). Contrasts between patients with affective disorders and patients with schizophrenia on a neuropsychological test battery. *American Journal of Psychiatry, 150*, 1355–1362.

Gur, R. (1978). Left hemisphere dysfunction and left hemisphere overactivation in schizophrenia. *Journal of Abnormal Psychology, 87*, 226–238.

Hagelthorn, K. M., Brown, W. S., Amano, S., & Asarnow, R. (2000). Normal development of the bilateral field advantage and evoked potential interhemispheric transfer time. *Developmental Neuropsychology, 18*, 11–32.

Hellige, J. B., Jonsson, J. E., & Michimata, C. (1988). Processing from LVF, RVF and BILATERAL presentations: Examination of metacontrol and interhemispheric interaction. *Brain and Cognition, 7*, 39–53.

Hellige, J. B., Taylor, A. K., & Eng, T. L. (1989). Interhemispheric interaction when both hemispehres have access to the same stimulus information. *Journal of Experimental Psychology: Human Perception and Performance, 15*, 711–722.

Hellige, J. B., Taylor, K. B., Lesmes, L., & Peterson, S. (1998). Relationships between brain morphology and behavioral measures of hemispheric asymmetry and interhemispheric interaction. *Brain & Cognition, 36,* 158–192.

Hines, M., Chui, L., McAdams, L. A., Bentler, P. M., & Lipcamon, J. (1992). Cognition and the corpus callosum: Verbal fluency, visuospatial ability, and language lateralization related to midsagittal surface areas of callosal subregions. *Behavioral Neuroscience, 106,* 3–14.

Holtzman, J. D. (1984). Interactions between cortical and subcortical visual areas: Evidence from human commissurotomy patients. *Vision Research, 24,* 801–813.

Holtzman, J. D., Sidtis, J. J., Volpe, B. T., Wilson, D. H., & Gazzaniga, M. S. (1981). Dissociation of spatial information for stimulus localization and the control of attention. *Brain, 104,* 861–872.

Jacobson, J. T., Deppe, U., & Murray, T. J. (1983). Dichotic paradigms in multiple sclerosis. *Ear and Hearing, 4,* 311–317.

Janowsky, J. S., Kaye, J. A., & Carper, R. A. (1996). Atrophy of the corpus callosum in Alzheimer's disease. *Journal of the American Geriatric Society, 44,* 798–803.

Jeeves, M. A. (1979). Some limits to interhemispheric integration in cases of callosal agenesis and partial commissurotomy. In I. S. Russell, M. W. van Hoff, & G. Berlucchi (Eds.), *Structure and function of the cerebral commissures* (pp. 449–474). New York: Macmillan.

Jeeves, M. A., & Lamb, A. (1988). Cerebral asymmetries and interhemispheric processes. *Behavioral Brain Research, 29,* 211–223.

Johnson, L. E. (1984). Bilateral visual cross-integration by human forebrain commissurotomy subjects. *Neuropsychologia, 22,* 167–175.

Kimchi, R., & Palmer, S. E. (1985). Separability and integrality of global and local levels of hierarchical patterns. *Journal of Experimental Psychology: Human Perception and Performance, 11,* 673–688.

Lamantia, A. S., & Rakic, P. (1990). Cytological and quantitative characteristics of four cerebral commissures in the rhesus monkey. *Journal of Comparative Neurology, 291,* 353–366.

Larson, E. B., & Brown, W. S. (1997). Bilateral field interactions, hemispheric specialization and evoked potential interhemispheric transmission time. *Neuropsychologia, 35,* 573–581.

Levin, S., High, W. M., Williams, D. J., Eisenberg, H. M., Amparo, E., Guinto, F., & Ewert, J. (1989). Dichotic listening and manual performance in relation to magnetic resonance imaging after closed head injury. *Journal of Neurology, Neurosurgery, and Psychiatry, 52,* 1162–1169.

Liederman, J., Merola, J., & Hoffman, C. (1986). Longitudinal data indicate that hemipsheric independence increases during early adolescence. *Developmental Neuropsychology, 2,* 183–201.

Luck, S. J., Hillyard, S. A., Mangun, G. R., & Gazzaniga, M. S. (1994). Independent attentional scanning in the separated hemispheres of split-brain patients. *Journal of Cognitive Neuroscience, 6,* 84–91.

Macmillan, N. A., & Creelman, C. D. (1991). *Detection theory: A user's guide*. New York: Cambridge University Press.

Marzi, C. A. (1999). The Poffenberger paradigm: A first, simple, behavioural tool to study interhemispheric transmission in humans. *Brain Research Bulletin, 50*, 421–422.

Marzi, C. A., Bisiacchi, P., & Nicoletti, R. (1991). Is interhemispheric transfer of visuomotor information asymmetric? Evidence from a meta-analysis. *Neuropsychologia, 29*, 1163–1177.

Michel, F., Henaff, M. A., & Intriligator, J. (1996). Two different readers in the same brain after a posterior callosal lesion. *NeuroReport, 7*, 786–788.

Milner, A. D., & Lines, C. R. (1982). Interhemispheric pathways in simple reaction time to lateralized light flash. *Neuropsychologia, 20*, 171–179.

Milner, B., Taylor, L., & Sperry, R. W. (1968). Lateralized suppression of dichotically presented digits after commissural section in man. *Science, 161*(3837), 184–186.

Mohr, B., Pulvermüller, F., Cohen, R., & Rockstroh, B. (2000). Interhemispheric cooperation during word processing: Evidence for callosal transfer dysfunction in schizophrenic patients. *Schizophrenia Research, 46*, 231–239.

Myers, J. J., & Sperry, R. W. (1985). Interhemispheric communication after section of the forebrain commissures. *Cortex, 21*, 249–260.

Nalçaci, E., Basar-Eroglu, C., & Stadler, M. (1999). VEP-interhemispheric transfer time in 20–32 Hz band in man. *NeuroReport, 10*, 3105–3109.

Pandya, D. N., & Seltzer, B. (1986). The topography of commissural fibers. In F. Lepore, M. Ptito, and H. Jasper (Eds.), *Two hemispheres—one brain: Functions of the corpus callosum* (pp. 47–73). New York: Liss.

Passarotti, A. M., Banich, M. T., Sood, R. K., & Wang, J. M. (2002). A generalized role of interhemispheric interaction under attentionally demanding conditions: Evidence from the auditory and tactile modalities. *Neuropsychologia, 40*, 1082–1096.

Pelletier, J., Habib, M., Lyon-Caen, O., Salamon, G., Poncet, M., & Khalil, R. (1993). Functional and magnetic resonance imaging correlates of callosal involvement in multiple sclerosis. *Archives of Neurology, 50*(10), 1077–1082.

Polster, M. R., & Rapcsak, S. Z. (1994). Hierarchical stimuli and hemispheric specialization: Two case studies. *Cortex, 30*, 487–497.

Preilowski, B. (1975). Bilateral motor interaction: Perceptual motor performance of partial and complete "split-brain" patients. In K. J. Zulch, O. Creutzfeldt, and G. C. Galbraith (Eds.), *Cerebral localization* (pp. 115–132). Berlin: Springer.

Preilowski, B. (1990). Intermanual transfer, interhemispheric interaction, and handedness in man and monkeys. In C. Trevarthen (Ed.), *Brain circuits, and functions of the mind* (pp. 168–180). New York: Cambridge University Press.

Quinn, K., & Geffen, G. (1986). The development of tactile transfer of information. *Neuropsychologia, 24*, 793–804.

Rao, S. M., Bernardin, L., Leo, G. J., Ellington, L., Ryan, S. B., & Burg, L. S. (1989). Cerebral disconnection in multiple sclerosis: Relationship to atrophy of the corpus callosum. *Archives of Neurology, 46,* 918–920.

Raye, C. L., Johnson, M. K., Mitchell, K. J., Nolde, S. F., & D'Esposito, M. (2000). fMRI investigations of left and right PFC contributions to episodic remembering. *Psychobiology Special Issue: Subregional Analysis of Prefrontal Cortex Mediation of Cognitive Functions in Rats, Monkeys, and Humans, 28*(2), 197–206.

Rayman, J., & Zaidel, E. (1991). Rhyming and the right hemisphere. *Brain and Language, 40,* 89–105.

Reuter-Lorenz, P. A., & Stanczak, L. (2000). Differential effects of aging on functions of the corpus callosum. *Developmental Neuropsychology, 18,* 113–137.

Reuter-Lorenz, P. A., Stanczak, L., & Miller, A. (1999). Neural recruitment and cognitive aging: Two hemispheres are better than one, especially as you age. *Psychological Science, 10,* 494–500.

Risse, G. L., Gates, J., Lund, G., Maxwell, R., & Rubens, A. (1989). Interhemispheric transfer in patients with incomplete section of the corpus callosum: Anatomical verification with magnetic resonance imaging. *Archives of Neurology, 46,* 437–443.

Robertson, L. C., Lamb, M. R., & Zaidel, E. (1993). Interhemispheric relations in processing hierarchical patterns: Evidence from normal and commissurotomized subjects. *Neuropsychology, 7,* 325–342.

Rugg, M. D., Lines, C. R., & Milner, A. D. (1984). Visual evoked potentials to lateralized visual stimuli and the measurement of interhemispheric transmission time. *Neuropsychologia, 22,* 215–225.

St. John, R., Shields, C., Krahn, P., & Tinney, B. (1987). The reliability of estimates of interhemispheric transfer times derived from unimanual and verbal response latencies. *Human Neurobiology, 6,* 195–202.

Salamy, A. (1978). Commissural transmission: Maturational changes in humans. *Science, 22,* 1409–1411.

Scarrone, S., Abbruzzese, M., & Gambini, O. (1993). Monaural and binaural recall of stories in schizophrenia: Neurofunctional hypotheses. *Neuropsychiatry, Neuropsychology & Behavioral Neurology, 6,* 154–158.

Schreiber, H., Stolz-Born, G., Heinrich, H., Kornhuber, H., & Born, J. (1992). Attention, cognition, and motor perseveration in adolescents at genetic risk for schizophrenia and control subjects. *Psychiatry Research, 44,* 125–140.

Sergent, J. (1990). Furtive incursions into bicameral minds. *Brain, 113,* 537–568.

Sergent, J. (1991). Processing of spatial relations within and between the disconnected cerebral hemispheres. *Brain, 114,* 1025–1043.

Shenker, J. I., & Banich, M. T. (submitted). The modulation of attentional capacity in the Stroop task by communication between the cerebral hemispheres.

Simon, J. H., Holtas, S. L., Schiffer, R. B., Rudick, R. A., Herndon, R. M., Kido, D. K., & Utz, R. (1986). Corpus callosum and subcallosal periventricular lesions in multiple sclerosis: Detection with MR. *Radiology, 160*, 363–367.

Sperry, R. W., Zaidel, E., & Zaidel, D. (1979). Self recognition and social awareness in the deconnected minor hemisphere. *Neuropsychologia, 17*, 153–166.

Suzuki, K., Yamadori, A., Endo, K., Fujii, T., Ezura, M., & Takahashi, A. (1998). Dissociation of letter and picture naming resulting from callosal disconnection. *Neurology, 51*, 1390–1394.

Trevarthen, C. (Ed.) (1990). *Brain circuits and functions of the mind.* Cambridge: Cambridge University Press.

Trevarthen, C., & Sperry, R. W. (1973). Perceptual unity of the ambient visual field in human commissurotomy patients. *Brain, 96*, 547–570.

Vuilleumier, P., & Assal, G. (1995). Complete callosal disconnection after closed head injury. *Clinical Neurology and Neurosurgery, 97*, 39–46.

Weissman, D. H., & Banich, M. T. (1999). Global-local interference modulated by communication between the hemispheres. *Journal of Experimental Psychology: General, 128*, 283–308.

Weissman, D. H., & Banich, M. T. (2000). The cerebral hemispheres cooperate to perform complex but not simple tasks. *Neuropsychology, 14*(1), 41–59.

Weissman, D. H., Banich, M. T., & Puente, E. I. (2000). An unbalanced distribution of inputs across the hemispheres facilitates interhemispheric interaction. *Journal of the International Neuropsychological Society, 6*, 313–321.

Woodruff, P. W., Pearlson, G. D., Geer, M. J., Barta, P. E., & Chilcoat, H. D. (1993). A computerized magnetic resonance imaging study of corpus callosum morphology in schizophrenia. *Psychological Medicine, 23*, 45–56.

Zoccolotti, P., Matano, A., Deloche, G., Cantagallo, A., Passadori, A., Leclercq, M., Braga, L., Cremel, N., Pittau, P., Renom, M., Rousseaux, M., Truche, A., Fimm, B., & Zimmermann, P. (2000). Patterns of attentional impairment following closed head injury: A collaborative European study. *Cortex, 36*(1), 93–107.

Marie T. Banich

9 Asymmetries in Encoding Spatial Relations

Bruno Laeng, Christopher F. Chabris, and Stephen M. Kosslyn

Our phenomenology seems to respect the Newtonian distinction between matter and space, in contrast with the view of modern physics (since Einstein) of space and matter as two indissoluble aspects of a whole (Smart, 1964). Intuitively, space appears as either an all-pervading stuff or some sort of receptacle filled by material bodies. In cognitive neuroscience, evidence has accumulated that the brain processes space and form as two independent aspects of reality; indeed, a ventral neuroanatomical pathway running from the occipital lobe to the inferior temporal lobe processes shape, color, and other "object properties," whereas a dorsal pathway running from the occipital lobe to the posterior parietal lobe processes location and other "spatial properties" (e.g., Ungerleider & Mishkin, 1982). Such a division of labor between brain areas appears to be a pervasive principle of neural organization, and since the 1800s (cf. Harrington, 1987, 1995) evidence has been growing within the neurosciences that complex mental abilities fractionate into sets of subsystems, each devoted to a specific computational task (Kosslyn & Koenig, 1995).

At the root of our spatial knowledge is the ability to register *locations*. Our proposal is that at least two different properties can be extracted from specifications of location. These properties may be logically independent; that is, knowledge of one may be neither necessary nor sufficient to know the other. Because the properties we are referring to essentially define relations between locations, we shall refer to them as different types of *spatial relations*. According to its original formulation (Kosslyn, 1987), there is an early split within the dorsal stream of visual information into two subnetworks that process qualitatively different types of spatial information. These two networks within the dorsal system are each concerned with one type of computation, and each type describes a different kind of spatial relation.

COORDINATE SPATIAL RELATIONS

One type of spatial relations representation captures coordinate relations. These sorts of relations occur within a metric space; that is, an order or collection of points on which distance between points is defined. A point could be the lowest level of resolution of the visual system. An order of such points creates a continuum. In other words, this form of representing space is analog or dense (Goodman, 1976), in the sense that two spatial forms can transform into one another through intermediate orders of points.

For example, orders of points constitute lines and areas in two dimensions, or volumes in three, and all possible objects of this kind can transform continuously into one another by simply adding or deleting intermediate points. Thus, the ability to encode coordinate relations would allow the perception and expression of space in a quantitative sense. Distance, size, and orientation between two locations or sets of locations (such as volumes) could be represented integrally in such an encoding system.

This coordinate mode of coding interrelations is most suitable for the control of movement of the body and its parts. Thus, although visual, this type of coding appears to be motor-based, in the sense that it provides a form of representation that can be used to guide movements, such as navigating within the near-to-the-body physical medium, tracking, reaching, and manipulating other external bodies. In general, spatial action would seem to be supported by encodings that specify distal locations as the end points of actions. At first glance, this formulation might seem to exclude the mappings of places and objects that are unreachable or not navigable (e.g., flying birds and stars). Many classes of spatially located objects imply a lack of bodily contact; however, we can point to or look at any visible object. Hence, anything in the line of vision can constitute a specific external target of a directed movement for the index finger or the eye.

CATEGORICAL SPATIAL RELATIONS

As proposed by Piaget and Inhelder (1956), there may be modes of perception that are alternative and qualitatively different from the one

B. Laeng, C. F. Chabris, and S. M. Kosslyn

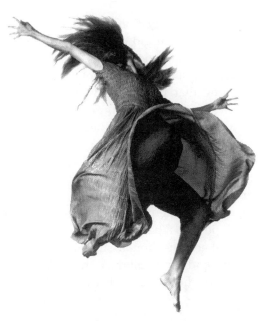

Figure 9.1 Contorted human body. (From Lois Greenfield, *Breaking Bounds*. London: Thames and Hudson, 1992.)

necessary to guide action, and each of these different formats may uniquely enrich the cognitive system's analysis of space. We have good reason to believe that for some tasks where spatial information seems useful, coordinate information is irrelevant and in fact may be counterproductive. For example, some problems of object recognition would seem to require integration of visual information about shape with spatial information about the arrangement of the object's parts. In particular, the recognition of nonrigid objects, when their parts are positioned in novel ways (e.g., a contorted human body; see figure 9.1), may depend heavily on being able to recover their spatial structure. Because the flexible object's parts may not be in their usual locations, a novel view could radically change an object's familiar global geometry and become, in essence, an unknown shape. If some parts are visible in the image and these suggest the presence of a specific object, then stored information about the spatial arrangement of the parts (i.e., a stored structural description) could guide a search for other parts of the object and confirm or discard such a perceptual hypothesis (e.g., Kosslyn, 1987).

However, using metric information would be irrelevant for such a recognition task, because nonrigid objects flex and bend, and therefore do not preserve constant metric relations between their parts. Therefore, another type of spatial description of the object's geometry seems more useful, one that preserves invariant spatial information by ignoring metric information. Indeed, many contemporary theories of object identification (e.g., Marr, 1982; Biederman, 1987) assume that objects are represented using such structural descriptions, which use abstract types of spatial representations to specify relations among parts (e.g., top-of, end-to-middle-connected, left-side-connected).

To offer another example (see figure 9.2), we can see a human hand as composed of many parts: the palm, the fingers, each finger with its nail and knuckles. Obviously, a hand can make gestures (that is, flex its fingers in several ways) and therefore assume many shapes, while only its boned parts remain rigid across all the transformations. Yet, the way the parts are arranged, or the specific constraints dictated by the structure of connectivity, remains invariant across these transformations and it is inherently spatial, albeit in an abstract sense. Consider that nails are the endpoint and topside of fingers and arc on the backside of the whole hand. When looking down at your hands' palms, the right hand is distinguishable from its left companion because the thumb (easily recognizable by the two, instead of three, phalanges) is attached to the right side of the palm. It is the specification of these connectivity relations that we believe provides a stable representation of the object's shape. The adaptive value of a spatial system that can provide encodings of such relations is not trivial. Its ability to aid the recognition of flexible objects (e.g., other living beings), especially in nonoptimal viewing conditions (when their bodies are contorted in novel ways), has obvious biological significance.

In addition, recognizing contorted objects may not be the only function of abstract, nonmetric, spatial encodings. Generally speaking, nonmetric relations can be described for completely disjointed objects or meaningless visual stimuli (e.g., two dots can be seen above or below a line). Within the more general account, whatever appears to be occupying space (i.e., a figure on a background) can in principle be encoded as being in some reciprocal spatial relation. Categorical encodings are mappings of abstract relations between locations; such processes can occur independently from, and in parallel with, the recognition or identification of shapes, objects, and parts of objects. Nevertheless, if the

B. Laeng, C. F. Chabris, and S. M. Kosslyn

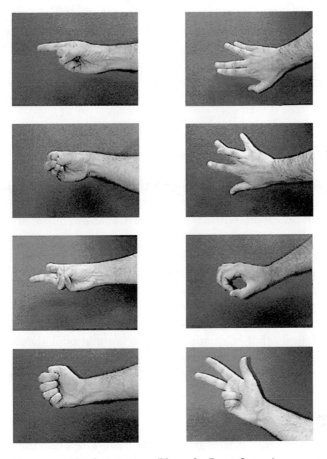

Figure 9.2 Hand contortions (Photos by Bruno Laeng.)

objects viewed have a complex geometry, higher-order spatial relations can emerge between them and can also be encoded (consider all the relations determined by the surfaces of the human body: front/back, top/bottom, and left/right sides).

Thus, close to Kosslyn's original formulation (1987), we define categorical encodings as groupings of locations that define an equivalence class. At the root of such encodings is the ability to delineate patches of space or to discover boundaries or limits that separate bins of space. Categorical encodings are abstract compared to coordinate ones, because a greater number of the latter can be comprised within a position described by the former (e.g., "anything to the left of that point"). Different categorical spatial relations are qualitatively disjoint, and therefore cannot transform into another (e.g., the relation "inside" cannot map onto "left of" in any formal sense); it is important that these spatial representations cannot support continuous rigid transformations of objects (e.g., spatial rotations), as can occur within a coordinate framework.

A Model of Spatial Relations Encodings: Lateralized Processing

In recent years, the use of computational theories in neuropsychology has become increasingly influential. Such theories make explicit how different processes work together to transform input to output in a given behavioral task, and thus have the advantage of being both specific enough to be implemented in a computer program and general enough to accomplish well-defined tasks (e.g., Kosslyn, 1987; Shallice, 1988; Farah, 1990; Behrmann et al., 1991; Humphreys et al., 1992; Kosslyn, 1994; Ivry & Robertson, 1998). We can distinguish the two hemispheres of the brain according to the type of information processing or computations that they support. A computational theory of cerebral asymmetry specifies what type of representation each hemisphere encodes most effectively. Thus, it differs from other theories of hemispheric specialization (cf. Bradshaw & Nettleton, 1983; for a review, see Springer & Deutsch, 1998) that either (1) focus on ill-defined distinctions, such as "cognitive style" or "strategies" (e.g., holistic versus analytical), or (2) equate each hemisphere's preferred function with specific tasks (e.g., spatial versus verbal versus musical).

Nevertheless, because all theories of cerebral lateralization must provide an account for the same data, there are analogies between different theories. For example, the present theory's distinction between categorical and coordinate encoding shows some relationship to the traditional verbal/nonverbal distinction between the processing of two hemispheres. Specifically, because we posit categorical spatial relations to be qualitative and discrete (often expressed in binary oppositions; e.g., on/off), we would expect that they should easily map onto spatial concepts and words. Indeed, all natural languages seem to have a special class in their grammar (i.e., prepositions) devoted to the expression of categorical spatial relations (cf. Miller & Johnson-Laird, 1976). In contrast, because we posit coordinate spatial relations to be quantitative and continuous, we would expect these relations to be difficult to verbalize (e.g., telling how many inches apart two objects are and verbally describing someone's face are notoriously difficult tasks).

Kosslyn (1987, 1994) hypothesized that although both hemispheres embody computational subsystems that encode the two types of spatial relations representations, the subsystem that encodes categorical spatial relations is more efficient in the left hemisphere, whereas the one that encodes coordinate spatial relations is more efficient in the right hemisphere. The theory is grounded on the idea that the two types of spatial relations are most efficiently computed by separate subsystems, a hypothesis that has been independently supported by computational simulations. For example, Kosslyn et al. (1992) showed that model neural networks encode the two types of spatial relations better if the networks are split, so that different partitions encode categorical and coordinate relations, than if a single, undifferentiated network must encode both types of relations (figure 9.3). One study with a large cohort of brain-damaged patients (Laeng, 1994) has shown that lesions to one hemisphere result in more impairment in one type of spatial encoding than in the other, and lesions to the other hemisphere result in the reverse impairment. This finding lends support to the idea that the human neural substrate separates the computations underlying each spatial encoding into split neural networks, each in one cerebral hemisphere.

DIFFERENCES IN RECEPTIVE VISUAL FIELDS

The theory has evolved over time, and the computational models have been developed in more detail (cf. Jacobs & Kosslyn, 1994; Kosslyn & Jacobs, 1994). In the current version of the theory, different processes accomplish the two kinds of spatial encoding, but these processes in turn regulate attention to facilitate encoding the appropriate aspects of the input. Specifically, according to this theory, the efficiency with which spatial relations are encoded depends critically on the receptive fields of the neurons that are being attended. A visual neuron's receptive field is the region in space from which that neuron receives stimulation, and neurons can differ in the sizes of their receptive fields. In addition, the receptive fields of different neurons may overlap to differing degrees.

Computational simulations showed that categorical spatial relations are encoded more effectively if the outputs being attended come from

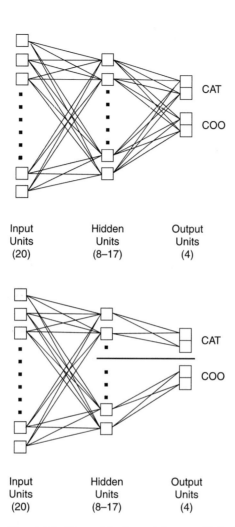

Figure 9.3 The architecture of the unsplit (*top*) and split (*bottom*) networks. (Numbers in parentheses indicate the size of the layers.) CAT, categorical spatial relations; COO, coordinate spatial relations. (From Kosslyn et al., 1992.)

neurons with relatively small, nonoverlapping receptive fields, as opposed to relatively large, overlapping receptive fields. For categorical relations, an observer can attend to one object and group the receptive fields for the surrounding space into "bins" that have specific spatial relations relative to the object being focused upon; it is then a small step to categorize the relation of a second object that falls into one of

B. Laeng, C. F. Chabris, and S. M. Kosslyn

these bins. Moreover, the models showed that coordinate spatial relations representations are encoded more effectively if the outputs from neurons with relatively large, overlapping receptive fields are attended, facilitating coarse-coding (e.g., Hinton et al., 1986; O'Reilly et al., 1990). According to this account, outputs from neurons with large, overlapping receptive fields allow a system to localize a stimulus precisely.

Empirical evidence from human studies has shown that the left cerebral hemisphere (LH) has a bias to filter visual input through small attended areas (or high spatial frequency processing), whereas the right cerebral hemisphere (RH) has a bias to filter visual input through large attended areas (low spatial frequencies; for a thorough review of the evidence, see Ivry & Robertson, 1998; see also Kitterle et al., 1990; Kitterle & Selig, 1991; Sergent, 1991a). For example, when "striped" stimuli, such as sinusoidal gratings with wide stripes (e.g., at a low spatial frequency of 1 cycle/degree) and narrow stripes (e.g., at a high spatial frequency of 9 cycles/degree) are presented in the left visual field (LVF) or in the right visual field (RVF), subjects identify the wide-striped stimuli better in the LVF than in the RVF. In contrast, narrow-striped stimuli are better identified in the RVF than in the LVF. This processing asymmetry appears to be mediated by attentional mechanisms, not hardwired differences in the population of receptors feeding into each hemisphere (Kosslyn et al., 1994; Ivry & Robertson, 1998).

The convergence and combination of outputs from neurons involved in early visual processing within each hemisphere could promote the encoding of higher-order spatial properties. However, these later encodings would be more or less easily computed, depending on properties of the early encodings. Specifically, we would expect that the large, overlapping receptive fields of the neurons in the RH would promote encoding fine-grained, precise, coordinate spatial relations through a coarse-coding strategy. In contrast, filtering visual input through small, nonoverlapping receptive fields in the LH would help to divide space around the center of attention into categorically distinct regions, which would promote encoding categorical spatial relations. Moreover, these hemispheric encoding biases should also affect the way each hemisphere process shapes (cf. Delis et al., 1986; Robertson & Delis, 1986; Robertson & Lamb, 1991; Jacobs & Kosslyn, 1994). Accordingly, we would expect exemplar or individual-level representations of shapes to be encoded more efficiently in the RH (Marsolek et al., 1992; Marsolek, 1995). In contrast, the LH's ability to focus attention over

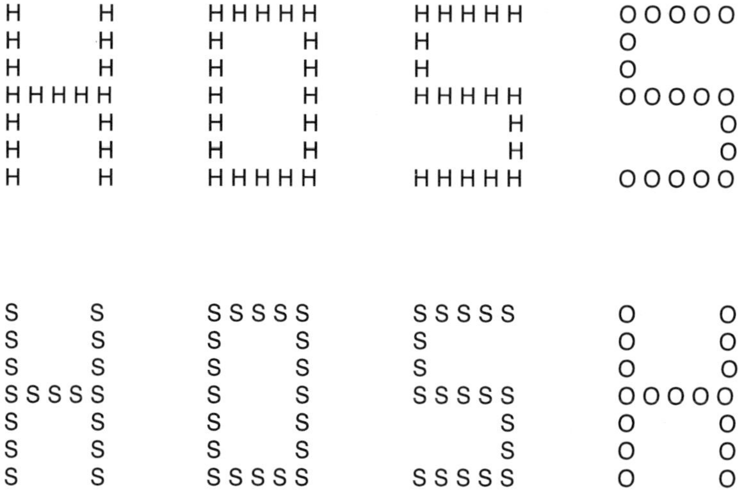

```
H       H       H H H H H       H H H H H       O O O O O
H       H       H       H       H               O
H       H       H       H       H               O
H H H H H       H       H       H H H H H       O O O O O
H       H       H       H               H               O
H       H       H       H               H               O
H       H       H H H H H       H H H H H       O O O O O


S       S       S S S S S       S S S S S       O       O
S       S       S       S       S               O       O
S       S       S       S       S               O       O
S S S S S       S       S       S S S S S       O O O O O
S       S       S       S               S       O       O
S       S       S       S               S       O       O
S       S       S S S S S       S S S S S       O       O
```

Figure 9.4 Hierarchical visual stimuli used by Van Kleeck (1989).

distinct and discrete regions may be better suited for "carving out" patterns contained within other patterns, or the extraction of parts from a global shape (Van Kleeck, 1989; figure 9.4).

The receptive field biases of the cerebral hemispheres may in part reflect differences in the use of information from two neural pathways: the transient, or magnocellular (M), and the sustained, or parvocellular (P). These pathways both begin at the retina and continue to high levels of the visual system; one of the differences between them is that neurons in the M pathway have larger receptive fields than those in the P pathway (Livingstone & Hubel, 1988). Kosslyn and colleagues (1992) proposed that the M pathway may provide more input to the RH than to the LH, whereas the P pathway has more connections with the LH than the RH. Alternatively, it may be that the LH is biased to encode information from the P pathway, and the RH is biased to encode information from the M pathway, rather than that there are actual anatomical distinctions between the connections of the two pathways in the two cerebral hemispheres.

THE "SNOWBALL" MECHANISM

At the initial formulation of the present theory (e.g., Kosslyn, 1987), other theoretical considerations had led us to expect that a specific

B. Laeng, C. F. Chabris, and S. M. Kosslyn

spatial encoding subsystem could develop more strongly in one hemisphere than in the other. Namely, the original idea was that an effective computational architecture will "yoke" subsystems that often operate together, facilitating their joint operation (cf. Jacobs & Kosslyn, 1994). Another way to express this relation between different but interdependent subsystems is that they exert reciprocal feedback training (Van Kleeck & Kosslyn, 1991); that is, to the extent that a process receives useful input, it reinforces the process that sends that input, thereby making the sending process operate more efficiently in the future (Kosslyn, Sokolov, et al., 1989). An interesting implication of this theory is that small initial differences between the hemispheres could compound during development, ultimately producing a wide range of functional asymmetries, via a "snowball" mechanism.

Of particular relevance for this account is the evidence that the speech output control system is genetically constrained to develop in the LH (Corballis, 1991). This constraint may derive from the fact that "action" in general may best originate from a unilateral source of control, as opposed to several potentially interfering, bilateral executive centers. Indeed, the evidence from neuropsychology indicates LH's dominance in speech as well as other complex motor behaviors or praxis (Heilman & Valenstein, 1985).

Our proposal is that LH's initial bias for the speech output control system may constitute the "seed" for the development in the same hemisphere of other interdependent, yoked subsystems. In turn, the knowledge database (semantic and verbal, containing facts and words) could become more dependent on processing in the LH than in the RH (cf. De Renzi et al., 1969; Warrington & Taylor, 1978; Gazzaniga, 1983; Gainotti et al., 1995; Damasio et al., 1996; Caramazza & Shelton, 1998). Moreover, if the LH generally possesses a richer representation of the lexical and semantic information than does the RH, then these systems in the LH will also exert better feedback training of the pattern recognition and spatial encoding subsystems in the same (LH) hemisphere, thereby providing them with the optimal input for access to conceptual and lexical representations of space.

In summary, according to the theory, complementary encoding subsystems develop in different hemispheres under the influence of different sources, such as early spatial frequency biases and unilateral feedback training from the speech control system. These sources contribute to channeling and grouping compatible types of information processing within one hemisphere while splitting and dividing, across the corpus callosum, the less compatible types.

EMPIRICAL EVIDENCE FOR CATEGORICAL AND COORDINATE SPATIAL RELATIONS ENCODING IN SEPARATE CEREBRAL HEMISPHERES

The theory is consistent with a large and varied body of empirical findings that rely on different methodologies and different subject populations. In this section, we briefly review these results.

Divided Visual Field Studies

Most of the evidence garnered for the theory relies on divided-visual-field studies (for a review of this methodology, see Beaumont, 1982, or Bryden, 1982). Specifically, the theory predicts an interaction between the visual field in which stimuli are presented and the way in which spatial relations must be encoded to perform the task: Subjects should be faster and more accurate when stimuli are presented in the LVF (to the RH initially) and coordinate spatial relations must be encoded, and faster and more accurate when stimuli are presented in the RVF (to the LH initially) and categorical spatial relations must be encoded.

In one of Kosslyn's (1987) initial experiments, subjects were shown stimuli like the blob and dot in figure 9.5. In one condition, the subjects were asked to verify whether the dot was on or off the blob, and in another condition they were asked whether the dot was within 2 mm of the blob (including being on its contour) or farther than 2 mm. As predicted, the on/off, categorical, spatial judgment was easier when the stimuli were presented initially to the LH, whereas the less/more than 2 mm, coordinate, judgment was easier when the stimuli were presented initially to the RH.

Hellige and Michimata (1989; see also Kosslyn, Koenig, et al., 1989) replicated these complementary hemispheric advantages for categorical and coordinate judgments with another simple perceptual task (figure 9.6). In the categorical condition, subjects were asked whether the dot was above or below the bar; in the coordinate condition, they were asked whether the dot was at a distance greater or less than 2 cm from the bar.

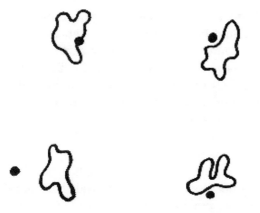

Figure 9.5 Blob and dot stimuli used in the original near/far, on/off task.

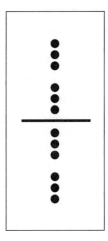

Figure 9.6 The standard dot-above/below-bar stimuli used by Hellige and Michimata (1989).

Several researchers criticized these initial experiments on both methodological and conceptual grounds. Sergent (1991a) had difficulty replicating Kosslyn and colleagues' findings, even with similar stimuli, unless the stimuli were presented with relatively low levels of luminance. She also challenged the validity of the categorical/coordinate distinction on methodological and conceptual grounds by proposing that a single, coordinate spatial representation was sufficient and logically prior to computing any other type of spatial relation. Specifically, if the exact locations of two objects in two-dimensional space are known, then it should be trivial to deduce which object is above the other. By contrast, knowing only that one object is above another does not provide the information needed to find the distance between them.

Kosslyn et al. (1992) replied by proposing a computational mechanism that could underlie the encoding of the two types of spatial relations. In these computational simulations (see also Jacobs & Kosslyn, 1994; Kosslyn & Jacobs, 1994), metric (coordinate) distance relations could be extracted directly from visual arrays by filtering visual input through large overlapping receptive fields, which enable coarse coding. In contrast, as we noted earlier, they showed that outputs from units with small, nonoverlapping receptive fields can divide visual space into patches corresponding to simple categorical relations. Moreover, they showed why these effects would be evident only at low levels of illumination, assuming that at higher levels the quantitative differences in the proportions of units with large vs. small receptive fields becomes irrelevant (due, essentially, to ceiling effects).

Cowin and Hellige (1994) used, together with the standard dot-above/below-bar paradigm of Hellige and Michimata (1989), a modified condition in which the stimuli were blurred. They found that blurring impaired categorical but not coordinate judgments. As Ivry and Robertson (1998) point out, it is not intuitive how a theory based on categorical and coordinate spatial relations accounts for such a selective effect. The key idea is that blurring does not affect the outputs from neurons with large receptive fields, but it degrades distinctions usually registered by neurons with small receptive fields. Hence, the theory does make the counterintuitive prediction that judgments of metric distance should be affected less by blurring than judgments of categorical relations, if in fact judgments of metric distance rely on outputs from neurons with large, overlapping receptive fields.

As noted earlier, information from the transient, or magnocellular (M), pathway may be tapped primarily by the coordinate spatial relations encoding process, whereas information from the sustained, or parvocellular (P), pathways may be used primarily by the categorical spatial relations encoding process (Kosslyn et al., 1992). One way to differentially activate the two pathways is to alter the color of stimuli: Diffuse red light reduces the response of some M pathway neurons, from the retina through the lateral geniculate nucleus, to primary visual cortex (Dreher et al., 1976). Accordingly, if the RH preferentially uses information from the M pathway, including red in a display should reduce LVF performance relative to a control condition with no red. Roth and Hellige (1998) directly tested this idea in two tasks, asking whether a line is above or below a pair of dots and whether it is short enough to fit between them (cf. Rybash & Hoyer, 1992). Critically, they varied the color (red/green) of the stimuli or the background. The results were consistent with Kosslyn and colleagues' (1992) predictions: The red background, which as the dominant color in the stimulus should inhibit the M pathway and reduce RH detection performance, slowed coordinate processing. Also, when red was the only color present in the display, coordinate processing was impaired and categorical processing was not.

Several other experiments, described below, have overall converged on finding the expected visual field differences. In some of these studies, the effects have been transient (e.g., Kosslyn et al., 1989), and there have also been clear failures to replicate some of the single visual field differences (cf. Sergent, 1991a; Rybash & Hoyer, 1992; Kogure & Hatta, 1999; Wilkinson & Donnelly, 1999). However, most important, the reverse pattern of dissociations has never been reported.

In addition, some studies have produced results that could not have been predicted by the theory. For example, Banich and Federmeier (1999) replicated the basic dot-bar task asymmetry only when the bar appeared unpredictably at one of several different vertical positions on each trial. Horner and Freides (1996) replicated the hypothesized asymmetries when stimuli were presented at 3 degrees of visual angle, but not at 1 or 9 degrees.

Bruyer et al. (1997) have shown that, at least with the standard dot-below/above-line paradigm, the expected task-by-visual-field interaction is fragile and influenced by several methodological factors. Bruyer and colleagues varied, in a series of experiments, either the mode of response (vocal versus manual), the presence or absence of feedback, whether there was a binary versus continuous response, and the age of the subjects. They were able to reveal the expected visual field effects and their double dissociation, but across all the experiments some of the single visual field differences appeared unstable.

Parrot et al. (1999) varied the level of difficulty of each spatial judgment, and observed an LH advantage for categorical spatial relations as well as "easy" coordinate processing, in contrast to an RH advantage for "difficult" coordinate decisions. Interestingly, other researchers have reported that the RH advantage for coordinate encoding may disappear before the end of the testing session (Kosslyn, Koenig, et al., 1989; cf. Rybash & Hoyer, 1992). Coordinate spatial relations encoding in the LH appears to improve over time, and eventually "catches up" with the RH. A possible explanation for this phenomenon is that new spatial categories get formed that allow the LH-based processes to perform more effectively. Consistent with this view, Koenig et al. (1992) have shown that the more complex and novel the categories a task calls for, the more time the LH needs to match the RH in performance. Chabris and Kosslyn (1998) have reported that practice in the coordinate task transfers to the categorical judgment, but not vice versa, again suggesting that the categorical system is gradually "tuned" when one performs a new coordinate task (and is thereby "primed" for operation).

A few divided-fields studies have made use of more "natural" stimuli than the initial studies. Michimata (1997) used figures of clocks and asked subjects to make categorical and coordinate decisions about the positions of the two hands. Laeng and Peters (1995) presented figures of animals that, given their geometric complexity, allow the testing of several high-order categorical relations (figure 9.7). Moreover, although studies have typically used distance for the coordinate judgments, Laeng and Peters (1995) tested other coordinate relations, such as size and tilt. Interestingly, this study revealed large visual field differences in response times for both spatial relation decisions (circa 100 ms), in contrast to the majority of studies in which differences between the hemispheres are on the order of a few tens of milliseconds. Possibly the increased computational complexity arising from the inferred 3-D geometry of depictions of natural objects, and the absence of a single, systematic relation manipulation in each spatial task, could have contributed to increase the strength of each hemisphere's encoding advantage and in reducing practice effects.

Servos and Peters (1990) used line drawings of objects in depth (such as the cubes of Shepard & Metzler, 1971) and asked subjects to decide whether the top or bottom part of the figure was closer to the observer (i.e., an in-front/behind categorical decision). They found a strong LH advantage, and also found such an advantage when the judgment involved simple flat figures occluding one another. The latter finding is in contrast to a study by Kogure and Hatta (1999), who also used flat, occluding stimuli, resembling playing cards, and a task that involved

B. Laeng, C. F. Chabris, and S. M. Kosslyn

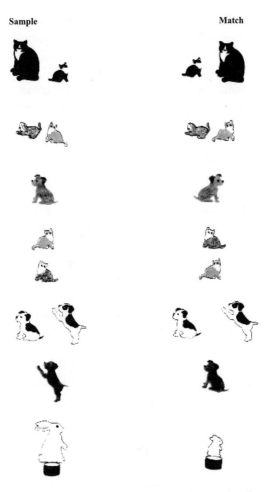

Sample   **Match**

Figure 9.7 Stimuli used by Laeng and Peters (1995).

reporting the number written on the leftmost/rightmost or front/rear card. An RH advantage was found with this task. The discrepancy between the two studies may arise from the fact that the latter experiment required subjects to find a number located on a specific card, which could have benefited from coordinate information.

Kosslyn et al. (1995) have tested the effects of categorical and coordinate processing within the imagery domain (see also Michimata, 1997). Subjects were asked to form images of uppercase letters and to judge whether a letter shape would cover a laterally presented probe. They found that in a condition where a grid was provided on which to form images, there was an RVF advantage, whereas in a condition without a grid there was an LVF advantage. They suggest that the grid supports arranging the parts according to categorical spatial relations (such as "left column, attached at top to right row"), whereas with no grid, subjects would have to rely on more precise metric information in order to generate the visual images.

Laeng et al. (1997) tested the hypothesis that the LH categorizes space into regions by studying the strength of each cerebral hemisphere's memory bias toward prototypical locations or centers of parsed regions of a display. They used a task developed by Huttenlocher et al. (1991) in which a dot appears within a circle at variable angular and radial positions, and subjects are later asked to indicate the dot's position on an empty circle. Huttenlocher and colleagues found that subjects make precise estimates but at the same time show a bias toward prototypical/canonical locations within regions of space (namely, the estimates regress toward the angular and radial center of each invisible quadrant in the circle). These effects demonstrate a double spatial coding of a point's location: (a) in terms of metrics (exactly where) and (b) in terms of the categorical location (where in relation to classes of locations corresponding to parsed regions of space). Laeng et al. (1997) found, in a divided-fields paradigm, that the regressions of spatial estimates toward each quadrant's canonical position were stronger after RVF presentation than LVF presentation, supporting the view that the LH is specifically engaged in parsing space into regions or classes of locations, and stores this spatial information.

Laeng, Shah, et al. (1999) have specifically tested the hypothesis that the LH's categorical spatial processing facilitates the recognition of difficult views of objects, particularly contorted poses of nonrigid objects (figure 9.8). Marr (1982) proposed that the brain stores "structural descriptions" composed of primitives such as generalized cones; Biederman (1987, 1995) has developed a theory of edge-based structural descriptions that specify the components (i.e., geons) of a shape and the qualitative (categorical) spatial relations between these parts (e.g., left-of, top-of, larger-than, end-to-end-connected). One key advantage conferred by the abstractness of these perceptual descriptions is that an object's structure can be captured in a way that remains invariant across a potentially infinite number of shapes or variations of projections.

B. Laeng, C. F. Chabris, and S. M. Kosslyn

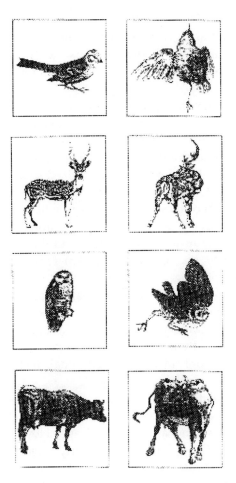

Figure 9.8 Conventional (*left*) and contorted poses (*right*) of animals. (From Laeng, Shah, et al., 1999.)

Based on the ideas that (a) overall shapes are encoded better by the RH, (b) categorical spatial relations are encoded better by the LH, and (c) categorical relations are used in structural descriptions, Laeng, Shah, et al. (1999) predicted and confirmed an RVF advantage when one first encodes the contorted pose of an animal and an LVF advantage for encoding the same shapes after they are familiar. Moreover, when correlation analyses between the time to match pictures of contorted animals to names and the time to encode categorical spatial relations (in an independent nonverbal task) were performed, they revealed that the degree and polarity of lateralization of categorical spatial encoding predicted the LH's initial advantage in the recognition of contorted shapes. This latter finding specifically supports the idea that the LH's categorical spatial encodings play a functional role in the recognition of nonrigid objects.

Divided visual field effects apply not only to lateral hemifields' differences but also to differences between the upper and lower visual fields (cf. Efron, 1990; Previc, 1990). The up/down asymmetry could derive from a greater accessibility of the cortical representations of the lower versus upper visual field with the specialized subsystems within the ventral versus dorsal stream (cf. Andersen et al., 1990; Rubin et al., 1996). The representation of these visual fields is split into disjoint portions of the cortical surface "sheet" so that, topographically, the upper visual field is represented near temporal areas and the lower field near parietal areas. Niebauer and Christman (1998) reasoned that if the upper visual field is specialized for visual search, whereas the lower visual field is specialized for visuomotor manipulations (see Previc, 1990), then it should be possible to observe an upper visual field advantage for categorical judgments and a lower visual field advantage for coordinate judgments. By using the standard dot-above/below-line task they were able to confirm these longitudinal, instead of lateral, differences.

A few divided visual field studies have examined specific subject populations. Koenig et al. (1990) replicated the visual fields' dissociations with children as young as 5 years of age. Hoyer and Rybash (1992) and Bruyer et al. (1997) have tested elderly subjects. Bruyer and colleagues found that the categorical, easier, task showed a visual field difference, whereas there was no field advantage for the coordinate task. They surmised that the disappearance of the LVF effect results from asymmetric aging effects on the brain. Kosslyn (1987), Hellige and colleagues (1994), and Laeng and Peters (1995) converged in showing a failure to reveal laterality effects in left-handers for either spatial relation encoding. Indeed, left-handers would not be expected to show the same pattern and degree of cerebral lateralization for spatial information as right-handers, if we assume that the localization of language areas as well as behavior asymmetries are highly variable in this group of subjects (cf. Bryden, 1982; Geschwind & Galaburda, 1987). Finally, Emmorey and Kosslyn (1996) found that deaf subjects who use American Sign Language as their primary language exhibited a strong RH advantage for image generation using either categorical or coordinate spatial relations representations. They suggested that the enhanced RH image generation abilities observed in deaf signers may be linked to a stronger RH involvement in processing imageable signs and linguistically encoded spatial relations.

To conclude this section, we present a meta-analysis of existing divided visual field experiments on the topic. To be included, an experiment had to test the encoding of both a categorical and a coordinate spatial relation using identical stimuli with normal human subjects (of any age group), and had to report sufficient information about the results to enable extraction of mean response times. Experiments testing categorical judgments that did not involve encoding a well-defined simple spatial relation under normal viewing conditions (e.g., the studies by Horner & Freides, 1996, and Cowin & Hellige, 1994) were not included. For many experiments, detailed accuracy data were not reported, usually because there were few errors, especially on categorical judgments. Although effects were sometimes found for error rates but not response times, speed-accuracy trade-offs were almost never reported.

The results of 24 experiments (with a total of 887 degrees of freedom) were considered. Twenty of these experiments used the above/below categorical judgment; of these, 16 used the distance coordinate judgment (with distances varying from 3 to 25 mm). For uniformity, we shall report only results based on response-time analyses from these 16 experiments (536 degrees of freedom), although the results from the other paradigms showed the same, predicted pattern. For the categorical judgments, subjects responded 8 ms faster when stimuli were presented initially to the LH (529 ms) than to the RH (537 ms), whereas for coordinate judgments subjects responded 14 ms faster when stimuli were presented initially to the RH (636 ms) than to the LH (650 ms). The overall effect size for this interaction was $d = .47$, the combined Z-value was 6.93, and the associated p-value was much smaller than .0001 (all calculations based only on experiments for which variability estimates could be extracted). Therefore, it is reasonable to conclude that although the hemispheric asymmetries predicted by the theory are small in absolute terms, they do exist.

Clinical Studies Laeng (1994) provided converging evidence for the distinction between the two types of spatial relations encoding on the basis of results from the study of patients with brain lesions. If categorical spatial relations are computed primarily in the LH, then damage to this hemisphere should cause the patient to become insensitive to changes in categorical relations between objects; in contrast, if coordinate spatial relations are computed primarily in the RH, then damage to this hemisphere should cause the patient to become insensitive to changes in the metric relations among the same objects. The experiment confirmed a "double dissociation" between the spatial impairments of the two neurological patient groups.

Specifically, 30 patients with damage confined to the LH, 30 with damage confined to the RH, and 15 controls matched by age and education saw a drawing of one or more versions of the same object (typically, animals; e.g., a large cat to the left of a small cat). After a short delay, they were asked to decide whether another drawing was the same or different. Half of the drawings were changed so that they incorporated either a different categorical spatial relation (e.g., a large cat to the left of a small cat) or a different coordinate spatial relation (the large cat was still to the left of the small cat but the distance separating them had changed; see figure 9.7).

In another task, the same subjects initially saw one drawing and, after a delay, two variations of the sample drawing: one that had altered categorical relations and one that had altered coordinate relations. They were asked to indicate which of the two drawings looked more similar to the sample one. Both tasks confirmed that LH-damaged patients had more difficulty in perceiving that categorical relations were altered, since they committed more errors on the first task in categorical than in coordinate trials, and showed an abnormal increase of choices for the categorical alterations in the second task (figure 9.9). In contrast, in both tasks RH-damaged patients showed the opposite pattern of difficulty, now having problems in perceiving alterations of coordinate relations.

This study also provided some information about the underlying functional neuroanatomy of the two types of spatial processing. Each stroke patient had been included in the study if clinical brain imaging evidence indicated a lesion within the parietal lobe area, which was relevant because Kosslyn's (1987) original hypothesis assigned each function to the dorsal area of each hemisphere (e.g., posterior parietal, Brodmann area 40). However, for some of these patients, the lesions included parts of the parietal lobe together with parts of neighboring

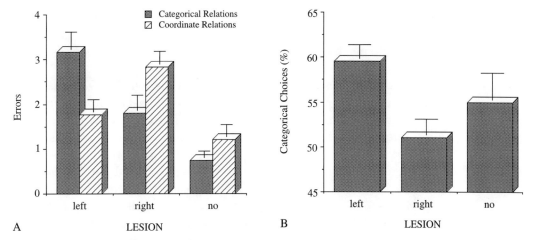

Figure 9.9 Performance of individuals with left or right unilateral lesions and without cerebral lesions in tasks requiring the encoding of categorical and coordinate spatial relations. (*A*) Error rates in a task requiring subjects to determine whether a drawing shown a short time after another one had categorical or coordinate relations, or was unchanged. (*B*) Percentage of choices in another task where the most similar picture to a sample picture had to be chosen from two versions, one showing a categorical relation change and another a coordinate relation change. (From Laeng, 1994.)

lobes, such as the frontal or temporal lobes. Thus patients could be subdivided into smaller groups and the relative contribution of parietal lobe lesions only could be compared with that of mixed lesions. The selective deficits in both tasks were largest for patients with damage to the parietal lobes per se.

LH patients were also given tasks to assess their language abilities (i.e., aphasia tests). There was no correlation between the language or verbal impairment and the degree of impairment in the spatial relations task. This evidence refutes the possibility that categorical spatial relations are simply easily labeled configurations (using prepositions and locatives), and that the categorical task could therefore be reduced to a verbal strategy of mentally naming and memorizing the verbal description (cf. Goodglass et al., 1974; Hannay et al., 1981). Indeed, if coordinate encodings are to support motor activity, they do not seem readily available to language. Although we are clearly able to discriminate quantitative differences in distance and we possess the ability to think and verbally express numerical quantities, we do not seem to be able to map these two types of knowledge onto one another. In contrast, a consequence of perceiving categorical relations is that verbal labels can be "directly" provided after a simple visual inspection and, in fact, they constitute much of our daily communications (e.g., "the book is on the table").

In addition, results on the "token test" (De Renzi & Vignolo, 1962) did not correlate with the degree of categorical spatial impairment. This aphasia test requires the patient to observe a display of wooden tokens of different colors and shapes, and to follow simple requests, such as "Point to the square to the left of the blue circle." Although sentences like these contain spatial predicates, several of the LH patients could follow these commands while showing clear impairments in the categorical spatial memory test, and some of the patients who failed the requests of the token test showed no impairment in the categorical spatial memory test. This situation suggests that for these posterior LH patients, the spatial problem is best characterized as affecting an encoding (bottom-up) stage; in contrast, these patients can access categorical spatial information in a top-down manner, possibly by translating the spatial predicative into a motor-based procedure (e.g., by looking leftward of the blue circle; see also Laeng, Kosslyn et al., 1999). Kemmerer and Tranel (2000) have also reported a subject with LH damage who was impaired in tasks requiring the assignment of the appropriate spatial prepositions but not in visual tasks hypothesized to require the encoding of categorical spatial information.

Sergent (1991b) used the divided visual field paradigm with three split-brain patients (N.G., A.A., and L.B.). These epileptic patients had their cerebral hemispheres surgically separated to relieve their seizures (cf. Trevarthen & Sperry, 1973). The patients were shown displays consisting of a dot within a circle, either at its center position or in 4 different angular and 2 different radial positions. The coordinate tasks were judging whether the dot was exactly on or off the circle's center, or in a near/far radial position from center. The categorical tasks consisted in judging whether the dot was above/below the circle's center or to the left/right of the center. One patient (N.G.) showed an LH advantage for the categorical tasks and an RH advantage for the coordinate tasks. However, another patient (L.B.) showed the reverse pattern—an RH advantage for the categorical task and an LH advantage for the coordinate tasks. The third patient (A.A.) showed no significant differences between visual fields.

B. Laeng, C. F. Chabris, and S. M. Kosslyn

Sergent concluded from these findings that the two hemispheres are equally competent at representing categorical and coordinate spatial relations. However, there are a few caveats to this conclusion. First, the findings showed the presence of significant complementary functional specialization, or division of labor between hemispheres, in two of the three patients. Moreover, none of the patients' performance supported a model in which the two spatial functions are performed by a single hemisphere (i.e., the RH). Second, and perhaps most important, localization data from a few split-brain patients cannot necessarily be generalized to the normal population. For example, some split-brain patients can respond verbally to stimuli presented to the RH; however, as pointed out by Gazzaniga (1983), the evidence for language function in the RH of a few split-brain patients exists for only 3 out of 28 cases (and it turns out that N.G. and L.B. are among these three "unusual" split-brain subjects). The variability in localization of function in these patients is interesting in other respects, but should not be incorrectly generalized to imply that RH language is a common feature of either the whole group of split-brain patients or of the normal population.

Animal Studies   It is well known that species other than man show asymmetries, either behaviorally (e.g., in handedness; Corballis & Morgan, 1978) or in terms of brain structure (e.g., songbirds; Nottebohm, 1979) as well as external body structures (e.g., the chela of crabs). In connection with the present topic, a few studies have investigated the processing of spatial information in nonhuman primates. For example, Hamilton and Vermeire (1988) proposed a complementary hemispheric specialization, on the basis of investigation on split-brain macaques (*Macaca mulatta*), between discriminations of line orientation and face identification. It would also seem that several species learn to distinguish spatial abstract relations. For example, Herrnstein et al. (1989) taught pigeons to distinguish two spatial categories, between a closed line and a dot, corresponding to the inside/outside relations. Depy et al. (1999) investigated the processing of above/below spatial relations in baboon subjects. The monkeys were able to transfer learning of the relation in a line-dot task to a task using a letter above/below a digit. However, in these studies, neither the pigeons nor the monkeys were tested for hemispheric differences.

Depy et al. (1998) specifically assessed the presence of lateralization in baboons (*Papio papio*) when processing distance categories. A matching-to-sample task was used with the divided visual field paradigm in which subjects, both human and baboon, had to decide whether the distance between a line and a dot belonged to one of two spatial categories. Humans initially showed an LVF advantage, which vanished with practice, but overall performance in this task was better for RVF presentations than for LVF ones. The same bias was found in baboons, but in a weaker way. Depy and colleagues concluded that initially distance is judged more efficiently by the RH than the LH, but the effect vanishes after practice—possibly because of a progressive involvement of the LH for spatial categorization (cf. Kosslyn, Koenig, et al., 1989; Chabris & Kosslyn, 1998).

Baboons do not possess a verbal system like humans. Yet, baboons seem to show the same LH specialization seen in humans for categorical spatial relations. If this finding is replicated and stable, it would clearly imply that lateralization models for categorical processing that are based on "feedback training" from lexical representation or spatial language (as we sketched it earlier) are inadequate to account for the development of laterality for categorical processing. Possibly hemispheric differences in receptive field size (spatial frequency filtering) could provide a more comprehensive explanation of hemispheric specialization of function for both human and nonhuman species.

Neuroimaging Studies Kosslyn et al. (1998) measured regional cerebral blood flow with PET while subjects performed separate blocks of categorical and coordinate spatial relations judgments on identical stimuli. In the control task, subjects simply viewed the stimuli (an X above/below a bar) without making any decision, whereas in the experimental task subjects viewed the X and the bar, and were requested to make categorical or coordinate spatial relations judgments. When subtracting measurements in the experimental tasks from those in the control task, Kosslyn and colleagues found activation within the RH's parietal lobe when subjects performed a coordinate decision, and within the LH's parietal lobe when subjects performed a categorical decision. Therefore, these results provide some converging evidence to those of Laeng (1994) on the effects of unilateral lesions to the parietal lobes on these same types of spatial judgments.

B. Laeng, C. F. Chabris, and S. M. Kosslyn

However, the subtractions of the activation patterns for the two tasks revealed differences in several additional areas. Particularly compared to each other (not to the baseline), the coordinate task appeared to activate areas in both the right and left parietal lobes, whereas the categorical task did not activate either parietal lobe (when the results from the two experimental tasks were subtracted from each other, rather than from a baseline). These effects are illustrated in figure 9.10.

One explanation for these results is that the categorical task, judging whether an X is above or below a large horizontal bar, is too easy to cause blood flow changes in the parietal lobes, whereas the coordinate task, judging whether the X is within a certain distance from the bar, is quickly converted into a categorical task as the brain gains practice with the stimuli and judgment involved (see Kosslyn, Koenig, et al., 1989; see also Goel et al., 1998), and thus both parietal lobes are activated within the duration of a single PET scan. However, there were clear lateralized differences in the dorsolateral prefrontal cortex, which is intimately connected with parietal cortex (Burnod et al., 1999).

A currently strong candidate area for the localization of the spatial relations encoding processes is the angular gyrus. Baciu et al. (1999) reported an fMRI study in which subjects first performed the categorical, then the coordinate, task with the dot-bar stimuli. Throughout the categorical task, the left angular gyrus was more active than the right, whereas over the course of the coordinate task, right angular gyrus activity decreased and left angular gyrus activity increased. Although these results are consistent with the predictions developed above (and, as Baciu and colleagues note, with the characteristics of lesions that cause Gerstmann's syndrome; cf. Heilman & Valenstein, 1985), it is important to note that no other brain regions were examined.

In another PET study, Kosslyn, Alpert, et al. (1994) found that subjects performing a picture-name matching task of canonical and noncanonical views of rigid objects showed massive activation of areas in the dorsal systems. Specifically, the inferior parietal lobe in the RH was active when objects were shown in noncanonical views. This brain-imaging evidence converges with the fact that brain damage has corresponding effects on the encoding of noncanonical views of rigid objects (e.g., Warrington & Taylor, 1973, 1978). In addition, Kosslyn and colleagues found no selective activation in the LH's parietal lobe when subjects saw noncanonical views of rigid objects in compar-

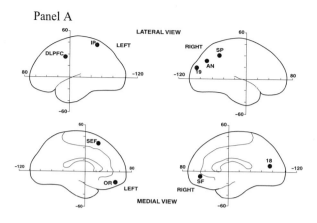

Panel A

LATERAL VIEW

LEFT — RIGHT

MEDIAL VIEW

LEFT — RIGHT

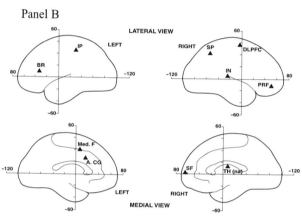

Panel B

LATERAL VIEW

LEFT — RIGHT

MEDIAL VIEW

LEFT — RIGHT

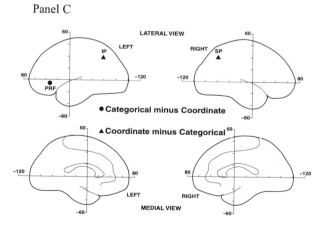

Panel C

LATERAL VIEW

LEFT — RIGHT

● Categorical minus Coordinate

▲ Coordinate minus Categorical

MEDIAL VIEW

LEFT — RIGHT

B. Laeng, C. F. Chabris, and S. M. Kosslyn

ison to the activation while judging the canonical views of the same objects.

If the brain uses a top-down hypothesis-testing process based on structural descriptions when recognizing objects seen in difficult views, and if structural descriptions involve the encoding of categorical spatial relations (cf. Laeng, Shah, et al., 1999), then we would expect to see activation of the LH's parietal areas when identifying noncanonical views. One possible way to account for the lack of activation in these subtractions is that top-down processing mechanisms run virtually all the time, reflexively and in parallel, even when their engagement is not essential, and other mechanisms terminate the processing before the top-down mechanisms can contribute to object recognition. If the whole visual system truly operates in such "cascade" manner, then brain imaging studies based on the subtraction method may fail to distinguish the activation of a cerebral area in conditions in which its processing is essential and contributes to the decision from those conditions in which it is not.

CONCLUSIONS

The value of a new theory must be measured by its ability to provide a systematic framework for organizing findings and to make new predictions that lead to additional empirical observations. To the extent that those predictions are counterintuitive, the theory accrues greater value. Partial reviews of the interrelations between previous theories of spatial relations encoding and the current theory are available in earlier

Figure 9.10 (*A*) Areas in which there was significantly greater blood flow in the categorical spatial relations encoding condition than in the baseline condition. 18 and 19, the respective Brodmann's areas; AN, angular gyrus; DLPFC, dorsolateral prefrontal cortex; IP, inferior parietal; OR, the orbital gyrus; SEF, supplementary eye fields; SF, superior frontal; SP, superior parietal. (*B*) Areas in which there was significantly greater blood flow in the coordinate spatial relations encoding condition than in the baseline condition. A.CG, anterior cingulated gyrus; BR, Broca's area; DLPFC, dorsolateral prefrontal cortex; IN, insula; IP, inferior parietal; TH(na), thalamus (nucleus accumbens); Med.F, medial frontal; PRF, prefrontal area; SF, superior frontal; SP, superior parietal. (*C*) Areas in which there was significantly greater blood flow in the categorical spatial relations encoding condition than in the coordinate spatial relations encoding condition (circles) or vice versa (triangles). IP, inferior parietal; PRF, prefrontal area; SP, superior parietal. (From Kosslyn et al., 1998.)

publications (e.g., Kosslyn, 1994; Laeng, 1994; Chabris & Kosslyn, 1998). The theory proposed here would seem to have the benefit of being sufficiently general to allow us to make sense of a wide range of findings, without the failing of being vague or unsubstantiated; moreover, the theory has generated a large number and variety of empirical tests and findings.

The meta-analysis of results from divided visual field studies provides strong evidence for the distinction between categorical and coordinate encoding of spatial relations, as do the basic dissociations that have been replicated with a variety of types of visual material, types of judgments, modes of response, subject populations, and measurement methods. The theory has also proved compatible with facts about neuroanatomy and neurophysiology, as well as results from simulation modeling and neuropsychological experimentation. Such converging factors have extended the model to account for otherwise unpredictable results, and apply it to other hemispheric asymmetries. Hence, the model outlined here goes far beyond the initial proposal (Kosslyn, 1987) and is certainly now more complex than one based on a direct assignment of subsystems or modules to encoding tasks. The incremental development of the theory is a good sign; if the foundations were not firm, it would not have been possible to build upon them.

ACKNOWLEDGMENTS

During the preparation of this chapter, Bruno Laeng was supported by a grant from the University of Tromsø; Christopher F. Chabris was supported by a postdoctoral fellowship from the National Institutes of Health through the MGH-NMR Center; and Stephen Kosslyn was supported by NIH grant no. 1 R01 MH60734-01 and AFOSR award no. F49620-98-1-0334. We thank Bill Thompson for assistance in preparing some of the pictures.

REFERENCES

Note: References marked with an asterisk indicate studies included in the meta-analysis.

Andersen, R. A., Asanuma, C., Essick, G., & Siegel, R. M. (1990). Corticocortical connections of anatomically and physiologically defined subdivisions within the inferior parietal lobule. *Journal of Comparative Neurology, 296,* 65–113.

Baciu, M., Koenig, O., Vernier, M.-P., Bedoin, N., Rubin, C., & Segebarth, C. (1999). Categorical and coordinate spatial relations: fMRI evidence for hemispheric specialization. *NeuroReport, 10*, 1373–1378.

*Banich, M. T., & Federmeier, K. D. (1999). Categorical and metric spatial processes distinguished by task demands and practice. *Journal of Cognitive Neuroscience, 11*, 153–166.

Beaumont, J. G. (Ed.). (1982). *Divided visual field studies of cerebral organisation*. London: Academic Press.

Behrmann, M., Moscovitch, M., & Mozer, M. C. (1991). Directing attention to words and nonwords in normal subjects and in a computational model: Implications for neglect dyslexia. *Cognitive Neuropsychology, 8*, 213–248.

Biederman, I. (1987). Recognition-by-components: A theory of human image understanding. *Psychological Review, 94*, 115–147.

Biederman, I. (1985). Human image understanding: Recent research and a theory. In S. M. Kosslyn and D. N. Osherson (Eds.), *Visual cognition: An invitation to cognitive science* (pp. 121–165). Cambridge, MA: The MIT Press.

Bradshaw, J. L., & Nettleton, N. C. (1983). *Human cerebral asymmetry*. Englewood Cliffs, NJ: Prentice-Hall.

Bruyer, R., Scailquin, J. C., & Coibon, P. (1997). Dissociation between categorical and coordinate spatial computations: Modulation by cerebral hemispheres, task properties, mode of response, and age. *Brain and Cognition, 33*, 245–277.

Bryden, M. P. (1982). *Laterality: Functional asymmetry in the intact brain*. New York: Academic Press.

Burnod, Y., Baraduc, P., Battaglia-Mayer, A., Guigon, E., Koechlin, E., Ferraina, S., Lacquaniti, F., & Caminiti, R. (1999). Parieto-frontal coding of reaching: An integrated framework. *Experimental Brain Research, 129*, 325–346.

Caramazza, A., & Shelton, J. R. (1998). Domain-specific knowledge systems in the brain: The animate-inanimate distinction. *Journal of Cognitive Neuroscience, 10*, 1–34.

Chabris, C. F., & Kosslyn, S. M. (1998). How do the cerebral hemispheres contribute to encoding spatial relations? *Current Directions in Psychological Science, 7*, 8–14.

Corballis, M. C. (1991). *The lopsided ape. Evolution of the generative mind*. New York: Oxford University Press.

Corballis, M. C., & Morgan, M. J. (1978). On the biological basis of human laterality: I. Evidence for a maturational left-right gradient. *Behavioral and Brain Sciences, 2*, 261–336.

*Cowin, E. L., & Hellige, J. B. (1994). Categorical versus coordinate spatial processing: Effects of blurring and hemispheric asymmetry. *Journal of Cognitive Neuroscience, 6*, 156–164.

Damasio, H., Grabowski, T. J., Tranel, D., Hichwa, R. D., & Damasio, A. R. (1996). A neural basis for lexical retrieval. *Nature, 380*, 499–505.

*David, A. S., & Cutting, J. C. (1990). Categorical-semantic and spatial-imagery judgments of non-verbal stimuli in the cerebral hemispheres. Unpublished manuscript, Institute of Psychiatry, London.

Delis, D. C., Robertson, L. C., & Efron, R. (1986). Hemispheric specialization of memory for visual hierarchical stimuli. *Neuropsychologia, 24,* 205–214.

Depy, D., Fagot, J., & Vauclair, J. (1998). Comparative assessment of distance processing and hemispheric specialization in humans and baboons (*Papio papio*). *Brain and Cognition, 38,* 165–182.

Depy, D., Fagot, J., & Vauclair, J. (1999). Processing of above/below categorical spatial relations by baboons (*Papio papio*). *Behavioural Processes, 48,* 1–9.

De Renzi, E., Scotti, G., & Spinnler, H. (1969). Perceptual and associative disorders of visual recognition. *Neurology, 19,* 634–642.

De Renzi, E., & Vignolo, L. (1962). The token test: A sensitive test to detect receptive disturbances in aphasics. *Brain, 85,* 665–678.

Dreher, B., Fukuda, Y., & Rodieck, R. W. (1976). Identification, classification, and anatomical segregation of cells with X-like and Y-like properties in the lateral geniculate nucleus of old-world primates. *Journal of Physiology* (London), *258,* 433–452.

Efron, R. (1990). *The decline and fall of hemispheric specialization.* Hillsdale, NJ: Lawrence Erlbaum Associates.

Emmorey, K., & Kosslyn, S. M. (1996). Enhanced image generation abilities in deaf signers: A right hemisphere effect. *Brain and Cognition, 32,* 28–44.

Farah, M. (1990). *Visual agnosia.* Cambridge, MA: MIT Press.

Gainotti, G., Silveri, M. C., Daniele, A., & Giustolisi, L. (1995). Neuroanatomical correlates of category-specific semantic disorders: A critical survey. *Memory, 3,* 247–264.

Gazzaniga, M. J. (1983). Right hemisphere language following brain bisection. *American Psychologist, 38,* 525–549.

Geschwind, N., & Galaburda, A. M. (1987). *Cerebral lateralization: Biological mechanisms, associations, and pathology.* Cambridge, MA: MIT Press.

Goel, V., Gold, B., Kapur, S., & Houle, S. (1998). Neuroanatomical correlates of human reasoning. *Journal of Cognitive Neuroscience, 10,* 293–302.

Goodglass, H., Denes, F., & Calderon, M. (1974). The absence of covert verbal mediation in aphasia. *Cortex, 10,* 264–269.

Goodman, N. (1976). *Languages of art: An approach to a theory of symbols.* Indianapolis, IN: Hackett.

Hamilton, C. R., & Vermeire, B. A. (1988). Complementary hemispheric specialization in monkeys. *Science, 242,* 1691–1694.

Hannay, H. J., Dee, H. L., Burns, J. W., & Masek, B. S. (1981). Experimental reversal of a left visual field superiority for forms. *Brain and Language, 3,* 54–66.

B. Laeng, C. F. Chabris, and S. M. Kosslyn

Harrington, A. (1987). *Medicine, mind, and the double brain: A study in nineteenth century thought*. Princeton, NJ: Princeton University Press.

Harrington, A. (1995). Unfinished business: Models of laterality in the nineteenth century. In R. J. Davidson & K. Hughdahl (Eds.), *Brain asymmetry* (pp. 3–27). Cambridge, MA: MIT Press.

Heilman, K. H., & Valenstein, E. (1985). *Clinical neuropsychology*. New York: Oxford University Press.

*Hellige, J. B., Bloch, M. I., Cowin, E. L., Eng, T. L., Eviatar, Z., & Sergent, V. (1994). Individual variation in hemispheric asymmetry: Multitask study of effects related to handedness and sex. *Journal of Experimental Psychology: General, 123*, 235–256.

*Hellige, J. B., & Michimata, C. (1989). Categorization versus distance: Hemispheric differences for processing spatial information. *Memory & Cognition, 17*, 770–776.

Herrnstein, R. J., Vaughan, W., Mumford, D. B., & Kosslyn, S. M. (1989). Teaching pigeons an abstract relational rule: Insideness. *Perception and Psychophysics, 46*, 56–64.

Hinton, G. E., McClelland, J. L., & Rumelhart, D. E. (1986). Distributed representations. In D. E. Rumelhart & D. L. McClelland (Eds.), *Parallel distributed processing: Explorations in the microstructure of cognition*. Volume 1: *Foundations* (pp. 77–109). Cambridge, MA: MIT Press.

*Horner, M. D., & Freides, D. (1996). Effects of retinal eccentricity on the lateralized processing of categorical and coordinate spatial relations. *International Journal of Neuroscience, 86*, 7–13.

*Hoyer, W. J., & Rybash, J. M. (1992). Age and visual field differences in computing visual-spatial relations. *Psychology and Aging, 7*, 339–342.

Humphreys, G. W., Freeman, T. A. C., & Muller, H. J. (1992). Lesioning a connectionist model of visual search: Selective effects on distractor groupings. *Canadian Journal of Psychology, 46*, 417–460.

Huttenlocher, J., Hedges, L. V., & Duncan, S. (1991). Categories and particulars: Prototype effects in estimating spatial location. *Psychological Review, 98*, 352–376.

Ivry, R. B., & Robertson, L. C. (1998). *The two sides of perception*. Cambridge, MA: MIT Press.

Jacobs, R. A., & Kosslyn, S. M. (1994). Encoding shape and spatial relations: The role of receptive field size in coordinating complementary representations. *Cognitive Science, 18*, 361–386.

Kemmerer, D., & Tranel, D. (2000). A double dissociation between linguistic and perceptual representations of spatial relationships. *Cognitive Neuropsychology, 17*, 393–414.

Kitterle, F., Christman, S., & Hellige, J. (1990). Hemispheric differences are found in the identification, but not detection, of low versus high spatial frequencies. *Perception and Psychophysics, 48*, 297–306.

Kitterle, F., & Selig, L. (1991). Visual field effects in the discrimination of sine-wave gratings. *Perception & Psychophysics, 50*, 15–18.

Koenig, O., Kosslyn, S. M., Chabris, C. F., & Gabrieli, J. D. E. (1992). Computational constraints upon the acquisition of spatial knowledge in the cerebral hemispheres. Unpublished manuscript, University of Lyon 2, Bron, France.

*Koenig, O., Reiss, L. P., & Kosslyn, S. M. (1990). The development of spatial relations representations: Evidence from studies of cerebral lateralization. *Journal of Experimental Child Psychology, 50*, 119–130.

Kogure, T., & Hatta, T. (1999). Hemisphere specialisation and categorical spatial relations representations. *Laterality, 4*, 321–331.

Kosslyn, S. M. (1987). Seeing and imagining in the cerebral hemispheres: A computational approach. *Psychological Review, 94*, 148–175.

Kosslyn, S. M. (1994). *Image and brain: The resolution of the imagery debate*. Cambridge, MA: MIT Press.

Kosslyn, S. M., Anderson, A. K., Hillger, L. A., & Hamilton, S. E. (1994). Hemispheric differences in sizes of receptive fields or attentional biases? *Neuropsychology, 8*, 139–147.

Kosslyn, S. M., Chabris, C. F., Marsolek, C. J., & Koenig, O. (1992). Categorical versus coordinate spatial relations: Computational analyses and computer simulations. *Journal of Experimental Psychology: Human Perception and Performance, 18*, 562–577.

Kosslyn, S. M., & Jacobs, R. A. (1994). Encoding shape and spatial relations: A simple mechanism for coordinating complementary representations. In V. Honavar & L. M. Uhr (Eds.), *Artificial intelligence and neural networks: Steps toward principled integration* (pp. 373–385). Boston: Academic Press.

Kosslyn, S. M., Alpert, N. M., Thompson, W. L., Chabris, C. F., Rauch, S. L., & Anderson, A. K. (1994). Identifying objects seen from different viewpoints: A PET investigation. *Brain, 117*, 1055–1071.

Kosslyn, S. M., & Koenig, O. (1995). *Wet mind*. New York: The Free Press.

*Kosslyn, S. M., Koenig, O., Barrett, A., Cave, C. B., Tang, J., & Gabrieli, J. D. E. (1989). Evidence for two types of spatial representations: Hemispheric specialization for categorical and coordinate relations. *Journal of Experimental Psychology: Human Perception and Performance, 15*, 723–735.

Kosslyn, S. M., Maljkovic, V., Hamilton, S. E., Horwitz, G., & Thompson, W. L. (1995). Two types of image generation: Evidence for left and right hemisphere processes. *Neuropsychologia, 33*, 1485–1510.

Kosslyn, S. M., Sokolov, M. A., & Chen, J. C. (1989). The lateralization of BRIAN: A computational theory and model of visual hemispheric specialization. In D. Klahr & K. Kotovsky (Eds.), *Complex information processing: The impact of Herbert Simon* (pp. 3–29). Hillsdale, NJ: Lawrence Erlbaum Associates.

Kosslyn, S. M., Thompson, W. T., Gitelman, D. R., & Alpert, N. M. (1998). Neural systems that encode categorical versus coordinate spatial relations: PET investigations. *Psychobiology, 26*, 333–347.

Laeng, B. (1994). Lateralization of categorical and coordinate spatial functions: A study of unilateral stroke patients. *Journal of Cognitive Neuroscience, 6,* 189–203.

Laeng, B., Kosslyn, S. M., Caviness, V. S., & Bates, J. (1999). Can deficits in spatial indexing contribute to simultanagnosia? *Cognitive Neuropsychology, 16,* 81–114.

Laeng, B., & Peters, M. (1995). Cerebral lateralization for the processing of spatial coordinates and categories in left- and right-handers. *Neuropsychologia, 33,* 421–439.

Laeng, B., Peters, M., & McCabe, B. (1997). Memory for locations within regions. Spatial biases and visual hemifield differences. *Memory and Cognition, 26,* 97–107.

Laeng, B., Shah, J., & Kosslyn, S. M. (1999). Identifying objects in conventional and contorted poses: Contributions of hemisphere-specific mechanisms. *Cognition, 70,* 53–85.

Livingstone, M. S., & Hubel, D. H. (1988). Segregation of form, color, movement, and depth: Anatomy, physiology, and perception. *Science, 240,* 740–749.

Marr, D. (1982). *Vision.* San Francisco: Freeman.

Marsolek, C. J. (1995). Abstract visual-form representations in the left cerebral hemisphere. *Journal of Experimental Psychology: Human Perception and Performance, 21,* 375–386.

Marsolek, C. J., Kosslyn, S. M., & Squire, L. R. (1992). Form-specific visual priming in the right cerebral hemisphere. *Journal of Experimental Psychology: Learning, Memory, and Cognition, 18,* 492–508.

Michimata, C. (1997). Hemispheric processing of categorical and coordinate spatial relations in vision and visual imagery. *Brain and Cognition, 33,* 370–387.

Miller, G. A., & Johnson-Laird, P. N. (1976). *Language and perception.* Cambridge, MA: Harvard University Press.

*Niebauer, C. L. (1996). A possible connection between categorical and coordinate spatial relation representations. Unpublished manuscript, University of Toledo, Toledo, OH.

*Niebauer, C. L., & Christman, S. D. (1998). Upper and lower visual field differences in categorical and coordinate judgments. *Psychonomic Bulletin & Review, 5,* 147–151.

Nottebohm, F. (1979). Origins and mechanisms in the establishment of cerebral dominance. In M. S. Gazzaniga (Ed.), *Handbook of behavioral neurology.* Volume 2: *Neuropsychology.* New York: Plenum Press.

O'Reilly, R. C., Kosslyn, S. M., Marsolek, C. J., & Chabris, C. F. (1990). Receptive field characteristics that allow parietal lobe neurons to encode spatial properties of visual input: A computational analysis. *Journal of Cognitive Neuroscience, 2,* 141–155.

Parrot, M., Doyon, B., Démonet, J. F., & Cardebat, D. (1999). Hemispheric preponderance in categorical and coordinate visual processes. *Neuropsychologia, 37,* 1215–1225.

Piaget, J., & Inhelder, B. (1956). *Le développement des quantités chez l'enfant.* Paris.

Previc, F. H. (1990). Functional specialization in the lower and upper visual fields in humans: Its ecological origins and neurophysiological implications. *Behavioral and Brain Sciences, 13,* 519–575.

Robertson, L. C., & Delis, D. C. (1986). "Part-whole" processing in unilateral brain-damaged patients: Dysfunctions of hierarchical organization. *Neuropsychologia, 24*, 363–370.

Robertson, L. C., & Lamb, M. R. (1991). Neuropsychological contributions to theories of part-whole organization. *Cognitive Psychology, 24*, 363–370.

*Roth, E. C., & Hellige, J. B. (1998). Spatial processing and hemispheric asymmetry: Contributions of the transient/magnocellular visual system. *Journal of Cognitive Neuroscience, 10*, 472–484.

Rubin, N., Nakayama, K., & Shapley, R. (1996). Enhanced perception of illusory contours in the lower versus upper visual hemifields. *Science, 271*, 651–653.

Rueckl, J. G., Cave, K. R., & Kosslyn, S. M. (1989). Why are "what" and "where" processed by separate cortical visual systems? A computational investigation. *Journal of Cognitive Neuroscience, 1*, 171–186.

*Rybash, J. M., & Hoyer, W. J. (1992). Hemispheric specialization for categorical and coordinate spatial representations: A reappraisal. *Memory & Cognition, 20*, 271–276.

*Sergent, J. (1991a). Judgments of relative position and distance on representations of spatial relations. *Journal of Experimental Psychology: Human Perception and Performance, 17*, 762–780.

Sergent, J. (1991b). Processing of spatial relations within and between the disconnected cerebral hemispheres. *Brain, 114*, 1025–1043.

Servos, P., & Peters, M. (1990). A clear left hemisphere advantage for visuo-spatially based verbal categorization. *Neuropsychologia, 28*, 1251–1260.

Shallice, T. (1988). *From neuropsychology to mental structure*. Cambridge: Cambridge University Press.

Shepard, R. N., & Metzler, J. (1971). Mental rotation of three-dimensional object. *Science, 171*, 701–703.

Smart, J. J. C. (1964). *Problems of space and time*. New York: Collier Macmillan.

Springer, S. P., & Deutsch, G. (1998). *Left brain, right brain: Perspectives from cognitive neuroscience*. Fifth edition. New York: Freeman.

Teuber, H. L. (1955). Physiological psychology. *Annual Review of Psychology, 6*, 267–296.

Trevarthen, C., & Sperry, R. W. (1973). Perceptual unity of the ambient visual field in human commissurotomy patients. *Brain, 96*, 547–570.

Ungerleider, L., & Mishkin, M. (1982). Two cortical visual systems. In D. J. Engle, M. A. Goodale, & R. J. Mansfield (Eds.), *Analysis of visual behavior* (pp. 549–586). Cambridge, MA: MIT Press.

Van Kleeck, M. H. (1989). Hemispheric differences in global versus local processing of hierarchical visual stimuli by normal subjects: New data and a meta-analysis of previous studies. *Neuropsychologia, 27*, 1165–1178.

Van Kleeck, M. H., & Kosslyn, S. M. (1989). Gestalt laws of perceptual organization in an embedded figures task: Evidence for hemispheric specialization. *Neuropsychologia, 27,* 1179–1186.

Van Kleeck, M. H., & Kosslyn, S. M. (1991). The use of computer models in the study of cerebral lateralization. In F. L. Kitterle (Ed.), *Cerebral laterality: Theory and research* (pp. 155–174). Hillsdale, NJ: Lawrence Erlbaum Associates.

Warrington, E. K., & James, M. (1991). A new test of object decision: 2D silhouettes featuring a minimal view. *Cortex, 27,* 370–383.

Warrington, E. K., & Taylor, A. M. (1973). The contribution of the right parietal lobe to object recognition. *Cortex, 9,* 152–164.

Warrington, E. K., & Taylor, A. M. (1978). Two categorical stages of object recognition. *Perception, 7,* 695–705.

*Wilkinson, D., & Donnelly, N. (1999). The role of stimulus factors in making categorical and coordinate spatial judgments. *Brain and Cognition, 39,* 171–185.

10 Complexities of Interhemispheric Communication in Sensorimotor Tasks Revealed by High-Density Event-Related Potential Mapping

Clifford D. Saron, John J. Foxe, Charles E. Schroeder, and Herbert G. Vaughan, Jr.

THE POFFENBERGER PARADIGM

Since the second decade of the twentieth century, a compellingly simple behavioral paradigm has been used to estimate the transit time of visuomotor information across the corpus callosum (Poffenberger, 1912; Marzi, 1999). Left- or right-hand simple reaction times (RTs) are obtained in response to brief left or right visual field stimuli, creating two types of task conditions: uncrossed—where visual input and response hand are on the same side—and crossed—where visual input and response hand are on opposite sides (figure 10.1). The logic of this paradigm has been that uncrossed conditions involve processing within one hemisphere, while crossed conditions require interhemispheric transfer in order to generate a motor response. Thus, the RT for crossed conditions should be, overall, longer than the RT for uncrossed conditions, owing to the additional conduction pathway length and synaptic delays imposed by callosal transfer (e.g., Poffenberger, 1912; Jeeves, 1969; Marzi et al., 1991; Berlucchi et al., 1995; Iacoboni & Zaidel, 2000).

Subtraction of the RT obtained during uncrossed conditions from the RT obtained during crossed conditions yields the crossed/uncrossed difference (CUD), which has been held to be the behavioral estimate of interhemispheric transfer time (IHTT). By this method, Poffenberger himself (1912) found the CUD to be 5–6 ms. Many determinations of the CUD have followed: 2 ms (Iacoboni & Zaidel, 2000), 2.5 ms (average of studies reviewed in Bashore, 1981), 4 ms (meta-analysis by Marzi et al., 1991; see also review by Braun, 1992), and 7.4 ms (St. John et al., 1987). The assertion that the CUD reflects callosal transfer time has

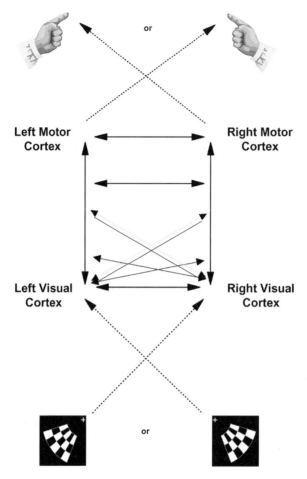

Figure 10.1 This diagram illustrates the design of the classic Poffenberger (1912) paradigm and includes schematic brain activation pathways. Hemiretinal stimuli are briefly presented in a simple reaction time (RT) task. Responses are made with the hand either ipsilateral or contralateral to the stimulated visual field. Ipsilateral task conditions have been thought to involve visuomotor integration within one hemisphere, while contralateral conditions require interhemispheric transfer (using visual and/or motor routes) via the corpus callosum for response execution. Diagonal arrows indicate heterotopic callosal pathways. The checkerboard wedges indicate the visual stimuli used in the reported experiments. RT responses were index finger lifts off an optical switch placed at body midline. (From Saron et al., 2002.)

C. D. Saron and colleagues

derived strong support from findings in patients with total agenesis (e.g., Tassinari et al., 1994 [CUD = 23 ms]; Milner et al., 1985; Di Stefano et al., 1992; Aglioti et al., 1993; Di Stefano & Salvadori, 1998; Lassonde et al., 1988, 2002) or complete transection of the corpus callosum (e.g., Clarke & Zaidel, 1989 [CUD = 48 ms]; Sergent & Myers, 1985; Aglioti et al., 1993; Forster & Corballis, 1998), where CUD is seen to increase dramatically.

VARIABLE INTERHEMISPHERIC TIMING RESULTS

Even in light of clear increases in IHTT assessed in populations lacking intact corpora callosa, two general inconsistencies in the literature argue against the straightforward interpretation of the CUD as reflecting callosal IHTT. The first concerns the variability of CUDs obtained at both the population and the individual levels, while the second refers to discrepancies between behavioral and electrophysiological methods of estimating interhemispheric transfer time (IHTT). In Braun's 1992 review of 41 studies using behavioral methods to estimate IHTT, 8 studies failed to find the crucial visual field by hand interaction predicted by the design of the Poffenberger task (also Thut et al., 1999). The range of CUDs for the studies included in the Marzi et al. (1991) meta-analysis was 1.0 to 10.3 ms, and the CUD range for earlier studies reviewed in Bashore (1981) was 1.0 to 28.5 ms. Saron and Davidson (1989) found that only 67% of subjects had CUDs in the direction of anatomic prediction, while Davidson et al. (1990), in a study of normal and reading disabled boys, found only 56% of 25 12-year-old normal readers had positive CUDs.

The unclear interpretation of a negative CUD prompted these authors to question the validity of RT methods for estimating IHTT, using typical numbers of stimuli (100–200). An important early study of the reliability of RT methods to estimate IHTT (St. John et al., 1987) used 5000 stimuli given over 20 experimental sessions per subject and found positive CUDs for each of the 12 subjects tested. However CUD values per session per subject were not presented in this study, leaving open the question of within subject variability of the CUD.

Iacoboni and Zaidel (2000) have demonstrated that the CUD is not a stable parameter within individuals across sessions. These authors tested three individuals across 12 to 15 sessions of 800 trials per session in the largest RT dataset per subject thus far collected. Although Iacoboni and Zaidel (2000) found that the overall estimate of IHTT was 2 ms, each subject showed a broad range of CUDs across sessions: −5 to +5 ms for subject 1, −9 to +7 ms for subject 2, and −3 to +10 ms for subject 3. CUD variability within an individual was not different from CUD variability across individuals in a group of 15 subjects tested once. This observation suggested to these authors that the variability of CUD findings in the literature reflects the instability of the measure within individuals rather than stable, but differing, callosal IHTTs between subjects.

PHYSIOLOGICAL PLAUSIBILITY OF THE CUD

Very short estimates of IHTT have been obtained in two recent studies. Ratinckx et al. (2001) obtained a mean CUD of 0.7 ms for right-hand conditions from a population of 48 subjects, while Marzi et al. (1999) found a CUD of 0.7 ms, combining the results of both hands. CUD values this short must prompt questioning of the physiological plausibility of such results. An anatomical interpretation of the 0.7 ms CUD as callosal IHTT would require conduction velocities of 214 m/s (assuming an occipitally mediated interhemispheric visuomotor integration and a pathway distance of 15 cm), which exceeds the conduction velocity of the largest 11 μm myelinated fibers seen by LaMantia and Rakic (1990) by a factor of 3.3 (Waxman & Bennett, 1972), discounting synaptic delays that would further add to the timing of interhemispheric neural transmission.

Considering a shorter motor-to-motor transcallosal route (4–6 cm)—for example, via the rich callosal connections between left and right supplementary motor area (SMA) (Rouiller et al., 1994)—a 0.7 ms CUD would also exceed the 66 m/sec conduction times of the largest callosal fibers. Further, estimates of mammalian synaptic delays range from 0.15 ms for rat cerebellar synapses (Sabatini & Regehr, 1996) to 0.43 ms for rat trigeminal neurons to the V motor nucleus (Appenteng et al., 1989), and 0.7 ms measured in slice preparations of the anteroventral cochlear nucleus (Oertel, 1983). Therefore, even in a "best case" scenario where interhemispheric transfer of visuomotor information is mediated solely by the very small population of largest callosal fibers (LaMantia & Rakic, 1990; Aboitiz et al., 1992, 1996), synaptic delays and their maximum conduction velocity impose timing requirements exceeded by very short CUDs.

The variability of obtained CUDs and the seeming physiological implausibility of many estimations point to an inescapable conclusion: that the underlying processes of visuomotor integration subserving generation of the motor response, even in this simple RT task, are more complex than the canonical anatomical interpretation of results from this paradigm. Exploration of these complexities as revealed by studies using high-density event-related potentials (ERPs) is the focus of this chapter (see also Saron et al., 2002).

PHYSIOLOGIC MEASURES VS. BEHAVIORAL MEASURES

A critical finding from event-related potential (ERP) studies is that there is no relationship between estimates of IHTT determined by electrophysiological measures and RT IHTT estimates (the CUD) obtained simultaneously in the same subjects (Saron & Davidson, 1989; Hoptman et al., 1996; Braun et al., 1999). ERPs can be simultaneously recorded over sensory cortices of both hemispheres and in the absence of motor output (e.g., Andreassi et al., 1975; Rugg et al., 1985), allowing for an assessment of the contributions of transfer between sensory cortices versus between motor cortices. This contrasts with the RT measure, which reflects the end point of visuomotor integration. The anatomical paths by which this integration takes place are varied, and presumably involve both visual and motor interhemispheric transfer (Bisiacchi et al., 1994; Forster & Corballis, 1998; Thut et al., 1999; Saron, 1999; Saron et al., 2002).

When ERPs are applied to the Poffenberger task, the latency differences of component peaks recorded occipitally over the directly and indirectly stimulated hemispheres can be compared. These differences have generally been found to be between 10 and 25 ms (e.g., Rugg et al., 1984, 1985; Lines et al., 1984; Saron & Davidson, 1989; Hoptman et al., 1996; see Brown et al., 1994), values that are considerably longer than CUD estimates of IHTT. Callosal mediation of the ipsilateral occipital sensory ERP response has been demonstrated by recordings from individuals with agenesis of the corpus callosum (e.g., Rugg et al., 1985; Saron et al., 1997; Brown et al., 1998, 1999), and from those with complete or partial collosotomies (Tramo et al., 1995; Brown et al., 1999).

One view of the differences between RT and ERP measures of IHTT is based upon an insensitivity of RT measures of IHTT to manipulations of the visual stimulus (intensity or eccentricity), which has been interpreted to reflect primarily motor-related transfer (Berlucchi, 1972; Milner & Lines, 1982). The discrepancy between RT and visual ERP measures of IHTT, derived as they generally have been from occipital scalp regions, has therefore been thought of as a contrast in IHTTs between motor and visual regions of the callosum. Initial ERP evidence for this came from short ERP estimates of IHTT recorded over central scalp regions, to which motor cortex activations project (Rugg et al., 1984, 1985; Ipata et al., 1997). Shorter (3–4 ms) ERP IHTT estimates obtained between ipsilateral and contralateral central scalp recordings, compared with differences from recordings over visual cortices (e.g., Rugg et al., 1984), have been used to suggest that the CUD reflects motor, rather than visual, interhemispheric transfer, since central ERP IHTT estimates are similar in value to the average CUD across studies (e.g., Berlucchi et al., 1995; Ipata et al., 1997; Forster & Corballis, 1998).

However, all of these studies reported scalp voltage measures that are susceptible to the effects of volume conduction. Due to the superposition of potentials produced by left and right hemisphere sources, volume conduction can result in decreased peak latency differences in scalp potential recordings (see Saron et al., 2002). Indeed, the short motor transfer time hypothesis is not supported by scalp current density (SCD) measures (see "Methods," below) recorded over central cortex. Such recordings show that central voltage waveforms reflect volume conducted potentials generated in visual areas (Saron et al., 2002). Further, when lateral central SCD measures *are* obtained, presumptive motor-to-motor IHTT ranges from 7 to 26 ms (Ilmoniemi et al., 1997; Saron, 1999; Komssi et al., 2000; Saron et al., 2002), values consistent with estimates of IHTT derived over occipital scalp. In support, magnetoencephalography (MEG) estimates of somatosensory IHTT have obtained values of ~11 ms (Tang et al., 2000).

Even noting regional differences in the preponderance of callosal fibers of different diameters (LaMantia & Rakic, 1990; Aboitiz et al., 1992), the overall similarity of occipital, and pre- and postcentral physiological estimates of IHTT points toward a basic correspondence of noninvasively measurable callosal transfer times across the caudal to rostral plane. Evidence in normals that the CUD does not reflect only motor-level transfer comes from a combined RT and transcranial magnetic stimulation (TMS) study (Marzi et al., 1998). Concurrent TMS over left or right occipital cortex facilitated RT during the Poffenberger task, but less so for crossed conditions. This finding was interpreted as relative interference with posterior callosal routes involved in the transfer of visual input to the opposite hemisphere necessary for response generation.

TMS STUDIES SHOW STABLE, AND NOT SHORT, MOTOR IHTT

TMS has been effectively used to determine the timing and examine the effects of callosal stimulation on human motor cortex activation. Ferbert et al. (1992) used stimulating coils placed over the hand motor region of each hemisphere. One coil was used to elicit movements in the contralateral hand (the test stimulus, TS) and the other coil was used to deliver a conditioning stimulus (CS) ipsilateral to the responding hand just prior to the test stimulation. Induced movements were measured using the first dorsal interosseous muscle (FDI) surface EMG. Conditioning stimuli presented 6–25 ms prior to the onset of the test stimulus consistently resulted in attenuation of the movement evoked by the test stimulus (CS–TS examined range was 5–30 ms). This finding was interpreted as transcallosally mediated inhibition of motor cortex contralateral to the responding hand. The cortical interhemispheric mediation of these effects was investigated, in part, by noting a lack of inhibitory effects of the conditioning stimulus when using electrical stimulation that is known to directly stimulate neurons of the pyramidal tract. Single motor-unit studies were used to derive an approximate IHTT of 13 ms, a value consistent with ERP measures of IHTT, and not with RT-based methods (see also Di Lazzaro et al., 1999).

A validation of the callosal mediation of this effect is presented in B. U. Meyer et al. (1995). In this study, a transient inhibition of tonic maximal contraction of the FDI ipsilateral to the TMS-stimulated hemisphere was absent or delayed in individuals lacking, or with abnormalities in, the anterior half of the corpus callosum, suggesting that the transcallosal fibers that mediated this effect obey the interhemispheric topography previously described (e.g., Pandya & Rosene, 1985; Pandya & Seltzer, 1986; B. U. Meyer et al., 1998). The estimated transcallosal delay in this study was also 13 ms (also Schnitzler et al., 1996; Boroojerdi et al., 1998, 1999). Further support for the transcallosal mediation of TMS-induced suppression of the FDI response comes from lesion studies (Boroojerdi et al., 1996; Liepert et al., 2000) and tests of individuals with multiple sclerosis (Boroojerdi et al., 1998). A more direct approach to investigating motor transcallosal transfer times has been to combine TMS with high-resolution EEG recordings (Ilmoniemi et al., 1997). Komssi et al. (2000) used TMS over the hand motor area and recordings from 60 scalp electrodes to estimate motor IHTT at 21 ± 4 ms. Taken together, the motor IHTT values across TMS studies, allied to the similar central ERP IHTT estimates cited above, amount to a strong case against the hypothesis that 2–4 ms CUDs simply reflect motor rather than visual transfer.

Although physiologically plausible transfer times based on a 13 cm path length in humans range from 1.5 ms to 433 ms, the largest populations of fibers are between 0.6 and 1.5 μm, which correspond to transfer times of 9.9 to 24.9 ms (Aboitiz et al., 1992), values well in agreement with the physiological results reviewed above. Clearly, with such a broad spectrum of possible transfer times, as has been pointed out by others (LaMantia & Rakic, 1990; Aboitiz et al., 1992; Ringo et al., 1994; Hoptman & Davidson, 1994; Berlucchi et al., 1995), the simple heuristic of *an* IHTT requires reexamination.

A LONGSTANDING CHALLENGE TO STRUCTURAL INTERPRETATION OF THE CUD

The Kinsbourne Model

Questioning of the assumptions underlying the CUD method of estimating IHTT is not new. Swanson et al. (1978) disputed the approach on both theoretical and empirical grounds. These authors, basing their argument on a model of lateral cerebral interactions put forward by Kinsbourne (e.g., Kinsbourne, 1974, in press), suggested that the CUD did not reflect IHTT, but rather reflected differential effects of response preparation due to the attentional bias produced by a unilateral stimulus. Two factors, independent of sensory relay via the corpus callosum, are seen to alter the speed with which visuomotor integration occurs for crossed and uncrossed conditions. The first, thought to facilitate response generation in uncrossed conditions, is a generalized activation of the hemisphere initially receiving the stimulus, which would then speed motor output via distributed activations of multiple cortical regions. The second is posited to be a complementary, callosally mediated, inhibitory influence of the activated hemisphere on the indirectly stimulated hemisphere, which would slow behavioral output in crossed conditions. Thus, the processing speed effects of stimulus and response compatibility inherent in the design of the Poffenberger paradigm are seen as an unavoidable confound in simple anatomical interpretations of the CUD. Evidence in support of these assertions follows this section.

Swanson et al. presage the physiologically based conclusions put forward in the present chapter: "In the context of the orientation model, either information is exchanged between the hemispheres in a time so short that it cannot reasonably or reliably be detected by RT methods, or *lateral processing takes place after interhemispheric integration of information and so a transfer time component is present in all response measures*" (Swanson et al., 1978, p. 278; italics added). In support, Kaluzny et al. (1994), using unilateral electrical stimulation of the finger and uni- and bimanual RT found highly inconsistent CUDs at the individual level; they attribute this variability to potential individual differences in the routes of interhemispheric transfer and to attentional factors (see also Braun et al., 1997). Kinsbourne (2002) has interpreted our evidence of early intrahemispheric stimulus-related activations in motor regions (Saron et al., 2002; Saron et al., 2001; data to be reported below) as consistent with the activation processes posited in Swanson et al. (1978).

Although the predicted effects of stimulus-response (S-R) spatial compatibility have been found in choice RT versions of the Poffenberger paradigm (Anzola et al., 1977; Ledlow et al., 1978), others have shown that the CUD obtained by simple RT measures is immune to S-R spatial compatibility effects (Anzola et al., 1977; Berlucchi et al., 1977; Di Stefano et al., 1992). There is, however, support for the two fundamental assertions of the Kinsbourne model: (1) distributed sensory-related activations of motor cortex and (2) callosally mediated inhibitory effects.

Evidence for Sensory-Related Activations of Motor Cortex

Single unit studies in monkeys have found visually responsive neurons that are widely distributed within "motor" cortices, including premotor cortex (PMC) (e.g., Riehle & Requin, 1989; Riehle, 1991; Boussaoud & Wise, 1993; Graziano et al., 1997; Fogassi et al., 1999; Fadiga et al., 2000), supplementary motor area (SMA) (D. F. Chen et al., 1991; Schall,

1991), primary motor cortex (M1) (Miller et al., 1992; Zhang et al., 1997), dorsolateral prefrontal cortex (DLPFC) (e.g., Ito, 1982; Funahashi et al., 1990, 1993), and frontal eye fields (FEF) (e.g., Schall et al., 1995; Ferrera et al., 1999).

These physiological findings are well supported by anatomical studies that describe inputs from visual cortices to these regions. Wise et al. (1997) summarize pathways from parieto-occipital visual areas (PO, V6A) that project both directly and indirectly to dorsal premotor regions. Extensive connections exist between PMC and SMA that can subserve sensory activation of SMA (Luppino et al., 1993; Rizzolatti et al., 1998). Visually responsive cells in dorsolateral prefrontal cortex are likely mediated by the extensive network of parietal-frontal pathways (e.g., Cavada & Goldman-Rakic, 1989; Petrides & Pandya, 1999). The FEF receives extensive projections from multiple extrastriate visual areas of both the dorsal and the ventral streams (Schall, 1997). Given these findings from animal studies, visual stimulation would be expected to result in activation of human frontocentral cortex. Several recent human studies have demonstrated such activation during perceptual tasks using fMRI (Culham et al., 1998; Toni et al., 1999), intracranial recording (Clarke et al., 1995), ERPs (Thut et al., 2000; Saron et al., 2001), and MEG (Kawamichi et al., 1998; Endo et al., 1999).

Evidence for Callosally Mediated Interhemispheric Inhibition

There is also considerable evidence for callosal inhibition. Although the bulk of callosally projecting cells are excitatory (Innocenti, 1986), two varieties of callosally mediated inhibition may occur: excitation of inhibitory interneurons or direct inhibitory influences of smaller populations of callosally projecting GABAergic cells (e.g., Conti & Manzoni, 1994; others reviewed in Saron et al., 2002). In addition to the TMS studies reported above, TMS of the ipsilateral hemisphere during unimanual movement delays or degrades motor activity, a finding interpreted as activation of interhemispheric inhibition of the contralateral motor cortex (R. Chen et al., 1997; Ziemann et al., 1997; B. U. Meyer & Voss, 2000).

Functional imaging (fMRI) has also provided evidence for callosally mediated inhibition (Tootell et al., 1998). Decreased activations were observed in medial calcarine cortex and regions associated with V2 of the hemisphere ipsilateral to stimulation. These areas were homologous to regions of marked increased activation in the hemisphere contralateral to the stimulus. The decreased ipsilateral activation was interpreted as evidence of transcallosal inhibition due to the corresponding activations of the contralateral hemisphere. Similarly, a recent fMRI investigation demonstrated that repetitive finger tapping resulted in activation of contralateral sensorimotor cortex (as expected) and *deactivation* of ipsilateral sensorimotor cortex (Allison et al., 2000). Such data are confirmatory of the predictions of the Kinsbourne interpretation of the Poffenberger task.

Recent Tests of the Model

An investigation of Kinsbourne's model, specifically focused on the notion of hemispheric activation balance by mutual transcallosal inhibition, was conducted by Oliveri et al. (1999). This study examined the effects of TMS over frontal or parietal regions of the intact hemisphere upon the detection of unilateral or bilateral cutaneous electrical stimulation for brain-damaged patients. In right-brain-damaged patients, TMS to the left frontal cortex 40 ms after tactile stimulation actually *reduced* the number of missed detections of left-hand stimulation in bimanual conditions. TMS, in this case, was interpreted as interfering with a hypothetical transcallosal left frontal-to-right parietal tonic inhibition of right parietal regions. In accord with Kinsbourne's model, in the absence of TMS, right parietal regions were assumed to be overly inhibited by the left hemisphere due to the lack of compensatory transcallosal left hemisphere inhibition from damaged regions of the right hemisphere. TMS was proposed to result in a net disinhibition of right parietal regions, thereby partially restoring left somatosensory neglect (contralesional extinction). Oliveri et al. (2000) replicated this effect with paired-pulse TMS, and demonstrated partial recovery of contralesional extinction by TMS over parietal regions with shorter delays from tactile stimulation than in 1999.

A modification of the Poffenberger task has been performed to specifically test the validity of structural versus asymmetrical activation interpretations of the CUD. Studying 138 normal individuals, Iacoboni and Zaidel (1998) embedded bilateral stimulus presentations on some trials of a simple RT task to "equilibrate" hemispheric activation, and compared the CUD obtained from lateralized stimuli during the embedded task against the CUD from conditions when only unilateral stimuli were presented. The CUD decreased from 3.0 to 0.3 ms when the embedded bilateral trials were added, consistent with results predicted by the Kinsbourne model.

CUD AS IHTT: ADDITIONAL IMPLICIT ASSUMPTIONS

The alternative view of the Poffenberger paradigm put forward by Kinsbourne and colleagues prompts mention of three additional assumptions inherent in viewing the CUD as meaningful.

(1) That there is a basic equivalence of visuomotor processing and brain areas involved for crossed vs. uncrossed conditions, save for the imposition of callosally mediated transfer.

This assumption is strongly questioned by a recent positron emission tomography (PET) examination of brain regions activated during performance of the Poffenberger task (Marzi et al., 1999). Here, a marked rostral/caudal asymmetry in activation between crossed and uncrossed conditions was found. The crossed condition resulted in activations of the right cuneus, precuneus, and temporoparieto-occipital junction as well as left superior parietal lobule. Uncrossed conditions showed activation generally of more anterior regions, including right superior and medial frontal gyri, left posterior cingulate, and right lingual gyrus. The near dichotomous mapping of crossed vs. uncrossed activations as posterior vs. anterior to the ventral plane passing through the anterior commissure prompted these authors to state: "Thus, a major thrust of this study is that a simple model of visuomotor interhemispheric transfer (as assessed by the Poffenberger paradigm), whereby the direct and indirect cortical routes are identical except for a callosal extra step, is no longer tenable" (p. 457).

(2) That measures of RT central tendency such as median or mean reflect the typical brain activation states required to execute the manual response.

The considerable trial-to-trial variability of RT, its non-Gaussian distribution (e.g., Luce, 1986; Miller, 1988), and the unclear contributions of variations in sensory or motor system activations to a population of RTs suggest that a single RT metric cannot adequately reflect the multiplicity of brain response profiles that actually characterize a population of such responses. Therefore, the RT subtraction method cannot yield a relatively fixed parameter of neural conduction analogous to simultaneous physiological measurement along a fiber tract, an observation that dates back to Donder's (1868–1869) critique of Helmholz (1850). This concern operationalizes into a conception of *intra*individual differences, where the functional connectivity of brain regions involved in visuomotor integration may differ from trial to trial, and characteristically by RT. One consequence of this view is the prediction that the predominant interhemispheric visuomotor route in crossed conditions for fast and slow RTs will differ.

(3) That RT is directly related to timing of movement-related cortical activations.

An open question concerns to the relation between timing and the magnitude of movement-related activations of motor cortex. RT is determined by the time required by one or more of the brain regions along the neural pathways between sensory input and response execution to reach a threshold of activation required to generate an overt motor response. This threshold will depend in part upon the magnitude of motor command signals, generated within cortical regions having direct corticospinal connections with the relevant motoneuron pools, and the level of activation of these motoneurons due to ongoing excitatory and inhibitory processes within the spinal cord at the segmental level of the responding muscles. The magnitude of motor command signals will depend upon the strength of sensory-related stimulation of motor cortical areas and the ongoing activity in these regions. In this view, trial-to-trial variation in RT may be mainly related to differences in strength of the corticospinal motor command from the cortical motor output regions that interact with the momentary activation level of the motoneuron pool.

Recent empirical support for an activation "threshold-to-movement" model of RT has come from single neuron recordings in macaque frontal eye fields during an anti-saccade task that showed an inverse linear relationship between the rate of growth of cell firing (spikes/sec^2) and RT (Hanes & Schall, 1996; K. G. Thompson et al., 1996; Schall & Thompson, 1999). These physiological data were consistent with a previous quantitative analysis of the statistical properties of human saccadic latencies (Carpenter & Williams, 1995) that was based on a "threshold-to-movement" model. Clearly, variability in stimulus-related inputs to motor cortex will, in part, determine the degree of motor cortex activation.

However, Hanes and Schall (1996) point toward stochastic processes within motor cortex that may result in differing RTs from indistinguishable sensory activations. Based on the threshold model, longer RTs may not reflect an increase in the activation onset time of motor output regions, and therefore may be misleading regarding a pathway-length interpretation of response times. These considerations, along with investigation of the critical intrahemispheric processing assumption of the uncrossed conditions, form the motivating framework for undertaking the electrophysiological studies of the Poffenberger paradigm reported below.

Four findings characterize the results: (1) the data demonstrate that, indeed, bilateral activations of motor cortex occur in uncrossed conditions; (2) the magnitude of these activations is inversely related to RT; (3) multiple regions of motor cortex appear to contribute differentially to movement generation for different RTs; and (4) for crossed conditions, central callosal pathways appear as predominant interhemispheric visuomotor routes for fast RTs, while posterior visual sensory routes appear to predominate for slow RTs.

METHODS

General Approach

As we have argued, ERP measures provide anatomically predicted IHTT estimates more in keeping with predictions based on transcallosal fiber conduction times than do behavioral estimates. However, in Saron and Davidson (1989) some subjects had ERP waveforms that lacked clearly defined components, or had negative or near zero IHTT values computed from well defined ERPs. These difficult-to-interpret data likely reflected normal variations of cortical geometry that produced temporally overlapping waveforms, given the scalp potential recordings and very limited spatial sampling used in that, and most, ERP IHTT studies.

The methodological approach we have used in the present studies (detailed in tutorial form in Saron et al., 2002) significantly redresses these limitations. These methods combine high spatial sampling (figure

10.2), large trial numbers, and analysis of spherically interpolated (Perrin et al., 1989) scalp current density (Perrin et al., 1987) of individual subjects to improve visualization of sensory- and movement-related electrocortical activity. Further, for each subject, separate sets of ERPs are derived based on 10 ms-wide bins of the RT distribution, affording a detailed examination of intraindividual differences as a function of RT while constraining the behavioral variability associated with a given set of physiological measures.

Analysis of Scalp Current Density

The topographic display of scalp *voltage* is of limited utility in relating scalp-recorded signals to their underlying electrocortical sources for two principal reasons. First, the apparent distribution of scalp potential is dependent on the reference electrode. Activity picked up by the reference alters the absolute value of the voltage at each scalp site. In addition, the conductive nature of the brain and its coverings disperses the volume currents generated within discrete brain areas, so the scalp potentials they generate are usually spatially and temporally overlapping. The widespread superposition of electrical fields generated by multiple intracranial sources greatly restricts the possibilities for differentiating and correctly identifying the contributions from each source using voltage mapping alone.

A simple analytic method that eliminates the influence of the reference electrode and emphasizes local contributions to the surface map, providing better visualization of approximate locations of intracranial generators, is provided by current source density (CSD) analysis. CSD (or Laplacian) analysis involves the estimation of the second spatial derivative of the field potential, which is proportional to the current density at each point. The two-dimensional application of current density analysis to scalp recordings (scalp current density or SCD) provides a method for estimating the component of current radial to the surface of the scalp, thus providing an estimate of local transcranial current flow (Perrin et al., 1987; Vaughan, 1987; Regan, 1989). SCD analysis mathematically eliminates the voltage gradients due to tangential current flows within the scalp, as well as the contribution of the reference. Thus, by sharpening the spatial resolution of scalp-recorded data, SCD facilitates the identification of activity generated by distinct intracranial sources.

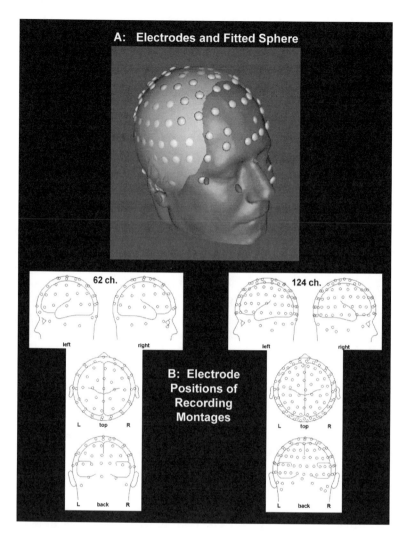

Figure 10.2 (*A*) 124-channel montage, fitted interpolation sphere, and fiduciary markers relative to a surface rendering obtained from a 3-D MRI of a subject's head. (*B*) Electrode positions of 62 (subjects 1 and 2) and 124 (subject 3) channel recording montages show the uniform distribution of electrode locations. (From Saron, 1999.)

C. D. Saron and colleagues

RESULTS AND DISCUSSION

General Remarks and Caveats

The detailed descriptions of the electrocortical response profiles that follow are motivated by the need to examine the complex and rapid interplay of multiple cortical regions, from initial sensory input to motor output, in order to conceptualize the dynamics of simple visuomotor integration. Although numerous references are made to specific scalp current foci and the probable brain areas and neural activations they represent, such assignments must be regarded somewhat cautiously. We take it as a given that the scalp-recorded data are contributed by multiple, simultaneously active brain regions, which the SCD method cannot unambiguously separate. The geometric orientation of underlying neuroelectric sources produces a variety of response patterns. Sources radial to the scalp surface generally produce focal patterns of a single polarity, while tangential sources produce bipolar patterns that covary over time. Of course, most foci are neither exactly radial nor exactly tangential, and therefore result in combinations of such patterns. Nevertheless, the general spatiotemporal profiles are interpretable in terms of known anatomy, expected contributions of multiple brain regions, and interareal connectivity.

The view here is necessarily "corticocentric." SCD analyses remove the widely distributed scalp potential fields generated by subcortical sources. However, the measured cortical responses undoubtedly reflect both cortical and subcortical influences. For instance, given the role of the basal ganglia in movement initiation (reviewed in Wise et al., 1996; Mink, 1996), the question arises as to whether the observed movement-related responses in the present studies are influenced by preceding activity in the basal ganglia relayed to motor cortex via pallidothalamocortical projections. It is unlikely that such circuitry directly influences visuomotor integration in the present experiment, since nonhuman primate studies have shown normal RTs with inactivation of the globus pallidus (Mink & Thach, 1991), and that movement-related activity in the putamen overlaps (Montgomery & Buchholz, 1991) or begins after activity in M1 (Alexander & Crutcher, 1990). However, the basal ganglia likely play an indirect role determining trial-to-trial variability.

Likewise, recent regional cerebral blood flow (rCBF) findings that correlate decreased choice RT to increased ipsilateral cerebellar activation (Horwitz et al., 2000) implicate a cerebellar role in rapid movement initiation. However, recent models of cerebellar function point toward a primary role in movement programming, with sensory-related cortical inputs providing a trigger for a preestablished movement program (Houk & Wise, 1995). The complexities of interactions between cortical and subcortical structures in movement generation are important considerations beyond the scope of the present chapter.

Finally, while quantification of electrocortical measures allows for direct comparison of findings between and within subjects, and affords a tractable reduction of the complexity of the spatiotemporal data, as will be shown, the importance of qualitatively considering the information derived from high temporal and spatial sampling should not be minimized. The individual electrophysiological case study approach typified here makes three fundamental suppositions. The first is that individual differences in brain morphology (e.g., Brindley, 1972; Stensaas et al., 1974; D. N. Kennedy et al., 1998) and functional organization (DeYoe et al., 1996; Hasnain et al., 1998) necessarily produce unique electrophysiological signatures that bear analysis. Second, the multiplicity of intra- and interhemispheric pathways interconnecting sensory and motor cortices creates a dynamic and distributed network that may accomplish very similar behaviors (i.e., the RT response) in a variety of ways, via a variety of routes, depending on ongoing activity in different brain regions, and thus creates *intra*individual differences that require assessment. Third, a somewhat inductive consideration of the regularities of these inter- and intraindividual differences, when based on data from sufficient numbers of trials, points toward the fundamental importance of considering *variability* in brain activation patterns related to similar behaviors as more "signal" than noise.

ELECTROCORTICAL ACTIVATION SEQUENCE FOR UNCROSSED CONDITIONS SHOWS BILATERAL OCCIPITAL, CENTRAL, AND FRONTAL RESPONSES

An orientation to the observed electrocortical response profile for uncrossed conditions, averaged across RT, is provided by the top and back view SCD maps shown in figure 10.3 and plate 4. These maps are based on 1407 trials for the LVF/LH condition and 1308 trials for the

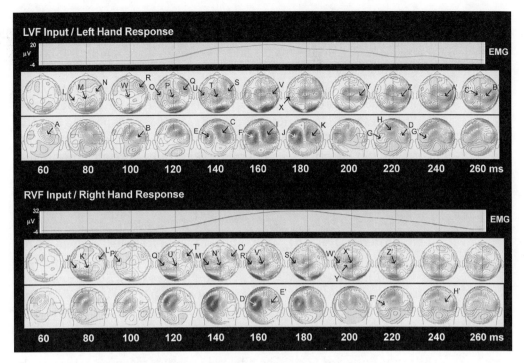

Figure 10.3 Top and back view SCD maps at 20 ms intervals and rectified EMG from 60 to 260 ms poststimulus for the LVF/LH and RVF/RH conditions for subject 1. Data are from averages collapsed across RT (120 to 600 ms). Red contours correspond to outward and blue (stippled) contours to inward scalp currents (plotted sensitivity 0.5 μV/cm²). See text for detailed descriptions of the visual and motor spatiotemporal activation patterns. (From Saron, 1999.) See plate 4 for color version.

RVF/RH condition for Subject 1 and are plotted every 20 ms from 60 to 260 ms. The RT range for these trials was between 120 ms and 600 ms. Red contours represent outward, and blue (stippled) inward, scalp current. Over each panel of SCD maps is a waveform of the averaged rectified EMG response of the left extensor indicus corresponding to the index finger lifts of the manual RT response.

Response to LVF Input

Right Posterior Regions The LVF/LH back view maps (lower row of upper panel of figure 10.3) depict a posterior response pattern that is, overall, characteristic across subjects. An initial focus of outward current over right posterior regions is evident by 60 ms (*A*), representing the direct projection from contralateral hemiretinae. This current focus moves laterally by 100 ms (*B*) and reverses in direction by 140 ms (*C*). The medial-to-lateral shift in this focus from (*A*) to (*B*) suggests that (*A*) may reflect, at least partially, the initial striate cortical activation, and that the later, more lateral activity at (*B*) represents the additional activation of extrastriate regions. Foci at (*B*) and (*C*) correspond to the P100 and N160 components of the visual ERP, and outward and inward currents will henceforth be referred to generally as relative positivities and negativities along the dimension of $\mu V/cm^2$. A late reactivation of right extrastriate regions is visible beginning at 220 ms (*D*), which is similar in location and polarity to (*B*).

Left Posterior Regions Activation of left posterior regions is not prominent until 140 ms (*E*). A strong inward current is present by 160 ms (*F*), followed by a late response pattern at 220 ms (*G*) that is weaker than the right hemisphere response (*D*). The large late positivity near the midline at 220 ms (*H*) likely reflects contributions of multiple visual regions from both hemispheres.

Bilateral Posterior Foci The bilateral posterior response pattern in the time range of 140 to 180 ms is asymmetrical in both extent and timing, and is presumed to represent the callosally mediated delayed activation of the posterior cortical regions ipsilateral to the stimulus. The asynchronous right, then left, activation sequence can be seen in the following observations. At 140 ms, the amplitude and extent of the right negativity is greater than the left (*C* > *E*). At 160 ms, the foci are roughly equal in strength (*F* ≡ *I*), but (*I*) is more extensive. By 180 ms, the left hemisphere focus has increased in magnitude (*J*) while the right focus (*K*) is reduced in strength. The interhemispheric visual delay is 15 ms, measured by N160 peak latency differences between SCD waveforms corresponding to the left and right posterior foci (best seen at *F* and *I*).

Left-Hand Response Patterns

Early Central and Prefrontal Activity The top view map sequences in the upper panel of figure 10.3 illustrate the sequential activation of several cortical regions of both hemispheres. By 80 ms there is indication of small distributed left and right central stimulus-evoked foci

(L–N) in regions that will subsequently show movement-related activity. This observation is based on the pattern of multifocal positivities that includes left postcentral (L), midline central (M), and right precentral (N) regions that are generally similar in location to the negativities seen in these regions at 120 ms (O–Q). Beginning at 100 ms there is a clear right frontal negativity (R). The early onset and location of this response suggest that this focus may correspond to stimulus-generated activation of dorsolateral prefrontal cortex (DLPFC) (see Saron et al., 2001).

The sensory-related nature of the activations at 80 ms is supported by the lack of any EMG activity until after 100 ms. Given that the recent CMD estimate for contraction of the extensor indicis forearm muscle (the primary muscle recorded by the EMG electrodes) is 21 ms (Salenius et al., 1997), electrocortical activity seen at 80 ms are unlikely to be associated with movement generation. The very small rise in EMG by 120 ms suggests that the right prefrontal focus at (R) is also sensory-related. These responses are in accord with the distributed sensory activations overlapping motor cortex predicted by the Kinsbourne model. The right prefrontal negativity shifts slightly posterolaterally between 120 (Q) and 140 ms (S), along with the emergence of a strong negative midline central response (T) and an increase in the magnitude of left laterocentral activity (U).

Putative Premotor and SMA Activity The posterolateral shift of right central activity from 100 to 140 ms (R, Q, and S) is considered to correspond to activation of right premotor cortex (PMC). The midline central focus at 120 ms (P) is presumably within the supplementary motor area (SMA). The medial location and demonstrated bilateral activation of this area during unimanual movements (e.g., Praamstra et al., 1996; Ikeda et al., 1995; Wiesendanger et al., 1996) does not permit an assignment of hemisphere of origin to this pattern.

Putative M1 Activation By 140 ms the central pattern indicates increased activation of the midline negativity (T) and further posterolateral spread of the right frontocentral focus (S), which is well localized to a right lateral central focus by 160 ms (V). The location of this focus, contralateral to the responding hand, is consistent with representing activation of primary motor cortex (M1). It is noteworthy that both the medial central and the lateral frontocentral foci may represent movement generation-related activity. Corticospinal projections to hand motoneurons have been demonstrated from multiple regions of motor cortex, including SMA (Dum & Strick, 1991, 1996; Tandon et al., 2000).

Since the marked increase in SMA activity from 100 to 120 ms (W to P) corresponds to the large EMG increase seen 20 ms later (from 120 to 140 ms), it is likely that SMA, and not M1, corticospinal efference (CE) results in movement initiation. This activation order is not an artifact of combining data across RTs, since SMA also precedes M1 activation for the fastest responses (RT range 215–225 ms) when considered separately (see figure 10.5), and is consistent with the finding of SMA activations preceding M1 activity for self-initiated movements (e.g., Deecke et al., 1999).

RT, EMG, and the ERP   It is useful to consider at this point relations between RT, EMG, and the ERP data. EMG activity follows motor command generation by a corticomuscular delay (CMD). RT, indicated by the optical switch signal, will follow EMG onset due to mechanical delay. A population estimate of RT such as the median bears only an indirect relation to the expected timing of electrocortical signs of motor output as seen in across-RT averaged data of figure 10.3. In Saron (1999) it is suggested that for data averaged across RT, the latency of the half-peak EMG amplitude (LHPA) is an appropriate EMG estimate of movement onset. The mechanical delay of the optical switch is shown to be ~100 ms. As mentioned, a recent CMD estimate for contraction of the extensor indicis forearm muscle (the primary muscle recorded by the EMG electrodes) is 21 ms (Salenius et al., 1997). Given the LHPA of 127 ms and median RT of 266 ms for the LVF/LH data in figure 10.3, electrocortical signs of motor output would then be expected to be visible as early as 106 ms. Notably, examination of ms-by-ms animations of the SCD map time series does show rapidly increasing magnitude of midline central foci beginning at 105 ms, consistent with this prediction.

Left Motor Cortex Responses   The left hemisphere lateral-central response increases in magnitude by 120 ms (O), and wanes by 180 ms (X). The importance of this focus is that it may reflect involvement of corresponding hand areas of the left hemisphere in movement generation, as predicted by numerous studies that demonstrate bilateral activation of motor cortex during unimanual responses (e.g., Urbano, Babiloni, Onorati, & Babiloni, 1998; Urbano, Babiloni, Onorati, Carducci, et al., 1998; studies reviewed in following section).

C. D. Saron and colleagues

Postcentral Reafferent Responses From 200 ms to 260 ms the right lateral central negativity spreads further posteriorly (Y–B') while the midline central focus wanes (C'). The shift away from putative SMA and M1 activation into a more posterior pattern by 240 ms likely represents postmovement reafferent activation of postcentral somatosensory cortex (e.g., Praamstra et al., 1996; Ball et al., 1999; Babiloni et al., 2000). The gradual transition to this pattern seen from 200 to 240 ms may represent the superimposition of activations related to generation of slow RTs and reafferent activations associated with faster RTs. However, the late postcentral focus is also obtained when fast RTs (e.g., 215–225 ms RT) are considered separately (see figure 10.5).

LVF/LH Summary

Overall, the major posterior and central foci show the expected lateralization of visual input to and primary motor output from the right hemisphere. Posterior stimulus-related activation is characterized by an initial right hemisphere positivity that becomes a bilateral negativity by 140 ms, reflecting visual interhemispheric transfer. Central foci show evidence of a sequence of activations that are presumably located within right PFC, PMC, SMA, and M1. Assuming that our resolution of the "true" onset of activity is comparable for M1 and SMA, the early onset timing and long duration of these activations suggest that SMA makes the predominant contribution to corticospinal outflow. Left hemisphere lateral central regions were also active prior to a shift to a right postcentral reafferent response pattern, suggesting ipsilateral cortical involvement in movement generation.

RVF vs. LVF Input: Contrast of Bilateral Activations

The lower panel of figure 10.3 presents the RVF input/right hand response data for Subject 1. The posterior patterns of response to RVF input are principally the anatomic converse of the pattern to LVF input. However, there are two differences that suggest visual field asymmetries in the responses to hemiretinal input. The bilateral negativity (D' and E') does not begin until 160 ms, 20 ms later than the LVF/LH condition (E and C). The interhemispheric delay measured between peaks of the SCD waveforms corresponding to the posterior map foci that represent the N160 component of the visual ERP is 35 ms (versus 15 ms for LVF input). This longer left-to-right than right-to-left IHTT asymmetry is often characteristic of ERP measures of IHTT (e.g., Saron & Davidson, 1989), and asymmetrical transfer times have now been inferred from meta-analyses using RT (Marzi et al., 1991; Braun, 1992) and ERP methods (Brown et al., 1994).

A second difference of RVF compared with LVF input is an increased magnitude of response in the directly stimulated hemisphere (LVF = 24 µV/cm²; RVF = 44 µV/cm² for N160 Laplacian peak amplitude measures). Finally, the late visual reactivation pattern (200–260 ms) to RVF input is very similar to that for LVF input. Within this similarity, the hemisphere showing the greater magnitude positivity reverses from LVF to RVF input (*D* vs. *F′*; *G′* and *H′*).

Right-Hand Response Patterns

The movement-related response pattern (top view maps of bottom panel) is not the simple converse of the left-hand response pattern. However, the basic scheme of motor area parcellation described for the LVF/LH data is the same.

Premotor and M1 Activity   As seen for the LVF/LH condition, by 80 ms there is a pattern of weak stimulus-related central and frontocentral positivity (*J′*, *K′*, and *L′*) in regions that will later show negative movement-related activity (e.g., *M′*, *N′* and *O′*). The broad left central negativity visible by 100 ms (*P′*) suggests a stimulus-related activation of motor regions, possibly including PMC. The small increase in the EMG trace at 120 ms suggests that this focus also represents the same contribution from the generation of corticospinal outflow associated with movement initiation for the fastest RTs. The more focal pattern in this location at 120 ms (*Q′*) presumably represents continued stimulus-related activation via parietocentral pathways as well as movement-related activity associated with the fastest RTs. The continued strong response in this region to 180 ms (*M′*, *R′*, and *S′*) is consistent with M1 contributions to the activity pattern.

Also visible at 120 ms is a right frontocentral focus (*T′*), with identical location but smaller magnitude than seen for the LVF/LH task condition (*Q*, putative right PMC, possibly including regions of right PFC). The observation of right frontocentral foci suggests that some regions of ipsilateral motor cortex are associated with right unimanual movement generation, as seen for the LVF/LH condition. The location of the ipsilateral foci for the LVF/LH condition (*O* and *U*) suggested

M1 activation, compared with ipsilateral PMC activation (foci at T' and O') for the RVF/RH condition. It is unclear from these data if greater ipsilateral motor cortex contributions to movement generation are found with left, compared to right, hand movements, since PMC and M1 both contain corticospinal projections (Dum & Strick, 1991, 1996), though Kim, Ashe, Hendrich, et al. (1993) found fMRI evidence for increased ipsilateral activation for left, compared with right, finger movements.

M1 vs. SMA Activations The medial spreading pattern of the left lateral central focus (U' and N') is identified as putative SMA activation by 160 ms (V'). This focus is slightly leftward of the LVF/LH SMA pattern, consistent with right-hand responses. In contrast to the left-hand response pattern, for which SMA preceded M1 activation, the reverse is true here. This is most likely due to contributions from both stimulus- and movement-related activity to the left lateral central negativity. The left lateral and medial central response pattern persists between 120 and 200 ms (Q', U' to W', X'), reflecting the distribution of RTs within this average and the broad peak of the EMG trace. With the 20 ms intermap interval, the midpoint of the duration of these foci is 160 ms, consistent with the median RT of 281 ms. The waning of the left lateral central focus (W') and posterior spread of the SMA focus (Y') that begins at 200 ms presumably represents the onset of reafference to postcentral somatosensory cortex related to earlier movement-related activations that produced the faster RTs. This pattern appears more medial than that seen for the LVF/LH condition. The continued midline response (e.g., Z') may also reflect, for the slowest RTs, the M1 → SMA activation delay seen for the bulk of RTs between 120 and 160 ms.

RVF/RH Summary

Although the major posterior and central foci again show the expected lateralization, there were several departures from a strict converse of the LVF/LH response pattern. Responses over posterior regions contralateral to the stimulus were increased in magnitude, and the ipsilateral posterior response was delayed and reduced. Responses over the left premotor region were more posterior than putative right PMC, possibly suggesting activation of superior parietal regions as well. Left M1 responses appeared to have a more direct contribution to corticospinal outflow for right-hand than for left-hand finger movements. Right PMC/PFC appeared to be the ipsilateral regions activated, and the reafferent pattern was more medial than for the LVF/LH condition.

ADDITIONAL SUBJECTS SHOW SIMILAR EFFECTS

Figure 10.4 shows the LVF/LH responses for Subjects 2 and 3 in the same format as figure 10.3. The number of trials for these data are Subject 2 = 737 and Subject 3 (124 channels) = 1093.

Occipital Responses

Both subjects show the prototypical unilateral → bilateral activation pattern to visual half-field stimulation. Right posterior positivities are seen by 80 ms (A and B), transitioning to right posterior negativities by 140 ms (E and F); clear bilateral foci (G/H and I/J) are well established by 160 ms. The occipital IHTT estimate was 21 ms for Subject 2 and 12 ms for Subject 3. Subject 3 shows a clear ipsilateral P1 (C) at 100 ms, which was notably absent in Subject 1 and is seen delayed to 120 ms (D) for Subject 2.

Frontocentral Responses

Although there are considerable spatiotemporal differences in the pattern of frontal and central foci between subjects, there are several shared features. These include a right frontocentral negativity at 100 ms (K and L), bilateral frontocentral foci by 140 ms (M/N and O/P), and right lateral central responses by 180 ms (presumptive M1) at (U) and (C'). The EMG traces show earlier motor output for Subject 2 (onset ~105 ms) than for Subject 3 (~134 ms), which is reflected in their median RTs (S#2 = 252 ms; S#3 = 309 ms). Subject 2 shows a sequence of increasing presumptive M1 activation as the amplitude of EMG rises (R–U), which precedes the presumptive SMA activation (V–X), in contrast to the activation sequence of Subject 1. Bilateral central foci are seen for Subject 2 beginning at 140 ms (V/S). For Subject 3, midline central responses with covarying positive and negative foci, suggestive of a tangential source configuration, increase markedly from 140 to 160 ms (small arrows at Z vs. A'), corresponding to the rise in EMG from 160 to 180 ms. The subsequent increase in the response of right

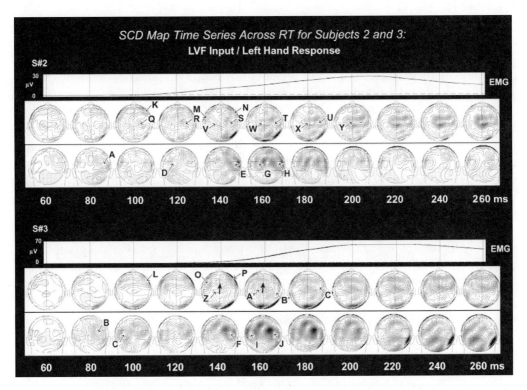

Figure 10.4 Top and back view SCD maps at 20 ms intervals and rectified EMG from 60 to 260 ms poststimulus for the LVF/LH conditions for subjects 2 and 3, as in figure 10.3. Stippled contours correspond to inward scalp currents (plotted sensitivity 0.8 μV/cm² for Subject 2 and 0.4 μV/cm² for subject 3). Both similarities and differences from the response profile of subject 1 are detailed in the text. (Modified from Saron, 1999.)

M1 from 160 to 180 ms (*B'* vs. *C'*) is consistent with medial motor structures initiating movement. There is an overall pattern of bilateral frontocentral activity for Subject 3 from 120 to 260 ms, both before and during movement.

BILATERAL MOTOR CORTEX ACTIVATION SHOULD BE EXPECTED IN AN INTRAHEMISPHERIC CONDITION

Of critical importance to the canonical interpretation of the Poffenberger paradigm is the assumption of unilateral premovement processing during uncrossed conditions. Numerous studies have now demonstrated a pattern of bilateral central activation prior to, and during, movements that violates this assumption. Further, these findings contribute to an emerging view of the cortical motor system as a highly distributed network of pre- and postcentral regions of both hemispheres that are involved in the control of even the simplest movements (e.g., Marsden et al., 2000). Tanji et al. (1988), recording intracranially in the macaque, showed that 25% of SMA neurons and 17% of premotor neurons showed activity prior to ipsilateral movements. The bilateral organization of SMA has been suggested (e.g., Wiesendanger et al., 1996), and the robust callosal pathways that have been found between left and right distal forelimb representations in SMA (Rouiller et al., 1994) are likely to have mediated the responses observed by Tanji et al. (1988). Connections between SMA and primary motor cortex (Tokuno & Tanji, 1993; Tanji, 1994), and premotor regions (e.g., Luppino et al., 1993) likely provide the pathways for bihemispheric activation of multiple motor regions observed in human studies.

Human Electrophysiology

A pattern of bilateral motor cortex activations for unilateral movements, including bilateral readiness fields for simple index finger flexions, has been shown using MEG (Salmelin et al., 1995; Cheyne et al., 1995; Hoshiyama et al., 1997; C. Babiloni et al., 1999) and steady-state ERPs (Gerloff et al., 1997). Praamstra et al. (1996) used spatiotemporal dipole modeling of ERPs and described bilateral activations before finger movement in putative locations corresponding to M1 and in SMA. The assumption of bilateral SMA activation was based on finding a radially oriented midline source dipole that could represent concurrent activity generated by left and right SMA, an interpretation supported by observation of bilateral SMA activation premovement seen in intracranial recordings (Ikeda et al., 1995) and SMA activations recorded with MEG (Erdler et al., 2000; Kaiser et al., 2000).

During brisk single-finger extensions similar to the movements performed in the RT task of the present studies, Urbano et al. (1996; Urbano, Babiloni, Onorati, Carducci, et al., 1998) used 128-channel EEG recordings and realistic head models obtained from the individual subjects' MRIs to compute the projection of the scalp-recorded Laplacian onto the cortical surface. Both left and right finger movements resulted in bilateral activation of nearly equal amplitude in left sensorimotor cortex (identified as M1-S1) during response preparation, movement initiation, and finger motion epochs. Right M1-S1 showed equal activations during response preparation, and about one-half response amplitude during right (ipsilateral) compared with left finger movements. The authors interpret the ipsilateral responses as reflecting transcallosal activations mediated by the SMA-M1 interactions referred to above.

A more global measure of bilateral movement-related activation has been demonstrated by Stančák and Pfurtscheller (1996). These authors used event-related desynchronization (ERD) of EEG recorded in response to index finger movements. There was bilateral premovement ERD for both left- and right-hand responses, with equal degrees of left and right hemisphere desynchronization for left-handed movements (see also C. Babiloni et al., 1999 for direct comparison of ERD and high-density ERP measures in the same subjects). Bilateral activation of motor cortex during unimanual finger movements was found by Urbano, Babiloni, Onorati, and Babiloni (1998), using lagged cross-covariance measures of EEG between selected electrodes as an index of functional coupling between different cortical regions (see also Gerloff et al., 1998; Crone et al., 1998).

Neuroimaging

Bilateral motor cortex activations have also been demonstrated using positron emission tomography (PET) (e.g., Jenkins et al., 2000) and fMRI. In a study using fMRI to investigate responses to finger movements, Kim, Ashe, Hendrich, et al. (1993) found a strong hemispheric asymmetry in bilateral motor cortex activation consistent with the ERD data of Stančák and Pfurtscheller (1996) and the ERP data of Urbano, Babiloni, Onorati, Carducci, et al. (1998) (see also Kim, Ashe, Georgopoulos, et al., 1993). Particularly for right-handers, left hemisphere motor regions showed nearly identical activations during left or right finger movements. Mattay et al. (1998) found a similar pattern, as well as increased activation of ipsilateral motor cortex for more complex motor sequences seen for the dominant hand. Activation of medial motor areas in response to self-initiated and visually triggered simple and sequenced finger oppositions were investigated by Deiber et al. (1998). Bilateral pre-SMA, SMA, and cingulate activations were found in both cases (also Baraldi et al., 1999).

Cramer et al. (1999) found the regions of ipsilateral motor cortex activated in response to paced unilateral finger taps were anterolateral and ventral compared with contralaterally activated regions, suggesting a functional distinction between ipsilateral and contralaterally activated areas. Lee et al. (1999) used event-related fMRI during a delayed, visually cued finger opposition task and observed bilateral SMA and premotor activations during movement preparation for both left and right finger movements.

Callosum Size and Bilateral Motor Activity

Recent evidence specifically relates bilateral motor cortex activations associated with unimanual movement to callosal function. Stančák et al. (2000) correlated measures of callosal cross-sectional area to the amplitude of the ipsilateral readiness (*Bereitshaftspotential*) potential elicited by self-initiated right finger movements. These authors found that the areas of the genu and anterior midbody were directly related to the amplitude difference between left and right Laplacian-derived central electrodes. The overall correlation between these areas (corrected for brain size) was 0.9 for the anterior midbody (from -4 to -0.7 s prior to movement) and 0.88 for the genu (from -3 to -0.7 s prior to movement). These findings suggest that movement preparation involves interhemispheric interaction in some proportion to the available interhemispheric connectivity as indexed by callosal size, specifically in those callosal regions associated with frontal and centrally projecting fibers. Further studies along these lines with more subjects and denser electrocortical sampling will be needed to determine if interhemispheric interactions closer to the time of movement generation also relate to callosum size.

ELECTROCORTICAL RESPONSES SORTED BY RT SHOW MAGNITUDE AS WELL AS TIMING DIFFERENCES

The spatiotemporal patterns described for figures 10.3 and 10.4 are a composite of brain response profiles due to the inclusion of trials from a broad range of reaction times (120–600 ms). To investigate differing response patterns within the distribution of RTs, the across-RT grand average was parceled into a number of subaverages. Each subaverage consisted of trials from one 10 ms wide RT bin. These RT bins

C. D. Saron and colleagues

where chosen after examining the RT distribution for each subject and condition.

Figure 10.5 displays top view SCD map time series from 75 ms to 255 ms poststimulus for the LVF/LH condition for subjects 1 and 2 (see also plate 5). The data are displayed for three of the 12 RT bins derived for each subject, with each indicated RT value the midpoint of a 10 ms range. The rectified extensor indicus EMG is displayed above each map row and shows the expected increasing response latency with increasing RT.

A general pattern of the stability of the posterior visual response across RT is evident. For example, both the initial lateralized positivity at 75 ms (A–F) and bilateral negativity seen at 155 ms (dual arrows at G–L) differ little by RT bin. In contrast, the patterns of central foci for both subjects markedly differ by RT bin. For Subject 1, the central response patterns for the 220 ms RT bin are characterized by a bilateral frontal negativity at 95 ms (dual arrows at M), which shows a right hemisphere increase by 115 ms (N). A midline central focus (presumptive SMA) is also visible by 115 ms (O), consistent with the rise of EMG seen by 135 ms. This response increases in magnitude until 155 ms (P). Also at that time, a right lateral-central negativity (presumptive M1; Q) is visible. The pattern of prior midline and frontal foci (O and N) suggests that M1 activation is subsequent to activations in these regions, as suggested by the pattern of the across-RT data. The late posterior shift of the broad right central negativity by 235 ms (R) is suggestive of responses of somatosensory cortex from postmovement reafference. Also of note in earlier responses are the left lateral-central foci seen at (S), (T), and (U). These foci, ipsilateral to the responding hand, are clear evidence of bilateral central involvement in motor output.

The timing and topography of the central response pattern for the 280 ms RT bin are similar to those seen for the 220 ms RT bin, though generally weaker in magnitude through 195 ms (see P and Q vs. V and W). This observation suggests that decreased *magnitude* of motor cortex activation, rather than timing of activation may be related to slower RT. This is also suggested by the slower rate of rise of the EMG response for the 280 ms, compared with the 220 ms, RT bin. The 320 ms RT bin pattern differs markedly from that of the 220 and 280 ms RT bins, and is more consistent with a pattern of delayed motor cortex activation for the slowest RTs. For instance, the absence of central foci and presence of right frontal activity at 155 (X) is similar to features of earlier response

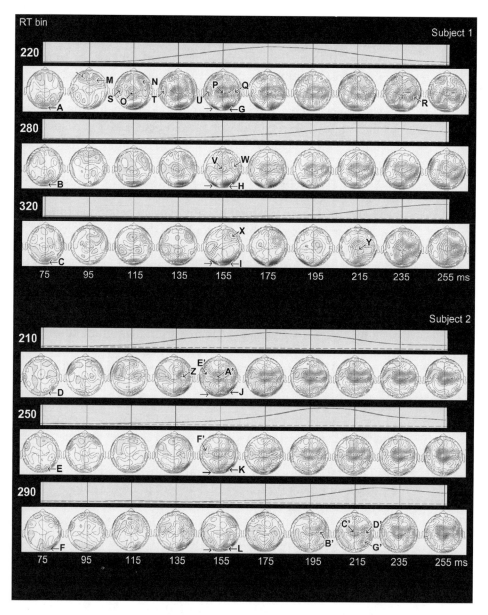

Figure 10.5 Top view LVF/LH SCD maps for subjects 1 and 2 displayed by RT. (Ns for subject 1 were 86, 105, and 55 for RT bins 220, 280, and 320 ms, respectively. Ns for subject 2 were 49, 76, and 37 for RT bins 210, 250, and 290.) The stability of the posterior visual response across RT is evident. The patterns of central activation for both subjects

patterns for the faster RTs (e.g., N). A rapid increase in central negativity does not occur until after 195 ms (Y), also consistent with a delayed motor activation pattern.

The spatiotemporal patterns of central foci for Subject 2 illustrate many of the same basic findings as Subject 1, with some notable individual differences. For example, in this subject, activation of presumptive M1 (focus at Z) precedes activation of presumed SMA (A'). However, the similar timing and topography of RT bins 210 and 250 replicate the observation from Subject 1 of decreased magnitude of motor cortex responses as associated with slower RTs. In addition, the 290 ms RT bin data show a late onset of rapidly increasing central negativity beginning at 195 ms (B'–D'), a pattern consistent with delayed activation of motor cortex for the slowest RTs. The left lateral-central negativities seen at 155 ms for RT bins 210 and 250 ms (E' and F') again demonstrate that bilateral motor cortex activations occur during unimanual intrahemispheric visuomotor simple RT tasks. The marked posterior spread of the right lateral central negativity at 215 ms (G') suggests a basis for a secondary visuomotor activation of right motor regions by a reactivation of superior parietal cortex at this time.

CORRELATIONS BETWEEN REGIONAL MOTOR CORTEX ACTIVITY AND EMG SHOW DIFFERENTIAL CONTRIBUTIONS TO MOTOR OUTPUT AS A FUNCTION OF RT

EMG and SCD Waveforms

Another way that differences in movement-related activity as a function of RT have been examined is shown in figure 10.6 and plate 6. In this approach, SCD waveforms calculated from the centers of presumed SMA and M1 foci ("virtrodes") were lag cross-correlated with

differ markedly by RT bin, with the two faster RT bins sharing similar overall activation patterns that are lower in magnitude than for the middle RT bin. For both subjects, the slowest RTs show a delayed activation pattern. These data illustrate the multiplicity of motor regions of both hemispheres active during performance of intrahemispheric task conditions and highlight individual differences in spatiotemporal activation patterns during performance of simple RT. Stippled (blue) regions correspond to inward scalp current, red to outward current. Plotted sensitivity is 0.5 μV/cm^2 for subject 1 and 0.8 μV/cm^2 for subject 2. See text for detailed explanation of activation patterns. (Modified from Saron et al., 2002.) See plate 5 for color version.

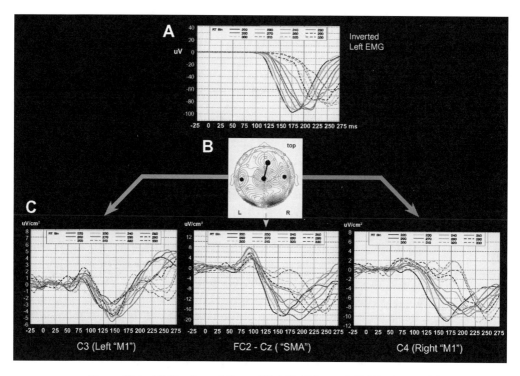

Figure 10.6 (*A*) Overlays of the rectified EMG for each RT bin, inverted for comparison with SCD waveforms for the LVF/LH condition for subject 1. (*B*) The locations from which SCD waveforms (*C*), indicating left and right lateral (presumed PMC/M1) and tangentially oriented midline (presumptive bilateral SMA) activations, placed on the across-RT 162 ms SCD map. (*C*) SCD waveforms derived from locations in (*B*), for each 10 ms RT bin. See text for description of sensory- and movement-related aspects of these waveforms. (Modified from Saron, 1999.) See plate 6 for color version.

the forearm EMG to estimate the corticomuscular delay (CMD) and to examine their relative contributions to motor output.

EMG Waveforms Figure 10.6A displays overlays of the rectified EMG for each RT bin, inverted for comparison with SCD waveforms. Four observations can be made regarding the EMG traces within the overall pattern of increasing response latencies as RT slows: (1) EMG onset times cluster for RT bins 220–280, compared with the more delayed responses for later bins; (2) within these faster bins, slower RTs are associated with decreased slope of EMG onset; (3) RT bins 290 and 300 show a two-step pattern of shallow onset slope until 175 ms, followed by a rapid descent; (4) the response pattern for RT bins 310–330 is consistent primarily with a delay in the onset of EMG, with the slowest RTs revealing a combined pattern of delay, shallower onset slope, and weaker peak response amplitude. The importance of these findings is to highlight the heterogeneity of behavioral response profiles within nonoutlying regions of the RT distribution. Overall, the patterns are suggestive of different response "modes" for motor output, which may include corticospinal efference from multiple regions of motor cortex whose activation time course and motor output efficacy differ. This possibility was explored by comparing waveforms derived from different central regions with the EMG traces.

SCD Waveforms The locations from which SCD waveforms were derived are depicted in figure 10.6B, which indicates left and right lateral (presumed M1) and tangentially oriented midline (presumptive bilateral SMA) foci. These are superimposed on the across-RT SCD map taken at 162 ms poststimulus. Figure 10.6C shows the SCD waveforms derived from these locations for each 10 ms RT bin. A striking feature of the C3 waveforms is the relative lack of relatedness to RT, and the early response onset. These waveforms show sensory-related activation throughout their time course until 200 ms. These later effects, related to RT, reflect positivities indicating reafferent activity associated with fast RTs, and negativities with late and more diffuse midline responses associated with slow RTs. Sensory-related activation of left central regions could be mediated by several pathways: (1) left extrastriate to central pathways following right-to-left interhemispheric transfer of the initial visual response; (2) heterotopic callosal connections between right visual and left frontocentral regions (e.g., Hedreen & Yin, 1981; Di Virgilio & Clarke, 1997); or (3) heterotopic right frontal-to-left central connections, since right frontal responses in this condition begin as early as 50 ms (see general view of callosal connectivity in H. Kennedy et al., 1991).

The SMA waveforms are the difference between two foci located at FC2 and Cz because the SCD maps showed a midline central response pattern consistent with a tangentially oriented source configuration. The striking feature of these waveforms is the presence of both a clearly defined stimulus-related positivity (~85 ms), followed by a movement-related negativity that varies as a function of RT. The amplitude of the early peak is clearly variable as a function of RT, but this relation is not entirely systematic, although the strongest positivities are RT bins 230–250, suggesting that these early differences may account in part for the magnitude and timing of subsequent movement-related activity in this region. The peak latencies of these later responses, but not necessarily their continuous shape, appear to closely precede the peak latencies of the EMG response for the different RT bins. The consistency of this pattern across RTs strongly suggests a direct relation between the observed electrocortical activity and subsequent behavior. As previously discussed, the plausibility of SMA responses directly initiating movement has been made clear by the finding of corticospinal fibers originating in this location in both monkeys (e.g., Dum & Strick, 1991, 1996; Rouiller et al., 1996; Wise, 1996) and humans (Tandon et al., 2000).

Three overall RT-related differences are present in the movement-related portion of these waveform overlays. The first, illustrated by the 220–250 ms RT bins, is characterized by a steep onset limb and similar amplitude of the movement-related negativity that is delayed 5–10 ms, as RT slows. The second, illustrated by the 260–290 ms RT bins, are decreases in slope and magnitude as RT slows, with onset times of the movement-related negativity similar to those for RT bins 220–250 ms. The third observation is of delayed onset that is best seen for the slowest RT bins, 320 and 330 ms. RT bins 300 and 310 ms show a transitional pattern of decreased initial slope and subsequent delayed response. Notably, the two-step amplitude sequence seen in the EMG for RT bins 290 and 300 is also present in these waveforms. The differing patterns of response are consistent with the global observation from the EMG traces of different *modes or classes* of visuomotor activation. The basic pattern of these magnitude and timing differences was consistently observed across subjects.

The waveforms from the C4 virtrode lack early stimulus-related activity, consistent with interpretation of this region as reflecting the activity of primary motor cortex. As would be expected, these waveforms are closely related to those from the EMG. This similarity is striking, with clustering of waveforms from different RT bins paralleling that seen in the EMG, particularly for the data from the 270–330 ms RT bins. In addition, for the 220 ms RT bin, the onset of the C4 negativity occurs prior to that seen for the SMA waveforms; and the peak of the C4 waveform is both similar in shape and earlier than the EMG waveform for this RT bin, suggesting that M1 corticospinal effer-

C. D. Saron and colleagues

ence contributes to these motor responses. However, the overall temporal relation between the movement-related C4 negativities and the EMG is less clear, particularly with respect to the timing of peak amplitudes. Inspection of the FC2-Cz versus C4 waveforms suggests that SMA responses more consistently precede movement by a plausible corticomuscular delay than does M1 activity.

In summary, left central responses were notably sensory-related and not movement-related, while both putative SMA and M1 appeared to contribute to motor output differentially as a function of RT. Visuomotor integration appeared most likely to involve SMA, with possible contributions from the sensory-related activations of left motor regions.

Quantitative Comparison of Electrocortical and Muscle Activity

The degree of similarity between the different SCD waveforms and the EMG was quantitatively assessed using a lag-to-maximum correlation procedure that computed the cross-correlation between SCD waveform segments and the EMG waveform at various bidirectional lags, and determined the lag that maximized the cross-correlation. The lag value at maximum correlation (lag max r) was taken as an estimate of corticomuscular delay (CMD). Relations between lag max r values and RT were examined by regression analyses for each virtrode location. The regression plot for the C3 SCD waveform versus EMG lagged correlation procedure, along with zero-lag correlations (0 lag r) and maximum correlations (max r) is presented in figure 10.7A.

The dashed lines represent 95% confidence intervals for the mean of the predicted values. The correlation window (80–200 ms, $\pm$175 ms test lag) was chosen to capture the full extent of the sensory-related negativity of these waveforms (figure 10.6C). The C3 waveforms and the EMG were uncorrelated at zero ms lag, which increased to maximum correlations at the plotted lag values. As would be expected when comparing stimulus-related responses with increasing RT, lag max r values increased with increasing RT. Inspection of the plotted lag values suggests a sigmoidal pattern. A cubic polynomial regression demonstrated a very high degree of fit as indicated by the r^2 of 0.99. The high degree of overlap of the 220 and 230 ms RT bin EMG responses, on the one hand, and the 320 and 330 ms EMG waveforms, on the other, most likely account for the small differences in lag values for the slowest and fastest RT bins.

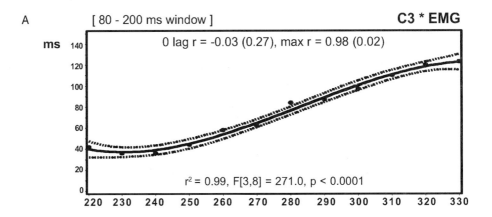

A [80 - 200 ms window]   C3 * EMG

ms 140   0 lag r = -0.03 (0.27), max r = 0.98 (0.02)

$r^2 = 0.99$, F[3,8] = 271.0, p < 0.0001

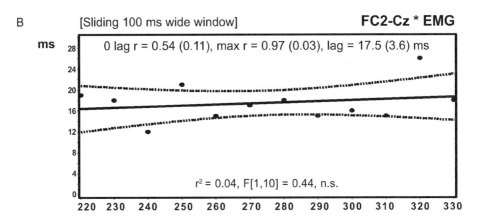

B [Sliding 100 ms wide window]   FC2-Cz * EMG

ms 28   0 lag r = 0.54 (0.11), max r = 0.97 (0.03), lag = 17.5 (3.6) ms

$r^2 = 0.04$, F[1,10] = 0.44, n.s.

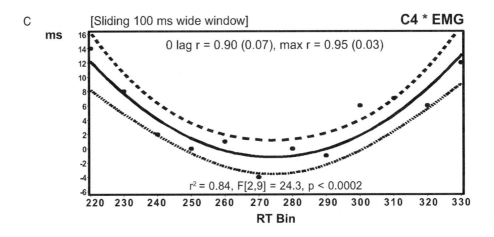

C [Sliding 100 ms wide window]   C4 * EMG

ms 16   0 lag r = 0.90 (0.07), max r = 0.95 (0.03)

$r^2 = 0.84$, F[2,9] = 24.3, p < 0.0002

RT Bin

Since both the movement-related putative SMA and M1 activations were in part delayed with increasing RT, the cross-correlation windows were systematically adjusted. A 100 ms wide window was used to compare the virtrode and EMG waveforms. For the 220 ms RT bin, this window began at 100 ms poststimulus and was lagged across the rectified, inverted EMG waveform $\pm$100 ms. The window start position was incremented 10 ms for each subsequent RT bin. This was done both to compensate for the later activity onsets associated with slower responses and to avoid compromise fits due to waveform asymmetries that result when using overly long correlation windows. As was seen for the C3 values, figure 10.7B shows the consistently large increase in correlation at the indicated lag values. The graph shows the overall stability of the lag max r values and the absence of any linear trend as a function of RT. These data therefore suggest a determinative role for SMA in generating the behavior, since SMA activity reliably precedes, and is closely related to, the EMG response. Given this interpretation, the 17.5 ms mean lag max r value would represent measurement of corticomuscular delay for this subject. This value is close to the average extensor indicis CMD of 21 ms found by Salenius et al. (1997), based on MEG/EMG measurement during isometric contraction. However, given multiple sources of corticospinal outflow, such estimates must be regarded with caution.

An identical lag correlation analysis was performed on the C4 and EMG waveforms and is presented figure 10.7C with a striking result. The lag max r values approach 0 ms for the middle RT bins and increase for *both* the fastest and slowest RTs. The curvilinear nature of this relation was assessed by a quadratic regression analysis, which was highly significant. While the activation time course of C4 activity closely followed motor output; its simultaneity with actual behavior

Figure 10.7 Regressions of lag at maximum correlation between central SCD waveforms and rectified EMG versus RT bin for the LVF/LH condition for Subject 1. (*A*) Cubic polynomial fit for the C3*EMG plot. Increasing lag values by RT bin is consistent with sensory activations that are invariant across RT. (*B*) The consistent CMD estimate for the FC2-Cz*EMG suggests SMA as the primary source of corticospinal efference across RT. (*C*) Quadratic fit for C4*EMG lag values suggests M1 contributions to movement for fast and slow RTs. EMG does not lag cortical activation for the middle of the RT distribution, suggesting unclear contributions to movement for the majority of RTs. (Modified from Saron, 1999.)

over the middle of the RT distribution (RT bins 240–290) suggests that this activity had little role in generating movement. Conversely, though still somewhat later than corresponding SMA activity, the larger temporal disparity between C4 and EMG for the fastest and slowest RTs *does* suggest a role in generating or sustaining movements. The implication of this pattern of results is that multiple motor areas contribute to actual movement generation, consistent with anatomical evidence (e.g., Wise, 1996) and human electrophysiological data (e.g., Cui & Deeke, 1999). Further, for a given timing of visuomotor activation, particular RTs may be determined in part by the degree of synchrony of SMA and M1 activations, which may act synergistically to produce the most rapid movements. Biphasic peaks in the EMG, such as seen for RT bin 290 (figure 10.6A) may correspond to sequential activation of these regions because the peak of the SMA negativity is earlier than that for M1 (figure 10.6C).

QUANTIFICATION OF MOVEMENT-RELATED SCD WAVEFORMS DEMONSTRATES DECREASED MOTOR CORTEX ACTIVATION AS RT SLOWS

Based on the analyses presented in figure 10.7, while both SMA and M1 appear to contribute to movement generation, SMA activity far more consistently preceded the EMG, and did so in a time range consistent within the range of the expected CMD (Salenius et al., 1997). As the SMA waveforms in figure 10.6C show, within the time range of about 100–175 ms there is a pattern of decreasing negativity as RT slows. This is also true for the slowest RT bins, for which subsequent strong movement-related responses occur. These observations are consistent with the notion that for a given trial, it is "how much" and not just "when" activations of motor cortex occur that determines behavioral response time.

In order to further examine this claim, the integrated amplitude of movement-related negativities was examined by RT bin. For all subjects and uncrossed conditions, medial and lateral central foci (presumptive SMA and M1), reflecting movement-related negativities contralateral to the responding hand, were identified visually from examination of the SCD map sequences. To determine which of these locations were most closely related to movement generation, SCD waveforms were derived from these foci and were lag cross-correlated with the EMG wave-

Table 10.1 Mean (SD) lagged cross-correlation values for correlations between SCD waveforms and inverted rectified forearm EMG for maximum lagged r, and lag times (in ms) to maximum r for LVF/LH and RVF/RH data averaged across subjects and conditions

	Max r	Lag at max r (CMD est.)
Unselected virtrodes	0.98 (0.02)	18.9 (24.2) ms
Selected virtrodes	0.98 (0.01)	20.5 (2.8) ms

forms. The lag to max r values were derived for each presumptive motor region for each RT bin and were used to estimate the CMD. For each subject and condition, the central region with lag values for the maximum correlations that approximated the expected physiological CMD estimate for finger movements (Salenius et al., 1997) was taken as the appropriate location for further analysis of movement-related activity.[1]

The results of this analysis, collapsed across conditions and subjects, are shown in table 10.1. The most notable feature of these data is the low variability of the CMD estimates from the selected virtrodes. Although the mean CMD estimates for the unselected and selected virtrodes are relatively close, the SDs differ widely. The mean lag value for the selected SCD waveforms was 20.5 ms, which is in very close agreement with the 21 ms CMD value found by Salenius et al. (1997).

Segments of the selected waveforms were quantified by computing values of integrated amplitude for each RT bin for each subject and condition. The onset time of the analysis interval was chosen to include the average onset of the movement-related negativity across conditions and subjects. The offset time was chosen to include the pattern of decreasing initial response with increasing RT, and excluded the delayed activation associated with the slowest responses. Thus, the analysis provides a measure of the initial responses that resulted in movement for faster RTs and that failed to elicit rapid movement for slower RTs. The analysis windows did not differ between conditions, and are indicated on the plots in figure 10.8. Linear regressions by RT were performed, and these are plotted in figure 10.8 by subject and condition.[2]

The results indicate a strong linear relationship between decreasing initial activation magnitude of motor output regions and increasing RT.

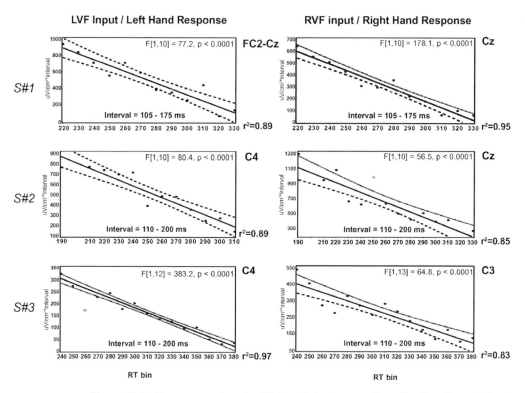

Figure 10.8 Linear regressions by RT bin of the integrated amplitude values obtained over the indicated intervals from the Laplacian waveforms of all RT bins. The dashed lines indicate the 95% confidence interval of the mean of predicted values. The F-statistic, *p*-value, and r² for each analysis are indicated. The results show a strong linear relation between decreasing initial activation magnitude of motor output regions and increasing reaction time, despite differences in the RT ranges for different subjects. (From Saron, 1999.)

MOTOR CORTEX EXCITABILITY AND RT

The relationship between motor cortex activation magnitude and RT may represent a macroscopic confirmation in humans of the results of Hanes and Schall (1996) and Hanes et al. (1998). These authors examined the behavior of single movement-related cells in Macaque frontal eye fields during a saccade generation task. They found that RTs were linearly related ($r^2 = 0.97$) to the slope of the activation function of the recorded cells. As described at the opening of this chapter, the model of

RT variability that they support involves a constant activation threshold to movement initiation. Different response times occur as activation functions of differing slope cross the threshold. Hanes and Schall (1996) conclude that the variability characteristic of RT distributions is "irreducible," and results from stochastic processes within response-generating circuits. The stability of the visual sensory responses in the current data set across RTs supports the notion that variations in the state of motor output regions may account for much of the RT differences within a task condition.

Two different lines of work have recently demonstrated that the state of ongoing neural activity interacts with stimulus-evoked responses. In one type of study, physiological variables recorded just prior to or at the time of sensory input predict later physiological or behavioral responses (e.g., Arieli et al., 1996; Ioannides et al., 1998; Everling et al., 1997, 1998; Everling & Munoz, 2000). In the other, electrical or magnetic stimulation presented close to the time of sensory input (−50 to +10 ms) facilitates simple RTs up to 50 ms (e.g., Pascual-Leone et al., 1992; Terao et al., 1997; Davey et al., 1998), and when presented just prior to muscle movements, it delays simple RT up to 100 ms (Ziemann et al., 1997; B. U. Meyer & Voss, 2000). Taken together, these studies suggest that multiple factors, such as the timing and strength of the previous movement, interstimulus interval (Uusitalo et al., 1996; Iacoboni et al., 1997), and stochastic processes may influence the strength of motor cortex activation in response to sensory-related input.

DIFFERENCES IN INTERHEMISPHERIC VISUOMOTOR ROUTING ARE ASSOCIATED WITH FAST AND SLOW RTs

A central question regarding interhemispheric visuomotor transfer concerns the callosal "level" at which this transfer occurs. Both visual and motor routes have been proposed, as reviewed at the opening of this chapter. An obvious way to approach this question is to examine the spatiotemporal profile of electrocortical responses in crossed conditions for fast versus slow RTs. Such an example is provided by the SCD map time series shown in figure 10.9 and plate 7. The top panel shows averages from trials with RTs between 215 and 235 ms (225 ms RT bin, N = 118). The bottom panel shows averages from trials 100 ms slower, with RTs between 315 and 335 ms (325 ms RT bin, N = 112).

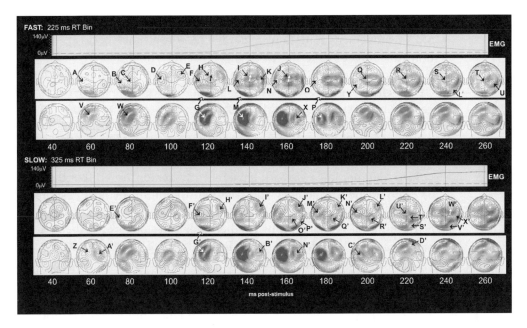

Figure 10.9 Rectified forearm EMG, and top and back view SCD maps at 20 ms intervals, from 40 to 260 ms poststimulus for fast and slow RTs from the RVF/LH condition for subject 1. Red contours correspond to outward, and blue (stippled) contours to inward scalp currents. From 80 to 180 ms, posterior responses differ little between response speeds, while central activations and EMG differ markedly over this interval. See text for explanation of the activations indicated by the lettered arrows. The data are displayed at sensitivity of 0.5 μV/cm². See plate 7 for color version.

Fast RTs

The back view map series (lower row of upper panel) depicts the characteristic unilateral → bilateral posterior focal pattern seen previously, and bears a close resemblance to the across-RT RVF/RH pattern of figure 10.3. This similarity demonstrates that response hand has little observable effect on the spatiotemporal pattern of electrocortical responses recorded over posterior regions. Conversely, overall, the top view map sequences are similar to the pattern of central activity for the LVF/LH data of figure 10.3, a correspondence that demonstrates the expected primacy of response hand, independent of input visual field, in determining the configuration of motor cortex activations.

Early Central Responses   Already beginning by 60 ms, there is a weak sensory-related left laterocentral positivity (*A*) that increases in magnitude at 80 ms for both lateral (*B*) and medial (*C*) regions, before any rise in the EMG at 100 ms (allowing for the CMD). The strength of the presumptive SMA sensory activation at this early latency may be related to the subsequent strength of motor output that results in fast RTs. This is an important observation for four reasons. First, the initial lateral and then medial activation sequence suggests a possible routing pathway, likely involving left premotor cortex (PMC), presumably by way of parietal-central pathways (e.g., Wise et al., 1997), followed by involvement of PMC to SMA pathways (e.g., Kurata, 1991). Second, early activation of presumed SMA establishes an interhemispheric route for subsequent activation of right motor output regions (Rouiller et al., 1994). Third, the increased central positivities at 80 ms correspond to the increase from 60 to 80 ms of the left occipital major positivity (*V* → *W*), suggesting a link between the degree of early response in visual cortex and the strength of subsequent motor output. Fourth, it supports the early distributed sensory-related activations of the directly stimulated hemisphere posited by the Kinsbourne model.

Movement-Related Responses   At 100 ms, bilateral frontocentral foci (negativities at *D* and *E*) and transitional midline pattern are associated with the onset of movement-related activity, indicated by the slight rise in EMG at 120 ms. The 120 ms SCD map shows a marked increase in central activity at several locations, reflecting the larger motor output shown in the EMG at 140 ms. The increase in the left lateral central focus (*F*) appears to be associated with the strong left posterior negativity (dual arrows at *G*), consistent with the action of parietal to central pathways. Also at 120 ms, the presumptive SMA response has shifted to the tangential focal pattern as described previously, with a positivity and negativity that appear to covary until the peak of movement-related activity seen at 160 ms (small arrows at *H–J*). By 140 ms, an additional right lateral central focus (*K*), taken to be M1, appears, replicating the SMA → M1 activation sequence seen for the LVF/LH condition (figure 10.3). It is of note that the strong M1 focus arises prior to the onset at 160 ms of the transcallosal right posterior response (*X*). This pattern is strongly suggestive of central, rather than posterior, callosal routes supporting activation of right motor cortex. Contributions from SMA and M1 were quantitatively assessed using lagged cross-correlations with the EMG in the same manner as described for the LVF/LH condition. The mean CMD estimate was 17 ms for the SMA focus and 5 ms for M1. The close correspondence between CMD estimates for LVF/LH and RVF/LH conditions suggests that overall, movement-related activations for left-hand finger lifts are independent of input visual field.

Also occurring at 140 ms is further increase in the magnitude of the left lateral central negativity (L), which appears to be associated with the increased magnitude of the left posterior negativity seen at (M). The stimulus-related nature of this left central focus is suggested by the diminution in this response at 160 and 180 ms (N and O), which corresponds to the decreased extent and magnitude of the left posterior negativity (P). Thus, as was seen for the analysis of the LVF/LH condition, left central regions appear to reflect sensory-related activation in this subject for left-hand responses, also independent of input visual field.

Both M1 and SMA responses are sustained from 140 ms through 180 ms, an interval that is centered on the peak of motor output as reflected in the EMG trace. This pattern is consistent with the suggested synergistic role of SMA and M1 contributing to corticospinal efference for the fastest responses (figure 10.7). As movement generation wanes, the SMA responses decrease, beginning at 200 ms and thereafter (Q–T). The posteromedial shift of the right central negativity likely reflects reafferent activation of somatosensory cortex (U). Also emerging at 200 ms is a sustained left postcentral positivity (Y), possibly of superior parietal origin, that appears to be associated with reactivation of left hemisphere visual regions.

Summary of Putative Visuomotor Routing   The sequence of activations detailed above suggests the following schematic account of right hemisphere motor output for left hemisphere visual input for fast RTs (CE: corticospinal efference):

$$L \text{ extrastriate} \rightarrow L \text{ PMC} \rightarrow L \text{ SMA} \dashrightarrow R \text{ SMA} \rightarrow R \text{ PMC} \rightarrow R \text{ M1} \Rightarrow CE$$

ctx

cc   CE

Since the strong movement-related foci at (I) and (K) occur prior to the appearance of the interhemispherically mediated right posterior negativity (X), the principal interhemispheric visuomotor activation

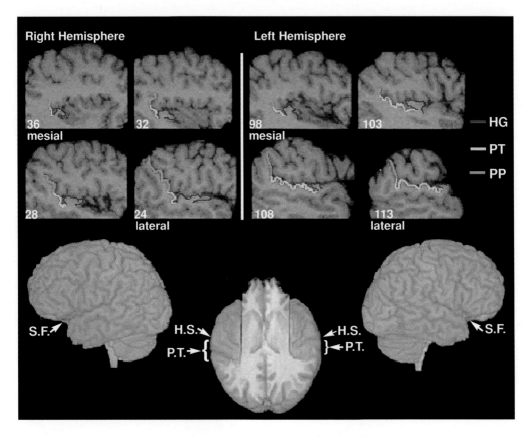

Plate 1 Example of delineated anatomical regions on the superior temporal plane of a representative brain. Tracing line in red indicates Heschl's gyrus (HG); in yellow, the planum temporale (PT); and in green, the planum parietale (PP). Reconstructed brain in the lower row indicates the position of Heschl's sulcus (H.S.) and the PT. (Courtesy of Gottfried Schlaug.) See chapter 6.

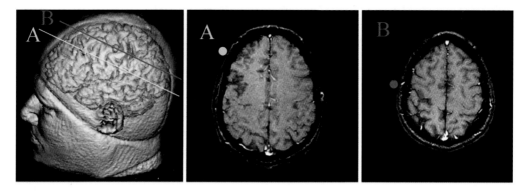

Plate 2 The results in a representative subject are presented. The 3-D reconstruction of the subject's head MRI (*left*) demonstrates the sites of TMS application and the level of the axial slices of fMRI displayed in the other two panels. The middle figure illustrates the statistically significant fMRI BOLD changes observed during the performance of the verbal fluency task, and marks on the scalp show the location of the TMS coil for induction of speech arrest. Note that speech arrest is induced by TMS over brain regions that are activated during the verbal fluency task. The figure at right shows the most representative slice of fMRI BOLD activity corresponding to a motor task consisting of opening and closing the right hand, which is shown to be directly under the TMS scalp position that evokes hand movements (but does not lead to speech arrest). Note that the changes corresponding to the motor areas appear more posterior than those responsible for the word generation task. The latter include the areas targeted by rTMS during speech arrest. (Modified from Bartres-Faz et al., 1998, with permission.) See chapter 7.

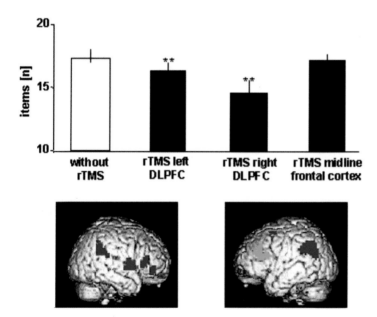

Plate 3 The bar histogram displays the number of correct items (n = 20) in the task depending on stimulation condition. The first bar represents the performance in the two-back working-memory task without rTMS; the second, with rTMS over the left dorsolateral prefrontal cortex; the third, with rTMS over the right dorsolateral prefrontal cortex; and the fourth, with rTMS over the midline prefrontal cortex. ** = $p < 0.01$ (paired t-test). The bottom part of the figure shows the spatial distribution of rCBF changes. Specifically, the deactivations induced by rTMS of the left (green) and the right (blue) dorsolateral prefrontal cortex are shown as an overlay on a 3-D surface-rendered anatomical MR ($p < 0.01$; k = 20) to illustrate the differences in TMS-induced changes in brain activity despite similar behavioral effects. (Modified from Mottaghy et al., 2000, with permission.) See chapter 7.

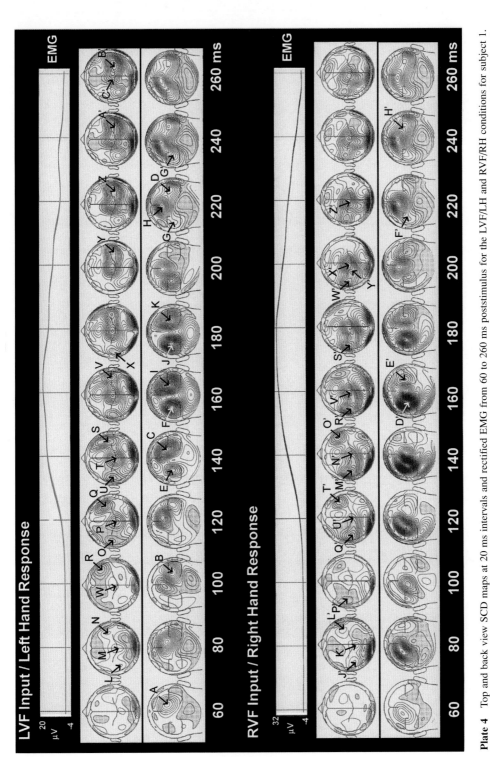

Plate 4 Top and back view SCD maps at 20 ms intervals and rectified EMG from 60 to 260 ms poststimulus for the LVF/LH and RVF/RH conditions for subject 1. Data are from averages collapsed across RT (120 to 600 ms). Red contours correspond to outward and blue (stippled) contours to inward scalp currents (plotted sensitivity 0.5 μV/cm²). See text for detailed descriptions of the visual and motor spatiotemporal activation patterns. (From Saron, 1999.) See chapter 10.

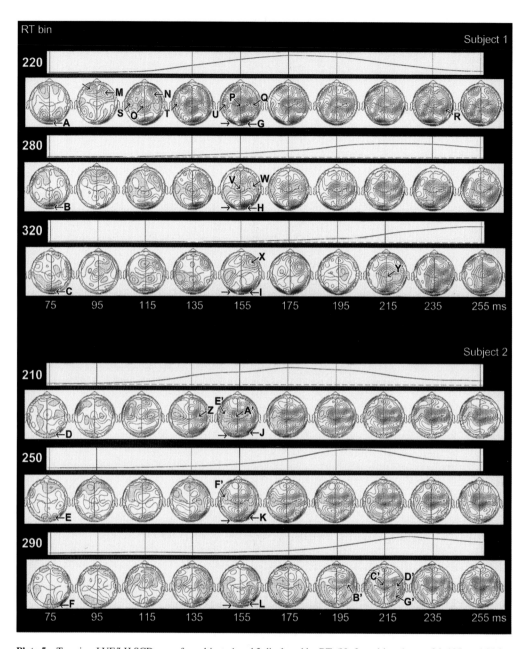

Plate 5 Top view LVF/LH SCD maps for subjects 1 and 2 displayed by RT. (Ns for subject 1 were 86, 105, and 55 for RT bins 220, 280, and 320 ms, respectively. Ns for subject 2 were 49, 76, and 37 for RT bins 210, 250, and 290.) The stability of the posterior visual response across RT is evident. The patterns of central activation for both subjects differ markedly by RT bin, with the two faster RT bins sharing similar overall activation patterns that are lower in magnitude for the middle RT bin. For both subjects, the slowest RTs show a delayed activation pattern. These data illustrate the multiplicity of motor regions of both hemispheres active during performance of intrahemispheric task conditions and highlight individual differences in spatiotemporal activation patterns during performance of simple RT. Stippled (blue) regions correspond to inward scalp current, red to outward current. Plotted sensitivity is 0.5 µV/cm² for subject 1 and 0.8 µV/cm² for subject 2. See text for detailed explanation of activation patterns. (Modified from Saron et al., 2002.) See chapter 10.

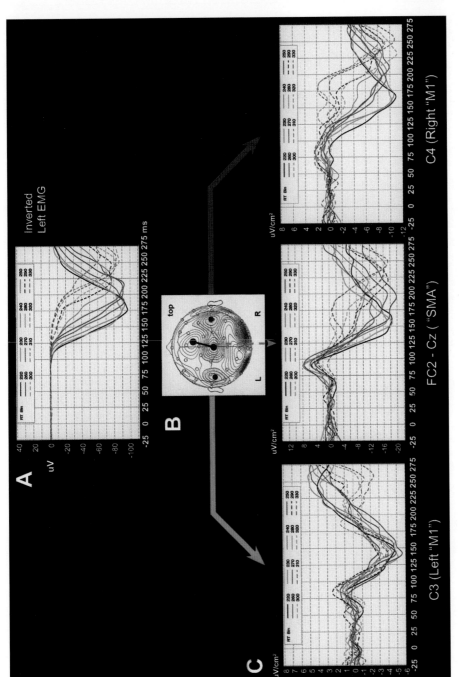

Plate 6 (*A*) Overlays of the rectified EMG for each RT bin, inverted for comparison with SCD waveforms for the LVF/LH condition for subject 1. (*B*) The locations from which SCD waveforms (*C*), indicating left and right lateral (presumed PMC/M1) and tangentially oriented midline (presumptive bilateral SMA) activations, were placed on the across-RT 162 ms SCD map. (*C*) SCD waveforms derived from locations in (*B*), for each 10 ms RT bin. See text for description of sensory- and movement-related aspects of these waveforms. (Modified from Saron, 1999.) See chapter 10.

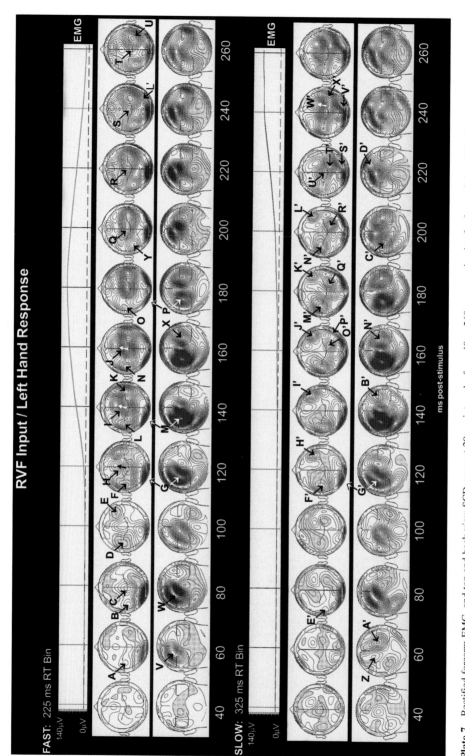

Plate 7 Rectified forearm EMG, and top and back view SCD maps at 20 ms intervals, from 40 to 260 ms poststimulus for fast and slow RT's from the RVF/LH condition for subject 1. Red contours correspond to outward, and blue (stippled) contours to inward scalp currents. From 80 to 180 ms, posterior responses differ little between response speeds, while central activations and EMG differ markedly over this interval. See text for explanation of the activations indicated by the lettered arrows. The data are displayed at sensitivity of 0.5 µV/cm². See chapter 10.

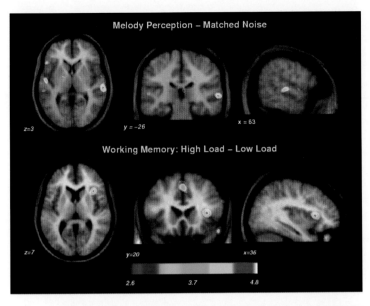

Melody Perception – Matched Noise

z=3   y=−26   x=63

Working Memory: High Load – Low Load

z=7   y=20   x=36

2.6   3.7   4.8

◀Plate 8 Selected PET CBF activation sites associated with processing of tonal melodies. The figures show averaged PET subtraction images superimposed on a corresponding section of an average anatomical MRI. (*Top*) Horizontal, coronal, and sagittal views through a focus located in the upper bank of the right superior temporal sulcus, representing a significant blood flow increase while subjects listened to a series of short, unfamiliar tonal melodies, as compared with a baseline condition in which they listened to noise bursts that were acoustically equated to the melodies. Also visible in the horizontal section is a region of significant activity in the left temporal cortex. (*Bottom*) Horizontal, coronal, and sagittal views through a focus in the right frontal/opercular region showing activity associated with making judgments about the pitch of the first and last notes of the tonal sequences (high working memory load) as compared to making judgments about the first two notes (low working memory load). (Data reanalyzed from Zatorre et al., 1994.) See chapter 11.

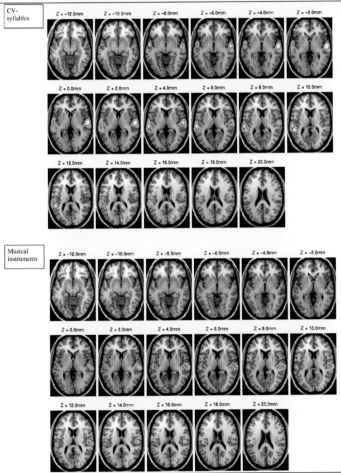

CV-syllables

Musical instruments

◀Plate 9 15O-PET activation images in 2 mm axial slices covering the planum temporale and adjacent inferior and superior areas. Note the absence of activation to the musical instruments stimuli in areas inferior to the planum temporale, while the CV syllable stimuli also activated areas in the vicinity of the superior temporal sulcus. Left in the image is left in the brain, following neurological conventions. (Data obtained in collaboration with Ian Law, Copenhagen University Hospital PET Center.) See chapter 12.

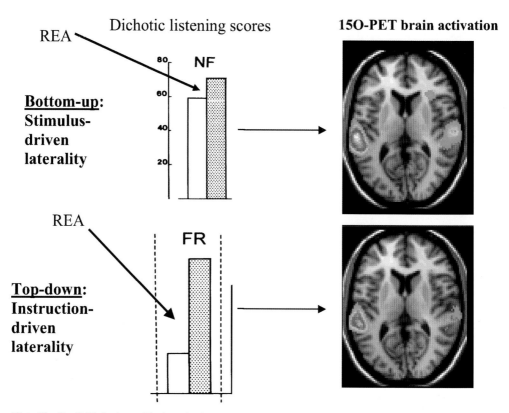

Plate 10 Parallel behavior and brain activation (PET) effects during nonforced and forced-right attention conditions. See chapter 12.

route for movement initiation appears to be via the callosal connections linking left and right SMA. A secondary, later visuomotor route may contribute to right M1 activation via right parietal to central pathways following from the right transcallosal visual response.

Slow RTs

Visual Cortex Responses The major features of the visual sensory responses associated with slow RTs do not differ from the fast RT pattern. However, there are a number of clear differences at specific points in time. The single most striking is the weak positivity at 60 ms (Z), compared with the strong response shown at V for fast RTs. The coincident negativity at (A') suggests a different, and likely weaker, configuration of early striate activation for slow RTs. Although this near-midline tangential pattern might suggest foveation of the hemi-retinal stimuli, the clear expected lateralization and similarity to the fast RT pattern from 80 to 180 ms argues against eye movements shifting the retinotopic location of the stimuli.

The interhemispherically delayed right posterior negativity appears to onset earlier for slow compared to fast RTs (B' at 140 ms). Conversely, at 200 ms, the persistence of the left posterior negativity at (C') indicates that a delayed offset of the contralateral N160 component of the VEP is associated with slow RTs, with presumed lengthening of the duration of active transcallosal input to right extrastriate cortex. In addition, beginning at 220 ms, there is a fingerlike projection of an anterior-spreading right superior parietal positivity at (D') that is not seen for fast RTs, and that appears to be associated with the right centroparietal negativity.

Motor Cortex Responses As expected, there are marked differences between central patterns for fast versus slow RTs. From 60 to 100 ms, early sensory-related central responses for slow RTs are less well organized and weaker than those for fast RTs. This is particularly evident at 80 ms, where the weak left lateral central positivity and medial spread at (E') is similar to the 60 ms fast RT pattern at (A). In contrast to the fast RT pattern, an early putative SMA activation does not subsequently develop. By 120 ms, the marked increase of the left lateral central negativity (F') is associated with appearance of the strong left posterior negativity at (G'), as seen for (G) and (F) foci for fast RTs. This finding serves as a check on the sensory-relatedness of this response, since the EMG is negligible at 140 ms. Although left lateral central foci are very similar for fast vs. slow RTs, the putative SMA activations at this time strongly differ, with only weak activation of SMA suggested by the medial spread of the focus at (F'). The failure of stimulus-related inputs to activate motor regions capable of generating corticospinal outflow is demonstrated by the lack of an increase in SMA or right M1 over the ensuing interval. Thus activation of motor output regions is delayed, rather than diminished, consistent with the pattern seen for the slowest RTs from the LVF/LH condition (figures 10.5 and 10.6).

From 120 to 200 ms there is a sustained right prefrontal negativity $(H'-L')$. The absence of this pattern for the fast RTs suggests the possibility that this activity, prior to the motor response for slow RTs, relates to a working memory trace of the stimulus within dorsolateral prefrontal cortex (e.g., Funahashi et al., 1990). Such activation could be maintained in part by the ongoing transcallosal right occipital input to right frontal regions via intrahemispheric parietocentral pathways (e.g., Cavada & Goldman-Rakic, 1989). Alternatively, or complementarily, because the sensory-related left lateral central foci are prolonged for slow compared to fast RTs $(M'$ vs. $O)$, frontocentral callosal pathways could contribute to maintenance of the right frontal response, particularly prior to the further activation of right posterior regions.

An additional response that appears to be associated with the growth of the right posterior negativity from 140 to 160 ms $(B'$ to $N')$ is the small 160 ms negativity at O'. This focus appears to be associated with the lateral and anterior spread of the right posterior negativity N' that can be seen at P'. The focus O' is adjacent to two positivities, one immediately posterior and the other anterolateral, that in turn are adjacent to the right posterior negativity. The gradual rise from 160 to 200 ms in the magnitude of the foci O', Q', and R' parallels the gradual EMG increase seen from 180 to 220 ms. At 220 ms, the anterior spread of the right posterior positivity S' (seen in the back view map at D') is associated with a marked increase in the magnitude of the movement-related right central negativity seen at T'. In addition, the anteromedial spread of this focus (U') suggests activation of midline central structures that likely include SMA.

The overall increase in right central response magnitude is reflected by the increase in EMG seen at 240 ms. The 240 ms SCD map shows a continued anterior spread of the right posterior positivity at V' and a

C. D. Saron and colleagues

further increase in the magnitude of right central activity. This develops into a pattern that is consistent with a tangential orientation of motor output regions, illustrated by the small arrow at W'. The lateral spread of the right central negativity from 220 to 240 ms (seen at X') suggests additional involvement of right M1. It is of note that the tangential focus W' is a lateral displacement of the midline SMA pattern seen, for example, at 140 ms (I) for fast RTs. This suggests that SMA activation for fast RTs may be more bilateral than for slow RTs, which is consistent with an SMA → SMA interhemispheric visuomotor route reflected in the cortical activations underlying fast RTs.

Regarding the slow RTs, the laterally displaced pattern may represent more unilateral activation of SMA, given the general medial central location of these foci compared to the putative M1 focus seen for the fast responses (i.e., K). Overall, it appears that the anterior spread of right posterior activity, associated with both the callosally mediated major negativity (e.g., N') and the late right hemisphere positivities seen at D' are the major stimulus-related responses that result in activations of motor cortex sufficient for movement generation.

Summary of Putative Visuomotor Routing The sequence of activations described above for slow RTs suggests the primacy of posterior callosal routes for activation of right motor output regions, as well as the following major pathway for movement generation:

L extrastr ctx ⇢ R extrastr ctx → R PMC → R SMA → R M1 ⇨ CE

                                                               ⇩

               cc   CE

Summary

The qualitative contrast of fast versus slow RTs just described provides intriguing evidence that slow and fast RTs differ in the callosal routes that are effective for interhemispheric visuomotor integration. Fast RTs appear to be associated with central interhemispheric routes, most likely via left and right SMA-to-SMA connections. The failure of sensory-related left central activation to result in comparable midline central activation for slow RTs, and a subsequent failure to find such midline responses during movement, suggests that other interhemispheric routes must be responsible for activation of right motor cortex.

The late anterior spread of the transcallosally mediated right posterior response suggested activation of right motor cortex via posterior transcallosal routes. Converging input to right motor cortex would likely also occur via prefrontal to central pathways, given the prolonged right putative PFC response. PFC activation in turn could be supported by further converging inputs from right posterior and transcallosal heterotopic connections from left premotor cortex, which also showed prolonged activation for slow compared to fast RTs. One further suggestion from these findings is that differences in early visual responses (well established by 60 ms) may result in large differences in subsequent visuomotor activation and produce delayed RTs. Supporting this hypothesis, early visual response magnitude has been found to correlate with RT (Saron, 1999).

An obvious question regarding these results concerns their generalizability across, and reliability within, subjects. In order to preliminarily address these issues, the peak latencies of major visual and motor foci for fast versus slow RTs were sequenced for all subjects and crossed conditions. To explore within-subject reliability for this analysis, ERPs were recomputed from alternate trial blocks to create two independent data sets for each subject, condition, and RT range (fast vs. slow). The same pattern of results was obtained from each data set. For Subject 1, the LVF/RH condition results were analogous to the results just described. Subjects 2 and 3 showed a pattern suggestive of central and posterior transcallosal routes converging to produce activation of motor output regions for fast RTs. For slow RTs, close temporal association of late ipsilateral posterior activations with onset of movement-related responses, and an average of 130 ms separating peaks of frontal and movement-related activations, strongly suggested greater contribution of posterior than central callosal pathways for these responses (Saron, unpublished observations).

MULTIPLE PATHWAYS SUPPORT MULTIPLE FUNCTIONAL ROUTES

The existence of *intra*hemispheric parietal-central (e.g., Wise et al., 1997) and parietal-frontal (e.g., Cavada & Goldman-Rakic, 1989) pathways suggests that stimulus-related central and frontal activations may serve to activate interhemispheric projections from these regions. Connections between left and right SMA likely subserve central interhemispheric transfer, since these regions are callosally well interconnected (Rouiller et al., 1994) and receive strong input from premotor regions (Luppino et al., 1993) that are interconnected with parietal cortex (Wise et al., 1997). Since Rouiller et al. (1994) found weak callosal projections between the hand areas of left and right primary motor cortices, connections between SMA and primary motor cortex are likely to provide additional pathways for central interhemispheric routes (Tokuno & Tanji, 1993; Tanji, 1994).

As mentioned, the observation that SMA is among the regions of motor cortex that contain corticospinal projections which activate motoneurons of the contralateral hand (Dum & Strick, 1991, 1996), and its bilateral organization (Wiesendanger et al., 1996), suggest a general importance of central interhemispheric routes via SMA. This seems particularly to be the case in the present task situation, since the relatively direct parietal $\rightarrow$ premotor $\rightarrow$ SMA $\rightarrow$ SMA pathway appears to result in movement generation prior to activation of M1. Thus, faster RTs will result to the extent that visual input is effective in activating ipsilateral premotor cortex.

When trial-to-trial variability in the degree of activation of visual cortex results in low-magnitude responses of ipsilateral premotor regions, subsequent weak activation of SMA will fail to initiate a rapid RT for at least two reasons: (1) weaker activations of motor output regions are associated with longer RTs (e.g., Hanes & Schall, 1996; figures 10.6 and 10.8) and (2) below some threshold, activation of SMA is too weak to generate corticospinal efference sufficient for overt movement generation.

Thus, the model that emerges from consideration of these data is one of parallel pathways in a race to activate motor output regions. The electrocortical response patterns for fast RTs best support a coactivation race model in which multiple interhemispheric routes contribute to movement-related activity, in a manner similar to redundancy gain observed in SRT to multimodal (auditory and visual) stimuli, compared to either modality alone (Hughes et al., 1994). The response sequence for slow RTs demonstrates that sustained late activity in visual cortex can provide stimulus-related activation of motor output regions when prior inputs to motor cortex fail to generate movement-related activity.

OVERALL SUMMARY

This chapter has presented an approach to the analysis of noninvasively recorded human electrophysiology and motor response speed that examines both *interindividual* differences in functional brain organization and dynamic *intraindividual* fluctuations in brain state indexed by differences in RT. The motivation for this effort stems from two sources: (1) compelling evidence of anatomical and functional variation in brain organization across individuals (e.g., Brindley, 1972; Stensaas et al., 1974; D. M. Thompson et al., 1996; Hasnain et al., 1998; see especially figures 1 and 2 of DeYoe et al., 1996) and (2) the need to delineate variation in the dynamic activation patterns of brain motor responses that are implied by response time variability in simple RT tasks (Swanson et al., 1978; McClelland, 1979; Milner, 1986; D. E. Meyer et al., 1988). These two aspects of inter- and intraindividual spatiotemporal cortical dynamics have been examined using the case study methodological strategy as outlined herein.

The data are results from a simple behavioral task, the Poffenberger paradigm (figure 10.1): detection of an unambiguous visual event presented to the left or right of central fixation, indicated by rapid finger lifts using either the left or the right hand. The subjects themselves have supplied the most important independent variable: the naturally occurring trial-to-trial variations in individual responses. This variability enabled investigation of systematic variation in electrocortical activity based on RT. Four major results have been presented in this chapter.

1. In uncrossed conditions, bilateral frontal, central, and occipital activations were found either before or during movement, thereby violating the intrahemispheric processing assumption of the crossed minus uncrossed RT difference in the Poffenberger paradigm.

2. The group of movement-related cortical regions that differentially contributed to movement generation as a function of RT included (in addition to M1) the supplementary motor area and premotor cortex, all of which have direct corticospinal efferent projections. The pattern of activation across the set of motor-related areas was seen to vary as a function of RT. This finding casts doubt on the idea that various visuomotor response latencies share a single common corticospinal pathway mechanism across a range of RTs.

C. D. Saron and colleagues

3. The degree of motor cortex activation, in terms of onset slope and magnitude, *but not onset timing*, was related to RT. A wide range of RTs were generated by movement-related cortical activations that differed little in onset timing, while the slowest RTs appeared to represent delayed activation of motor output regions.

4. Interhemispheric routes of visuomotor activation differ across RT values. Overall, central routes of interhemispheral transfer were found for faster, and posterior routes for slower, RTs in crossed conditions.

IMPLICATIONS FOR THE POFFENBERGER PARADIGM

It seems clear that the notion that IHTT can be inferred from the difference in RT for crossed versus uncrossed conditions (the CUD) is no longer sustainable. The consistent bilateral activation of motor cortex with similar timing in intrahemispheric as well as interhemispheric conditions suggests that *subtracting the uncrossed from the crossed RT may actually contrast one form of interhemispheric interaction with another, rather than the presence versus absence of callosal mediation.* Further, the assumption that interhemispheric versus intrahemispheric differences in RT represent the sum of activation delays from visual to motor cortex also appears to be problematic, inasmuch as changes in RT are closely related to the slope and magnitude, rather than to the onset timing, of movement-related activation of motor cortex. Thus, it appears that RT is determined by the action of summed distributed inputs to motor cortex, the effects of which in turn depend on the current state of the motor system and the degree of activation of visual cortex. As such, RT cannot serve as a simple index of uncrossed versus callosally mediated visuomotor integration.

The primacy of central callosal routes for interhemispheric visuomotor transfer for fast RTs, as argued above, is in accord with the general claims of motor-related interhemispheric transfer made by Milner and Lines (1982) and Forster and Corballis (1998). However, the present results further weaken the basic assumptions underlying straightforward interpretation of the CUD due to the heterogeneity of physiological response profiles that comprise the crossed condition RT distribution. Further studies that examine more precisely the temporal relations between multiple cortical regions throughout the RT spectrum will be required to assess the relative contributions of different interhemispheric routes for the bulk of responses.

Finally, the most often cited validation of this experimental design is the increase in IHTT obtained in patients who have undergone callosal section (e.g., Sergent & Myers, 1985; Clarke & Zaidel, 1989; Iacoboni & Zaidel, 1995). Rather than providing accurate estimates of transcallosal transfer time in normal individuals, it would seem this paradigm is best suited for estimating *subcortical* transfer in patients lacking cortical commissures. Even then, the physiological interpretation of simple RT remains problematic, given the evidence for multiple activation routes to movement-related output.

In moving beyond an oversimplified model of interhemispheric transfer, the opportunity arises for investigation of the rich complexity and dynamics of brain function as revealed by the functional activity underlying the simplest of discrete tasks. Further studies based on close examination of intra- and interindividual differences, yet performed on larger numbers of subjects, will be necessary to characterize, and generalize more fully, the multiplicity of activation sequences and response profiles that have been explored here. Although the resources and analytic tools required to approach single individuals as populations within themselves are daunting, such an approach appears fruitful for meeting the challenge of developing more realistic models of interhemispheric interaction.

ACKNOWLEDGMENTS

The authors wish to thank Dr. Seppo Ahlfors, Beth Higgins, Dr. Jan Hrabe, James Long Company, Megis Software, and Neuroscan Corporation for technical and software support. This work was supported by grants from NICHD (HD001799), NIMH (MH15788, MH11431, and MH60358) and NINDS (NS027900).

NOTES

1. This comparison was not made in two instances: RVF/RH for subject 1 and LVF/LH for subject 2. For subject 1, the waveforms for the left lateral central activation were clearly stimulus- rather than movement-related, consistent with the SCD maps in figure 10.3 ($Q'-W'$). For subject 2, the medial central waveforms did not resemble the shape of the EMG waveforms. A comparison between these waveforms and the EMG would have resulted in uninterpretable max r and lag values. Examination of the SCD map sequences suggested that the SCD waveforms were reflecting activations that were not centered at the selected virtrode location. Both subjects did, however, have foci that were clearly

movement-related, and the virtrode waveforms from these locations were lag cross-correlated with the EMG.

2. The bin 250 data point for the RVF/RH condition of Subject 2 was excluded because of a slow potential offset in that waveform. The bin 260 data from the LVF/LH condition of Subject 3 was excluded from the analysis to demonstrate the high colinearity of the remaining points.

REFERENCES

Aboitiz, F., Rodriguez, E., Olivares, R., & Zaidel, E. (1996). Age-related changes in fibre composition of the human corpus callosum: Sex differences. *NeuroReport, 7*, 1761–1764.

Aboitiz, F., Scheibel, A. B., Fisher, R. S., & Zaidel, E. (1992). Fiber composition of the human corpus callosum. *Brain Research, 98*, 143–153.

Aglioti, S., Berlucchi, G., Pallini, R., Rossi, G. F., & Tassinari, G. (1993). Hemispheric control of unilateral and bilateral responses to lateralized light stimuli after callosotomy and in callosal agenesis. *Experimental Brain Research, 95*, 151–165.

Alexander, G. E., & Crutcher, M. D. (1990). Neural representations of the target (goal) of visually guided arm movements in three motor areas of the monkey. *Journal of Neurophysiology, 64*, 164–168.

Allison, J. D., Meador, K. J., Loring, D. W., Figueroa, R. E., & Wright, J. C. (2000). Functional MRI cerebral activation and deactivation during finger movement. *Neurology, 54*, 135–142.

Andreassi, J. L., Okamura, H., & Stern, M. (1975). Hemispheric asymmetries in the visual cortical evoked potential as a function of stimulus location. *Psychophysiology, 12*, 541–546.

Anzola, G. P., Bertoloni, G., Buchtel, H. A., & Rizzolatti, G. (1977). Spatial compatibility and anatomical factors in simple and choice reaction time. *Neuropsychologia, 15*, 295–302.

Appenteng, K., Conyers, L., & Moore, J. A. (1989). The monosynaptic excitatory connections of single trigeminal interneurones to the V motor nucleus of the rat. *Journal of Physiology* (London), *417*, 91–104.

Arieli, A., Sterkin, A., Grinvald, A., & Aertsen, A. (1996). Dynamics of ongoing activity: Explanation of the large variability in evoked cortical responses. *Science, 27*, 1868–1871.

Babiloni, C., Carducci, F., Pizzella, V., Indovina, I., Romani, G. L., Rossini, P. M., & Babiloni, F. (1999). Bilateral neuromagnetic activation of human primary sensorimotor cortex in preparation and execution of unilateral voluntary finger movements. *Brain Research, 827*, 234–236.

Babiloni, F., Carducci, F., Cincotti, F., Del Gratta, C., Roberti, G. M., Romani, G. L., Rossini, P. M., & Babiloni, C. (2000). Integration of high resolution EEG and functional magnetic resonance in the study of human movement-related potentials. *Methods of Information in Medicine, 39*, 179–182.

Ball, T., Schreiber, A., Feige, B., Wagner, M., Lucking, C. H., & Kristeva-Feige, R. (1999). The role of higher-order motor areas in voluntary movement as revealed by high-resolution EEG and fMRI. *Neuroimage, 10,* 682–694.

Baraldi, P., Porro, C. A., Serafini, M., Pagnoni, G., Murari, C., Corazza, R., & Nichelli, P. (1999). Bilateral representation of sequential finger movements in human cortical areas. *Neuroscience Letters, 269,* 95–98.

Bashore, T. R. (1981). Vocal and manual reaction time estimates of interhemispheric transmission time. *Psychological Bulletin, 89,* 352–368.

Berlucchi, G. (1972). Anatomical and physiological aspects of visual functions of corpus callosum. *Brain Research, 37,* 371–392.

Berlucchi, G., Aglioti, S., Marzi, C. A., & Tassinari, G. (1995). Corpus callosum and simple visuomotor integration. *Neuropsychologia, 33,* 923–936.

Berlucchi, G., Crea, F., Di Stefano, M., & Tassinari, G. (1977). Influence of spatial stimulus-response compatibility on reaction time of ipsilateral and contralateral hand to lateralized light stimuli. *Journal of Experimental Psychology: Human Perception and Performance, 3,* 505–517.

Bisiacchi, P., Marzi, C. A., Nicoletti, R., Carena, G., Mucignat, C., & Tomaiuolo, F. (1994). Left-right asymmetry of callosal transfer in normal human subjects. *Behavioural Brain Research, 64,* 173–178.

Boroojerdi, B., Diefenbach, K., & Ferbert, A. (1996). Transcallosal inhibition in cortical and subcortical cerebral vascular lesions. *Journal of Neurological Science, 144,* 160–170.

Boroojerdi, B., Hungs, M., Mull, M., Topper, R., & Noth, J. (1998). Interhemispheric inhibition in patients with multiple sclerosis. *Electroencephalography and Clinical Neurophysiology, 109,* 230–237.

Boroojerdi, B., Topper, R., Foltys, H., & Meincke, U. (1999). Transcallosal inhibition and motor conduction studies in patients with schizophrenia using transcranial magnetic stimulation. *British Journal of Psychiatry, 175,* 375–379.

Boussaoud, D., & Wise, S. P. (1993). Primate frontal cortex: Effects of stimulus and movement. *Experimental Brain Research, 95,* 28–40.

Braun, C. M., Collin, I., & Mailloux, C. (1997). The "Poffenberger" and "Dimond" paradigms: Interrelated approaches to the study of interhemispheric dynamics? *Brain and Cognition, 34,* 337–359.

Braun, C. M. J. (1992). Estimation of interhemispheric dynamics from simple unimanual reaction time to extrafoveal stimuli. *Neuropsychology Review, 3,* 321–364.

Braun, C. M. J., Achim, A., & Villeneuve, L. (1999). Topography of averaged electrical brain activity relating to interhemispheric dynamics in normal humans: Where does the critical relay take place? *International Journal of Psychophysiology, 32,* 1–14.

Brindley, G. S. (1972). The variability of the human striate cortex. *Journal of Physiology* (London), *225,* 1–3.

Brown, W. S., Bjerke, M. D., & Galbraith, G. C. (1998). Interhemispheric transfer in normals and acallosals: Latency adjusted evoked potential averaging. *Cortex, 34,* 677–692.

Brown, W. S., Jeeves, M. A., Dietrich, R., & Burnison, D. S. (1999). Bilateral field advantage and evoked potential interhemispheric transmission in commissurotomy and callosal agenesis. *Neuropsychologia, 37,* 1165–1180.

Brown, W. S., Larson, E. B., & Jeeves, M. A. (1994). Directional asymmetries in interhemispheric transmission time: Evidence from visual evoked potentials. *Neuropsychologia, 32,* 439–448.

Carpenter, R. H., & Williams, M. L. (1995). Neural computation of log likelihood in control of saccadic eye movements. *Nature, 377,* 59–62.

Cavada, C., & Goldman-Rakic, P. S. (1989). Posterior parietal cortex in rhesus monkey: II. Evidence for segregated corticocortical networks linking sensory and limbic areas with the frontal lobe. *Journal of Comparative Neurology, 287,* 422–445.

Chen, D. F., Hyland, B., Maier, V., Palmeri, A., & Wiesendanger, M. (1991). Comparison of neural activity in the supplementary motor area and in the primary motor cortex in monkeys. *Somatosensory and Motor Research, 8,* 27–44.

Chen, R., Cohen, L. G., & Hallett, M. (1997). Role of the ipsilateral motor cortex in voluntary movement. *Canadian Journal of Neurological Science, 24,* 284–291.

Cheyne, D., Weinberg, H., Gaetz, W., & Jantzen, K. J. (1995). Motor cortex activity and predicting side of movement: Neural network and dipole analysis of pre-movement magnetic fields. *Neuroscience Letters, 188,* 81–84.

Clarke, J. M., Halgren, E., Scarabin, J. M., & Chauvel, P. (1995). Auditory and visual sensory representations in human prefrontal cortex as revealed by stimulus-evoked spike-wave complexes. *Brain, 118,* 473–484.

Clarke, J. M., & Zaidel, E. (1989). Simple reaction times to lateralized light flashes: Varieties of interhemispheric communication routes. *Brain, 112,* 849–870.

Conti, F., & Manzoni, T. (1994). The neurotransmitters and postsynaptic actions of callosally projecting neurons. *Behavioural Brain Research, 64,* 37–53.

Cramer, S. C., Finklestein, S. P., Schaechter, J. D., Bush, G., & Rosen, B. R. (1999). Activation of distinct motor cortex regions during ipsilateral and contralateral finger movements. *Journal of Neurophysiology, 81,* 383–387.

Crone, N. E., Miglioretti, D. L., Gordon, B., Sieracki, J. M., Wilson, M. T., Uematsu, S., & Lesser, R. P. (1998). Functional mapping of human sensorimotor cortex with electrocorticographic spectral analysis. I. Alpha and beta event-related desynchronization. *Brain, 121,* 2271–2299.

Cui, R. Q., & Deecke, L. (1999). High resolution DC-EEG analysis of the Bereitschafts-potential and post movement onset potentials accompanying uni- or bilateral voluntary finger movements. *Brain Topography, 11,* 233–249.

Culham, J. C., Brandt, S. A., Cavanagh, P., Kanwisher, N. G., Dale, A. M., & Tootell, R. B. (1998). Cortical fMRI activation produced by attentive tracking of moving targets. *Journal of Neurophysiology, 80*, 2657–2670.

Davey, N. J., Rawlinson, S. R., Maskill, D. W., & Ellaway, P. H. (1998). Facilitation of a hand muscle response to stimulation of the motor cortex preceding a simple reaction task. *Motor Control, 2*, 241–250.

Davidson, R. J., Leslie, S. C., & Saron, C. D. (1990). Reaction time measures of interhemispheric transfer time in reading disabled and normal children. *Neuropsychologia, 28*, 471–485.

Deecke, L., Lang, W., Uhl, F., Beisteiner, R., Lindinger, G., & Cui, R. Q. (1999). Movement-related potentials and magnetic fields: New evidence for SMA activation leading M1 activation prior to voluntary movement. *Electroencephalography and Clinical Neurophysiology Supplement, 50*, 386–401.

Deiber, M. P., Ibanez, V., Honda, M., Sadato, N., Raman, R., & Hallett, M. (1998). Cerebral processes related to visuomotor imagery and generation of simple finger movements studied with positron emission tomography. *Neuroimage, 7*, 73–85.

DeYoe, E. A., Carman, G. J., Bandettini, P., Glickman, S., Wieser, J., Cox, R., Miller, D., & Neitz, J. (1996). Mapping striate and extrastriate visual areas in human cerebral cortex. *Proceedings of the National Academy of Sciences, USA, 93*, 2382–2386.

Di Lazzaro, V., Oliviero, A., Profice, P., Insola, A., Mazzone, P., Tonali, P., & Rothwell, J. C. (1999). Direct demonstration of interhemispheric inhibition of the human motor cortex produced by transcranial magnetic stimulation. *Experimental Brain Research, 124*, 520–524.

Di Stefano, M., & Salvadori, C. (1998). Asymmetry of the interhemispheric visuomotor integration in callosal agenesis. *NeuroReport, 9*, 1331–1335.

Di Stefano, M., Sauerwein, H. C., & Lassonde, M. (1992). Influence of anatomical factors and spatial compatibility on the stimulus-response relationship in the absence of the corpus callosum. *Neuropsychologia, 30*, 177–185.

Di Virgilio, G., & Clarke, S. (1997). Direct interhemispheric visual input to human speech areas. *Human Brain Mapping, 5*, 347–354.

Donders, F. C. (1868–1869). Over de snelheid van psychische processen. *Onderzoekingen Gedann in het Physiologish Laboratorium der Utrechtsche Hoogeshool*, Tweed Reeks, series 2, 92–120. In W. G. Koster (Ed. and Transl.), *Attention and Performance II*. Amsterdam: North-Holland, 1969. (Reprinted from *Acta Psychologica, 30* [1969], 412–431).

Dum, R. P., & Strick, P. L. (1991). The origin of corticospinal projections from the premotor areas in the frontal lobe. *Journal of Neuroscience, 11*, 667–689.

Dum, R. P., & Strick, P. L. (1996). Spinal cord terminations of the medial wall motor areas in macaque monkeys. *Journal of Neuroscience, 16*, 6513–6525.

Endo, H., Kizuka, T., Masuda, T., & Takeda, T. (1999). Automatic activation in the human primary motor cortex synchronized with movement preparation. *Cognitive Brain Research, 8*, 229–239.

Erdler, M., Beisteiner, R., Mayer, D., Kaindl, T., Edward, V., Windischberger, C., Lindinger, G., & Deecke, L. (2000). Supplementary motor area activation preceding voluntary movement is detectable with a whole-scalp magnetoencephalography system. *Neuroimage, 11,* 697–707.

Everling, S., Dorris, M. C., & Munoz, D. P. (1998). Reflex suppression in the anti-saccade task is dependent on prestimulus neural processes. *Journal of Neurophysiology, 80,* 1584–1589.

Everling, S., Krappmann, P., Spantekow, A., & Flohr, H. (1997). Influence of pre-target cortical potentials on saccadic reaction times. *Experimental Brain Research, 115,* 479–484.

Everling, S., & Munoz, D. P. (2000). Neuronal correlates for preparatory set associated with pro-saccades and anti-saccades in the primate frontal eye field. *Journal of Neuroscience, 20,* 387–400.

Fadiga, L., Fogassi, L., Gallese, V., & Rizzolatti, G. (2000). Visuomotor neurons: Ambiguity of the discharge or "motor" perception? *International Journal of Psychophysiology, 35,* 165–177.

Ferbert, A., Priori, A., Rothwell, J. C., Day, B. L., Colebatch, J. G., & Marsden, C. D. (1992). Interhemispheric inhibition of the human motor cortex. *Journal of Physiology* (London), *453,* 525–546.

Ferrera, V. P., Cohen, J. K., & Lee, B. B. (1999). Activity of prefrontal neurons during location and color delayed matching tasks. *NeuroReport, 10,* 1315–1322.

Fogassi, L., Raos, V., Franchi, G., Gallese, V., Luppino, G., & Matelli, M. (1999). Visual responses in the dorsal premotor area F2 of the macaque monkey. *Experimental Brain Research, 128,* 194–199.

Forster, B., & Corballis, M. C. (1998). Interhemispheric transmission times in the presence and absence of the forebrain commissures: Effects of luminance and equiluminance. *Neuropsychologia, 36,* 925–934.

Funahashi, S., Bruce, C. J., & Goldman-Rakic, P. S. (1990). Visuospatial coding in primate prefrontal neurons revealed by oculomotor paradigms. *Journal of Neurophysiology, 63,* 814–831.

Funahashi, S., Chafee, M. V., & Goldman-Rakic, P. S. (1993). Prefrontal neuronal activity in rhesus monkeys performing a delayed anti-saccade task. *Nature, 365,* 753–756.

Gerloff, C., Richard, J., Hadley, J., Schulman, A. E., Honda, M., & Hallett, M. (1998). Functional coupling and regional activation of human cortical motor areas during simple, internally paced and externally paced finger movements. *Brain, 121,* 1513–1531.

Gerloff, C., Toro, C., Uenishi, N., Cohen, L. G., Leocani, L., & Hallett, M. (1997). Steady-state movement-related cortical potentials: A new approach to assessing cortical activity associated with fast repetitive finger movements. *Electroencephalography and Clinical Neurophysiology, 102,* 106–113.

Graziano, M. S., Hu, X. T., & Gross, C. G. (1997). Visuospatial properties of ventral premotor cortex. *Journal of Neurophysiology, 77,* 2268–2292.

Hanes, D. P., Patterson, W. F., & Schall, J. D. (1998). Role of frontal eye fields in counter-manding saccades: Visual, movement, and fixation activity. *Journal of Neurophysiology, 79,* 817–834.

Hanes, D. P., & Schall, J. D. (1996). Neural control of voluntary movement initiation. *Science, 274,* 427–430.

Hasnain, M. K., Fox, P. T., & Woldorff, M. G. (1998). Intersubject variability of functional areas in the human visual cortex. *Human Brain Mapping, 6,* 301–315.

Hedreen, J. C., & Yin, T. C. (1981). Homotopic and heterotopic callosal afferents of caudal inferior parietal lobule in *Macaca mulatta. Journal of Comparative Neurology, 197,* 605–621.

Helmholtz, H. L. F. von. (1850). Über die methoden, kleinste zeittheile zu messen, und ihre anwendung für physiologische zwecke. Original work translated in *Philosophical Magazine, 6* (sec. 4) (1853), 313–325.

Hoptman, M. J., & Davidson, R. J. (1994). How and why do the two cerebral hemispheres interact? *Psychological Bulletin, 116,* 195–219.

Hoptman, M. J., Davidson, R. J., Gudmundsson, A., Schreiber, R. T., & Ershler, W. B. (1996). Age differences in visual evoked potential estimates of interhemispheric transfer. *Neuropsychology, 10,* 263–271.

Horwitz, B., Deiber, M., Ibanez, V., Sadato, N., & Hallett, M. (2000). Correlations between reaction time and cerebral blood flow during motor preparation. *Neuroimage, 12,* 434–441.

Hoshiyama, M., Kakigi, R., Berg, P., Koyama, S., Kitamura, Y., Shimojo, M., Watanabe, S., & Nakamura, A. (1997). Identification of motor and sensory brain activities during uni-lateral finger movement: Spatiotemporal source analysis of movement-associated magnetic fields. *Experimental Brain Research, 115,* 6–14.

Houk, J. C., & Wise, S. P. (1995). Distributed modular architectures linking basal ganglia, cerebellum, and cerebral cortex: Their role in planning and controlling action. *Cerebral Cortex, 5,* 95–110.

Hughes, H. C., Reuter-Lorenz, P. A., Nozawa, G., & Fendrich, R. (1994). Visual-auditory interactions in sensorimotor processing: Saccades versus manual responses. *Journal of Experimental Psychology: Human Perception and Performance, 20,* 131–153.

Iacoboni, M., Rayman, J., & Zaidel, E. (1997). Does the previous trial affect lateralized lexical decision? *Neuropsychologia, 35,* 81–88.

Iacoboni, M., & Zaidel, E. (1995). Channels of the corpus callosum: Evidence from simple reaction times to lateralized flashes in the normal and split brain. *Brain, 118,* 779–788.

Iacoboni, M., & Zaidel, E. (1998). Context effects in simple reaction times to lateralized flashes. *Society for Neuroscience Abstracts, 25* (Part 2), 1263.

Iacoboni, M., & Zaidel, E. (2000). Crossed-uncrossed difference in simple reaction times to lateralized flashes: Between- and within-subjects variability. *Neuropsychologia, 38,* 535–541.

Ikeda, A., Luders, H. O., Shibasaki, H., Collura, T. F., Burgess, R. C., Morris, H. H. III, & Hamano, T. (1995). Movement-related potentials associated with bilateral simultaneous and unilateral movements recorded from human supplementary motor area. *Electroencephalography and Clinical Neurophysiology, 95*, 323–334.

Ilmoniemi, R. J., Virtanen, J., Ruohonen, J., Karhu, J., Aronen, H. J., Naatanen, R., & Katila, T. (1997). Neuronal responses to magnetic stimulation reveal cortical reactivity and connectivity. *NeuroReport, 10*, 3537–3540.

Innocenti, G. M. (1986). General organization of callosal connections in the cerebral cortex. In E. G. Jones & A. Peters (Eds.), *Cerebral cortex. Vol. 5: Sensory-motor areas and aspects of cortical connectivity* (pp. 291–354). New York: Plenum Press.

Ioannides, A. A., Taylor, J. G., Liu, L. C., Gross, J., & Muller-Gartner, H. W. (1998). The influence of stimulus properties, complexity, and contingency on the stability and variability of ongoing and evoked activity in human auditory cortex. *Neuroimage, 8*, 149–162.

Ipata, A., Girelli, M., Miniussi, C., & Marzi, C. A. (1997). Interhemispheric transfer of visual information in humans: The role of different callosal channels. *Archives Italiennes de Biologie, 135*, 169–182.

Ito, S. I. (1982). Prefrontal unit activity of macaque monkeys during auditory and visual reaction time tasks. *Brain Research, 247*, 39–47.

Jeeves, M. A. (1969). A comparison of interhemispheric transmission times in acallosals and normals. *Psychonomic Science, 16*, 245–246.

Jenkins, I. H., Jahanshahi, M., Jueptner, M., Passingham, R. E., & Brooks, D. J. (2000). Self-initiated versus externally triggered movements. II. The effect of movement predictability on regional cerebral blood flow. *Brain, 123*, 1216–1228.

Kaiser, J., Lutzenberger, W., Preissl, H., Mosshammer, D., & Birbaumer, N. (2000). Statistical probability mapping reveals high-frequency magnetoencephalographic activity in supplementary motor area during self-paced finger movements. *Neuroscience Letters, 283*, 81–84.

Kaluzny, P., Palmeri, A., & Wiesendanger, M. (1994). The problem of bimanual coupling: A reaction time study of simple unimanual and bimanual finger responses. *Electroencephalography and Clinical Neurophysiology, 93*, 450–458.

Kawamichi, H., Kikuchi, Y., Endo, H., Takeda, T., & Yoshizawa, S. (1998). Temporal structure of implicit motor imagery in visual hand-shape discrimination as revealed by MEG. *NeuroReport, 9*, 1127–1132.

Kennedy, D. N., Lange, N., Makris, N., Bates, J., Meyer, J., & Caviness, V. S., Jr. (1998). Gyri of the human neocortex: An MRI-based analysis of volume and variance. *Cerebral Cortex, 8*, 372–384.

Kennedy, H., Meissirel, C., & Dehay, C. (1991). Callosal pathways and their compliancy to general rules governing the organization of corticocortical connectivity. In B. Reher & S. R. Robinson (Eds.), *Neuroanatomy of the visual pathways and their development* (pp. 324–359). Boca Raton, FL: CRC Press. (Vol. 3 of J. R. Cronly-Dillon [Ed.], *Vision and visual dysfunction*.)

Kim, S. G., Ashe, J., Georgopoulos, A. P., Merkle, H., Ellermann, J. M., Menon, R. S., Ogawa, S., & Ugurbil, K. (1993). Functional imaging of human motor cortex at high magnetic field. *Journal of Neurophysiology, 69,* 297–302.

Kim, S. G., Ashe, J., Hendrich, K., Ellermann, J. M., Merkle, H., Ugurbil, K., & Georgopoulos, A. P. (1993). Functional magnetic resonance imaging of motor cortex: Hemispheric asymmetry and handedness. *Science, 261,* 615–617.

Kinsbourne, M. (1974). Lateral interactions in the brain. In M. Kinsbourne & W. L. Smith (Eds.), *Hemispheric disconnection and cerebral function* (pp. 239–259). Springfield, IL: Charles C. Thomas.

Kinsbourne, M. (2002). The corpus callosum equilibrates the cerebral hemispheres. In E. Zaidel & M. Iacoboni (Eds.), *The parallel brain: The cognitive neuroscience of the corpus callosum.* Cambridge, MA: MIT Press.

Komssi, S., Aronen, H. J., Kesäniemi, M., Soinne, L., Nikouline, V. V., Ollikainen, M., Roine, R. O., Huttunen, J., Savolainen, S., & Ilmoniemi, R. J. (2000). Transcallosal connectivity revealed by transcranial magnetic stimulation and high-resolution EEG. *Neuroimage, 11,* S766. (Abstract.)

Kurata, K. (1991). Corticocortical inputs to the dorsal and ventral aspects of the premotor cortex of macaque monkeys. *Neuroscience Research, 12,* 263–280.

LaMantia, A. S., & Rakic, P. (1990). Cytological and quantitative characteristics of four cerebral commissures in the rhesus monkey. *Journal of Comparative Neurology, 291,* 520–537.

Lassonde, M., Sauerwein, H. C., & Lepore, F. (2002). Agenesis of the corpus callosum. In E. Zaidel & M. Iacoboni (Eds.), *The parallel brain: The cognitive neuroscience of the corpus callosum.* Cambridge, MA: MIT Press.

Lassonde, M., Sauerwein, H., McCabe, N., Laurencelle, L., & Geoffroy, G. (1988). Extent and limits of cerebral adjustment to early section or congenital absence of the corpus callosum. *Behavioral Brain Research, 30,* 165–181.

Ledlow, A., Swanson, J. M., & Kinsbourne, M. (1978). Differences in reaction time and average evoked potentials as a function of direct and indirect neural pathways. *Annals of Neurology, 3,* 525–530.

Lee, K. M., Chang, K. H., & Roh, J. K. (1999). Subregions within the supplementary motor area activated at different stages of movement preparation and execution. *Neuroimage, 9,* 117–123.

Liepert, J., Hamzei, F., & Weiller, C. (2000). Motor cortex disinhibition of the unaffected hemisphere after acute stroke. *Muscle and Nerve, 23,* 1761–1763.

Lines, C. R., Rugg, M. D., & Milner, A. D. (1984). The effect of stimulus intensity on visual evoked potential estimates of interhemispheric transmission time. *Experimental Brain Research, 57,* 89–98.

Luce, R. D. (1986). *Response times.* Oxford Psychology Series, no. 8. New York: Oxford University Press.

Luppino, G., Matelli, M., Camarda, R., & Rizzolatti, G. (1993). Corticocortical connections of area F3 (SMA-proper) and area F6 (pre-SMA) in the macaque monkey. *Journal of Comparative Neurology, 338,* 114–140.

Marsden, J. F., Werhahn, K. J., Ashby, P., Rothwell, J., Noachtar, S., & Brown, P. (2000). Organization of cortical activities related to movement in humans. *Journal of Neuroscience, 20,* 2307–2314.

Marzi, C. A. (1999). The Poffenberger paradigm: A first, simple, behavioural tool to study interhemispheric transmission in humans. *Brain Research Bulletin, 50,* 421–422.

Marzi, C. A., Bisiacchi, P., & Nicoletti, R. (1991). Is interhemispheric transfer of visuomotor information asymmetric? Evidence from a meta-analysis. *Neuropsychologia, 29,* 1163–1177.

Marzi, C. A., Miniussi, C., Maravita, A., Bertolasi, L., Zanette, G., Rothwell, J. C., & Sanes, J. N. (1998). Transcranial magnetic stimulation selectively impairs interhemispheric transfer of visuo-motor information in humans. *Experimental Brain Research, 118,* 435–438.

Marzi, C. A., Perani, D., Tassinari, G., Colleluori, A., Maravita, A., Miniussi, C., Paulesu, E., Scifo, P., & Fazio, F. (1999). Pathways of interhemispheric transfer in normals and in a split-brain subject: A positron emission tomography study. *Experimental Brain Research, 126,* 451–458.

Mattay, V. S., Callicott, J. H., Bertolino, A., Santha, A. K., Van Horn, J. D., Tallent, K. A., Frank, J. A., & Weinberger, D. R. (1998). Hemispheric control of motor function: A whole brain echo planar fMRI study. *Psychiatry Research, 83,* 7–22.

McClelland, J. L. (1979). On the time relations of mental processes: An examination of systems of processes in cascade. *Psychological Review, 80,* 287–330.

Meyer, B. U., Roricht, S., Grafin von Einsiedel, H., Kruggel, F., & Weindl, A. (1995). Inhibitory and excitatory interhemispheric transfers between motor cortical areas in normal humans and patients with abnormalities of the corpus callosum. *Brain, 118,* 429–440.

Meyer, B. U., Roricht, S., & Niehaus, L. (1998). Morphology of acallosal brains as assessed by MRI in six patients leading a normal daily life. *Journal of Neurology, 245,* 106–110.

Meyer, B. U., & Voss, M. (2000). Delay of the execution of rapid finger movement by magnetic stimulation of the ipsilateral hand-associated motor cortex. *Experimental Brain Research, 134,* 477–482.

Meyer, D. E., Osman, A. M., Irwin, D. E., & Yantis, S. (1988). Modern mental chronometry. *Biological Psychology, 26,* 3–67.

Miller, J. (1988). A warning about median reaction time. *Journal of Experimental Psychology: Human Perception and Performance, 14,* 539–543.

Miller, J., Riehle, A., & Requin, J. (1992). Effects of preliminary perceptual output on neuronal activity of the primary motor cortex. *Journal of Experimental Psychology: Human Perception and Performance, 18,* 1121–1138.

Milner, A. D. (1986). Chronometric analysis in neuropsychology. *Neuropsychologia, 24,* 115–128.

Milner, A. D., Jeeves, M. A., Silver, P. H., Lines, C. R., & Wilson, J. (1985). Reaction times to lateralized visual stimuli in callosal agenesis: Stimulus and response factors. *Neuropsychologia, 23,* 323–331.

Milner, A. D., & Lines, C. R. (1982). Interhemispheric pathways in simple reaction times to lateralized light flashes. *Neuropsychologia, 20,* 171–179.

Mink, J. W. (1996). The basal ganglia: Focused selection and inhibition of competing motor programs. *Progress in Neurobiology, 50,* 381–425.

Mink, J. W., & Thach, W. T. (1991). Basal ganglia motor control. III. Pallidal ablation: Normal reaction time, muscle cocontraction, and slow movement. *Journal of Neurophysiology, 65,* 330–351.

Montgomery, E. B., Jr., & Buchholz, S. R. (1991). The striatum and motor cortex in motor initiation and execution. *Brain Research, 549,* 222–229.

Oertel, D. (1983). Synaptic responses and electrical properties of cells in brain slices of the mouse anteroventral cochlear nucleus. *Journal of Neuroscience, 3,* 2043–2053.

Oliveri, M., Caltagirone, C., Filippi, M. M., Traversa, R., Cicinelli, P., Pasqualetti, P., & Rossini, P. M. (2000). Paired transcranial magnetic stimulation protocols reveal a pattern of inhibition and facilitation in the human parietal cortex. *Journal of Physiology, 529,* 461–468.

Oliveri, M., Rossini, P. M., Traversa, R., Cicinelli, P., Filippi, M. M., Pasqualetti, P., Tomaiuolo, F., & Caltagirone, C. (1999). Left frontal transcranial magnetic stimulation reduces contralesional extinction in patients with unilateral right brain damage. *Brain, 122,* 1731–1739.

Pandya, D. N., & Rosene, D. L. (1985). Some observations on trajectories and topography of commissural fibers. In A. G. Reeves (Ed.), *Epilepsy and the corpus callosum* (pp. 21–40). New York: Plenum Press.

Pandya, D. N., & Seltzer, B. (1986). The topography of commissural fibers. In F. Lepore, M. Ptito, & H. H. Jasper (Eds.), *Two hemispheres—one brain: Functions of the corpus callosum* (pp. 47–73). New York: Alan R. Liss.

Pascual-Leone, A., Valls-Sole, J., Wassermann, E. M., Brasil-Neto, J., Cohen, L. G., & Hallett, M. (1992). Effects of focal transcranial magnetic stimulation on simple reaction time to acoustic, visual and somatosensory stimuli. *Brain, 115,* 1045–1059.

Perrin, F., Bertrand, O., & Pernier, J. (1987). Scalp current density mapping: Value and estimation from potential data. *IEEE Transactions on Biomedical Engineering, 34,* 283–288.

Perrin, F., Pernier, J., Bertrand, O., & Echallier, J. F. (1989). Spherical splines for scalp potential and current density mapping. *Electroencephalography and Clinical Neurophysiology, 72,* 184–187.

Petrides, M., & Pandya, D. N. (1999). Dorsolateral prefrontal cortex: Comparative cytoarchitectonic analysis in the human and the macaque brain and corticocortical connection patterns. *European Journal of Neuroscience, 11,* 1011–1036.

Poffenberger, A. T. (1912). Reaction time to retinal stimulation with special reference to the time lost in conduction through nerve centers. *Archives of Psychology*, *23*, 1–73.

Praamstra, P., Stegeman, D. F., Horstink, M. W., & Cools, A. R. (1996). Dipole source analysis suggests selective modulation of the supplementary motor area contribution to the readiness potential. *Electroencephalography and Clinical Neurophysiology*, *90*, 468–477.

Ratinckx, E., Brysbaert, M., & Vermeulen, E. (2001). CRT screens may give rise to biased estimates of interhemispheric transmission time in the Poffenberger paradigm. *Experimental Brain Research*, *136*, 413–416.

Regan, D. (1989). *Human brain electrophysiology: Evoked potentials and evoked magnetic fields in science and medicine*. New York: Elsevier Science Publishing.

Riehle, A. (1991). Visually induced signal-locked neuronal activity changes in precentral motor areas of the monkey: Hierarchical progression of signal processing. *Brain Research*, *540*, 131–137.

Riehle, A., & Requin, J. (1989). Monkey primary motor and premotor cortex: Single-cell activity related to prior information about direction and extent of an intended movement. *Journal of Neurophysiology*, *61*, 534–549.

Ringo, J. L., Doty, R. W., Demeter, S., & Simard, P. Y. (1994). Time is of the essence: A conjecture that hemispheric specialization arises from interhemispheric conduction delay. *Cerebral Cortex*, *4*, 331–343.

Rizzolatti, G., Luppino, G., & Matelli, M. (1998). The organization of the cortical motor system: New concepts. *Electroencephalography and Clinical Neurophysiology*, *106*, 283–296.

Rouiller, E. M., Babalian, A., Kazennikov, O., Moret, V., Yu, X. H., & Wiesendanger, M. (1994). Transcallosal connections of the distal forelimb representations of the primary and supplementary motor cortical areas in macaque monkeys. *Experimental Brain Research*, *102*, 227–243.

Rouiller, E. M., Moret, V., Tanne, J., & Boussaoud, D. (1996). Evidence for direct connections between the hand region of the supplementary motor area and cervical motoneurons in the macaque monkey. *European Journal of Neuroscience*, *8*, 1055–1059.

Rugg, M. D., Lines, C. R., & Milner, A. D. (1984). Visual evoked potentials to lateralized visual stimuli and the measurement of interhemispheric transfer time. *Neuropsychologia*, *22*, 215–225.

Rugg, M. D., Lines, C. R., & Milner, A. D. (1985). Further investigation of visual evoked potentials elicited by lateralized stimuli: Effects of stimulus eccentricity and reference site. *Electroencephalography and Clinical Neurophysiology*, *62*, 81–87.

Sabatini, B. L., & Regehr, W. G. (1996). Timing of neurotransmission at fast synapses in the mammalian brain. *Nature*, *384*, 170–172.

Salenius, S., Portin, K., Kajola, M., Salmelin, R., & Hari, R. (1997). Cortical control of human motoneuron firing during isometric contraction. *Journal of Neurophysiology*, *77*, 3401–3405.

Salmelin, R., Forss, N., Knuutila, J., & Hari, R. (1995). Bilateral activation of the human somatomotor cortex by distal hand movements. *Electroencephalography and Clinical Neurophysiology, 95*, 444–452.

Saron, C. D. (1999). Spatiotemporal electrophysiology of intra- and interhemispheric visuomotor integration: Relations with behavior. Ph.D. dissertation, Albert Einstein College of Medicine, New York.

Saron, C. D., & Davidson, R. J. (1989). Visual evoked potential measures of interhemispheric transfer time in humans. *Behavioral Neuroscience, 103*, 1115–1138.

Saron, C. D., Foxe, J. J., Simpson, G. V., & Vaughan, H. G., Jr. (2002). Interhemispheric visuomotor activation: Spatiotemporal electrophysiology related to reaction time. In E. Zaidel & M. Iacoboni (Eds.), *The parallel brain: The cognitive neuroscience of the corpus callosum.* Cambridge, MA: MIT Press.

Saron, C. D., Lassonde, M., Vaughan, H. G., Jr., Foxe, J. J., Alfhors, S. P., & Simpson, G. V. (1997). Interhemispheric visuomotor interaction in callosal agenesis: Spatiotemporal patterns of cortical activation. *Society for Neuroscience Abstracts, 23* (Part 2), 1949.

Saron, C. D., Schroeder, C. E., Foxe, J. J., & Vaughan, H. G., Jr. (2001). Visual activation of frontal cortex: Segregation from occipital activity. *Cognitive Brain Research, 12*, 75–88.

Schall, J. D. (1991). Neuronal activity related to visually guided saccadic eye movements in the supplementary motor area of rhesus monkeys. *Journal of Neurophysiology, 66*, 530–558.

Schall, J. D. (1997). Visuomotor areas of the frontal lobe. In K. S. Rockland, J. H. Kaas, & A. Peters (Eds.), *Cerebral cortex.* Vol. 12: *Extrastriate cortex in primates* (pp. 527–638). New York: Plenum Press.

Schall, J. D., Hanes, D. P., Thompson, K. G., & King, D. J. (1995). Saccade target selection in frontal eye field of macaque. I. Visual and premovement activation. *Journal of Neuroscience, 15*, 6905–6918.

Schall, J. D., & Thompson, K. G. (1999). Neural selection and control of visually guided eye movements. *Annual Review of Neuroscience, 22*, 241–259.

Schnitzler, A., Kessler, K. R., & Benecke, R. (1996). Transcallosally mediated inhibition of interneurons within human primary motor cortex. *Experimental Brain Research, 112*, 381–391.

Sergent, J., & Myers, J. J. (1985). Manual, blowing, and verbal simple reactions to lateralized flashes of light in commissurotomized patients. *Perception and Psychophysics, 37*, 571–578.

St. John, R., Shields, C., Krahn, P., & Timney, B. (1987). The reliability of estimates of interhemispheric transmission times derived from unimanual and verbal response latencies. *Human Neurobiology, 6*, 195–202.

Stančák, A., Jr., Lucking, C. H., & Kristeva-Feige, R. (2000). Lateralization of movement-related potentials and the size of corpus callosum. *NeuroReport, 11*, 329–332.

Stančák, A., Jr., & Pfurtscheller, G. (1996). Event-related desynchronisation of central beta-rhythms during brisk and slow self-paced finger movements of dominant and non-dominant hand. *Cognitive Brain Research, 4*, 171–183.

Stensaas, S. S., Eddington, D. K., & Dobelle, W. H. (1974). The topography and variability of the primary visual cortex in man. *Journal of Neurosurgery, 40*, 747–755.

Swanson, J., Ledlow, A., & Kinsbourne, M. (1978). Lateral asymmetries revealed by simple reaction time. In M. Kinsbourne (Ed.), *Asymmetrical function of the brain* (pp. 274–291). Cambridge: Cambridge University Press.

Tandon, N., Fox, P., Narayana, S., Iyer, M., & Lancaster, J. (2000). Evidence for the existence of direct corticospinal projections from the human supplementary motor area. *Society for Neuroscience Abstracts, 27* (part 2), 1580. (Abstract.)

Tang, A. C., Phung, D. B., & Pearlmutter, B. A. (2000). Direct measurement of interhemispherical transfer time for natural somatosensory stimulation during voluntary movement using meg and blind source separation. *Society for Neuroscience Abstracts, 26* (part 2), 1461. (Abstract.)

Tanji, J. (1994). The supplementary motor area in the cerebral cortex. *Neuroscience Research, 19*, 251–268.

Tanji, J., Okano, K., & Sato, K. C. (1988). Neuronal activity in cortical motor areas related to ipsilateral, contralateral, and bilateral digit movements of the monkey. *Journal of Neurophysiology, 60*, 325–343.

Tassinari, G., Aglioti, S., Pallini, R., Berlucchi, G., & Rossi, G. F. (1994). Interhemispheric integration of simple visuomotor responses in patients with partial callosal defects. *Behavioural Brain Research, 64*, 141–149.

Terao, Y., Ugawa, Y., Suzuki, M., Sakai, K., Hanajima, R., Gemba-Shimizu, K., & Kanazawa, I. (1997). Shortening of simple reaction time by peripheral electrical and submotor-threshold magnetic cortical stimulation. *Experimental Brain Research, 115*, 541–545.

Thompson, K. G., Hanes, D. P., Bichot, N. P., & Schall, J. D. (1996). Perceptual and motor processing stages identified in the activity of macaque frontal eye field neurons during visual search. *Journal of Neurophysiology, 76*, 4040–4055.

Thompson, P. M., Schwartz, C., Lin, R. T., Khan, A. A., & Toga, A. W. (1996). Three-dimensional statistical analysis of sulcal variability in the human brain. *Journal of Neuroscience, 16*, 4261–4274.

Thut, G., Hauert, C. A., Blanke, O., Morand, S., Seeck, M., Gonzalez, S. L., Grave de Peralta, R., Spinelli, L., Khateb, A., Landis, T., & Michel, C. M. (2000). Visually induced activity in human frontal motor areas during simple visuomotor performance. *NeuroReport, 11*, 2843–2848.

Thut, G., Hauert, C. A., Morand, S., Seeck, M., Landis, T., & Michel, C. (1999). Evidence for interhemispheric motor-level transfer in a simple reaction time task: An EEG study. *Experimental Brain Research, 128*, 256–261.

Tokuno, H., & Tanji, J. (1993). Input organization of distal and proximal forelimb areas in the monkey primary motor cortex: A retrograde double labeling study. *Journal of Comparative Neurology, 333*, 199–209.

Toni, I., Schluter, N. D., Josephs, O., Friston, K., & Passingham, R. E. (1999). Signal-, set- and movement-related activity in the human brain: An event-related fMRI study. *Cerebral Cortex, 9,* 35–49.

Tootell, R. B., Mendola, J. D., Hadjikhani, N. K., Liu, A. K., & Dale, A. M. (1998). The representation of the ipsilateral visual field in human cerebral cortex. *Proceedings of the National Academy of Sciences, USA, 95,* 818–824.

Tramo, M. J., Baynes, K., Fendrich, R., Mangun, G. R., Phelps, E. A., Reuter-Lorenz, P. A., & Gazzaniga, M. S. (1995). Hemispheric specialization and interhemispheric integration: Insights from experiments with commissurotomy patients. In A. G. Reeves & D. W. Roberts (Eds.), *Epilepsy and the corpus callosum.* Vol. 2 (pp. 263–295). New York: Plenum Press.

Urbano, A., Babiloni, C., Onorati, P., & Babiloni, F. (1996). Human cortical activity related to unilateral movements: A high resolution EEG study. *NeuroReport, 8,* 203–206.

Urbano, A., Babiloni, C., Onorati, P., & Babiloni, F. (1998). Dynamic functional coupling of high resolution EEG potentials related to unilateral internally triggered one-digit movements. *Electroencephalography and Clinical Neurophysiology, 106,* 477–487.

Urbano, A., Babiloni, C., Onorati, P., Carducci, F., Ambrosini, A., Fattorini, L., & Babiloni, F. (1998). Responses of human primary sensorimotor and supplementary motor areas to internally triggered unilateral and simultaneous bilateral one-digit movements: A high-resolution EEG study. *European Journal of Neuroscience, 10,* 765–767.

Uusitalo, M. A., Williamson, S. J., & Seppa, M. T. (1996). Dynamical organisation of the human visual system revealed by lifetimes of activation traces. *Neuroscience Letters, 213,* 149–152.

Vaughan, H. G., Jr. (1987). Topographic analysis of brain electrical activity. *Electroencephalography and Clinical Neurophysiology Supplement, 39,* 137–142.

Waxman, S. G., & Bennett, M. V. L. (1972). Relative conduction velocities of small myelinated and non-myelinated fibres in the central nervous system. *Nature, New Biology, 238,* 217–219.

Wiesendanger, M., Rouiller, E. M., Kazennikov, O., & Perrig, S. (1996). Is the supplementary motor area a bilaterally organized system? *Advances in Neurology, 70,* 85–93.

Wise, S. P. (1996). Corticospinal efferents of the supplementary sensorimotor area in relation to the primary motor area. *Advances in Neurology, 70,* 57–69.

Wise, S. P., Boussaoud, D., Johnson, P. B., & Caminiti, R. (1997). Premotor and parietal cortex: Corticocortical connectivity and combinatorial computations. *Annual Review of Neuroscience, 20,* 25–42.

Wise, S. P., Murray, E. A., & Gerfen, C. R. (1996). The frontal cortex-basal ganglia system in primates. *Critical Reviews in Neurobiology, 10,* 317–356.

Zhang, J., Riehle, A., Requin, J., & Kornblum, S. (1997). Dynamics of single neuron activity in monkey primary motor cortex related to sensorimotor transformation. *Journal of Neuroscience, 17,* 2227–2246.

Ziemann, U., Tergau, F., Netz, J., & Homberg, V. (1997). Delay in simple reaction time after focal transcranial magnetic stimulation of the human brain occurs at the final motor output stage. *Brain Research, 744,* 32–40.

IV Auditory Laterality

11 Hemispheric Asymmetries in the Processing of Tonal Stimuli

Robert J. Zatorre

How can we characterize the functional differences between the two cerebral hemispheres? This question has occupied a central place in human cognitive neuroscience since well before the field even had that name. In the auditory domain, this issue has been largely dealt with from the perspective of the processing of speech signals. Given the ecological value of vocal communication to human behavior, this focus is not surprising. In fact, some of the earliest observations of human cerebral asymmetry stem from disturbances of speech perception and production. Nevertheless, such a relatively narrow approach may lead to a more restricted understanding than could be achieved by comparing speech-related hemispheric asymmetries to those of other domains of auditory information processing. In this spirit, the study of musical tonal processing may offer a more comprehensive view of the division of hemispheric labor; it is in this context that the present chapter will review the findings of recent studies, with the aim of integrating information to achieve a better synthesis.

Music is increasingly recognized in the scientific community as an important component of human activity that may help us to gain insight into the functional organization of the human brain (Zatorre & Peretz, 2001). It may be argued that the perception, encoding, and reproduction of musical sounds requires at least as complex neural mechanisms as those for speech; indeed, it seems likely that speech and music must engage the most cognitively demanding aspects of auditory processing. It may further be argued that these two classes of stimuli are uniquely human (but see Gray et al., 2001 for another view), making it particularly relevant to study them in the context of understanding those aspects of brain organization which are most relevant to human cognition and behavior.

Music is a very complex phenomenon, however, with many possible levels of analysis. To address something like music in a scientifically rigorous fashion, it is necessary, at least to start, to focus on one particular aspect. Tonal pitch would seem like a good choice, inasmuch as it appears to be a central aspect of all music. Although other aspects of music, such as temporal organization for rhythm, may play an equally important role, it is difficult to conceive of a musical system of any type that does not involve some kind of patterning of tonal elements. Moreover, pitch processing is amenable to study not only because the physical parameters of sounds associated with pitch are relatively well-understood and easily manipulated, but also because it affords the opportunity to analyze different levels of processing.

In this chapter, therefore, I will concentrate on studies from my laboratory and from others that have examined hemispheric asymmetries in pitch processing. I will first discuss relatively low-level aspects of pitch processing, such as pitch discrimination; second, higher-order aspects, including pitch patterns and melodies will be reviewed. The research to be discussed includes both behavioral-lesion studies and functional neuroimaging findings. Finally, we will consider some anatomical findings that may help us to understand the functional asymmetries.

PROCESSING OF LOW-LEVEL PITCH INFORMATION

In this context, the idea of low-level information processing merely refers to the cognitive requirements associated with pitch processing in the absence of relational information (such as would be present in pitch patterns) or heavy working memory demands, and does not necessarily imply low-level neural processes. The question to be addressed most directly in what follows is simply whether hemispheric differences exist at the level of cortical contributions to simple pitch processing.

One of the salient features of the auditory nervous system is that a tonotopic organization exists from the periphery up to various auditory cortical fields. The important role of stimulus frequency in tonotopically organized cortex would suggest that the cortex plays an important role in the processing of frequency, and hence of pitch. However, the relation between pitch and frequency is not a simple one, since pitch is a perceptual entity that is affected by many different stimulus parameters. Thus, the effects of lesions of auditory cortex on pitch depend on the nature of the task and stimuli used.

In many animal studies, for example, it has been shown that even after complete destruction of primary auditory cortex (A1) and surrounding areas bilaterally, only transient difficulties in simple frequency discrimination tasks are seen (Evarts, 1952; Heffner & Masterton, 1978; Jerison & Neff, 1953). Similar results have been demonstrated in human patients with unilateral temporal-lobe lesions of auditory areas who have been tested with simple discrimination tasks (Milner, 1962; Zatorre, 1988). The conclusion to be drawn from these studies is not that auditory cortex plays no role in pitch perception, but rather that these simple discrimination tasks do not require the processes carried out by cortical structures.

More complex pitch processing does recruit cortical mechanisms. Consider, for example, the phenomenon of residue pitch, or missing fundamental pitch, which arises when a complex tone is presented with little or no energy at the fundamental frequency (Schouten, 1938). Under certain conditions, it is possible to hear the pitch corresponding to the fundamental even in its absence, as a consequence of the frequencies of the remaining harmonics that are multiples of the fundamental. This percept, which requires integration of information coming from several harmonics to abstract the missing element, is affected by bilateral ablation of A1 in cats (Whitfield, 1980).

This finding thus raises the question of whether a similar effect can be observed in humans and, more relevant for the present discussion, whether there is any evidence of lateralization of function at this level of cortical processing. The answer to both questions appears to be positive, based on a study by Zatorre (1988), in which patients with unilateral temporal-lobe resection were studied. The patients were subdivided according to whether or not the excision encroached upon Heschl's gyrus (figure 11.1), the medial portion of which contains the human primary auditory cortex (Liégeois-Chauvel et al., 1991; Rademacher et al., 1993). A simple discrimination task was administered in which a pair of different complex tones was presented, and the subject indicated if the first was higher in pitch than the second, or vice versa. Stimuli consisted either of control tones with energy at the fundamental frequency, or missing-fundamental tones, with harmonics spanning the same spectral range within a pair, but having different implied fundamental. The evidence indicated that in certain of the more difficult missing-fundamental conditions, only those patients with excisions invading Heschl's gyrus (HG) on the right side were significantly im-

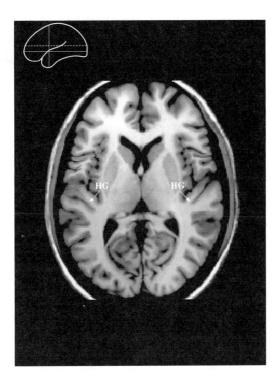

Figure 11.1 Magnetic resonance image of a normal human brain showing a horizontal section through the region of Heschl's gyrus, marked HG. The orientation and level of the horizontal section are indicated by the dashed line in the inset.

paired, while patients with more restricted right anterior temporal lobe damage, or those with left temporal lobe removals, performed as well as control subjects. Moreover, with the control stimuli that contained energy at the fundamental, all subjects performed well, indicating no generalized pitch processing deficit or inability to understand the task. These findings therefore implicate specific subfields within the right auditory cortical system in some type of pattern analysis that is required in order to abstract missing fundamental pitch. This process may involve analysis of the spectral information resolved at more peripheral levels.

Further evidence for an asymmetric contribution of right auditory cortices to spectral processes comes from a number of other lesion studies that have examined a variety of aspects of spectral processing, including timbre. Many of these studies have demonstrated that damage to the right temporal neocortex often leads to greater disturbance than equivalent damage to the left side when stimuli differ in terms of the distribution of energy across the spectrum, or in number of harmonics (Milner, 1962; Samson & Zatorre, 1988, 1994). Similarly, Sidtis and Volpe (1988) tested patients with right or left hemisphere strokes on a binaural and a dichotic complex pitch task using a match to sample technique. Although the site of the lesion was not well specified, they found a significant disturbance for the dichotic task, which requires segregation of one tone from the other, among the patients with right-sided damage, whereas the binaural task was performed well by both groups. Additional evidence in the same direction was presented by Robin et al. (1990), who showed a double dissociation such that damage to association cortices in the right hemisphere resulted in spectral but not temporal processing deficits, while the converse was observed after left hemisphere damage. Contrary to the conclusion drawn above, that simple pitch discrimination is unaffected by cortical damage, these authors did report that right hemisphere-damaged patients were severely impaired in a pitch discrimination task. However, these data are most likely not contradictory with other findings. The task used by Robin et al. was a match to sample, in which a target tone was first presented, followed by two additional tones, one of which matched the target. The working memory load and/or the relational nature of the task may have been sufficient to require a contribution from the right temporal cortex.

A striking example of how a seemingly subtle aspect of a task may strongly influence the degree to which the cortex may be necessary is provided by Johnsrude et al. (2000). They tested patients similar to those described above, in whom a unilateral temporal lobe resection was carried out with or without encroachment onto Heschl's gyri. An MRI-based anatomical method was used to document and quantify the extent of removal (see Penhune et al., 1999 for further details). An adaptive psychophysical discrimination procedure was used; pairs of pure tones were presented on each trial to determine the threshold, or minimal frequency separation, needed to achieve a certain level of performance. Two separate tasks were administered. In the first, the two tones either were identical or differed in pitch. In the second task, the two tones were always different in pitch, and the subject's task was to indicate if the second tone was higher *or* lower than the first. The tones themselves were identical in the two tasks. The idea here is that whereas

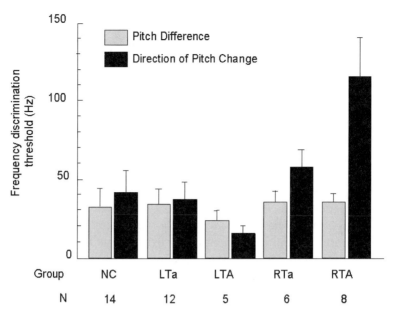

Figure 11.2 Mean frequency difference discrimination thresholds observed in two pitch discrimination tasks in patients with right or left (RT or LT) temporal lobe excision, extending into the region of Heschl's gyrus (A) or sparing this area (a). The simple discrimination thresholds were not different across the groups. Thresholds in the direction-of-pitch-change task were significantly higher in the RTA group than in any of the other groups. See text for additional details. (Figure adapted from Johnsrude et al., 2000.)

the simple pitch discrimination task merely requires that a difference be noted, the second, pitch-direction task requires that the tones be discriminated and ordered along some underlying pitch scale.

The findings indicated several interesting dissociations (figure 11.2). The group of subjects with right Heschl's gyrus damage, showed a fourfold increase in their pitch thresholds, but only for the pitch-direction task; they were normal on the simple pitch discrimination task. In contrast, the patients with damage in the right anterior temporal lobe but sparing Heschl's gyrus, or those with left temporal lobe resection, showed normal thresholds as compared to control participants on both tasks. The findings are thus quite specific in indicating that only a certain restricted lesion on the right side has an effect, and then only on a particular task. Thus, one may conclude that the right primary auditory area plays a special role not simply in discriminating one pitch from another, but also in some aspect of organizing the sounds according to their pitch. This aspect of pitch organization would be essential for any musical use of pitch information. An additional detail worthy of note is that all but one of the patients with right Heschl's gyrus damage were actually able to perform the task itself; it was only the threshold that was abnormally high. This aspect of the result suggests that a much coarser level of pitch organization still exists in these patients which may be mediated by left auditory cortex, a point to be taken up below. Note that this latter finding explains why patients with similar lesions were able to perform well in the control test series of Zatorre (1988), since the pitch differences used in that study were all much greater than the near-threshold differences used by Johnsrude et al. (2000).

The findings of Johnsrude et al. (2000) are also, broadly speaking, in agreement with conclusions drawn from the animal literature, at least as far as the nature of the cortical contribution is concerned. These studies have concluded that a cortical contribution to the processing of pitch is required when the task cannot be accomplished on the basis of a simple change detection. For example, lesions of at least some portions of auditory cortex impair the ability to respond to the cessation of a pitch from a set (e.g., detecting that ABAB has changed to AAAA), whereas the reverse order is not affected by such lesions (Diamond et al., 1962). The important factor here is that it is easier to detect a change when a new element is added than when some of the same stimulation remains in both cases. Similarly, cortical lesions impair cats' ability to discriminate simple pitch patterns (e.g., ABA from BAB), whereas there is no difficulty in discriminating AA from AB (Whitfield, 1985). The one clear difference between the human and animal studies, of course, is the lateralization of function so evident in the human studies (but see also Wetzel et al., 1998 for evidence of a remarkably similar asymmetry for processing of frequency modulation in the Mongolian gerbil).

Functional imaging studies have also been employed to examine various aspects of tonal processing. These techniques provide critical complementary evidence for the data derived from more traditional behavioral studies because they are a noninvasive means to obtain anatomically accurate information about how and where neural activity changes as a function of stimulus or task parameters. However, whereas activation studies can identify the sites of neural activity associated with a particular function, they cannot determine the degree to which essential computations are carried out. Conversely, only lesion techniques or stimulation techniques (such as transcranial magnetic stimulation), can provide information about essential areas, but they are constrained by various other limitations (Steinmetz & Seitz, 1991). The optimal situation, clearly, is to obtain converging evidence from a variety of methods whenever possible.

One recent study used positron emission tomography (PET) to examine a relatively simple aspect of pitch processing: maintaining a steady pitch during vocalization. Perry et al. (1999) compared a condition in which subjects repeatedly produced a single vocal tone of constant pitch to a control condition in which they heard synthetic tones at the same rate. Increased cerebral blood flow (CBF) was noted in several motor areas, but of greatest relevance to the present review, only right-sided activations were noted in both primary and secondary auditory cortices, again reflecting the specialization of the right auditory cortex for pitch perception. Additional findings in favor of this conclusion come from regression analyses in which the accuracy of the subjects' sung output was covaried against CBF in the whole brain volume (Perry et al., 1996). In this analysis a region of covariation was identified in right Heschl's gyrus, such that increased CBF was observed with increasing pitch deviation. This result confirms the special role played by this region in pitch processing, and suggests that a feedback mechanism may be operative to maintain consistency of vocalized pitch.

PROCESSING OF HIGHER-ORDER TONAL INFORMATION

As one may readily discern from the above discussion, the contribution of specific neural systems to tonal processing, and the degree to which they may be functionally lateralized, depends to a great extent on the specific nature of the process in question. A common failing in the literature on this topic, and indeed in many other domains of cognitive neuroscience, is that the nature of the processes under study is not fully elucidated, or even understood well enough to be specified. Nonetheless, it is possible to draw certain conclusions from reviewing the literature, though it may be wise to keep in mind that many of today's conclusions are likely to be overturned by tomorrow's data.

Moving, therefore, from the relatively simpler situation of processing of simple pitches to the processing of tonal patterns entails a jump in complexity. Many experimental studies have been carried out with brain-damaged patients that explore their abilities to perceive and discriminate melodic patterns. A variety of perceptual disorders have been described following unilateral damage to one or the other hemisphere (for a review, see Marin & Perry, 1999), although for the reasons outlined above, it is often not clear how to interpret the observed effects. One conclusion that can be drawn from a series of recent studies is that although unilateral hemispheric lesions do often lead to serious perceptual disturbance, the most severe deficits are seen after bilateral damage (Peretz et al., 1994). Peretz and her colleagues, for example, have shown that "amusia," a complete inability to perform even the simplest of tonal processing tasks (such as recognizing a familiar tune), is generally associated with bilateral damage to the temporal cortices. These findings therefore remind us that whatever the magnitude of the hemispheric differences which are the focus of this chapter, these asymmetries are probably best characterized as relative and not absolute.

Having said that, the preponderance of the evidence from systematic studies of behavioral-lesion effects does suggest a relative hemispheric asymmetry favoring the right temporal cortex in processing melodic patterns (Milner, 1962; Samson & Zatorre, 1988; Zatorre, 1985; Liégeois-Chauvel et al., 1998), although most studies also indicate that left temporal lobe damage can result in disturbances on certain tasks. This result is, of course, in keeping with the studies reviewed in the previous section on simpler pitch processing tasks. It stands to reason that if basic mechanisms of pitch analysis are disturbed, this will likely lead to disorders of more complex processes as well.

Whenever a series of tones is presented, a pattern is formed by the relationships between the pitches. These patterns form the basis for melodies, which are essential to many aspects of music throughout the world. Melodic patterns may be investigated at many different levels of analysis, from the basic interval relationships between tones to the semantic networks that are important for long-term representations of familiar tunes and the output mechanisms necessary for singing or playing them. In the present discussion I have chosen to concentrate on the way in which the auditory cortex is engaged in perceiving melodies. One critical consideration in this respect is that melodic perception (all auditory perception, in fact) involves working memory mechanisms. Sounds unfold over time, and once a sound is finished, it disappears from the environment; hence, in order to compute the relationships between successive events, an on-line retention system would clearly be necessary. Even in the case of a brief melody, relationships between tones have to be computed and maintained over periods ranging from seconds to minutes, in order to achieve a relatively stable and coherent internal representation.

There is some evidence from experimental psychology that working memory for pitch information is at least partially independent from working memory for other types of sounds. For example, Deutsch (1970) showed that memory for tones was relatively specific because it was not disrupted by the presence of other sounds during an interference period, but only by other tones (see also Semal et al., 1996). In a lesion study from our laboratory (Zatorre & Samson, 1991) this task was adapted to test patients with unilateral temporal lobe excision. It was found that pitch discrimination was significantly worse following damage to the right than to the left temporal cortex when interfering tones were interposed during the time interval between a target and a comparison tone. No significant deficits emerged among the patient groups when a silent time interval was used, again indicating that basic pitch discrimination was not significantly affected by the temporal lobe excision. In this study, unlike the studies of basic pitch processing discussed above (Johnsrude et al., 2000; Zatorre, 1988), there was no difference in degree of behavioral deficit as a function of encroachment onto Heschl's gyrus. Thus, areas of auditory cortex outside of the primary zone are most likely to be involved in this function. Converging evidence for this latter conclusion comes from behavioral studies in monkeys which show that temporal lobe damage results in deficits in tonal retention (Colombo et al., 1990; Stepien et al., 1960); this region is implicated in auditory short-term memory by single-unit data as well (Gottlieb et al., 1989).

Zatorre and Samson (1991) also observed that damage to the right frontal lobe resulted in poor performance on the interference task. The latter result may reflect a disruption of functional connectivity between frontal and temporal cortices (Petrides & Pandya, 1988; Romanski et al., 1999), which may be involved in maintenance of pitch in working memory (Marin & Perry, 1999). These data therefore extend the findings of hemispheric asymmetry to a specific type of task involving tonal working memory, and suggests that there may be a specialized neural substrate for this function that involves right superior temporal cortex and right frontal regions as well.

The above findings lead to the prediction that it should be possible to demonstrate the recruitment of specialized neural circuitry for tonal working memory. This aim was part of the rationale behind a study of melodic processing using PET (Zatorre et al., 1994). Four conditions were run in which a group of 12 nonmusician volunteers were asked to (1) listen to noise bursts equated acoustically to melodies; (2) listen to a series of novel tonal melodies, without explicit instruction; (3) listen to the same melodies and compare the pitch of the first and second notes; and (4) listen to the melodies and compare the pitch of the first and last notes. It is to be noted that the last condition approximates the working memory requirements of the Deutsch pitch retention task, used in Zatorre & Samson (1991). Comparing conditions (2) and (1) yielded areas of activation in the superior temporal gyri, more prominently on the right. A reanalysis of these results (Zatorre & Binder, 2000) indicated that the activity is most likely located in the inferior portion of the superior temporal gyrus, near the superior temporal sulcus (figure 11.3 and plate 8), a brain area that has also been shown to be sensitive to complex spectral and temporal features such as are contained within human voices (Belin et al., 2000). The finding of an activation within the right temporal cortex while listening to melodies fits in well with the lesion data, and likely reflects the specialization of neuronal networks within the right secondary auditory cortices for perceptual analysis of tonal information.

Tonal working memory was evaluated by comparing conditions (4) and (3) to the baseline (1). Both comparisons elicited activity in a similar location, within the right inferior frontal cortex, but condition (4) also showed recruitment of a large number of other cortical and subcortical areas. Comparing conditions (4) and (3) directly to one another also showed activity within the right frontal lobe, within the opercular portion of the frontal cortex (figure 11.3 and plate 8). These findings therefore support the idea that the right frontal cortex is involved in tonal working memory processing, in accord with previous PET data on pitch judgments on syllables (Zatorre et al., 1992). The data from the melody study also indicate that the more complex and cognitively demanding pitch retention task elicits a greater range of neural activity in both hemispheres, perhaps reflecting various subprocesses associated with the task. The findings of Perry et al. (1993) are directly relevant to this issue; they observed CBF increases with a rightward asymmetry in dorsolateral frontal areas when subjects were engaged in

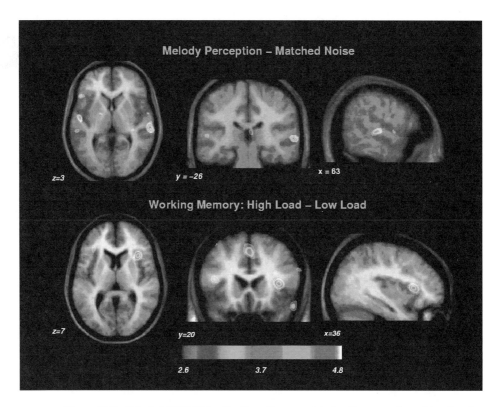

Figure 11.3 Selected PET CBF activation sites associated with processing of tonal melodies. The figures show averaged PET subtraction images superimposed on a corresponding section of an average anatomical MRI. (*Top*) Horizontal, coronal, and sagittal views through a focus located in the upper bank of the right superior temporal sulcus, representing a significant blood flow increase while subjects listened to a series of short, unfamiliar tonal melodies, as compared with a baseline condition in which they listened to noise bursts that were acoustically equated to the melodies. Also visible in the horizontal section is a region of significant activity in the left temporal cortex. (*Bottom*) Horizontal, coronal, and sagittal views through a focus in the right frontal/opercular region showing activity associated with making judgments about the pitch of the first and last notes of the tonal sequences (high working memory load) as compared to making judgments about the first two notes (low working memory load). (Data reanalyzed from Zatorre et al., 1994.) See plate 8 for color version.

an auditory-tonal working memory task that required them to monitor a sequence of tones. This finding therefore suggests a functional dissociation between the cognitive process of monitoring information and holding sensory information in working memory, with the former associated with dorsolateral frontal activity, and the latter recruiting inferior frontal systems (see also Petrides 1995).

Additional data relevant to tonal processes were provided in a PET study of rhythm by Penhune et al. (1998). Rather than explore tonal relationships formed by pitch differences, these investigators used tone sequences whose elements differed only in the temporal dimension. They contrasted perception and reproduction of tonal sequences with a perceptual baseline and found CBF increases in the right superior temporal gyrus (STG), among many other areas, which might be consistent with a strategy of using tonal imagery (see below). The right-sided STG activity would be in keeping with the important role for right auditory cortical areas in tonal processing already discussed, and extends this finding to temporal aspects of the stimulus. It is important to note that evidence converging toward this conclusion was obtained in a parallel study using similar tasks with patients who had undergone temporal lobe resection (Penhune et al., 1999). In that study, patients with excision that encroached upon HG in the right but not the left temporal lobe were impaired in reproducing auditory temporal sequences, but were unimpaired in reproducing visually presented stimuli. Thus, these data extend the conclusions about right temporal cortex predominance for tonal sequences to the temporal domain.

Binder et al. (1997), investigated an active tone judgment task using fMRI. This task, which required subjects to discriminate two pitches during a series of tones (which ranged from three to seven tones in length) and then to make a judgment pertaining to the entire series of tones, emphasized not only pitch perception but also maintenance of simple pitch information in working memory. Compared to a resting state, this task activated extensive auditory regions bilaterally, including HG, the superior temporal plane anterior to HG, planum temporale (PT), and much of the lateral surface of the STG. Temporal lobe activation was confined to the STG in the left hemisphere, but in the right hemisphere spread ventrally into the posterior half of the middle temporal gyrus (MTG), consistent with the first/last pitch condition of Zatorre et al. (1994). Notably, there was no activation of the anterior superior temporal sulcus (STS) in either hemisphere. In both hemispheres, superior temporal activation spread posteriorly into the planum parietale and surrounding supramarginal gyrus. This supramarginal activation was much more extensive in the right hemisphere. Activation also involved frontal cortex bilaterally. In the left hemisphere, this was primarily confined to premotor cortex, whereas right frontal activation also extended anteriorly to involve prefrontal cortex in inferior and middle frontal gyri, findings that are partly in accord with the results of Zatorre et al. (1994) and Perry et al. (1993) implicating frontal mechanisms in auditory tonal working memory, particularly on the right.

Other activated areas included the anterior insula bilaterally, the supplementary motor area bilaterally, the anterior putamen and thalamus bilaterally, and the dorsal midbrain. Activation in these structures was also somewhat more prominent on the right side. The posterior and lateral cerebellum was activated bilaterally, more extensively on the left. When this task was compared to an active task involving semantic categorization of words, stronger activation associated with the tone task was observed in the planum temporale bilaterally, the supramarginal region bilaterally (but much more on the right), the right posterior middle temporal gyrus, premotor cortex bilaterally (also much more on the right), and right superior parietal cortex. These right temporoparietal foci are in very close agreement with the right posterior STG, middle temporal, and inferior parietal foci reported by Démonet in their tones-speech comparisons (1992, 1994). These studies thus provide additional evidence for a special role of the right hemisphere in various aspects of pitch processing. Since the tone tasks also made additional demands on short-term memory, it is not yet clear which of the differentially activated regions might be involved in pitch perception and which in short-term memory for pitch information. But it seems likely that the premotor, STG, and supramarginal areas are involved in maintaining pitch information in working memory, since these regions in the left hemisphere appeared to comprise a functional network for auditory verbal information in many studies of verbal working memory.

Another relevant imaging study to examine pitch processing was carried out by Griffiths et al. (1998) using iterated noise patterns. These investigators took advantage of the phenomenon that when random noise is passed through a cascade of delay-and-add networks, a pitch is heard corresponding to the reciprocal of the time delay constant used.

This pitch sensation is of particular interest because it does not result from resolvable spectral components at the periphery, as would be the case with a typical complex tone, but rather must be the outcome of the central nervous system's capacity to encode temporal regularity in the neural firing pattern. Subjects were scanned with PET while listening to a series of such stimuli varying in the number of iterations. The resulting pitches either conformed to a diatonic melodic pattern or formed a nonmelodic scale pattern. Griffiths et al. analyzed CBF changes as a function of increasing number of iterations of the noise-delay stimulus (each of which produces a stronger phenomenological sense of pitch), and found linear CBF increases bilaterally in the STG, near the primary auditory cortex, lateral and inferior to Heschl's gyrus. These results directly implicate a region within or adjacent to the true koniocortical region in processing temporal fine structure, and indicate that temporal integration occurs at or before the cortical level, though the results would not be incompatible with such processes also happening at subcortical levels, especially at the inferior colliculus or medial geniculate.

The two types of stimuli (resulting in a percept of a diatonic melodic pattern or not) allowed the authors to investigate the emergence of longer-term structure in the stimulus by seeking areas that showed an interaction between number of iterations (and hence pitch salience) and the presence or absence of a melodic pattern. Four such areas were identified that increased their response as a function of iteration much more for tonal melodic patterns than for nonmelodic pitch patterns. The regions were located symmetrically in the two hemispheres: two in the STG posterior to HG, and two in the superior temporal sulcus/middle temporal gyrus. These four regions were spatially distinct from the periprimary areas identified in the previous analysis, indicating a functional dissociation between regions involved in fine temporal processing related to pitch extraction, and other areas that process emergent temporal properties that would be relevant for melodic pattern processing.

This carefully controlled study challenges the conclusions reached above concerning the right auditory cortical functional specialization for pitch processing. However, the findings may not be contradictory, if the various studies in question have in fact been examining different aspects of a complex mechanism. Pitch processing may require partially independent spectral and temporal mechanisms, each of which may have dissociable neural correlates. Thus, the right-side bias that has emerged from imaging and from behavioral-lesion studies reviewed earlier may reflect a predominant spectral pattern analysis process, whereas fine-grained temporal analysis of periodicity may be a more bilaterally distributed function. Moreover, as reviewed above, simple pitch discrimination tasks have not generally been found to yield much evidence for lateralization. Thus, the bilateral nature of the imaging results of Griffiths et al. may simply reflect a relatively low-level analysis of pitch, with lateralization emerging only for more complex pattern-matching processes.

The other interesting feature of the findings of Griffiths et al. is the distinction between low-level pitch extraction, which occurs in primary or adjacent areas, and higher-order pitch-pattern analysis, which is associated with belt areas more distant from the auditory core. This aspect of their results is in partial agreement with the results reviewed earlier (Démonet et al., 1994; Binder et al., 1997; Zatorre et al., 1994) insofar as these data agree on a functional distinction between primary areas that respond to simple stimuli and secondary areas in the STG surrounding HG that are important in processing of various stimulus features, some of which are particularly pertinent for melodic patterns.

Taken together, these studies of various aspects of frequency processing seem to point to distinct, functionally specialized cortical fields. In particular, the evidence is beginning to indicate dissociable regions concerned with spectral as opposed to temporal aspects of stimulus processing. What remains to be done, however, is to specify which areas in particular are involved, what their boundaries are, what their precise functional contribution to different types of auditory processing may be, and to what extent these subprocesses may be handled differently in the two cerebral hemispheres. This topic will be taken up again below.

MUSICAL IMAGERY

An intriguing aspect of musical processing that is worth discussing is musical imagery. Many people, whether musically trained or not, report a strong subjective experience of being able to imagine music or musical attributes in the absence of real sound input. Subjective reports are of limited use, of course, to assess the characteristics of cognitive representations in a scientifically rigorous manner. Therefore, in recent years, psychologists have tried to find more objective means of evaluating the nature of imagery processes. In our laboratory we have examined this phenomenon, using both a behavioral lesion approach (Zatorre & Halpern, 1993) and via PET functional imaging (Halpern & Zatorre, 1999; Zatorre et al., 1996). We adapted a paradigm originally developed by Halpern (1988), in which musically untrained subjects compared the pitch of two lyrics from a familiar, imagined song. (For instance, is the pitch corresponding to "sleigh" higher or lower than that of "snow" in the song "Jingle Bells"?). The aim was to examine to what extent perceptual processes and imagery relied on a shared neural substrate and, of greatest relevance to the present chapter, whether hemispheric asymmetries would emerge in imagery that parallel those seen in perception.

In the first neuropsychological study (Zatorre & Halpern, 1993), a modification of the tune scanning task was presented to patients who had undergone right or left temporal lobe excision. A perceptual version of the task was devised in which the listener made pitch judgments while actually hearing the song. Subjects also participated in an imagery condition in which judgments of pitch were made to imagined tunes indexed by the lyrics. The results of that study were very clear and striking. While all subjects did better on the perception task compared to the imagery task, patients with left temporal excisions showed performance just as good as that of normal controls, whereas those with damage to the right temporal area were significantly worse than the other groups on both tasks, and by about the same amount on each task. The conclusion drawn was that structures in the right temporal lobe were crucial for successful performance of both imagery and perception tasks, suggesting the same kind of neuroanatomical parallelism (and by extension functional parallelism) shown by Kosslyn et al. (1999) and others for visual imagery and perception.

A second experiment to investigate the putative similarity between perceptual and imagery mechanisms was carried out using PET (Zatorre et al., 1996). Three tasks were presented to normal participants: a visual baseline condition and two active tasks, one termed "perception" and the other, "imagery." The latter two were similar to those used by Zatorre and Halpern (1993): Two words from a familiar tune were presented on a screen, and the task was to decide if the pitch corresponding to the second word was higher or lower than the pitch corresponding to the first word. In the perceptual task, participants actually heard the song being sung, while in the imagery task they carried out the task with no auditory input. In a baseline task, subjects viewed the words and performed a visual length judgment. The most salient finding was that for nearly every region demonstrating CBF change in the perceptual condition, there was a corresponding CBF peak in the imagery condition. The similarity in CBF distribution across the two conditions supports the idea that the two processes share a similar neural substrate.

Not surprisingly, highly significant CBF increases were found within the superior temporal gyrus bilaterally when subjects were processing the auditory stimuli for the perceptual task, as compared to the baseline task, in which no auditory stimulation was provided. More interesting is the finding that regions within the superior temporal gyrus were also activated, albeit at a much weaker level, when subjects imagined hearing the stimulus, again as compared to the baseline condition. Note that this latter subtraction entails two entirely silent conditions, so that positive CBF changes in the superior temporal gyri (associative auditory cortices) cannot be due to any external stimulation, but are most likely attributable to endogenous processing.

It is of interest to note that the temporal lobe activation in the perceptual-baseline comparison incorporated primary auditory cortex and extended well into association cortical regions along most of the length of the superior temporal cortices. In contrast, this was not the case for the imagery-baseline comparison: CBF increases in that case occurred exclusively in association cortex (and were of lower relative magnitude). This distinction may be important, and supports the idea that primary sensory regions are responsible for extracting stimulus features from the environment, whereas secondary regions are involved in higher-order processes, which might include the internal representation of complex familiar stimuli.

Because Zatorre et al. (1996) observed bilateral STG activity in their imagery condition, their finding could not support the conclusion derived from prior studies for a more important contribution of right STG areas in tonal processing. This was particularly notable given that Zatorre and Halpern (1993) had earlier shown that right temporal lobe excision resulted in deficits on a similar imagery task, whereas left temporal lesions did not. The bilateral STG activity may simply reflect the fact that the stimuli used contained both verbal and tonal information, however. In order to test this idea, a further PET study was

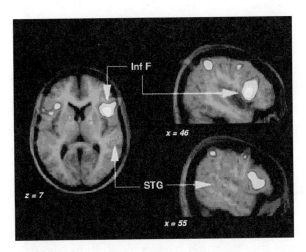

Figure 11.4 Merged PET/MRI images illustrating selected regions of significant increase in CBF in a musical imagery task. Subjects imagined the continuation of a melody upon hearing a cue, and the activation in this condition was compared to that in a baseline condition in which a similar stimulus was presented but without imagery. The leftmost image corresponds to a horizontal section and shows activity in the right superior temporal gyrus (STG), as well as right and left inferior frontal gyri (inf F). The right frontal and temporal areas of activity are also shown in the two parasagittal sections through the right hemisphere shown on the right. The positions of the dotted lines indicate corresponding planes of section in the figures. (Halpern & Zatorre, 1999.)

carried out, involving strictly nonverbal materials (Halpern & Zatorre, 1999). In this study subjects were presented with a tonal cue, consisting of the first few notes of a familiar tune devoid of verbal content (e.g., the first four notes of Beethoven's Fifth Symphony), and asked to generate, using imagery, the remainder of the tune. This task was contrasted to one in which subjects heard a similar set of notes that did not correspond to any known tune. The results (figure 11.4) indicated significant activity in the right STG, as predicted, in a region posterior to HG quite close to the sites associated with other tonal processing studies (Zatorre et al., 1994, 1996; Perry et al., 1999), thus confirming the role of this lateralized region in the re-evocation of tonal patterns in the absence of acoustic input, and consistent with the behavioral-lesion data (Zatorre & Halpern, 1993). Taking the findings of the PET studies together with the behavioral lesion study of imagery (Zatorre & Halpern, 1993), we conclude that there is good evidence that perception and imagery share partially overlapping neural mechanisms, and that these include superior temporal auditory regions, particularly on the right.

Spectral vs. Temporal Processes in the Auditory Cortices

Much of the evidence presented above converges toward the conclusion that a considerable degree of hemispheric specialization exists in the processing of pitch information, with right auditory cortical areas playing a more prominent role than those on the left, although this is not a universal finding. Moving beyond the fact that differences do exist, one might want to address the question of *why* such lateralization might have evolved. If one assumes that hemispheric processing advantages emerged because they confer some advantage over bilaterally shared processing, then it is reasonable to think about how a complementary specialization of auditory functional processing might reflect different types of features of the auditory environment that are important and that require specialized analysis mechanisms.

The specialization of right auditory cortices for tonal processes is, of course, mirrored by the well-established specialization of left auditory areas for speech processing. Several investigators have proposed that the analysis of speech sounds requires good temporal resolution in order to be able to process the rapidly changing energy peaks (formants) that are characteristic of many speech consonants (see, e.g., Tallal et al., 1993; Phillips & Farmer, 1990). In addition, it has been shown that behaviorally, speech recognition can be accomplished with primarily temporal cues (Shannon et al., 1995). The hypothesis that the left hemisphere specialization for speech derives from a temporal processing advantage has not always received universal support, but considerable evidence now exists in its favor.

For example, relevant findings regarding this idea come from a PET study by Belin et al. (1998), in which the rate of formant transitions in a pseudospeech syllable was varied from 40 to 200 ms. CBF changes in the left auditory region were found for both types of stimuli, indicating a capacity for processing spectral change over a wide range of durations; in contrast, regions in the right auditory cortex responded only to the slower rates, and not to the faster rate (figure 11.5). Thus, the right auditory cortex seems unable to respond to fast formant transitions, whereas the homologous area on the left is better able to track rapidly changing acoustic information that would be relevant for speech pro-

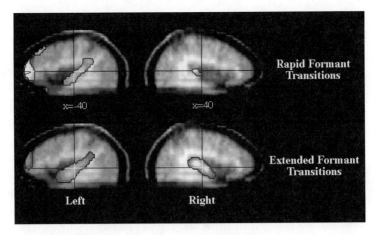

Figure 11.5 Brain activity (gray contour) induced by passive listening to pseudo sylla-bles with either rapid (40 ms) or extended (200 ms) formant transitions, overlaid on mean anatomical MR image. Left auditory cortex (*left panels*) was found to respond similarly to rapid and extended formant transitions. In contrast, right auditory cortex showed con-siderably reduced activity for the rapid as compared to the extended stimuli, thus show-ing functional asymmetry in auditory temporal processing. (Figure adapted from Belin et al., 1998.)

cessing. Results pointing toward a similar conclusion were obtained by Johnsrude et al. (1997).

In this context, the specialization of right auditory areas for tonal analysis might be seen to be the inverse of the specialization of the left auditory cortex for temporal anaysis. This idea may be related to the fact that in a linear system, temporal resolution is inversely propor-tional to spectral resolution. High temporal resolution can be achieved only at the expense of degrading spectral resolution, and vice versa. The auditory nervous system is, of course, a highly nonlinear and dis-tributed system; yet, it may also reflect this fundamental computational constraint, such that the high temporal resolution required to process speech efficiently imposes an upper limit on the ability to resolve spec-tral information in the left auditory cortex, and vice versa for the right auditory cortex. Thus, it is possible to hypothesize that there may be a trade-off to some extent in processing in temporal and spectral domains, and that auditory cortical systems in the two hemispheres have evolved a complementary specialization, with the left having better temporal resolution and the right better spectral resolution.

According to this idea, the hemispheric differences observed in the literature reviewed above reflect this fundamental level of functional organization; thus, rather than being specialized for speech or for tonal patterns per se, the auditory cortices are perhaps better viewed as optimized for certain types of acoustic information processing, which in turn lead to higher-order types of specialization for certain classes of signals. Because it so happens that many musically relevant types of sounds exploit the fine spectral resolution afforded by mechanisms within right auditory cortices, it is consequently often observed that musical processes recruit right-hemisphere mechanisms. To the extent that musical tasks may not always require access to this level of spectral processing, however, one might predict that musical processing might often result in some degree of bilateral hemispheric involvement, and this indeed appears to be the case in much of the literature (Marin & Perry, 1999).

If the foregoing idea is correct, then it should be possible to obtain evidence for differential responses within left and right auditory cortices by manipulating temporal and spectral parameters of an auditory stimulus, independently of whether it is speech or music. A functional imaging study (Zatorre & Belin, 2001) attempts to examine this question using a parametric approach. Rather than looking for differences in cerebral blood flow between a control and an activation condition, functional changes that correlated with a given input parameter were measured. This approach can be particularly powerful because it helps to isolate brain activity that is specifically related to the parameter of interest (see also Paus et al., 1996; Price et al., 1996). Nonverbal stimuli were synthesized that varied independently and systematically along two dimensions: one temporal, the other spectral. The stimuli consisted of a series of pure tones that varied in frequency and duration; in one set of conditions the frequency change was held constant and the temporal rate became faster across scans, while in the other set of conditions the rate was held constant and the frequency differences became finer across scans. The prediction was that increasing rate of temporal change would preferentially recruit left auditory cortical areas, while increasing rate of spectral change would engage right auditory cortical regions.

The results were twofold. First, distinct areas of auditory cortex were identified that responded to each parameter, with the primary cortex being mostly related to the temporal feature, while areas anterior to primary cortex responded best to the spectral feature. Of greatest relevance for the present discussion, cerebral blood flow in a region of the left auditory cortex showed a greater response to increasing temporal than spectral variation, whereas a symmetrical area on the right showed the reverse pattern. A third area, located in the right superior temporal sulcus, also showed a significant response to the spectral parameter, but no change to the temporal parameter. Thus, the data supported the hypothesis that corresponding regions of the auditory cortex in the two hemispheres have different sensitivity to temporal and spectral information. Neurophysiological recordings in macaque monkeys have shown that auditory cortical neurons are highly sensitive to both spectral and temporal features of sounds (deCharms et al., 1998; Phillips, 1993; Steinschneider et al., 1995). Furthermore, Eggermont (1998) noted that in two primary fields of the cat there was an inverse relation between bandwith and temporal resolution, consistent with the suggestion made above.

Additional electrophysiological evidence bearing on this question has been obtained from direct depth-electrode recordings within Heschl's gyri in patients undergoing neurosurgical intervention. Liégeois-Chauvel and colleagues (1999) showed that left auditory cortical units have higher temporal resolution because they are able to encode the voice-onset time of a consonant, whereas the right auditory cortex does not show sensitivity to this temporal parameter. Even more striking consistency is offered by further data from the same investigators (Liégeois-Chauvel et al., 2001), who showed that intracortically recorded auditory evoked potentials were more sharply tuned to frequency in the right auditory cortex than in the left, as predicted by the hypothesis that resolution in the frequency and time domains is different in the two hemispheres.

Anatomical Considerations

An advantageous feature of the hypothesis presented above is that it offers a unifying framework to understand some of the functional characteristics of the auditory nervous system that are relevant for processing speech and tonal patterns. Rather than being seen as two independent phenomena, the complementary specialization of the auditory cortices in the two hemispheres would be seen as arising from a single underlying principle. This model does raise the question, however, of how such functional differences might be instantiated in the brain. Is it possible to find any evidence in the structure of the auditory cortex that might not only support the existence of processing differences, but perhaps also suggest how these differences are implemented?

The findings of several anatomical studies are directly relevant to this question. Penhune et al. (1996) carried out an MRI investigation to characterize the structural features (shape, volume, and position) of the human primary auditory cortical region in vivo. They used interactive three-dimensional pixel-marking software to label the region of Heschl's gyrus (figure 11.1) in MRI scans from groups of normal right-handed volunteer subjects. The volume of Heschl's gyrus was found to be significantly greater on the left than on the right in two independent samples. Perhaps of greatest pertinence for the present discussion, when the labeled volumes were subdivided into white and gray matter, the left-right differences were confined to the white matter underlying Heschl's gyrus, and not to the cortical tissue (gray matter) within the structure (figure 11.6). This finding therefore suggests that the anatomical asymmetry arises not at the level of cortex, but rather that it stems from a difference in the volume of fibers that carry information to and from the primary auditory cortex, and surrounding regions. MRI measures are not able to distinguish what the neural organization might be that specifically accounts for this effect. However, one possibility that immediately comes to mind is that greater white matter volume might reflect a greater degree of myelination, which would in turn be consistent with the idea of faster conduction times in the left auditory cortex. Confirmation that the left auditory cortical regions are indeed more heavily myelinated comes from a postmortem electron microscopy study showing that the myelin sheath is significantly thicker in the left than in the right posterior temporal cortex (Anderson et al., 1999). These authors also confirmed that there is a greater volume of white matter in the left temporal region (figure 11.6), although their study concentrated on the posterior aspect of the superior temporal gyrus rather than Heschl's gyrus.

In addition to the idea that left auditory cortical fibers are more heavily myelinated, there is also evidence for other hemispheric differences in the structural organization of the human auditory cortex that

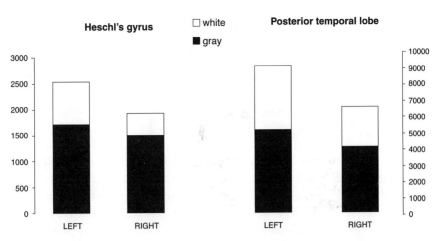

Figure 11.6 Histograms showing volumes of gray and white matter tissue in Heschl's gyrus (*left*) and posterior temporal lobe (*right*). Data from the left panel refer to the left scale and are taken from in vivo MRI volumetric measures after conversion into standardized stereotaxic space. (Penhune et al., 1996.) Data from the right panel refer to the right scale, and are taken from volume measures in postmortem brain samples. (Anderson et al., 1999.) (Units in mm³.)

are broadly consistent with the hypothesis presented above. For example, Hutsler and Gazzaniga (1996) reported larger left than right layer IV pyramidal cells in the primary auditory cortex, which would also lead to faster time constants. Two other studies have reported on the relative spacing of cortical columns in auditory regions. Seldon (1981) observed that cortical columns in the left auditory cortex were more widely spaced than those on the right, and Galuske et al. (2000) found wider intrinsic connections on the left, possibly indicating greater integration across the frequency domain.

These latter features might be consistent with a greater degree of integration across tonotopically organized cortical areas on the left than on the right, hence leading to a relative degradation of spectral resolution on the left. Conversely, neurons in the right auditory cortex would have structural features that would enhance spectral resolution (as observed directly by Liégeois-Chauvel et al., 2001), because these neurons would be smaller, with less myelinated inputs, and therefore perhaps more tightly packed together, which in turn would lead to integration over narrower frequency regions. These characteristics would of course also result in poorer temporal resolution.

CONCLUSION

Although it is clear that our knowledge of hemispheric functional asymmetries has advanced in the past several years, it is even clearer that much remains to be understood. The discussion offered in this chapter is meant to contribute to this discussion by pointing out the relevance of studying processes that have not been the subject of a great deal of exploration, but that may hold potential for uncovering some fundamental properties of the nervous system. The other important aspect of the research approach described in this chapter is that it points to the type of integration of evidence from multiple types of studies (behavioral, functional, structural) that will become more feasible in the near future, thanks to advances in functional imaging, the development of new in vivo structural imaging technologies (e.g., diffusion tensor imaging), and more traditional physiological and anatomical knowledge.

REFERENCES

Anderson, B., Southern, B. D., & Powers, R. E. (1999). Anatomic asymmetries of the posterior superior temporal lobes: A postmortem study. *Neuropsychiatry, Neuropsychology, and Behavioral Neurology, 12*, 247–254.

Belin, P., Zatorre, R., Lafaille, P., Ahad, P., & Pike, B. (2000). Voice-selective areas in human auditory cortex. *Nature, 403*, 309–312.

Belin, P., Zilbovicius, M., Crozier, S., Thivard, L., Fontaine, A., Masure, M.-C., & Samson, Y. (1998). Lateralization of speech and auditory temporal processing. *Journal of Cognitive Neuroscience, 10*, 536–540.

Binder, J., Frost, J., Hammeke, T., Cox, R., Rao, S., & Prieto, T. (1997). Human brain language areas identified by functional magnetic resonance imaging. *Journal of Neuroscience, 17*, 353–362.

Colombo, M., D'Amato, M. R., Rodman, H. R., & Gross, C. G. (1990). Auditory association cortex lesions impair auditory short-term memory in monkeys. *Science, 247*, 336–338.

deCharms, R. C., Blake, D. T., & Merzenich, M. M. (1998). Optimizing sound features for cortical neurons. *Science, 280*, 1439–1443.

Démonet, J.-F., Chollet, F., Ramsay, S., Cardebat, D., Nespoulous, J.-L., Wise, R., Rascol, A., & Frackowiak, R. (1992). The anatomy of phonological and semantic processing in normal subjects. *Brain, 115*, 1753–1768.

Démonet, J.-F., Price, C., Wise, R., & Frackowiack, R. S. J. (1994). A PET study of cognitive strategies in normal subjects during language tasks. *Brain, 117*, 671–682.

Deutsch, D. (1970). Tones and numbers: Specificity of interference in short-term memory. *Science, 168*, 1604–1605.

Diamond, I., Goldberg, J., & Neff, W. (1962). Tonal discrimination after ablation of auditory cortex. *Journal of Neurophysiology, 25*, 223–235.

Eggermont, J. (1998). Representation of spectral and temporal sound features in three cortical fields of the cat. Similarities outweigh differences. *Journal of Neurophysiology, 80*, 2743–2764.

Evarts, E. V. (1952). Effect of auditory cortex ablation on frequency discrimination in monkey. *Journal of Neurophysiology, 15*, 443–448.

Galuske, R., Schlote, W., Bratzke, H., & Singer, W. (2000). Interhemispheric asymmetries of the modular structure in human temporal cortex. *Science, 289*, 1946–1949.

Gottlieb, Y., Vaadia, E., & Abeles, M. (1989). Single unit activity in the auditory cortex of a monkey performing a short term memory task. *Experimental Brain Research, 74*, 139–148.

Gray, P. M., Krause, B., Atema, J., Payne, R., Krumhansl, C., & Baptista, L. (2001). The music of nature and the nature of music. *Science, 291*(5501), 52–54.

Griffiths, T. D., Büchel, C., Frackowiak, R. S. J., & Patterson, R. D. (1998). Analysis of temporal structure in sound by the human brain. *Nature Neuroscience, 1*, 422–427.

Halpern, A. R. (1988). Mental scanning in auditory imagery for tunes. *Journal of Experimental Psychology: Learning, Memory and Cognition, 14*, 434–443.

Halpern, A. R., & Zatorre, R. J. (1999). When that tune runs through your head: A PET investigation of auditory imagery for familiar melodies. *Cerebral Cortex, 9*, 697–704.

Heffner, H. E., & Masterton, B. (1978). *Contribution of auditory cortex to hearing in the monkey (Macaca mulatta)*. Vol. 1. New York: Academic Press.

Hutsler, J., & Gazzaniga, M. (1996). Acetylcholinesterase staining in human auditory and language cortices—regional variation of structural features. *Cerebral Cortex, 6*, 260–270.

Jerison, H. J., & Neff, W. D. (1953). Effect of cortical ablation in the monkey on discrimination of auditory patterns. *Federation Proceedings, 12*, 237.

Johnsrude, I. S., Penhune, V. B., & Zatorre, R. J. (2000). Functional specificity in right human auditory cortex for perceiving pitch direction. *Brain, 123*, 155–163.

Johnsrude, I. S., Zatorre, R. J., Milner, B. A., & Evans, A. C. (1997). Left-hemisphere specialization for the processing of acoustic transients. *NeuroReport, 8*, 1761–1765.

Kosslyn, S. M., Pascual-Leone, A., Felician, O., Camposano, S., Keenan, J. P., Thompson, W. L., Ganis, G., Sukel, K. E., & Alpert, N. M. (1999). The role of area 17 in visual imagery: Convergent evidence from PET and rTMS. *Science 284*, 167–170.

Liégeois-Chauvel, C., de Graaf, J., Laguitton, V., & Chauvel, P. (1999). Specialization of left auditory cortex for speech perception in man depends on temporal coding. *Cerebral Cortex, 9*, 484–496.

Liégeois-Chauvel, C., Giraud, K., Badier, J.-M., Marquis, P., & Chauvel, P. (2001). Intra-cerebral evoked potentials in pitch perception reveal a functional asymmetry of the human auditory cortex. *Annals of the New York Academy of Sciences*, *930*, 117–132.

Liégeois-Chauvel, C., Musolino, A., & Chauvel, P. (1991). Localization of the primary auditory area in man. *Brain*, *114*, 139–153.

Liégeois-Chauvel, C., Peretz, I., Babaï, M., Laguitton, V., & Chauvel, P. (1998). Contribution of different cortical areas in the temporal lobes to music processing. *Brain*, *121*, 1853–1867.

Marin, O. S. M., & Perry, D. W. (1999). Neurological aspects of music perception and performance. In D. Deutsch (Ed.), *The psychology of music*. Second edition (pp. 653–724). New York: Academic Press.

Milner, B. A. (1962). Laterality effects in audition. In V. Mountcastle (Ed.), *Interhemispheric relations and cerebral dominance* (pp. 177–195). Baltimore: Johns Hopkins University Press.

Paus, T., Perry, D. W., Zatorre, R. J., Worsley, K., & Evans, A. C. (1996). Modulation of cerebral blood-flow in the human auditory cortex during speech: Role of motor-to-sensory discharges. *European Journal of Neuroscience*, *8*, 2236–2246.

Penhune, V. B., Zatorre, R. J., & Evans, A. C. (1998). Cerebellar contributions to motor timing: A PET study of auditory and visual rhythm reproduction. *Journal of Cognitive Neuroscience*, *10*, 752–765.

Penhune, V. B., Zatorre, R. J., and Feindel, W. (1999). The role of auditory cortex in retention of rhythmic patterns in patients with temporal-lobe removals including Heschl's gyrus. *Neuropsychologia*, *37*, 315–331.

Penhune, V. B., Zatorre, R. J., MacDonald, J. D., & Evans, A. C. (1996). Interhemispheric anatomical differences in human primary auditory cortex: Probabilistic mapping and volume measurement from magnetic resonance scans. *Cerebral Cortex*, *6*, 661–672.

Peretz, I., Kolinsky, R., Tramo, M., Labrecque, R., Hublet, C., Demeurisse, G., & Belleville, S. (1994). Functional dissociations following bilateral lesions of auditory cortex. *Brain*, *117*, 1283–1301.

Perry, D., Zatorre, R., & Evans, A. (1996). Co-variation of CBF during singing with vocal fundamental frequency. *Neuroimage*, *3*(3), S315.

Perry, D. W., Petrides, M., Alivisatos, B., Zatorre, R. J., Evans, A. C., & Meyer, E. (1993). Functional activation of human frontal cortex during tonal working memory tasks. *Society for Neuroscience Abstracts*, *19*, 843.

Perry, D. W., Zatorre, R. J., Petrides, M., Alivisatos, B., Meyer, E., & Evans, A. C. (1999). Localization of cerebral activity during simple singing. *NeuroReport*, *10*, 3979–3984.

Petrides, M. (1995). Functional organization of the human frontal cortex for mnemonic processing: Evidence from neuroimaging studies. *Annals of the New York Academy of Sciences*, *769*, 85–96.

Petrides, M., & Pandya, D. N. (1988). Association fiber pathways to the frontal cortex from the superior temporal region in the Rhesus monkey. *Journal of Comparative Neurology*, *273*, 52–66.

Phillips, D. P. (1993). Representation of acoustic events in the primary auditory cortex. *Journal of Experimental Psychology: Human Perception and Performance*, *19*(1), 203–216.

Phillips, D. P., & Farmer, M. E. (1990). Acquired word deafness and the temporal grain of sound representation in the primary auditory cortex. *Behavioral Brain Research*, *40*, 84–90.

Price, C. J., Wise, R. J. S., Warburton, E. A., Moore, C. J., Howard, D., Patterson, K., Frackowiak, R. S. J., & Friston, K. J. (1996). Hearing and saying: The functional neuroanatomy of auditory word processing. *Brain*, *119*, 919–931.

Rademacher, J., Caviness, V. S., Steinmetz, H., & Galaburda, A. M. (1993). Topographical variation of the human primary cortices: Implications for neuroimaging, brain mapping and neurobiology. *Cerebral Cortex*, *3*, 313–329.

Robin, D. A., Tranel, D., & Damasio, H. (1990). Auditory perception of temporal and spectral events in patients with focal left and right cerebral lesions. *Brain and Language*, *39*, 539–555.

Romanski, L., Tian, B., Fritz, J., Mishkin, M., Goldman-Rakic, P., & Rauschecker, J. (1999). Dual streams of auditory afferents target multiple domains in the primate prefrontal cortex. *Nature Neuroscience*, *2*, 1131–1136.

Samson, S., & Zatorre, R. J. (1988). Melodic and harmonic discrimination following unilateral cerebral excision. *Brain and Cognition*, *7*, 348–360.

Samson, S., & Zatorre, R. J. (1994). Contribution of the right temporal lobe to musical timbre discrimination. *Neuropsychologia*, *32*, 231–240.

Schouten, J. (1938). The perception of subjective tones. *Proceedings of the Koninklijke Nederlandse Akademie van Wetenschappen 41*, 1086–1093.

Seldon, H. (1981). Structure of human auditory cortex. II: Axon distributions and morphological correlates of speech perception. *Brain Research*, *229*, 295–310.

Semal, C., Demany, L., Ueda, K., & Halle, P.-A. (1996). Speech versus nonspeech in pitch memory. *Journal of the Acoustical Society of America*, *100*, 1132–1140.

Shannon, R. V., Zeng, F.-G., Kamath, V., Wygonski, J., & Ekelid, M. (1995). Speech recognition with primarily temporal cues. *Science*, *270*, 303–304.

Sidtis, J. J., & Volpe, B. T. (1988). Selective loss of complex-pitch or speech discrimination after unilateral lesion. *Brain and Language*, *34*, 235–245.

Steinmetz, H., & Seitz, R. (1991). Functional anatomy of language processing: Neuroimaging and the problem of individual variability. *Neuropsychologia*, *29*(12), 1149–1161.

Steinschneider, M., Schroeder, C., Arezzo, J., & Vaughan, H. (1995). Physiologic correlates of the voice onset time boundary in primary auditory cortex of the awake monkey: Temporal response patterns. *Brain and Language*, *48*, 326–340.

Stepien, L. S., Cordeau, J. P., & Rasmussen, T. (1960). The effect of temporal lobe and hippocampal lesions on auditory and visual recent memory in monkeys. *Brain, 83,* 470–489.

Tallal, P., Miller, S., & Fitch, R. (1993). Neurobiological basis of speech: A case for the preeminence of temporal processing. *Annals of the New York Academy of Sciences, 682,* 27–47.

Wetzel, W., Ohl, F., Wagner, T., & Scheich, H. (1998). Right auditory cortex lesion in Mongolian gerbils impairs discrimination of rising and falling frequency-modulated tones. *Neuroscience Letters, 252,* 115–118.

Whitfield, I. (1980). Auditory cortex and the pitch of complex tones. *Journal of the Acoustical Society of America, 67,* 644–647.

Whitfield, I. (1985). The role of auditory cortex in behavior. In A. Peters and E. Jones (Eds.), *Cerebral cortex* (pp. 329–351). Vol. 4 of *Association and auditory cortices.* New York: Plenum Press.

Zatorre, R. J. (1985). Discrimination and recognition of tonal melodies after unilateral cerebral excisions. *Neuropsychologia, 23,* 31–41.

Zatorre, R. J. (1988). Pitch perception of complex tones and human temporal-lobe function. *Journal of the Acoustical Society of America, 84*(2), 566–572.

Zatorre, R., & Belin, P. (2001). Spectral and temporal processing in human auditory cortex. *Cerebral Cortex, 11,* 946–953.

Zatorre, R., & Binder, J. (2000). Functional and structural imaging of the human auditory system. In A. Toga and J. Mazziota (Eds.), *Brain mapping: The systems* (pp. 365–402). Los Angeles: Academic Press.

Zatorre, R. J., Evans, A. C., & Meyer, E. (1994). Neural mechanisms underlying melodic perception and memory for pitch. *Journal of Neuroscience, 14*(4), 1908–1919.

Zatorre, R. J., Evans, A. C., Meyer, E., & Gjedde, A. (1992). Lateralization of phonetic and pitch processing in speech perception. *Science, 256,* 846–849.

Zatorre, R. J., & Halpern, A. R. (1993). Effect of unilateral temporal-lobe excision on perception and imagery of songs. *Neuropsychologia, 31*(3), 221–232.

Zatorre, R. J., Halpern, A. R., Perry, D. W., Meyer, E., & Evans, A. C. (1996). Hearing in the mind's ear: A PET investigation of musical imagery and perception. *Journal of Cognitive Neuroscience, 8*(1), 29–46.

Zatorre, R. J., & Peretz, I. (Eds.). (2001). The biological foundations of music. *Annals of the New York Academy of Sciences, 930.*

Zatorre, R. J., & Samson, S. (1991). Role of the right temporal neocortex in retention of pitch in auditory short-term memory. *Brain, 114,* 2403–2417.

12 Dichotic Listening in the Study of Auditory Laterality

Kenneth Hugdahl

The present chapter is an update on the use of dichotic listening (DL) for the study of auditory laterality, focusing on research at the University of Bergen, Norway. The dichotic listening technique used in our laboratory was described in detail in the first edition of *Brain Asymmetry* volume (Davidson & Hugdahl, 1995). The basic features of the dichotic listening test developed at the University of Bergen (the Bergen DL test) (see also Hugdahl, 1995) will be described, together with psychometric data from the Bergen Dichotic Listening Database. The database currently includes 1018 cases ranging from 6 to 88 years of age. In addition, it is suggested that DL is an important method for the study of auditory laterality, with particular focus on (1) hemispheric asymmetry for the processing of phonetic stimuli (Hugdahl, 1995, 1997), (2) temporal lobe function and memory processing (Wester et al., 1998; Wester & Hugdahl, 1995; Hugdahl et al., 1993), (3) vigilance and attention (Asbjørnsen & Hugdahl, 1995; Løberg et al., 1999), and (4) interhemispheric interaction and callosal function (Hugdahl, 1998, in press; Reinvang et al., 1994).

Cowell and Hugdahl (2000) suggested that the controversy surrounding the reproducibility of different measures of laterality may partly be due not to the measures being insensitive to the underlying phenomenon of laterality—quite the contrary, the measures may be too sensitive. For example, in the area of human sex differences research, very few stable effects have been found in studies of corpus callosum anatomy (Bishop & Wahlsten, 1997) or behavioral measures such as dichotic listening (Hiscock et al., 1994) or the visual half-field technique (McKeever, 1986). Consequently, it has sometimes been suggested that the measures lack validity and the need for further research has been questioned. An alternative view is that these measures are highly sensitive to many developmental, physiological, and behavioral factors, which makes them ideal, rather than problematic, for use in the investigation of, for example, individual differences in laterality.

AUDITORY LATERALITY

The study of auditory laterality, or laterality in the auditory domain, has several advantages with respect to a general theoretical and methodological approach to hemispheric asymmetry. The terms "laterality" and "asymmetry" will be used interchangeably in this chapter, although laterality in a strict sense may relate more to the use of lateralized stimulus presentations, while asymmetry denotes more of a general theoretical approach to how the two cerebral hemispheres process information. In contrast to the visual domain, the auditory domain permits the study of a correspondence between functional and structural asymmetry. Interestingly, there is no known asymmetry of any visual area in the occipital cortex that would correspond to functional asymmetries involving the presentation of visual stimuli of any kind, using whatever known methodology. Despite the important breakthroughs with regard to differences in function between the two cerebral hemispheres since the 1970s (see Gazzaniga, 2000 for an overview of research on the split-brain patient), there are few overlapping findings where functional asymmetry corresponds with structural asymmetry, meaning that the two hemispheres also differ anatomically or structurally in a way that theoretically corresponds to a given functional asymmetry.

Anatomical differences between the hemispheres in cortical organization and connectivity are scarcely reported in the literature. In 1995, Galaburda wrote that despite extensive research with regard to anatomical differences between the hemispheres:

by and large ... we have only found side differences in the amount of brain substrate devoted to a particular architectonic area or a particular gross anatomical landmark. In other words, despite the fact that the left hemisphere is significantly different in function from the right, there appears to be no structure or chemical constituent that is present in one hemisphere but not in the other.... There are gyri with the same names and general structure on both sides. All architectonic areas are present in both hemispheres. There are no cell types found in one hemisphere but not in the other. There is no known pattern of connections that appears to be specific to the dominant hemisphere. And as far as has been determined, there are no physiologic properties in neurons of one hemisphere that are not present in the other. This leaves quantitative differences as the only difference between areas present in both hemispheres. (pp. 51–52)

However, within the domain of auditory laterality, the small triangular area in the posterior superior temporal gyrus (i.e., the planum temporale) is structurally different on the left and right sides. This seems to correlate with a functional difference related to language processing—or, to be more specific, to speech perception and phonological processing. In a classic paper, Geschwind and Levitsky (1968) found that the left planum temporale was longer in a majority of the brains they investigated. They investigated 100 brains postmortem, and found that the left planum was larger in 65 of them. Eleven brains showed a reverse pattern, with longer planum in the right hemisphere, and 24 brains did not show any difference between the left and right sides. Although Geschwind and Levitsky were not the first to report anatomical differences between the hemispheres, their paper gained widespread recognition and boosted interest in hemispheric asymmetry research (see historical account by Springer & Deutsch, 1989).

The recent interest in the asymmetry of the planum temporale may be not only because of its apparent asymmetry, but also because of the location of the planum in the axial plane in the upper portion of the superior temporal gyrus. The upper posterior surface of the temporal lobe functionally overlaps Wernicke's area (Brodmann areas 22/42), which is considered the primary cortical area for speech perception and language comprehension. The planum temporale is also located just behind the posterior wall of Heschl's gyrus (Brodmann area 41), which makes up the primary auditory cortex in man. Thus, a larger left planum temporale could be a structural correlate to the functional specialization of the left hemisphere for language, especially for language comprehension and speech perception, overlapping with the major auditory areas in the brain.

Although, the planum temporale area has been extensively studied since the 1990s (e.g., Steinmetz & Galaburda, 1991; Jäncke et al., 1994; Foundas et al., 1994; see also Beaton, 1997 for review), its exact anatomical demarcation still is a matter of some controversy (see, e.g., Ide et al., 1999; see also chapter 19, this volume), especially the delineation of the posterior border. Ide et al. (1999) have suggested that it may not be a true asymmetry of area between the left and right planum temporale, but rather that the two sides are displaced with regard to localization in relation two each other. Similarly, Binder and his colleagues (e.g., Binder et al., 1996, 2000) have argued, on the basis of fMRI brain imaging, that the planum temporale may be more responsive to the extraction of higher-order acoustical features of speech sounds, whereas the phonetic features are processed more anterior and ventrally along the superior temporal sulcus. Binder et al. (2000) found that when brain activation caused by tones was subtracted from the corresponding activation caused by words, the remaining activation was seen in the medial temporal lobe. The opposite contrast showed remaining activation in the upper posterior part of the temporal lobe, overlapping with the planum temporale area.

On the other hand, a magnetoencephalography (MEG) study Shtyrov et al. (2000) found increased response amplitudes from the upper part of the left temporal plane when phonological stimuli were used; it was not seen in response to nonphonological stimuli (see also Tervaniemi et al., 2000). In still another study, Mazoyer et al. (1999) found that the left planum temporale surface area correlated positively with increase in blood flow, measured with PET, to the same area when subjects listened to a factual story being read to them. Following up on these results, we reanalyzed data from the Hugdahl et al. (1999) ^{15}O-PET study with dichotic listening to consonant-vowel (CV) syllables and looked at activation in consecutive axial slices of 2 mm thickness from 12 mm below the anterior-posterior commissure (AC-PC) midline to 20 mm above the midline (covering a range from the medial temporal lobe to the superior end of the planum temporale) (figure 12.1 and plate 9). This analysis showed activations already at the level of the superior temporal sulcus to CV syllables. This would argue against a unique role for the planum temporale in speech perception. However, the activations below the planum temporale were clearly bilateral in nature,

Figure 12.1 15O-PET activation images in 2-mm axial slices covering the planum temporale and adjacent inferior and superior areas. Note the absence of activation to the musical instruments stimuli in areas inferior to the planum temporale, while the CV syllable stimuli also activated areas in the vicinity of the superior temporal sulcus. Left in the image is left in the brain, following neurological conventions. (Data obtained in collaboration with Ian Law, Copenhagen University Hospital PET Center.) See plate 9 for color version.

CV-
syllables

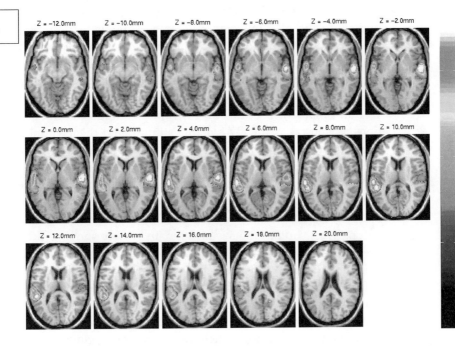

Musical
instruments

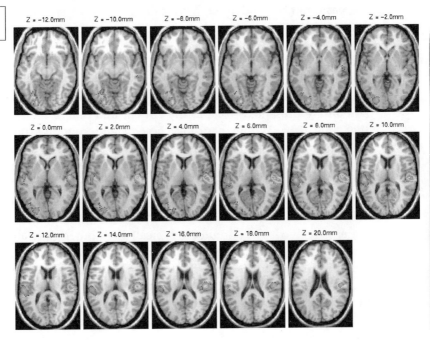

Dichotic Listening and Auditory Laterality

while a left-larger-than-right asymmetry appeared when moving upward into the planum temporale area. Thus, it may be that both the medial and the superior temporal gyri respond to phonological stimuli, but it is only in the superior temporal gyrus that a leftward asymmetry is observed. This interpretation is further strengthened in the activation patterns seen for the musical instrument stimuli (lower part of figure 12.1 and plate 9). The musical instrument stimuli did not show activations as ventral as the CV syllable stimuli, and the asymmetry pattern was also very different, particularly in the planum temporale region (+6 mm to +18 mm).

Another argument for the study of hemispheric asymmetry within the auditory domain is that, unlike the visual domain, processing of auditory input is neutral, or independent, of the subject's spatial orientation. Thus, unlike the visual domain, where moving the head and eyes shifts stimulus input to the left or right visual field, auditory input is independent of the spatial positioning of the head or the eyes. This makes it possible to study dynamic interactions between lateralized stimulus presentations (e.g. with the DL technique) and covert shifts of attention to either the left or right side of auditory space. Moving the head or the eyes during a dichotic listening experiment does not affect the basic right ear advantage typically seen in DL studies (Asbjørnsen et al., 1990).

DICHOTIC LISTENING: THE BASICS

Dichotic listening literally means that two (di-) different auditory (-otic) stimuli are presented—one to the left ear and one to the right ear—at the same time. Within neuropsychology and cognitive neuroscience, DL represents an easy to use technique to study brain asymmetry for phonetic processing (Kimura, 1961a, 1961b; Bryden, 1988; Hugdahl, 1995). In the dichotic listening situation, the subject is presented with, for example, the syllable /ba/ in the right ear, and simultaneously the syllable /da/ in the left ear, and required to report the one stimulus better perceived. The stimuli are typically computer-generated to allow for optimal synchronization between the output channels. Thus, the basic feature of the dichotic situation is to provide more elements to be processed at any moment in time than the brain is capable of. That is, more stimulus components are presented at the same time than can be consciously analyzed. The question then becomes which elements or components of the stimulus input will be selected (cf. Holender, 1986).

A typical finding in normal, right-handed, subjects is the so-called right ear advantage (REA), which means that more items are correctly reported from the right, compared to the left, ear. The REA in dichotic listening is inferred to reflect the linguistic specialization of the left hemisphere. Conversely, absence of an REA or a left ear advantage (LEA) may indicate a left temporal lobe dysfunction (Hugdahl, 1995). The DL technique has frequently been used in both adult and child neuropsychology, from the pioneering work by Kimura (1961a, 1961b) and Bryden (1963) to modern use of the DL technique in both basic brain science (Tervaniemi et al., 2000; Hugdahl et al., 1999) and clinical practice (Hugdahl & Carlsson, 1994; Hugdahl & Wester, 1992; Carlsson, et al., 1992; Roberts et al., 1990).

The explanation for the REA effect that has received most empirical support is the so-called structural, or neuroanatomical, model suggested by Kimura (1967; see also Sparks & Geschwind, 1968; Sidtis, 1988), which posits that the REA is caused by several interacting factors. First, the auditory input to the contralateral hemisphere is more strongly represented in the brain. Second, the left hemisphere (for right-handers) is specialized for language processing. Third, auditory information that is sent along the ipsilateral pathways is suppressed, or blocked, by the contralateral information. Fourth, information that reaches the ipsilateral right hemisphere has to be transferred cross the corpus callosum to the left hemisphere language-processing areas. A study by Pollmann et al. (2002) provides further support for the structural model. Pollmann et al. (2002) had patients with lesions in various portions of the corpus callosum (from the anterior genu to the posterior splenium) undergo testing with the Bergen DL test. It was found that patients with lesions in the posterior parts of the corpus callosum, including parts of the isthmus (where the auditory fibers cross over), showed an almost perfect left ear extinction effect, and a corresponding almost perfect 100% REA effect. This important study shows that the left ear stimulus is not processed in the right hemisphere but has to be transferred over the corpus callosum in order to be processed in the temporal lobe in the left hemisphere.

VALIDITY

It has been argued that dichotic listening lacks functional validity because it is sometimes hard to find correlations between dichotic listening and other laterality measures (like the visual half-field technique).

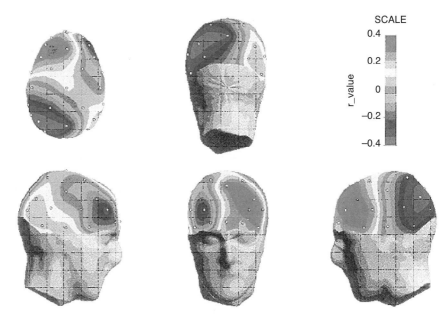

Figure 12.2 Correlation maps between EEG residualized alpha power and dichotic listening laterality index. (From Davidson & Hugdahl, 1996.)

However, auditory lateralization is probably not related to a single mechanism (cf. Jäncke & Steinmetz, 1993). This means that it should not be a surprise when dichotic listening shows low intercorrelations with other laterality tasks, like the visual half-field technique, since these tasks probably index different laterality modules. There is no such thing as *the* laterality function that can be assessed with whatever laterality task or test. Each hemisphere subserves multiple functions that need not correlate with each other. What should correlate, however, are measures of general activation of a hemisphere and tasks that tap specific functions within that hemisphere. This was exemplified in data reported by Davidson and Hugdahl (1996). It was found that the magnitude of the REA in the dichotic listening task significantly correlated with resting EEG asymmetry. Subjects with larger left than right EEG resting activation also had better recall from the right as compared to the left ear in dichotic listening (figure 12.2).

Hugdahl et al. (1997) attempted to validate the Bergen DL test against invasive injections of amobarbital (the Wada test; Wada & Rasmussen, 1960) in 13 children/adolescents who were to undergo surgical treatment for epilepsy. All subjects had symptomatic epilepsy with

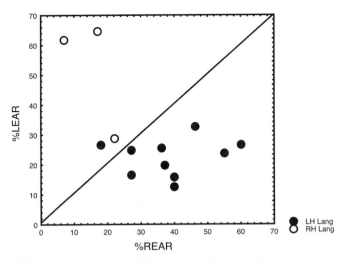

Figure 12.3 Scatter plot of dichotic listening performance in individuals with known language localization in either the right (open circles) or left (black circles) hemisphere, as determined from Wada testing. (From Hugdahl et al., 1997.)

partial seizures, and they were studied with the DL test both before and after surgery. The Wada test results before surgery revealed that 10 subjects had left hemisphere language, and 3 subjects had right hemisphere language. All 3 right hemisphere language subjects showed an LEA on the dichotic listening test, both pre- and postoperatively; 8 and 7 of the 10 left hemisphere dominant subjects showing an REA, pre- and postoperatively, respectively. Using a discriminant analysis, knowledge of the dichotic listening results led to correct classification according to the Wada test results in 92.31% of all subjects. Thus, a quantitative classification procedure like discriminant analysis may be even more sensitive when predicting hemisphere speech dominance from dichotic listening data than a qualitative procedure based solely on the ear advantage dichotomy, although both statistical procedures provided clear evidence for a correspondence between an invasive test and the DL test (figure 12.3).

THE BERGEN DL TEST

The stimuli used in the Bergen DL test are paired presentations of the six stop-consonants /b, d, g, p, t, k/ together with the vowel /a/ to form consonant-vowel (CV) syllable pairs of the type /ba-ga/, /ta-ka/, and so on. The syllables are paired for all possible combinations, thus yielding 36 dichotic pairs, including the homonymic pairs. The homonymic pairs are used as test trials, and are not included in the statistical analyses. The standard test consists of a CD that contains a digitized version of the stimuli, that can be played from any standard CD player or from a computer equipped with a CD unit. A computerized version also exists with each stimulus pair stored as audio files in the Wav format. The CD version of the Bergen DL test exists in English, Spanish, and German, in addition to all the Nordic languages except Icelandic. Each CV pair is recorded three times on the CD, with three different randomizations of the 36 basic pairs. Thus, the total number of trials on the CD is 108. The 108 trials are divided into 3×36 trial blocks, one trial block for each instructional condition: nonforced attention (NF), forced right (FR), and forced left (FL). (See below for details.) In some studies only the NF condition is used. For each condition, the analysis is based on 30 trials. Each subject is given a standardized set of instructions prior to the test.

You should listen to the six different sounds which are given on this page. (Show the six syllables on a page of paper.) After each presentation, you should repeat whichever sound you hear. Say the sound loud and clear directly after it has been presented. Sometimes it will seem as if you hear two different sounds at the same time. Don't worry about this, but say the sound you seemed to hear best or most clearly. Don't spend time thinking, but just repeat the sound as soon as it has been presented.

In some instances, such as when testing patients with expressive language difficulties, the experimenter asked the patient to point to a sheet of paper where the syllables were written in capital letters (e.g., Hugdahl et al., 1990).

The syllables are read by a male voice with constant intonation and intensity. Mean duration was approximately 350–400 ms, and the intertrial interval was about 4 s. The syllables were originally read through a microphone and digitized for computer editing on a computer equipped with a standard audio board. After digitization, each CV pair was edited for onset synchronization with the help of a standard audio editing software (Goldwave or Cool Edit).

In most of the studies reviewed in this chapter, the subjects were tested for differences between the ears in hearing acuity. Hearing thresholds were determined for each ear for the frequencies 500, 1000, 2000, 3000 and 5000 Hz. Subjects with larger threshold differences than

5 dB between the ears on any of the frequencies tested were excluded from the study. The 500 to 5000 Hz range was chosen because most of the spectral energy in the CV syllables is in this range.

The data presented were collected with a common procedure involving three different attentional instructions: nonforced (NF), forced right (FR), and forced left (FL). In the NF condition, which always is presented first so as not to confuse the subject, the subject is told that he/she will hear repeated presentations of the six CV syllables (ba, da, ga, pa, ta, ka), and that he/she should report which one he/she hears after each trial. The subjects are also told that "on some occasions there seems to be two sounds coming simultaneously." They should not bother about this, just report the one they hear first, or best. Subjects are instructed not to think about the syllables but to give the answer that spontaneously comes into their mind after each presentation. They are usually shown a cardboard sheet with all six syllables written before the experiment starts. They are advised that a single answer should be given on each trial, irrespective of whether they perceived one or both items. The main reason is that this procedure does not put the demands on short-term memory that a double-answer procedure would do, requiring that one item is held in memory while the subject answers with the other item (see Bryden, 1988 for a discussion of single versus double answers).

THE BERGEN DICHOTIC LISTENING DATABASE

Over the years, we have collected data with the CV syllables dichotic listening technique as described above from a large number of subjects. The Bergen Dichotic Listening Database[1] currently contains data from 1018 subjects ranging from 6 to 88 years of age, including both right- and left-handers, males and females. The Bergen database is based on data from many laboratories. All laboratories have used the same DL test, with the same instructions and scoring and analysis routines. What has differed between laboratories are the CD player and the type of headphones used. The database includes NF, FR, and FL attentional conditions. (The effects of attention on dichotic listening performance will be discussed later.)

A first series of analysis focused on the basic statistical properties with regard to ear advantage, effects of gender, handedness, and age, as well as comparing laterality index scores with analysis of the scores

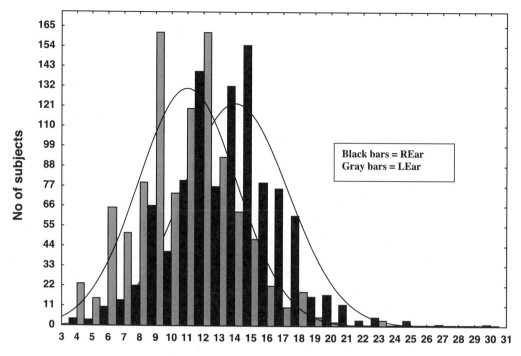

Figure 12.4 Histogram of number of subjects (y-axis) against number of correct reports (x-axis), separated for the right and left ear scores. N = 1018. Note the clear right shift of the distribution for the right ear scores.

from each ear separately. All analyses presented below were performed on the total sample (N = 1018), which included 825 right-handers and 193 left-handers.

The Ear Advantage

Figure 12.4 shows the distribution of subjects (y-axis) across the entire range of possible scores on the Bergen DL test (0–30) on the x-axis. A one-way analysis of variance with ear input as the dependent variable showed a highly significant effect of higher frequency of correct reports from the right compared with the left ear, $F(1,1017) = 338.76$, $p < .00001$. Thus, there was a highly significant REA effect in the total sample. Further analyses showed that 74% of the total sample showed an REA, with 20% showing an LEA, and 6% without a clear ear advantage (NEA, no ear advantage). Figure 12.4 shows that the distributions with

Table 12.1 Mean correct reports from the right and left ears

	A. Nonforced attention		B. Forced-right attention		C. Forced-left attention	
	Right ear	Left ear	Right ear	Left ear	Right ear	Left ear
Males	13.98	11.09	16.36	8.61	11.12	13.29
Females	14.00	10.87	16.58	8.45	10.68	14.01
Right-handers	14.01	10.71	18.00	8.53	13.52	14.97
Left-handers	13.92	12.13	16.33	8.51	10.91	10.85

regard to both right and left ear performance are fairly normal, but with a clear shift to the right for the right ear scores.

Effects of Gender

Table 12.1 shows the effects of gender when comparing performance for the males and females in the nonforced, forced-right, and forced-left attention situations. There were 483 males and 535 females in the total sample. As is obvious from panel A there are no significant sex effects. Actually, the two sexes have almost identical scores from both the right and left ears. Both sexes showed, however, a significant REA. Furthermore, there were no significant interactions with handedness or age. Thus, there are no sex differences in the Bergen DL test.

Effects of Handedness

Table 12.1, panel A also shows right and left ear performance when separating the total sample into right-handers (N = 825) and left-handers (N = 193). Both groups showed a significant REA. However, there was a significant two-way interaction between ear input and handedness, $F(1,1016) = 13.17$, $p < .0003$. The interaction was caused by a significantly higher mean left ear score in the left-handed group, thus reducing the magnitude of the REA in this group. It is interesting to note the almost complete overlap of the right ear scores for the two groups. Thus, the left-handers showed a reduction in the REA compared with the right-handed group, caused by a significant increase in number of items reported from the left ear.

Figure 12.5 shows a scatter plot of the data for the right- and left-handers. Number of correct reports from the right ear are shown along

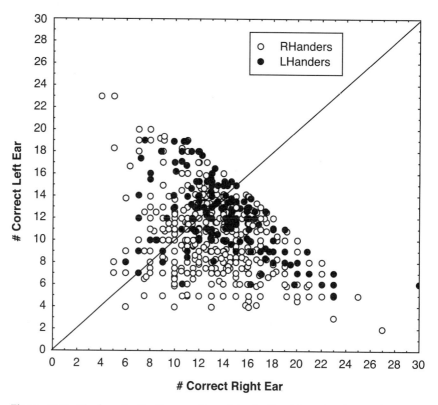

Figure 12.5 Nonforced attention: scatter plot of all subjects in the total database (N = 1018). Note the 45° symmetry-line. All subjects below the line show an REA; all subjects above the line show an LEA. Right-handers: open dots, left-handers: black dots. NB: Each dot may contain overlapping values from several individuals.

the x-axis, and number of correct reports from the left ear along the y-axis. Each dot in the scatter plot represents a single individual (some dots may cover several individuals occupying the same x and y coordinates). The diagonal line represents the 45^0 symmetry line (cf. Hugdahl, 1995). All individuals falling below the symmetry line by definition show an REA; all individuals falling above the symmetry line similarly show an LEA; and all individuals falling on the line show an NEA. Figure 12.5 shows that the left-handers (black dots) clustered toward the mid region of the scatter plot while the right-handers had a more widespread distribution within the response space provided by the scattergram.

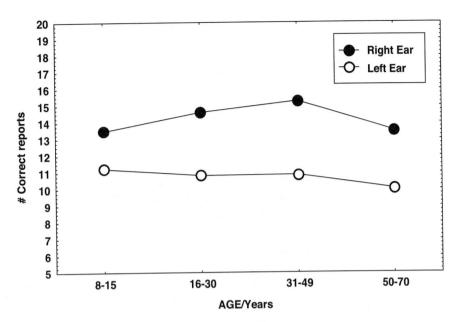

Figure 12.6 Nonforced attention: Effects of age.

Effects of Age

Figure 12.6 shows performance on the DL test split for four age groups (8–15, 16–30, 31–49, 50–70 years). All age groups showed a significant REA. However, there was also a significant interaction between age and ear input $F(3,1014) = 8.32$, $p < .0000$. The interaction was due to an increase in the REA with increasing age up to the 31–49 group, with a decline in the oldest group. The increase in the REA was entirely due to better performance on the right ear stimulus with increasing age. Thus, a clear age effect was seen in the data with optimal performance in the adult groups below the age of 50. (Note that there are different group sizes in the various age groups.)

Laterality Index

A laterality index was calculated on the total sample according to the formula [(REar − LEar)/(REar + LEar)]*100. A positive index would thus indicate an REA, while a negative index would indicate an LEA.

The laterality index for the right-handers was 17.61, and for the left-handers 6.52. The difference was statistically significant. Thus, the right-handers showed a much more marked laterality effect on the Bergen DL test compared with the left-handers. No interactions with sex was observed.

FORCED-RIGHT ATTENTION

A similar analysis as was done for the NF condition was performed for the FR condition. The sample was, however, reduced to 656 subjects, since not all subjects in the total sample had been tested with the FR and FL attention conditions.

The Ear Advantage

There was a significant increase of the REA during the FR condition, with a laterality index of 30.84 during it, compared to 15.52 during the NF condition, collapsing both right- and left-handers.

Effects of Gender

Table 12.1, panel B, shows the data split for gender. As with the NF condition, there were no significant effects of gender; males and females performed almost identically with respect to both the right and left ear reports.

Effects of Handedness

Table 12.1, panel B, also shows the effect of handedness. Although there was a tendency for a larger REA for the right-handers, the difference betwenn the handedness groups was not significant. No other effects of handedness on the ability to shift attention to the right ear was found.

Effects of Age

Figure 12.7 shows the effect of age on the ability to shift attention to the right ear. As with the NF condition, there was again a significant two-way interaction between age and ear input. The interaction was due to an increase in correct reports from the right ear stimulus with increas-

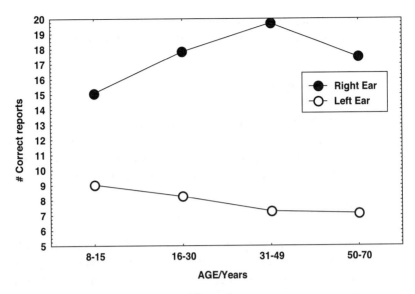

Figure 12.7 Forced-right attention: Effects of age.

ing age up to the age of 50; then there was a decline in the oldest group. All groups showed an REA, and the REA was overall larger than the corresponding REA during the NF condition, caused by more correct reports from the right ear during the FR condition compared with the NF condition.

FORCED-LEFT ATTENTION

The Ear Advantage

During the FL attention condition, the ear advantage was shifted to a significant left ear advantage (LEA), thus showing a clear effect of top-down attention to change an REA to an LEA as a consequence of active effort to monitor only the left ear stimulus. The laterality index during the FL condition was −10.08, which was significantly different from the laterality index during the NF (+15.54) and FR (+30.84) conditions.

Effects of Gender

The effects of gender are seen in table 12.1, panel C. As for the other two attentional conditions, there was no clear effect of gender, although

Dichotic Listening and Auditory Laterality

there was a tendency for the females to have more correct reports from the left ear, and fewer reports from the right ear, compared with the males.

Effects of Handedness

Table 12.1, panel C, shows the effect of handedness during the FL condition. The left-handed subjects had a tendency, although non-significant, to report more items from the left ear compared with the right-handers in the overall analysis of variance.

Effects of Age

Figure 12.8 shows the effect of age with regard to the ability to shift attention to the left ear stimulus. There was a highly significant two-way interaction between age and ear input, with the youngest and oldest age groups being unable to reverse to a significant LEA. All the other age groups showed a significant LEA with follow-up tests ($p < .05$).

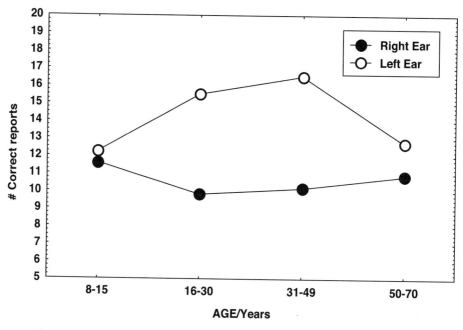

Figure 12.8 Forced-left attention: Effects of age.

VIGILANCE AND ATTENTION

Based on a large set of empirical findings, it could be argued that dichotic listening is a method also for the study of both bottom-up (stimulus driven) and top-down (instruction-driven) information processing. A synonym for bottom-up processing is "automatic" processing, versus "controlled" processing, which sometimes is used as a synonym for top-down processing. In the present context, I will denote this as "stimulus-driven" versus "instruction-driven" laterality effects. The basic idea is that certain stimuli are directly processed in specialized areas of the brain without conscious recollection or attentional awareness, while other stimuli, or stimulus settings, require allocation of attentional resources in order to be processed. An example of automatic processing is the REA typically found in DL studies in response to speech stimuli (see Bryden 1988; Hugdahl, 1995 for reviews). The neurological basis for the REA may be the anatomical asymmetry found in the planum temporale area in the superior temporal gyrus (Steinmetz et al., 1989), where the left side is larger than the right side. This may provide a biological foundation for the automatic perception of speech stimuli in the left side of the brain, which in turn causes the right ear advantage. If the subject, however, is required to focus attention to either the right or the left ear, the "stimulus-driven" REA can be either increased or decreased (sometimes shifted to an LEA), depending on which ear the subject is instructed to attend (Asbjørnsen & Hugdahl, 1995). Similarly, Mondor and Bryden (1991) showed that presenting an auditory cue in either the left or right ear a few milliseconds before the dichotic stimuli also affects the ear advantage on a trial-by-trial basis, by having the subject shift attention between the ears from trial to trial.

The change in ear advantage as a function of shifting attention to the left or right ear is illustrated in figure 12.9 and plate 10, illustrated for the forced right condition only, for the sake of simplicity. The increase in the right ear advantage seen in the FR condition is mainly caused by a decrease in the left ear score, rather than an increase in the right ear score. Thus, the effect of attention on dichotic listening performance is to inhibit, or suppress, the processing of the irrelevant signal, thereby increasing the overall right-left difference.

A similar result was found by Asbjørnsen and Hugdahl (1995) when instructing the subjects to focus attention to either the right or the left

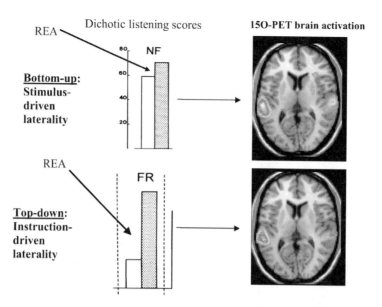

Dichotic listening scores

15O-PET brain activation

REA

NF

Bottom-up:
Stimulus-
driven
laterality

REA

FR

Top-down:
Instruction-
driven
laterality

Figure 12.9 Parallel behavior and brain activation (PET) effects during nonforced and forced-right attention conditions. See plate 10 for color version.

ear. The major finding was that the changes in ear advantage after forced attention was based on a suppression of the nonattended ear score, combined with a smaller facilitation of the attended ear scores. This is a somewhat surprising finding, considering that it would be more natural to have expected the effect of selective processing to result in at least a small gain in the total amount of information processed, and thus reported under the DL condition. However, several other studies have presented similar data, with a possible suppression effect. A closer inspection of the findings by Bryden et al. (1983) shows that the results support an interpretation of suppression of the nonattended ear input as the basic effect. Moreover, Obrzut and Boliek (1988), and Hugdahl and Anderson (1986) showed a suppression effect of attentional instructions in their studies on children. Thus, giving instructions to the subject to direct attention to either ear input basically will have the effect of inhibiting intrusive errors from the irrelevant, nonfocused signal. A possible explanation for this may be through blocking of the ipsilateral pathways of the nonattended channel. Blocking of the ipsilateral pathway from the nonattended channel will result in reduction of information passing through from the nonattended ear, and thus cause a suppression effect.

Figure 12.9 also shows that there is a corresponding change in the local distribution of cerebral blood flow in the superior temporal gyrus on the right and left sides. The PET-data presented to the right in figure 12.9 (and plate 10) are from Hugdahl et al. (2000) and show that the increase in the REA during the FR as a consequence of response suppression is accompanied by a corresponding decrease in blood flow on the right side, rather than an increase in blood flow on the left side. Thus, there seems to be a physiological mechanism that resembles the change observed at the behavioral level. It may be speculated whether the suppression effect is related to the functioning of the corpus callosum, in the sense that the irrelevant, nonattended signal is filtered when traversing the corpus callosum from the nonattended ear. Such an explanation is partly supported by an analysis of the correlations between the left and right ear scores during the three attentional conditions. If the nonattended ear stimulus is inhibited from being processed in the left hemisphere (and no processing occurs in the right hemisphere), one would expect the correlations between the left and right ear scores to become more negative compared to the NF condition.

This was studied by correlating the left and right ear scores for all three attentional conditions from the data in the Bergen Dichotic Listening Database. During the NF condition, the correlation was $-.30$. During the FR and FL conditions the correlations increased to $-.80$ ($p < .05$) and $-.84$ ($p < .05$), respectively, for the FR and FL attention conditions. Again, there were no significant differences between the sexes; both males and females showed the same basic suppression effect. However, children showed a much smaller correlation effect compared with the adults, indicating that children at the age of 8–9 years of age lack the ability to actively suppress a stimulus-driven laterality effect that is caused by speech stimuli such as CV syllables. Thus, the better the right ear stimulus was processed, the less was the left ear stimulus processed, and vice versa, during the FR and FL attention conditions. During the NF condition, the right ear stimulus was processed more or less independently of the processing of the left ear stimulus, indicating a bottom-up, stimulus-driven laterality effect from the right ear signal. The different age groups, however, contributed to the reduced correlation in the NF condition.

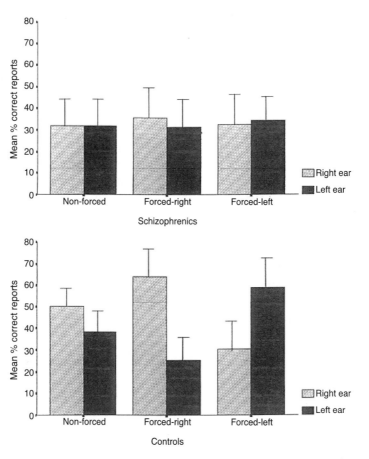

Figure 12.10 Mean percentage correct reports (small bars = SD) in schizophrenic and control subjects, for the NF, FR, and FL attention conditions. (From Løberg et al., 1999.)

APPLICATIONS TO SCHIZOPHRENIA

Applying the model of dichotic listening as an indicator of automatic versus controlled processing, Løberg et al. (1999) showed that schizophrenic patients suffered from both automatic and controlled processing skills, which the authors named "a dual deficits" model for the study of neurocognitive deficits in schizophrenia. This is shown in figure 12.10. The subjects were 33 schizophrenic inpatients and 33 healthy comparison subjects with the same age, handedness, and gender distribution as the patient subjects. The standard variant of the Bergen DL test was used, with the three attentional instructions: the nonforced, the forced-right, and the forced-left.

The results showed an absence of the expected right ear advantage in the schizophrenic group during the nonforced attention condition, and a failure to modify DL performance through shifting of attention to either the right or the left ear. The comparison group showed a right ear advantage during the nonforced and forced-right attention conditions (increased right ear advantage during the forced-right condition), and a left ear advantage during the forced-left attention condition. Thus, the schizophrenic group showed both impairment of left hemisphere processing of the CV syllable stimuli, and impairment of the ability to recruit cognitive processes to restore the impaired bottom-up laterality function (figure 12.10). Some recent data from our laboratory have, however, shown that this occurs only in chronic, older patients.

APPLICATIONS TO BRAIN LESIONED PATIENTS

Preliminary data suggest that the attentional modulation of an REA to the CV syllables also may involve frontal lobe functions. Recent functional brain imaging data (e.g., Posner et al., 1988) have shown that Broca's area in the left frontal lobe is also activated when listening to speech sounds. Thus, it may be hypothesized that left frontal lobe damage may affect the REA in the dichotic listening situation. Left frontal lobe patients may, furthermore, be more impaired on such tests than right frontal lobe patients, which would follow from left hemisphere language dominance.

The patients were inpatients of the University Clinic of Neurology, Innsbruck, Austria, in collaboration with Thomas Benke. Inclusion criteria were CT- or MR-documented frontal lesion and the absence of significant coexisting neurological or psychiatric disease or substance abuse. Moreover, the patients could not have aphasia or major hearing loss, and they should have the necessary physical and concentration ability to participate in testing for 1–2 hours. Twenty-six frontal lobe damaged patients, most of them in their chronic state, fulfilled the inclusion criteria and gave their informed consent to participating in the study.

Sixteen subjects had lesions in the left frontal lobe and 10 subjects had lesions in the right frontal lobe. Five of the patients had bilateral lesions, however, with a clearly leading pathology on one side (either

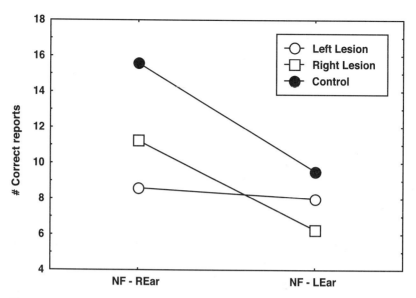

Figure 12.11 Mean correct reports for the NF attention conditions, separated for left and right frontal lesion patients. (Data obtained in collaboration with Thomas Benke, University of Innsbruck, Austria.)

left or right). Handedness was assessed using the Edinburgh Handedness Inventory (Oldfield, 1971). Premorbid IQ was estimated using a multiple choice vocabulary test.

The results showed that the patients with left-side lesions failed to show the expected REA during the nonforced attention condition. The right frontal lobe lesioned patients were overall reduced in their performance compared to a healthy control group. However, they showed an REA similar to the control group (figure 12.11).

The left frontal lobe patients also showed evidence of a dual-deficit, involving impairment of both stimulus processing and attentional modulation, while the right frontal patients showed evidence of impairment of attentional modulation only when their FR and FL performance scores were analyzed as well (data not shown in the figure). Thus, the left frontal cortex seems to be involved in both the bottom-up and top-down analysis of the stimulus, while the right frontal cortex is involved only in the top-down modulation. The frontal lobes obviously are also involved in the organization of language perception, and not only in speech output as previously demonstrated (see Stuss & Benson, 1984 for review), possibly through frontotemporal association fibers. The results from the frontal lobe patients thus seem to lend themselves to an interpretation of dichotic listening as tapping into a neuronal circuitry that also involves the frontal lobes. Thus, dichotic listening is not an exclusive test of temporal lobe function (cf. Spreen & Strauss, 1991).

To sum up this section, it is suggested that the dichotic listening method taps several other neurocognitive functions besides the "classic" laterality function, and that these other functions relate to attention, arousal, and higher cognitive processes. It is also suggested that the DL method may tap frontal lobe function, possibly related to the role played by the frontal lobes in speech perception and the receptive aspects of language processing. Hemodynamic neuroimaging methods have shown increased activation in the prefrontal cortex during word generation tasks (e.g., Posner et al., 1988; Petersen et al., 1988). In a PET study, Frith et al. (1991) found significantly increased blood flow in Brodmann area 46 in the dorsolateral prefrontal cortex during covert word generation. Thus, the frontal lobes seems to be involved in the initiation of both language and divergent thinking (cf. Stuss & Benson, 1984).

TEMPORAL LOBE FUNCTION AND MEMORY PROCESSING

The Bergen DL test has also been used in various other clinical populations (e.g., Bø et al., 1989; Carlsson et al., 1992; Hugdahl et al., 1990; Cohen et al., 1992; Green et al., 1994; Hugdahl & Wester, 1994; Reinvang et al., 1994; Løberg et al., 1999; Cacioppo et al., 2000). In addition, Hugdahl et al. (1990) developed a dichotic memory test based on a study by Christianson et al. (1987) with lists of 10 common nouns being presented dichotically, with the reversed word played in one ear and the correct word played in the other ear. After each list the subject had to recall as many words as possible. The reversed and correct words alternated between the left and right ear on successive lists.

The dichotic memory test has been applied to various neurological and neurosurgical patient groups (see Hugdahl & Wester, 2000 for review). In a first study (Hugdahl et al., 1993), the lateralized memory test was used to study memory impairment in patients with Parkinson's disease (PD). The PD patients were studied for memory performance before they were subjected to surgery, and compared to age-matched nondemented, and younger control subjects (19–30 years). Thus, both effects of age and PD could be evaluated in the same study. The age-matched controls were screened with a shortened version of the Mini Mental State (MMS) test, and had to show a score of 17 or higher, with a maximum of 21 (excluding the last item in the MMS). By using a memory version of the dichotic listening procedure, it could be evaluated whether the PD patients were more impaired for left or right ear stimulus presentations, and this could be compared to whether they had predominantly left- or right-sided symptomatology. We argued that if PD patients have a deficit in verbal memory (e.g., Sagar et al., 1988; Saint-Cyr et al., 1988), they should be particularly vulnerable to right ear (left hemisphere) word presentations. Finally, we compared performance on the early, middle, and late portions of the word lists, plotting the data according to serial position effects.

There were 21 patients with idiopathic PD and 64 neurologically intact controls. There were 32 subjects in each of the two control groups. In the PD group, 14 patients were males and 7 were females. Mean age for the PD patients was 67 years (range = 52–73 years). All subjects were tested for normal hearing with a standard screening audiometer. In order to be included in the study, each subject had to correctly identify the stimulus with a minimum of 20 dB for the frequency range 500–4000 Hz. They also were not allowed to have a difference in detection between the ears of more than 5 dB.

There were three versions of the memory test (to prevent learning effects). The ear to which the words were presented alternated between lists; thus there were three lists with the words presented to the right ear (and consequently the reversed words presented to the left ear), and three lists with the words presented to the left ear. Order of presentation of the lists was counterbalanced across subjects. The stimuli were read at a rate of one word every 2 seconds.

There was a significant effect of group, with the PD patients overall performing worst, followed by the age-matched controls, and the youngest subjects performing best. There was also a strong serial position effect in all three groups. More items were recalled from the early and late portions of the list, compared to the middle portion. There was, however, no interaction with group. Finally, no significant effects of laterality was observed, although the PD patients had a tendency for impaired reports from the left compared with the right ear, particularly for the last items in the lists. It was concluded that PD clearly manifest a short-term memory deficit that is not explained by age alone, since the PD patients also were significantly reduced in their recall of the items compared with the healthy age-matched group.

ARACHNOID CYSTS

A second application of the dichotic memory test has been to patients with arachnoid cysts, particularly patients with cysts in the left temporal lobe (see Wester & Hugdahl, 1995). The mechanisms underlying arachnoid cysts are far from clear. The intracranial pressure is seldom raised enough for reduced tissue perfusion to be the mechanism underlying loss of function. Since clinical improvement may occur following decompression, it would seem likely that the neurological deficit is related to processes which, while impairing neuronal function, do not necessarily result in cell death. Arachnoid cysts are thought to be due to a maldevelopment of the cerebral meninges (Starkman et al. 1958). They may be present at birth or develop soon after. After an initial growth in early life, most cysts are believed to remain stable over many years, having reached a permanent size that may well be substantial. Very few cysts have been reported to disappear spontaneously. Moreover, some seem to continue to grow in adult life, though rather slowly. The symptoms associated with arachnoid cysts vary according to the site of the lesion and the neural structures surrounding them. In adults, subjective complaints such as headache and dizziness are common. Major neurological symptoms such as motor or sensory deficits, epilepsy, or language problems may also occur, although they are often slight and tend to develop late in life. The lack of dramatic symptoms, even in patients with large arachnoid cysts, probably reflects the brain's ability to compensate for the presence of a slowly growing or stable expansion. A clear majority of the patients have the cyst localized to the middle cranial fossa (Rengachary & Watanabe, 1981), with a clear preference for left side localization (Wester et al., 1999).

It is unclear what, if any, cognitive deficits are caused by arachnoid cysts. It may, however, be hypothesized that if most cysts grow in the left perisylvian region, possibly affecting left temporal lobe development, typical left hemisphere functions may be affected, including hippocampal function. This was addressed in the study by Wester and Hugdahl (1995) where we applied the dichotic memory technique to six adult patients who were successfully operated on for arachnoid cysts in the left temporal fossa. Before surgery, the expected REA was absent in the memory test. Surgical treatment of the cysts with internal shunting procedures led to clinical improvement. It was also associated with a rapid normalization of the dichotic memory test, with a postoperative

REA and enhanced overall memory performance. These ameliorations appeared shortly after the operation, in some cases within hours. The results indicate that arachnoid cysts in the left temporal fossa may impair cognitive functions, and that neuropsychological tests may be necessary to reveal these impairments. A dramatic improvement was recorded shortly after surgery, even after many years of functional impairment. It is concluded that test batteries for cognitive functions should be developed and routinely included in the preoperative assessment of patients with middle fossa arachnoid cysts. This may broaden the indications for operative treatment of these cysts.

INTERHEMISPHERIC INTEGRATION AND CALLOSAL FUNCTION

As stated at the opening of this chapter, dichotic listening may reveal aspects of callosal transfer of information, and hence callosal functioning. This has been elaborated in detail in a recent paper by Hugdahl (in press), and will be summarized in the present chapter. The classic anatomical model for the explanation of the ear advantage in DL (Kimura, 1967) predicts that the left ear score should be positively correlated with efficiency of callosal transfer (see also Clarke et al., 1993). In other words, the size of callosal area should correlate positively with left ear performance, particularly for the posterior sectors of the corpus callosum. The reason for this is that the left ear score has to be transferred across the corpus callosum from the right to the left hemisphere in order to be processed, following recent data (e.g., Pollmann et al., 2002) that the right hemisphere does little, if any, processing of the left ear stimulus. Callosal transfer was investigated by Clarke et al. (1993), who determined callosal area size from magnetic resonance images where the callosum was sectioned into five areas in the rostral to caudal axis. The dichotic listening procedure involved manual identification (pointing) of left and right ear presentations of the CV syllables [bee, dee, gee, pee, tee, kee]. Clarke et al. only included a nonforced attention (divided attention) condition, with no specific instructions to focus attention to either side in space. The results showed the expected significant right ear advantage, with about 55% correctly identified items from the right ear, and 45% correctly identified items from the left ear. Importantly for the present discussion, callosum area did not correlate with left ear performance, that is, the expected positive correlation between larger callosal area size and better left ear reports was not found. Instead, they found that right ear performance was negatively correlated with callosum size, which was explained with reference to functional interhemispheric inhibition.

In the Hugdahl (in press) paper, a two-channel threshold model of callosal transfer was suggested that also included transfer of attentional resources (see also Hugdahl, 1998). The model is empirically founded on the results in Reinvang et al. (1994) on the relationship between callosal sector size and left ear performance in multiple sclerosis (MS) patients. The corpus callosum often shows atrophic changes in MS patients, and measures of the corpus callosum are often included in the diagnosis of this disease. The study by Reinvang et al. (1994) were similar to the Clarke et al. (1993) study in that both used the CV syllables dichotic listening test. However, Reinvang et al. had their subjects undergo a magnetic resonance imaging investigation, and images from the corpus callosum were analyzed for callosal size (dividing the corpus callosum into four different sectors along the rostral-caudal axis). The results showed a significant right ear advantage in both the MS patients and a healthy control group during the NF condition. The findings for the left ear scores during the NF condition were quite similar to the Clarke et al. (1993) results, with no correlation between the left ear scores and callosal size. However, when the subjects were instructed to focus their attention to the left ear, the correlations between left ear performance and callosal size were clearly significant, particularly for the three most posterior sectors (including the auditory sector just anterior to the splenium where the auditory fibers pass).

From this Hugdahl (1998) suggested that an attention amplification factor was needed in order to enhance callosal transfer of the left ear score. More specifically, this may indicate the existence of a two-channel threshold model of callosal transfer with a sensory modality-specific channel involving the large-diameter myelinated fibers, and a diffuse sensory, nonspecific channel involving the small-diameter non-myelinated fibers that are responsible for transfer of cognitive information. The model may act in a thresholded way in the sense that in many instances the recruitment of the cognitive channel may not be necessary, the sensory channel being enough for efficient transfer. However, in situations of increasing cognitive load (as in the "cocktail party" situation), or when the callosum may be degenerated (as in the case of the MS patient), attention may be recruited to facilitate or amplify the sensory transfer. The point is that attention may be recruited only when the sensory transfer falls below a threshold value which defines the interaction between different means of information transfer across the callosum (cf. Kinsbourne, 1974, discussing cognitive factors in callosal functioning).

SUMMARY AND CONCLUSIONS

In the present chapter I have reviewed new data from our laboratory on the use of dichotic listening as a vehicle to study auditory laterality. A new database with 1018 subjects has been established at the University of Bergen that includes such factors as handedness, gender, and age. The database also contains data on shifting of attention to either the right or the left ear. The general findings are that dichotic listening with CV syllables yields a robust right ear advantage that is modulated by attention, either increasing or decreasing the right ear advantage depending on which side attention is focused on. There were significant handedness and age effects in the data, but no sex effects were observed. Dichotic listening is discussed in relation to four specific topics in laterality research: asymmetry for speech perception and phonology, temporal lobe function, attention, and interhemispheric integration. It is concluded that dichotic listening may be a valuable tool for investigating not only language function in the two hemispheres but also top-down modulation of a stimulus-driven laterality, as well as callosal function.

ACKNOWLEDGMENTS

The present research was financially supported by grants from the Norwegian Research Council and from Innovest/Haukeland University Hospital, Bergen, Norway. The contributions of Ian Law, Thomas Benke, Kolbjørn Brønnick, Stefan Pollman, Michael Green, Knut Wester, Else Marie Løberg, Ivar Reinuang, Göran Carlsson, and Astri Lundervold are gratefully acknowledged.

NOTE

1. A CD version of the Bergen DL test with manual and more detailed psychometric properties of the test can be obtained from the author or from Psykologiförlaget AB in Stockholm, Sweden, which has acquired the marketing rights for the Bergen DL test in Scandinavia. The database is regularly updated and the latest version (May 2002) contains data from 1466 subjects.

REFERENCES

Asbjørnsen, A., & Hugdahl, K. (1995). Attentional effects in dichotic listening. *Brain and Language, 49*, 189–201.

Asbjørnsen, A., Hugdahl, K., & Hynd, G. W. (1990). The effects of head- and eye-turns on the right ear advantage in dichotic listening. *Brain and Language, 39*, 447–458.

Beaton, A. A. (1997). The relation of planum temporale asymmetry and morphology of the corpus callosum to handedness, gender, and dyslexia: A review of the evidence. *Brain and Language, 60*, 255–322.

Binder, J. R., Frost, J. A., Hammeke, T. A., Bellgowan, P. S. F., Springer, J. A., Kaufman, J. N., & Possing, E. T. (2000). Human temporal lobe activation by speech and non-speech sounds. *Cerebral Cortex, 10*, 512–528.

Binder, J. R., Frost, J. A., Hammeke, T. A., Rao, S. M., & Cox, R. W. (1996). Function of the left planum temporale in auditory and linguistic processing. *Brain, 119*, 1239–1247.

Bishop, K. M., & Wahlsten, D. (1997). Sex differences in the human corpus callosum: Myth or reality? *Neuroscience and Biobehavioral Reviews, 21*, 581–601.

Bø, O., Hugdahl, K., & Marklund, E. (1989). Dichotic listening in children with serious language problems. *Perceptual and Motor Skills, 68*, 1291–1301.

Bryden, M. P. (1963). Ear preference in auditory perception. *Journal of Experimental Psychology, 65*, 103–105.

Bryden, M. P. (1988). An overview of the dichotic listening procedure and its relation to cerebral organization. In K. Hugdahl (Ed.), *Handbook of dichotic listening: Theory, methods, and reseaarch* (pp. 1–44). Chichester, UK: John Wiley & Sons.

Bryden, M. P., Munhall, K., & Allard, F. (1983). Attentional biases and the right-ear effect in dichotic listening. *Brain and Language, 18*, 236–248.

Cacioppo, J. T., Ernst, J. M., Burleson, M. H., McClintock, M. K., Malarkey, W. B., Hawkley, L. C., Kowalewski, R. B., Paulsen, A., Hobson, J. A., Hugdahl, K., Spiegel, D., & Berntson, G. G. (2000). Lonely traits and concomitant physiological processes: The MacArthur social neuroscience studies. *International Journal of Psychophysiology, 35*, 143–154.

Carlsson, G., Hugdahl, K., Uvebrant, P., Wiklund, L., & von Wendt, L. (1992). Pathological handedness revisited: Dichotic listening in left vs. right congenital hemiplegia children. *Neuropsychologia, 30*, 471–481.

Christianson, S. Å., Nilsson, L., & Silfvenius, H. (1987). Initial memory deficits and subsequent recovery in two cases of head trauma. *Scandinavian Journal of Psychology, 28*, 267–280.

Clarke, J. M., Lufkin, R. B., & Zaidel, E. (1993). Corpus callosum morphometry and dichotic listening performance: Individual differences in functional interhemispheric inhibition. *Neuropsychologia, 31*, 547–557.

Cohen, M., Hynd, G. W., & Hugdahl, K. (1992). Dichotic listening performance in subtypes of developmental dyslexia and a left temporal lobe brain tumor contrast group. *Brain and Language*, *42*, 187–202.

Cowell, P., & Hugdahl, K. (2000). Individual differences in neurobehavioral measures of laterality and interhemispheric function as measured by dichotic listening. *Developmental Neuropsychology*, *18*, 95–112.

Davidson, R. J., & Hugdahl, K. (1996). Brain asymmetry in brain electrical activity predicts dichotic listening performance. *Neuropsychology*, *10*, 241–246.

Davidson, R. J., & Hugdahl, K. (Eds.) (1995). *Brain asymmetry*. Cambridge, MA: MIT Press.

Foundas, A. L., Leonard, C. M., Gilmore, R., Fennell, E. B., & Heilman, K. M. (1994). Planum temporale asymmetry and language dominance. *Neuropsychologia*, *32*, 1225–1231.

Frith, C. D., Friston, K. J., Liddle, P. F., & Frackowiak, R. S. J. (1991). A PET study of word finding. *Neuropsychologia*, *29*, 1137–1148.

Galaburda, A. M. (1995). Anatomical basis of cerebral dominance. In R. J. Davidson & K. Hugdahl (Eds.), *Brain asymmetry* (pp. 51–73). Cambridge, MA: MIT Press.

Gazzaniga, M. (2000). Cerebral specialization and interhemispheric communication— Does the corpus callosum enable the human condition? *Brain*, *123*, 1293–1326.

Geschwind, N., & Levitsky, W. (1968). Left-right asymmetries in temporal speech region. *Science*, *161*, 186–187.

Green, M. F., Hugdahl, K., & Mitchell, S. (1994). Dichotic listening during auditory hallucinations in schizophrenia. *American Journal of Psychiatry*, *151*, 357–362.

Hiscock, M., Inch, R., Jacek, C., Hiscock-Kalil, C., & Kalil, K. M. (1994). Is there a sex difference in human laterality? I. An exhaustive survey of auditory laterality studies from six neuropsychology journals. *Journal of Clinical and Experimental Neuropsychology*, *16*, 423–435.

Holender, D. (1986). Semantic activation without conscious identification in dichotic listening, parafoveal vision, and visual masking: A survey and appraisal. *Behavioral and Brain Sciences*, *9*, 1–66.

Hugdahl, K. (1995). Dichotic listening: Probing temporal lobe functional integrity. In R. J. Davidson & K. Hugdahl (Eds.), *Brain asymmetry* (pp. 123–156). Cambridge MA: MIT Press.

Hugdahl, K. (1997). Brain lateralization: Dichotic listening studies. In *Encyclopedia of Neuroscience*. Elsevier Science, Electronic CD version.

Hugdahl, K. (1998). The corpus callosum: More than a "passive corpus." *Behavioral and Brain Sciences*, *21*, 335. (Commentary.)

Hugdahl, K. (in press). Attentional modulation of interhemispheric transfer of auditory information: A "two-channel threshold" model. In E. Zaidel & M. Iacoboni (Eds.), *The parallel brain: The cognitive neuroscience of the corpus callosum*. Cambridge, MA: MIT Press.

Hugdahl, K., & Andersson, L. (1986). The "forced-attention paradigm" in dichotic listening to CV-syllables: A comparison between adults and children. *Cortex, 22,* 417–432.

Hugdahl, K., Law, I., Kyllingsbaek, S., Brønnick, K., Gade, A., & Paulson, O. B. (2000). Effects of attention on dichotic listening: An 15O-PET study. *Human Brain Mapping, 10,* 87–97.

Hugdahl, K., Asbjørnsen, A., & Wester, K. (1993). Memory performance in Parkinson's disease. *Neuropsychiatry, Neuropsychology, and Behavioral Neurology, 6,* 170–176.

Hugdahl, K., Brønnick, K., Law, I., Kyllingsbaek, S., & Paulson, O. B. (1999). Brain activation during dichotic presentations of consonant-vowel and musical instruments stimuli: A 15O-PET study. *Neuropsychologia, 37,* 431–440.

Hugdahl, K., & Carlsson, G. (1994). Dichotic listening and focused attention in children with hemiplegic cerebral palsy. *Journal of Clinical and Experimental Neuropsychology, 16,* 84–92.

Hugdahl, K., Carlsson, G., Uvebrant, P., & Lundervold, A. J. (1997). Dichotic listening performance and intracarotid amobarbital injections in children/adolescents: Comparisons pre- and post-operatively. *Archives of Neurology, 54,* 1494–1500.

Hugdahl, K., & Wester, K. (1992). Dichotic listening studies of brain asymmetry in brain damaged patients. *International Journal of Neuroscience, 63,* 17–29.

Hugdahl, K., & Wester, K. (1994). Auditory neglect and the ear extinction effect in dichotic listening: A reply to Beaton & McCarthy. (1993). *Brain and Language, 46,* 166–173.

Hugdahl, K., & Wester, K. (2000). Neurocognitive correlates of stereotactic thalamotomy and thalamic stimulation in Parkinson patients. *Brain and Cognition, 42,* 231–252.

Hugdahl, K., Wester, K., & Asbjørnsen, A. (1990). The role of the left and right thalamus in language asymmetry: Dichotic listening in Parkinson-patients undergoing stereotactic thalamotomy. *Brain and Language, 39,* 1–13.

Ide, A., Dolezal, C., Fernandez, M., Labbe, E., Mandujano, R., Montes, S., Segura, P., Verschae, G., Yarmuch, P., & Aboitz, F. (1999). Hemispheric differences in variability of fissural patterns in perasylvian and cingulate regions of human brains. *Journal of Comparative Neurology, 410,* 235–242.

Jäncke, L., Schlaug, G., Huang, Y., & Steinmetz, H. (1994). Asymmetry of the planum parietale. *NeuroReport, 5,* 1161–1163.

Jäncke, L., & Steinmetz, H. (1993). Auditory lateralization and planum temporale asymmetry. *NeuroReport, 5,* 169–172.

Kimura, D. (1961a). Cerebral dominance and the perception of verbal stimuli. *Canadian Journal of Psychology, 15,* 166–171.

Kimura, D. (1961b). Some effects of temporal-lobe damage on auditory perception. *Canadian Journal of Psychology, 15,* 156–165.

Kimura, D. (1967). Functional asymmetry of the brain in dichotic listening. *Cortex, 3,* 163–168.

Kinsbourne, M. (1974). Mechanisms of hemispheric interaction in man. In M. Kinsbourne & W. L. Smith (Eds.), *Hemispheric disconnection and cerebral function*. Springfield, IL: Thomas.

Løberg, E. M., Hugdahl, K., & Green, M. F. (1999). Hemispheric asymmetry in schizophrenia: A "dual deficits" model. *Biological Psychiatry, 45*, 76–81.

Mazoyer, N., Papathanassiou, D., Crivello, F., Beaudouin, V., Lochon, P., & Mazoyer, B. (1999). Left planum temporale surface correlates with language areas functional variability. Paper presented at the Fifth International Conference on Functional Mapping of the Brain, Düsseldorf, Germany.

McKeever, W. F. (1986). Tachistoscopic methods in neuropsychology. In J. Hannay (Ed.), *Experimental techniques in human neuropsychology* (pp. 167–211). New York: Oxford University Press.

Mondor, T. A., & Bryden, M. P. (1991). The influence of attention on the dichotic REA. *Neuropsychologia, 29*, 1179–1190.

Obrzut, J. E., & Boliek, C. A. (1988). Dichotic listening: Evidence from learning and reading disabled children. In K. Hugdahl (Ed.), *Handbook of dichotic listening: Theory, methods, and research* (pp. 475–512). Chichester, UK: John Wiley & Sons.

Oldfield, R. C. (1971). The assessment and analysis of handedness. The Edinburgh inventory. *Neuropsychologia, 9*, 97–113.

Petersen, S. E., Fox, P. T., Posner, M. I., Mintun, M., & Raichle, M. E. (1988). Positron emission tomographic studies of the cortical anatomy of single-word processing. *Nature, 331*, 585–589.

Pollmann, S., Maertens, M., von Cramon, D. Y., Lepsien, J., & Hugdahl, K. (2002). Dichotic listening in patients with splenial and nonsplenial callosal lesions. *Neuropsychology, 16*, 56–64.

Posner, M. I., Petersen, S. E., Fox, J. M., & Raichle, M. E. (1988). Localization of cognitive operations in the human brain. *Science, 240*, 1627–1631.

Reinvang, I., Bakke, S. J., Hugdahl, K., Karlsen, N. R., & Sundet, K. (1994). Dichotic listening performance in relation to callosal area on MRI-scan. *Neuropsychology, 8*, 445–450.

Rengachary, S. S., & Watanabe, I. (1981). Ultrastructure and pathogenesis of intracranial arachnoid cysts. *Journal of Neuropathology and Experimental Neurology, 40*, 61–83.

Roberts, R. J., Varney, N. R., Paulsen, J. S., & Richardson, E. D. (1990). Dichotic listening and complex partial seizures. *Journal of Clinical and Experimental Neuropsychology, 12*, 448–458.

Sagar, H. J., Cohen, N. J., Sullivan, E. V., Corkin, S., & Growdon, J. H. (1988). Remote memory function in Alzheimer's disease and Parkinson's disease. *Brain, 111*, 185–206.

Saint-Cyr, J. A., Taylor, A. E., & Lang, A. E. (1988). Procedural learning and neostriatal dysfunction in man. *Brain, 111*, 941–959.

Shtyrov, Y., Kujala, T., Palva, S., Ilmoniemi, R. J., & Näätänen, R. (2000). Left hemisphere's dominance in speech processing is not entirely based on acoustic structure of speech: MEG evidence. Paper presented at the Annual Meeting of the Cognitive Neuroscience Society, San Francisco.

Sidtis, J. J. (1988). Dichotic listening after commissurotomy. In K. Hugdahl (Ed.), *Dichotic listening: Theory, methods, and research.* Chichester, UK: John Wiley & Sons.

Sparks, R., & Geschwind, N. (1968). Dichotic listening in man after section of neocortical commissures. *Cortex, 4,* 3–16.

Spreen, O., & Strauss, E. (Eds.). (1991). *A compendium of neuropsychological tests: Administration, norm, commentary.* New York: Oxford University Press.

Springer, S., & Deutsch, G. (Eds.). (1989). *Left brain, right brain.* San Francisco: Freeman.

Starkman, S. P., Brown, T. C., & Linell, E. A. (1958). Cerebral arachnoid cysts. *Journal of Neuropathology and Experimental Neurology, 17,* 484–500.

Steinmetz, H., & Galaburda, A. M. (1991). Planum temporale asymmetry: In-vivo morphometry affords a new perspective for neuro-behavioral research. *Reading and Writing, 3,* 331–343.

Steinmetz, H., Rademacher, J., Huang, Y., Hefter, H., Zilles, K., Thron, A., & Freund, H. J. (1989). Cerebral asymmetry: MR planimetry of the human planum temporale. *Journal of Computer Assisted Tomography, 13,* 996–1005.

Stuss, D. T., & Benson, D. F. (1984). Neuropsychological studies of the frontal lobes. *Psychological Bulletin, 95,* 3–28.

Tervaniemi, M., Medvedev, S. V., Alho, K., Pakhomov, S. V., Roudas, M. S., van Zuijen, T. L., & Näätänen, R. (2000). Larealized autonomic auditory processing of phonetic versus musical information: A PET study. *Human Brain Mapping, 10,* 74–80.

Wada, J., & Rasmussen, T. (1960). Intracarotid injections of sodium amytal for the lateralization of cerebral speech dominance. *Journal of Neurosurgery, 17,* 266–282.

Wester, K., & Hugdahl, K. (1995). Arachnoid cysts of the left temporal fossa: Impaired preoperative cognition and postoperative improvement. *Journal of Neurology, Neurosurgery, and Psychiatry, 59,* 293–298.

Wester, K., Lundervold, A. J., Taksdal, I., & Hugdahl, K. (1998). Dichotic listening and dichotic memory. Paradoxical effect of removing a left frontal gyrus. *International Journal of Neuroscience, 93,* 279–286.

Wester, K., Svendsen, F., & Hugdahl, K. (1999). Intrakraniale araknoidale cysterlokalisasjon, kjønn, sidefordeling. *Tidsskrift for den Norske Laegeforening, 28,* 4162–4164.

13 Effects of Attention on Hemispheric Asymmetry

Daniel S. O'Leary

Differences in the neuronal architecture of the two hemispheres provide the fundamental basis of perceptual and motor asymmetries. But it is clear that attention also influences asymmetries, as may strategy, arousal, and priming. This chapter will discuss the effects of attention on dichotic listening measures. Behavioral and electrophysiological studies will be briefly reviewed, with an emphasis on more recent findings. Functional imaging data relevant to the effects of attention on visual and auditory processing will then be discussed, followed by a review of recent functional imaging studies that have explored the neural basis of dichotic listening asymmetries and/or the effects of auditory attention.

DICHOTIC LISTENING: BEHAVIORAL AND ELECTROPHYSIOLOGICAL STUDIES

The most frequently used dichotic listening paradigm involves simultaneous presentation of consonant-vowel (CVs) pairs with instructions to report either both syllables or the CV pair that was heard most clearly. This "free report" CV task has been widely used because it reliably generates a large right ear advantage (REA) (Studdert-Kennedy & Shankweiler, 1970), and because it lacks the possible semantic component of consonant-vowel-consonant (CVC) stimuli (Hugdahl et al., 1997). An REA for speech stimuli is typically observed in 65–90% of neurologically normal subjects. This has classically been interpreted to result from (1) left hemispheric specialization for language, (2) suppression at brain stem levels of left ear input to the left hemisphere by the prepotent contralateral pathway from the right ear, and (3) transmission of left ear input over the corpus callosum, resulting in degradation of left ear stimuli (Kimura, 1961). The first point is generally accepted as valid, but points (2) and (3) are controversial. In particular, attentional strategies have been shown to influence performance asymmetries on dichotic tasks, indicating that the REA is not entirely a result of neuroanatomical connections.

Kinsbourne (1970, 1973) offered an explanation of performance asymmetries that was based explicitly on the role of attention. He suggested that limited attentional resources are allocated to the hemisphere that is specialized for processing differing types of stimuli. The REA for linguistic stimuli emerges because the processing of verbal stimuli predominantly activates the left hemisphere, which biases attention to the right side of space. Even the expectation that stimuli will be linguistic can elicit an REA, whereas expectation that stimuli will be nonlinguistic can elicit an LEA (Spellacy & Blumstein, 1970). Bryden and Murray (1985) offered a different explanation of attention effects. They argued that attention acts at a late stage to select the stimuli that will be reported, but only after the right ear perceptual advantage has had its effect.

Directing subjects to attend exclusively to one ear typically enhances the REA when attention is directed to the right for dichotically presented CV stimuli. A left ear advantage (LEA) is frequently observed when attention is directed left (for a review, see Hugdahl, 1995). This effect results in part from enhancement of processing in the attended ear, but Asbjørnsen & Hugdahl (1995) found that the largest effect of directing attention involves suppression of intrusions from the nonattended ear. Asbjørnsen and Hugdahl argue that their data indicate that attention may act prior to response selection by surpressing input from the ear ipsilateral to the direction of attention.

There is evidence that attention may have little effect on the REA for some types of linguistic material. Asbjørnsen and Bryden (1996) assessed the effects of directed attention on two different dichotic tasks, the CV task and the fused dichotic word test (FDWT). The FDWT utilizes pairs of rhyming CVC words that have been empirically found to fuse to form a single percept (Wexler & Hawles, 1983, 1985). In line with previous studies (e.g., Hugdahl & Andersson, 1986; Asbjørnsen & Hugdahl, 1995) Asbjørnsen and Bryden (1996) found that the CV task was sensitive to directed attention. When attending right, subjects correctly reported many more stimuli from the right (mean = 42.9) than from the left (12.4) ear, but this asymmetry reversed with attend-left instructions (right ear = 16.2, left ear = 36.9). The FDWT showed a strong REA in both attend right (right ear = 70.2, left ear = 46.0) and attend left (right ear = 64.0, left ear = 49.9) conditions, although accuracy was marginally better when subjects attended to the right ear. Asbjørnsen and Bryden (1996) note that the FDWT shows greater resistance to attention effects than does the CV test. It seems likely that the perceptual fusing which is the basis of the FDWT occurs early in the auditory pathway, prior to the stage at which attention can bias processing. In conjunction with functional imaging (see below) the FDWT may provide a valuable tool for identifying the brain mechanisms involved in the dichotic effect and its interaction with focused attention.

For reasons that are not yet clear, the effects of instructing subjects to attend left or right are not always robust for CV stimuli. Mondor (1994) reviews dichotic studies using CV stimuli that failed to show significant effects of directed attention. He utilized a cueing technique developed by Mondor and Bryden (1991) in which a tone in the left or right ear cues the subject as to the "to-be-attended ear." The cue occurred at varying intervals prior to the dichotic stimuli. Mondor and Bryden found that in right-handed subjects, left ear performance improved as the interval between cue and dichotic pairs increased for left ear cues. There was no such effect for right ear cues. Utilizing the cueing technique with left-handed subjects, Mondor (1994) found the opposite pattern of results. That is, for left-handers the cue had little effect on left ear performance, but right ear cues significantly improved performance for the right ear. Mondor concludes that an attentional bias in the direction of the dominant hand contributes significantly to the ear asymmetry in dichotic performance. For both right- and left-handers the cueing effect was minimal at 150 ms and had its largest effect at 450 ms. This suggests that shifting attention may require several hundred milliseconds, and that attention can enhance performance at a relatively late stage of processing.

Wood et al. (2000) utilized another dichotic technique to explore whether attention acts at an early perceptual stage or at a later, response selection phase of processing. It had previously been found that the REA was decreased when a left ear stimulus was lagged behind a right ear stimulus by at least 20 ms (Berlin et al., 1973; Studdert-Kennedy & Shankweiler, 1970). In a nicely designed study containing three experiments, each performed with the same 60 subjects, Wood et al. used a variation of the dichotic CV task in which stimuli were lagged from 0 to 135 ms to assess whether selective attention alters the lag effect. An initial experiment replicated Berlin et al.'s lag effect with a larger sample and over a larger range of stimulus onset asynchronies (SOAs) than in the previous experiments. They then explored the effects of directed attention on identification and localization utilizing a dichotic lag design.

Despite the fact that attention increased accuracy, the lag effects observed in the initial study were replicated whether attention was focused on the left or right ear or was divided. As in the initial experiment, the lag effect was seen as a steeper SOA for the lagging signal than for the leading signal, and the SOA had a stronger effect on left ear than on right ear performance. A third experiment assessed the effects of attention and lag using a detection rather than an identification paradigm. On each trial, subjects received a visual cue indicating which of the six possible CVs was the target 1 s prior to onset of the auditory stimuli. Subjects responded with a key press to indicate whether the target was present in the L, R, or neither ear. Separate analyses were carried out for correct detections of the target irrespective of whether it was correctly localized, and for detections in the correct ear. The lag effect was significant for both measures, although the strongest effect was seen earlier for localization (45–60 ms) than for detection (75–90 ms). SOA had a larger effect on left than on right ear performance for detection but not for localization. Detection hits had an REA but localization did not. As in Hiscock and Beckie (1993), directed attention influenced localization but not detection. Wood et al. interpreted their findings to indicate that the lag effect operates at an automatic, preattentional stage of auditory processing. However, while attention did not alter the lag effect or improve subjects' ability to detect the stimuli, it improved their ability to localize stimuli to either ear. This suggests that attentional biases exert their effects at a late stage of processing in which stimuli are either selected or rejected after being labeled according to ear of entry.

Evidence that attention can influence auditory processing at a very early stage comes from electrophysiological studies utilizing event-related potentials (ERPs) and event-related magnetic fields (ERFs) recorded from the scalp. Although not addressing perceptual asymmetries, a large number of studies have assessed early versus late attention effects using nonlinguistic dichotic stimuli, typically tone pips with different frequencies presented to the two ears. The task usually requires detection of a "deviant" tone slightly louder or fainter than the standards. Brain electrical or magnetic field activity that is evoked by the standard tones is averaged, and comparisons are made between the attended and unattended conditions.

A classic finding has been that attention amplifies a negative wave in the ERP that is elicited by attended stimuli in comparison to the ERP for the same stimuli when they are unattended (Hillyard et al., 1973; Näätänen et al., 1978; Hansen & Hillyard, 1980). The negative difference (Nd) wave can onset as early as 60 ms, and often overlaps the "exogenous" N1 (a negative wave evoked by sounds that has peak amplitude about 100 ms after a stimulus). A long-standing debate has been whether the attention effect seen in the Nd involves modulation of the exogenous N1, or is a completely different negative wave from another source that just happens to overlap N1 at the scalp. Woldorff (1995) reviews a number of his own studies and those of others that have attempted to answer this question, and to determine the earliest stage of processing at which attention might have an effect.

In a series of studies using monaural tone pips presented randomly to the two ears at a very fast rate (four–five stimuli per second), no evidence of attention effects was found in very early evoked responses (0–20 ms) that index auditory processing in the brain stem (Woldorff & Hillyard, 1991). However, attention did enhance a positive component in the 20–50 ms range that appears to reflect processing in primary auditory cortex. Woldorff argues that this strongly supports an "early selection" model of attention, and suggests that processing of a stimulus can be tuned or biased prior to its full analysis. The fast-rate dichotic listening paradigm also revealed a number of attention-related ERP effects that occurred at different scalp locations and were a mixture of enhanced exogenous potentials and overlapping endogenous, attention-related waves. Thus, the highly focused attention required by the paradigm resulted in changes at different latencies in differing brain regions, some of which modulated normal auditory processes and some of which appeared to be generated by attentional processes.

In Woldorff's studies a "mismatch negativity" that is evoked by infrequent deviant stimuli (onset at 100 ms with a peak at 200 ms) was found to be present in both the attended and the nonattended channel. This supported a claim by Näätänen and colleagues that the mismatch negativity is an indicator of an automatic mismatch detection process (Näätänen et al., 1978). However, in the fast-rate dichotic paradigm the mismatch negativity in the nonattended channel was much smaller than is typically found. Woldorff (1995) argues that this result indicates that one of the effects of focused attention is to attenuate gate processing in unattended channels at an early sensory level.

Summary

In summary, findings from recent dichotic studies indicate that the REA for dichotically presented linguistic stimuli results at least partially from the hardwired structure of the auditory system. That focused attention does not alter the lag effect (Woods et al., 2000), and has relatively little effect on the fused dichotic word test (Asbjørnsen and Bryden, 1996), indicates that perceptual asymmetries can result from automatic, preattentional processing. But attention also clearly influences ear asymmetries. Wood et al. (2000) noted that "the question regarding attention in dichotic listening, then, is not whether attentional shifts influence the frequency with which right and left ear signals are reported, but whether attention acts to alter early (perceptual) or late (response selection) processes" (p. 374).

The studies reviewed above suggest that the answer to this question is that attention can act at both early and late stages. Asbjørnsen & Hugdahl (1995) interpreted their finding that attention suppresses intrusions from the unattended ear to indicate that attention acts prior to response selection. This is in line with a large body of electrophysiological data (reviewed by Woldorff, 1995) indicating that focused auditory attention can result in a preset biasing of early sensory processing that begins in primary auditory cortex. On the other hand, the relatively long latencies at which cueing had its maximal effects in Mondor's studies (Mondor, 1994; Mondor & Bryden, 1991) indicate that attention can influence asymmetries at a relatively late stage of processing. A late effect of attention on perceptual asymmetries is also suggested by the finding of Wood et al. and others that attention enhances localization of stimuli but not of detection.

BRAIN-BASED ATTENTIONAL MODELS

The possibility that attention may affect asymmetries at both early and late stages of processing is problematic for most information-processing models of cognition that continue to provide the primary theoretical basis for studies of dichotic listening. This view of cognition is based upon the computer metaphor and assumes that the brain, at its highest levels, operates according to the principles of a formal computational device (Marr, 1992). Just as a software program can be run on computers with different physical architectures, so in the mainstream cognitive tradition higher-level computations such as attention are independent of the lower-level biological circuitry that implements the computations.

Allport (1992) reviews the history of information-processing models of attention and notes that there have been two major themes. The first involves the question of whether attention acts at an early processing stage (also called sensory filter, precategorical, perceptual, or presemantic stage) or at a later stage (e.g., pigeonhole, post-categorical, response-selection, or semantic stage). The second theme concerns the relationship between automatic processes and capacity limitations involved in controlled processing. Allport notes that most approaches assume attentional selection takes place to protect a limited capacity computational resource that must be selectively allocated. Related assumptions in this approach are that attention is unitary, but can be divided with effort, and that attention is required for "controlled" but not for "automatic" processing.

Information-processing cognitive models were based almost exclusively upon behavioral studies with normal adults. Allport (1992) notes that extensive data concerning the neuroanatomy and neurophysiology of sensory and motor processing are now available, and that they offer a new perspective on attention. The new field of cognitive neuroscience is founded on the assumption that the hardwired architecture of the nervous system provides important constraints upon information processing. It should be noted that studies of perceptual and motor asymmetries have always embraced this assumption (at least implicitly), although borrowing theoretical perspectives from traditional cognitive approaches. As discussed in this section, emerging brain-based models of spatial attention offer an explanation of how attention can enhance processing at multiple locations/stages in the brain.

Attention to a spatial location typically results in enhanced processing of stimuli from the attended location and impaired processing at ignored locations (Posner et al., 1980). Most brain-based models of spatial attention emphasize that the "bottom-up" enhancement of attended sensory features is mediated by a "top-down" system that is anatomically separate from the sensory systems which are modulated by attention (Posner & Peterson, 1990; Näätänen, 1992; Crick, 1984; Desimone et al., 1990). The neural basis of the top-down attentional mechanisms was originally explored by assessing attentional deficits following brain damage.

Based on lesion studies, Mesulam (1990) viewed spatial orientation in humans as a complex process involving the posterior parietal cortex (spatial encoding of stimuli), the dorsolateral premotor/prefrontal cortex (planning eye and hand movements in relationship to stimuli), and the cingulate gyrus (motivational tone). Posner and colleagues (Posner & Peterson, 1990; Posner & Dhaene, 1994) similarly proposed a multi-faceted system involving a number of brain regions. In Posner's model a "posterior attention system" involves the posterior parietal lobe, the pulvinar nucleus of the thalamus, and the superior colliculus. This system is proposed to mediate attentional shifts by first disengaging attention from the current object of interest (parietal lobe), moving attention to a new location (superior colliculus), and engaging the new location (pulvinar). In Posner's model the posterior system is "supervised" by an anterior attention system involving the anterior cingulate gyrus and the basal ganglia (ventral striatum).

Functional imaging studies using positron emission tomography (PET) and functional magnetic resonance imaging (fMRI) in humans have begun to supplement the data available from human lesion studies and from neurophysiological studies in animals to provide insight into the mechanisms underlying both bottom-up and top-down attentional processes. Most of the work to date with spatial attention has involved the visual system (Corbetta et al., 1993, 2000; Haxby et al., 1994; Heinze et al., 1994; Hopfinger et al., 2000; Nobre et al., 1997; Vandenberghe et al., 1996; Woldorff et al., 1996). General principles derived from this work are likely to be relevant for auditory processing also, since two explicit comparisons of visual and auditory attentional systems have found overlap in brain systems mediating these modalities (Bushara et al., 1999; O'Leary et al., 1997). There have also been several auditory studies that have utilized dichotic listening paradigms and/or investigated auditory attention (Hugdahl et al., 1999, 2000; O'Leary et al., 1996a, 1996b, 1997, 1999; Alho et al., 1999; Tzourio et al., 1997; Woodruff et al., 1995). These will be discussed below.

Chelazzi and Corbetta (2000) review PET imaging studies in which subjects covertly directed attention to visual stimuli in peripheral locations (Corbetta et al., 1998; Haxby et al., 1994; Heinze et al., 1994; Nobre et al., 1997; Vandenberghe et al., 1996; Woldorff et al., 1996). Regions of activation that are consistent across studies include areas of parietal cortex (the postcentral and intraparietal sulcus) and frontal lobe (the precentral sulcus/gyrus and the posterior tip of the superior frontal sulcus). Regions that have been activated in some but not all studies are the cingulate gyrus, the medial frontal gyrus, and the superior temporal gyrus (STG). Chellazzi and Corbetta conclude that attention directed to peripheral visual stimuli recruits a common network of parietal and frontal regions that is independent of eye movements. They note that similar regions are recruited when attention is shifted to different locations or is maintained for a prolonged time at the same location.

Two very recent studies have utilized the powerful new technology of event-related fMRI to explore the brain systems that mediate attention to cued locations (Corbetta et al., 2000; Hopfinger et al., 2000). Event-related fMRI is similar to ERP in allowing trial-by-trial analysis of specific components of the brain's response to a stimulus, although fMRI measures the much slower (3–10 s) hemodynamic response rather than immediate electrical activity. Corbetta et al. and Hopfinger et al. utilized event-related fMRI in very similar visual attention studies in which a central stimulus cues the subject to covertly orient attention to the left or right. Event-related fMRI allowed independent analysis of the hemodynamic response to the cue and to the subsequent target.

Hopfinger et al. (2000) found that superior frontal, inferior parietal, and superior temporal cortices were activated by the cues, indicating that these regions participate in a network involved in voluntary control of attention. This voluntary system biased activity in a number of extrastriate regions. Corbetta et al. (2000) tested hypotheses based upon studies of brain-damaged patients. They investigated whether the temporal-parietal junction is involved in reorienting attention to stimuli at new, unexpected locations, whereas the region around the intraparietal sulcus mediates voluntary orientation and maintenance of attention at cued locations. Their results supported these hypotheses. Both studies found that retinotopically organized extrastriate regions processing cued locations had increased rCBF in anticipation of the stimuli. The two studies thus provide complementary findings that strongly support a model in which top-down attentional mechanisms enhance bottom-up processing of stimuli at attended spatial locations.

Bushara et al. (1999) assessed the frontal and parietal regions that are uniquely activated during auditory and visual spatial localization tasks. Rather than using binaural (Griffiths et al., 1998) or dichotic (O'Leary et al., 1997) stimuli that are perceived as internal, they created a "virtual auditory space" by presenting synthesized sounds through headphones that mimicked sounds coming from the free field. They argue that this allows true auditory localization rather than the lateralization of sounds that results from using binaural or dichotic stimuli. In both auditory and visual modalities, Bushara et al. used a delayed matching to sample task (subjects indicated whether each successive stimulus was in the same location as the previous one) as well as a task requiring a joystick movement in the direction of the stimulus.

Bushara et al. found regions in the frontal and parietal lobes that were uniquely activated during auditory and visual tasks, as well as "supramodal" regions that responded to both modalities. Both auditory and visual localization tasks activated bilateral regions of superior and inferior parietal lobules. Bushara et al. argue that superior parietal cortex contains modality-specific regions involved in early spatial processing. They further propose that this sensory input is relayed to the inferior parietal lobe for additional processing of both spatial and nonspatial supramodal aspects of perception. In prefrontal cortex, caudal aspects of the superior frontal sulcas were bilaterally activated during visual localization, and a more ventrolateral region of this sulcus was activated by auditory localization tasks. An additional region of left inferior frontal gyrus was more active during auditory tasks than visual tasks.

The inferior temporal gyrus (BA 20) is typically considered to be part of the ventral stream for object recognition, but was activated by both auditory and visual localization tasks. Regions responsive during both auditory and visual tasks were also found in right mesial frontal lobe (BA 6), bilateral inferior parietal lobe (BA 40), right thalamus, and left and right cerebellum. Bushara et al. conclude that there are separate subsystems for spatially selective attention for visual and auditory modalities in the parietal and frontal lobes. However, there are also "amodal" or multimodal regions that may be part of a higher-order system involved in both spatial and nonspatial cognitive processes.

A "bottom up" model of spatial attention (Desimone & Duncan, 1995) suggests that attention arises as an emergent property of interactions at each level of the neural hierarchy. Desimone and Duncan suggest that neural circuitry mediating working memory in the frontal lobes may hold the representation of attentional "templates" that guide the top-down selection of sensory features for attentional enhancement. Since all forms of spatial attention require memory of the location that is being attended, similar frontal mechanisms may mediate spatial working memory and spatial attention. Awh and colleagues (1998) also have discussed interactions between brain regions mediating working memory and those mediating attention. They have provided evidence that spatial selective attention may act as a rehearsal mechanism for spatial working memory. Thus, the interaction between spatial attention and spatial working memory is of interest, as is the possible overlap of the frontal and other brain mechanisms that mediate these processes.

We have recently completed a PET study that directly compared a condition requiring spatially selective attention to memory for a spatial location (O'Leary et al., 1999). In two conditions subjects had identical instructions to fixate a central "x" and to attend to the upper left or upper right visual quadrant for a target (a briefly appearing asterisk) against a background of a flashing checkerboard. In a spatial working memory condition the target appeared within the first few seconds of the trial, requiring memory for location for the remainder of the 40 s interval. In the spatial attention condition the target appeared in the last few seconds of the interval, so that the majority of the 40 s trial required spatial attention. Subtraction of a passive viewing baseline from the two active conditions largely replicated previous studies of spatially directed attention and spatial working memory, with activations in parietal and frontal lobes. All active condition minus baseline subtractions also showed activations in the cerebellum.

A spatial memory minus spatial attention subtraction showed memory activations in left and right parietal lobes (BA 40), cerebellar cortex, and precuneus. Activations unique to attention were found in the right thalamus, right striate, right lenticular nucleus, and anterior cingulate, with no significant rCBF differences between tasks in the frontal lobes. Failure to see rCBF differences in the frontal lobes in the memory minus attention tasks suggests that the same frontal executive mechanism may mediate both memory for a static spatial location and attention to that location (Desimone & Duncan, 1995; Awh et al., 1998). However, the different pattern of rCBF in parietal lobes, cerebellum, thalamus, and other brain regions during attention and memory processing indicate that there are differences in the functional connectivity of the frontal executive with other brain regions during these processes.

Most cognitive approaches conceptualize the representations that generate and maintain selective attention as abstract spatial maps. Chelazzi and Corbetta (2000) note that in these types of models, the parietal cortex may be conceptualized to contain a map of extrapersonal space in which potential locations of interest are activated or selected by working memory signals from prefrontal cortex. The parietal representation of space is abstract in the sense that it is not tied to any specific action system, and because it can be applied to a variety of perceptual and motor tasks. For example, spatially specific signals from the parietal lobe might be used to gate sensory responses in the ventral visual system during object recognition (Desimone & Duncan, 1995), or to guide saccades for reaching and grasping movements.

An alternative view is that frontal and parietal regions mediating spatially selective attention are nodes of specific sensorimotor systems that are necessary to perform stimulus-guided actions. Rizzolatti et al. (1994) have offered an "attention for action" approach, and argue that it is possible to consider spatially selective attention as a variety of systems, some of which are tied to specific motor systems, rather than as a unitary mechanism. They suggest that spatially selective attentional processes are embedded within multiple areas of the brain which are involved with carrying out eye, arm, hand, and other motor movements. For example, Corbetta and colleagues (1998) have provided evidence that there is a tight functional relationship between mechanisms for spatial attention and oculomotor control in humans. Subjects were scanned during a task in which eye movements were performed toward several sequential locations in order to detect visual probe stimuli, or while fixation was centrally maintained but attention was moved to the same locations. All regions that were active during overt eye movements were also active during the covert attention task, and no region was uniquely active in one condition or the other. Active regions in both conditions included the frontal eye fields (precentral sulcus region), supplementary eye field (medial frontal gyrus), and intraparietal sulcus (BA 7a).

Summary

A number of models of attention based upon brain lesion studies assume that location is used as a feature to select for further processing; that is, "spotlight of attention" models (Crick, 1984; Posner et al., 1980). Recent functional imaging data has strongly supported such models. But recent neuroanatomical and neurophysiological data also indicate that spatial location is not a simple physical characteristic. Rather, spatial location is encoded by many different parallel retinotopic, body-centered, object-centered, and possibly environment-centered coordinate systems. Coding of visual-spatial relations and attentional modulation of spatial encoding may, therefore, take place at many different levels of visual processing and visual-motor control. Allport (1992) noted that "where" effects of spatially selective attention in the dorsal stream may be early, but are in parallel with "what" effects in the ventral stream. Bushara et al. (1999), discussed above, indicates that some regions of the "what" system in the inferior temporal lobe are also involved in spatial attention/localization. It seems likely, therefore, that spatially selective attention may influence processing at many different locations in the brain, ranging from enhancement of attended stimuli in early sensory regions to attention-based selection of action-related systems that are thought to be late stage processes.

The relevance of these models for studies of dichotic asymmetries is that the effects of attention may be seen both early and late, depending upon task demands. Enhancement of stimuli in the attended ear may occur early, possibly in primary auditory cortex, or later, as attention is consciously shifted to a cued location, and/or at the stage of response selection. The early versus late controversy was based upon a computer model that did not consider the possibility of parallel pathways that can be modulated by attention. Comprehensive cognitive models based upon the biological reality of the brain rather than the metaphor of a computational device are only beginning to emerge. Functional imaging studies, in concert with neurophysiological studies in animals, are providing data that will permit the rapid development of brain-based models of cognition. Functional imaging studies of perceptual asymmetries will contribute significantly to this effort because they provide an intrinsic contrast of information processing that takes place in the differing neuronal architectures of the left and right hemispheres.

FUNCTIONAL IMAGING STUDIES USING AUDITORY STIMULI

Several recent studies have utilized functional imaging techniques to explore the brain mechanisms that underlie dichotic listening asymmetries or the effects of auditory attention. As discussed below, our group has used PET to assess the effects on rCBF of dichotic presentation of words, CVCs, and environmental sounds, and has also assessed the effects of monaural and binaural presentation of these stimuli (Kesler, 1997; O'Leary et al., 1996a, 1996b, 1997). We have consistently used focused attention instructions during dichotic conditions. Hugdahl has recently extended his pioneering explorations of dichotic behavioral measures to the measurement of cerebral blood flow during dichotic listening tasks with differing attentional instructions (Hugdahl et al., 1999, 2000). Hugdahl and colleagues (1999) performed the first PET imaging study that assessed rCBF during the "free report" paradigm with CV stimuli; it has been the most widely used behavioral dichotic measure. They also assessed focused attention for CV and music stimuli, and carried out the first functional imaging study with dichotic stimuli that assessed the effects of divided attention (Hugdahl et al., 2000). Several other studies have assessed the effects of focused auditory attention using tones presented to the left or right ears (Alho et al., 1999; Tzourio et al., 1997).

To our knowledge our group was the first to utilize functional imaging to explore regional cerebral blood flow during dichotic listening tasks in normal volunteers (O'Leary et al., 1996a), and in patients with schizophrenia (O'Leary et al., 1996b). In our initial studies we utilized nonsense CVC stimuli (e.g., /dak/), CVCs that were English words (e.g., "dog") and environmental sounds (e.g., a dog bark), presented either binaurally or dichotically. CVCs were used rather the more commonly used dichotic CV stimuli in order to have meaningless speech stimuli with physical characteristics identical to the words. All tasks required detection of a specified target within a sequence of stimuli. The environmental sounds and CVC conditions required detection of a specific target, but in order to force semantic processing of the word stimuli, subjects were required to make a category judgement (i.e., "Is the word an animal name?").

There were ten normal volunteers (nine males) in the O'Leary et al. (1996a) study, all right-handed with no first-degree relatives who were left-handed. Since PET studies use relatively small numbers of subjects in comparison to behavioral studies, we wanted the subjects to be as homogeneous as possible in terms of hemispheric asymmetries. To this end we also selected only subjects who had a strong REA on a dichotic CVC behavioral screening test (a right ear score at least 33% greater than their left ear score). A series of 40 trials was presented with each trial consisting of seven stimuli (in binaural conditions) or pairs of stimuli (in dichotic conditions), followed by a tone burst cueing the subject to make a manual response. Subjects responded by pressing a thumb switch, mounted in a small device held in the right hand, either away from the palm ("a target was detected") or toward the palm ("no target"). The yes/no response indicated whether a target had been detected in the preceding sequence (the tone bursts and the interval between them were the same as in the baseline reaction time task). This forced-choice design ensured that all subjects made the same number of motor responses. The baseline task consisted of a 1000 Hz tone burst of 50 ms duration that occurred with an interstimulus interval (ISI) that varied randomly from 10 to 12 s. The subject was instructed to respond as fast as possible to the tone with an "upward" thumb press on a manipulandum held in the right hand. Each trial lasted 400 s, beginning 90 s prior to the 100 s image acquisition period and continuing for another 210 s.

Because PET studies expose subjects to ionizing radiation, the number of conditions was limited to eight. We wanted to maximize the information gained about auditory processing in this initial study, and the conditions were selected to allow assessment of the effects on regional cerebral blood flow (rCBF) of (1) binaural versus dichotic presentation, (2) differing types of stimuli, and (3) the effects of attention directed to the left and right ears. The baseline RT task was presented first and last to allow assessment of possible changes in task performance and rCBF over the course of the study, which took several hours. Four conditions were used to present words and environmental sounds both binaurally and dichotically. In the dichotic conditions subjects were instructed to focus attention in a manner consistent with the expected ear advantage (i.e., to the right for words and to the left for environmental sounds) in order to maximize ear asymmetries. The remaining two conditions were used to explore the effects of directed attention. Subjects were instructed to attend to their right ear in one condition and to the left ear in the other during the dichotic presentation of CVCs.

All PET images were spatially normalized to each individual's MR images. Within-subject subtractions of the final RT baseline condition were then made for each of the binaural and dichotic conditions, followed by across-subject averaging of the subtraction images. Voxel-by-voxel t-tests were then computed and significant regions of activation were identified, using a technique that corrects for the large number of t-tests performed, the lack of independence between voxels, and the resolution of the processed PET images (Worsley et al., 1992).

The binaural word and environmental sound conditions showed a very similar pattern of bilateral rCBF activations in left and right temporal lobe regions surrounding Heschl's gyrus. Based upon studies using the lesion-deficit correlation approach (Caplan, 1992), we had expected to see greater left hemisphere than right hemisphere activation in temporal lobe regions for the word stimuli and perhaps activations in Broca's area. However, our finding of similar bilateral temporal lobe activations for word and nonword stimuli is consistent with several studies from other centers (Wise et al., 1991; Howard et al., 1992). Wise et al. noted the possibility that superior temporal gyrus (STG) circuitry involved with semantic processing in the left hemisphere may be organized in parallel with right hemisphere circuitry involved in acoustic or phonological analysis.

The effect of focusing attention to the right ear for word stimuli was dramatic. For binaurally presented words, activation (defined as significantly greater rCBF in the condition of interest than in the baseline condition) was bilateral: the left STG had a 3.7 cc "blob" (volume of contiguous voxels with a t-value threshold greater than 3.61) with a maximal t-value (t-max) of 5.2, and the right hemisphere had a 3.9 cc blob with a t-max of 5.0. In comparison to the binaural minus baseline subtraction, the attend right for words minus baseline subtraction showed a greater magnitude and volume of activation in the STG contralateral to the attended ear in left STG (10.0 cc, t-max = 7.0). Activation in the right STG ipsilateral to attention was smaller in volume than in the binaural condition (0.7 cc blob, t-max = 4.6).

A similar but opposite pattern of rCBF was observed during binaural and dichotic presentation of common environmental sounds (CES). Binaural presentation resulted in nearly equal activation of left and right STG (left, 3.5 cc blob, t-max = 5.3; right, 4.2 cc blob, t-max = 5.1). Dichotic presentation of CES with attend left instructions resulted in decreased activation in left STG in comparison to the binaural condition (0.2 cc blob, t-max = 4.1), but increased activation in right STG (two blobs totaling 4.8 cc with a t-max of 5.2).

The two CVC conditions provided a direct assessment of the effects of focused attention upon rCBF asymmetries during dichotic listening conditions. Attention to the left and right during presentation of CVC stimuli caused a reversal of rCBF asymmetries in STG. Attention to the right ear resulted in a pattern very similar to that seen in the attend right for words condition (left STG 11.1 cc blob, t-max = 6.6; right STG 1.8 cc blob, t-max = 4.7), but attention to the left reversed this asymmetry (left STG 1.5 cc blob, t-max = 5.2; right STG 5.5 cc blob, t-max = 5.1). A similar pattern of increased rCBF in auditory temporal lobe regions contralateral to the direction of attention was reported by Alho et al. (1999). In that study, tone stimuli were rapidly presented in the left and right ears along with concurrent foveal visual stimuli. As in our studies, attention-related enhancement of rCBF was seen exclusively in the STG contralateral to the direction of attention.

The same stimuli and conditions used in O'Leary et al. (1996a) were used in a PET study in 10 individuals with schizophrenia (O'Leary et al., 1996b). For the patient group the binaural conditions showed a strong asymmetry with a much smaller region of activation in right STG than in the normal volunteer group. The dichotic words condition showed no difference in the pattern of rCBF from the binaural words condition. Additionally, during the dichotic conditions requiring attention to the left ear, the patients failed to show the increase in the activated region of right STG, and the decrease in left STG activation, exhibited by the control group. We concluded that schizophrenia might involve deficits in temporal lobe processing mechanisms as well as a deficit in the mechanisms that mediate selective attention. A similar conclusion was reached by Loberg et al. (1999), who utilized behavioral dichotic measures with free report and focused attention instructions in a group of 33 schizophrenic patients and 33 comparison subjects. They found that the patients did not show the normal REA during the free report condition and were unable to modify their dichotic performance through attentional shifts to the left or right. They concluded that schizophrenia may be characterized by a dual deficit involving both automatic and controlled processing.

We performed a second PET study in an independent group of 11 normal volunteers (5 males 6 females) to more directly assess the effects of directed attention on differing types of linguistic and nonlinguistic stimuli. Subjects again were strongly right-handed with no first degree left-handed relatives, and had a strong REA on a behavioral screening test. In this study the baseline RT task was again administered first and last, and the remaining six conditions used attend left and attend right

Table 13.1 Significant activation foci for the last baseline subtracted from dichotically presented words, CVCs, and environmental sounds

t-value	Size (cc)	Right/left	Ant/post	Sup/inf	Location
Dichotic words—Attend right minus baseline					
9.4	14.9	−50	−23	3	Left STG (BA 42/22)[1]
7.4	6.3	54	−19	2	Right STG (BA 42/22)
Dichotic words—Attend left minus baseline					
7.9	7.5	−54	−25	2	Left STG (BA 42/22)
8.7	11.4	50	−26	6	Right STG (BA 42/22)
5.1	1.1	−2	10	43	Left cingulate (BA 32)
Dichotic CVCs—Attend right minus baseline					
8.8	20.2	−51	−23	4	Left STG (BA 42/22)
7.8	7.7	53	−20	3	Right STG (BA 42/22)
Dichotic CVC—Attend left minus baseline					
7.5	10.5	−53	−27	6	Left STG (BA 42/22)
8.6	13.8	49	−24	4	Right STG (BA 42/22)
Dichotic environmental sounds—Attend right minus baseline					
6.3	6.5	−51	−30	7	Left post. STG (BA 42)
5.0	2.5	−45	2	−5	Left ant. STG (BA 22)
5.3	2.0	54	−25	7	Right STG (BA 42/22)
Dichotic environmental sounds—Attend left minus baseline					
7.3	12.7	−51	−27	4	Left STG (BA 42/22)
6.8	12.7	50	−21	4	Right STG (BA 42/22)

Note: BA, Brodmann areas 22, 41, 42.
Sources: Hurtig et al. (submitted). Reported are the highest t-values and their x, y, and z coordinates in regions in which all t-values are positive (i.e., higher flow in activation condition) and are greater than 3.61. Stereotaxic coordinates are from Talairach & Tournoux (1988).

instructions for dichotically presented environmental sounds, CVCs, and words. Table 13.1 presents the results of the PET imaging analyses in which the final baseline RT task is subtracted from each of the dichotic conditions.

The pattern of results for the CVC stimuli was very similar to that observed in our initial study. Attention to the right ear again resulted in a large asymmetry in rCBF, with left STG showing both a higher t-value and a greater volume of activated voxels in the attend right condition. The asymmetry reversed when subjects attended to the left ear (see table 13.1). This pattern of attention-related shifts in rCBF was very similar for word stimuli. As in our initial study, the pattern for words and for meaningless CVCs was very similar. That may have resulted from a semantic "lookup" process for CVCs based upon their phonetic similarity to words (Wise et al., 1991; Hugdahl et al., 1997). For unclear reasons the environmental sounds did not show the same pattern of attention effects as in the initial study. Attention to the left ear resulted in a large bilateral activation that did, however, shift to greater left than right STG activation with attention to the right ear.

In all of our dichotic listening studies we had anticipated that an attentional network including parietal and frontal regions would be activated, but failed to observe significant rCBF differences from the baseline task in any region but STG (except for the anterior cingulate finding in one condition in Hurtig et al.). It seemed possible that the t-map analyses did not have enough power to detect subtle changes in attention-related brain regions. Kesler (Kesler et al., 1995; Kesler 1997) utilized correlational analyses on rCBF values within regions of interest (ROIs) traced on each individual's MR image to further investigate attentional effects.

Based upon review of attentional effects in the neuroscience literature, Kesler traced bilateral volumetric ROIs in the pulvinar nucleus of the thalamus, posterior parietal lobe (BA 39/40), dorsal prefrontal cortex (portions of BA 46/10/9/8), anterior cingulate gyrus (BA 24/33), and STG (Heschl's gyrus and the planum temporale were traced separately, BA 22/41/42), and in the right precentral gyrus (BA 4/6). All traces were placed on MR images without reference to the PET images, using locally developed BRAINS software (Andreasen et al., 1993) that generates three orthogonal views of the brain and telegraphs traces across views.

Each individual's MRI was coregistered with his/her PET images, using an automated two-stage process. To obtain an initial coarse fit, an adaptation of the surface-fitting program developed by Pelizzari and colleagues (1989) was applied. The resulting surface fit was then used as a starting point for the automatic image registration program developed by Woods et al. (1992). This was performed independently for each of the eight PET scans per subject, with each scan visually checked for goodness of fit. Correlational analyses utilized rCBF measured within these ROIs in the attend left and right CVC and baseline RT conditions for subjects in the O'Leary et al. and Hurtig et al. studies, since subjects in both studies had these conditions. The mean blood flow for each ROI for each condition was divided by whole brain flow to obtain a measure of normalized flow to reduce the effects of intersubject variability in whole brain blood flow.

An initial analysis was performed to corroborate the attention effects found in O'Leary et al. and Hurtig et al., studies that used t-map analyses. Using mean normalized flow values within the manually traced STG regions, a repeated measures analysis of variance (ANOVA) was applied, with hemisphere and condition (CVC attend left and right) as the repeated measures. The dependent variable was normalized flow during one CVC condition with normalized flow during the second baseline subtracted. For the STG, the repeated measures ANOVA showed a significant hemisphere by condition interaction ($F = 8.0$, $(pr > F) = 0.01$) which supported the t-map analysis. There was also a significant main effect of hemisphere, with right STG having greater flow than left ($F = 7.4$, $(pr > F) = 0.015$).

In an analysis utilizing normalized flow within Heschl's gyrus, excluding the remainder of STG, the hemisphere by condition interaction did not reach significance ($F = 0.39$, $(pr > F) = 0.54$). Primary auditory cortex is thought to lie within Heschl's gyrus on the supratemporal plane (Liégeois-Chauvel et al., 1991). Thus, the attentional modulation of rCBF within STG during the attend left and attend right conditions did not appear to result from changes in primary auditory cortex within Heschl's gyrus. However, several of the activation conditions in the PET multiple injection protocol employed the same attention instructions. In order to increase the signal-to-noise ratio, the rCBF measures from all conditions with the same attention instructions (attend to the right ear, attend to the left ear, or no directed attention instruction) were averaged together. With this averaging, a significant reversal in the blood flow asymmetry was seen in Heschl's gyri as a function of the attention instructions. This suggests that attention-related changes occur in primary auditory cortices, although these changes may be more subtle than the changes in STG as a whole.

Following the analyses of rCBF changes within temporal lobe auditory regions in STG, several correlational approaches were utilized to explore relationships between STG and other regions of the brain. The first correlational analysis utilized Spearman correlation coefficients that were computed between mean rCBF measures from each pair of regions across subjects (as suggested by Horwitz, 1991). The resulting correlation matrices were examined for pairs of regions whose flows were correlated during a selective attention condition, but not during

Daniel S. O'Leary

the baseline condition. Because highly localized rCBF changes could be obscured by averaging flow within large ROIs, a second analysis used automated methods to identify regions of maximal flow within the traced ROIs of each individual. Spearman correlations were again computed for pairs of regions using these maximal flow values. A third approach involved placing a "seed" at the voxel within STG that showed the largest rCBF change with attention. Normalized flow within the entire PET image was then correlated with the seed pixel.

These analyses found several brain regions in which correlations with STG were higher during both dichotic conditions than during the baseline. There were positive correlations between right STG and right dorsolateral frontal cortex, and between left STG and right medial temporal regions. Negative correlations were found between left STG and left pulvinar regions. In addition, the STG region contralateral to the direction of attention was negatively correlated with parietal regions. Outside of STG, parietal regions were positively correlated with pulvinar and dorsolateral frontal cortex (DLFC) regions in a manner dependent on the direction of attention, and both pulvinar nuclei were negatively correlated with DLFC regions. Finally, during both attend right and attend left conditions, positive correlations were seen between the right parietal and right precentral gyrus regions and between right DLFC and left anterior cingulate regions. These results indicate that the attentional network of frontal, parietal, and thalamic regions identified in a number of studies is also engaged in a complex fashion in dichotic paradigms with focused attention instructions.

Kesler (1997) notes that the target detection dichotic tasks with focused attention instructions used in these studies are similar to conjunction search tasks, in that both spatial and nonspatial stimulus features are important in detecting a target. In a discussion of the manner in which attention acts within auditory cortices to enhance processing she speculates that

certain cells in the STG, or inputs to cells in the STG, are gated on or off, so that a particular CVC (the target) in a particular location (right ear or left ear) produces an enhanced response. The reversal in the pattern of asymmetry in the STG ... specifically relates to the gating which is based on spatial location. Perhaps suppression column cells for which input from the attended ear is dominant, show increased firing relative to other suppression column cells (for which input from the unattended ear is dominant) and relative to summation column cells (which respond more to binaural input than to monaural input). The selected suppression column cells may show both a sustained elevation of firing and an increase in responding to a target stimulus. Both of these changes, in addition to the possible inhibition of the activity of cells selective for nontargets, would require greater energy consumption and a concomitant increase in rCBF (p. 21).

One further study from our group utilized both dichotic stimuli and bilaterally presented visual stimuli to assess cross-modal attention effects (O'Leary et al., 1997). In four conditions of a PET study, dichotic CVC stimuli were presented synchronously with vertically oriented CVC stimuli presented in the left and right visual fields. In different conditions subjects were instructed to attend to their left or right ear or to their left or right visual field. An analysis that contrasted the two visual attention conditions with the two auditory attention conditions found higher rCBF in BA 7 of the left parietal lobe and BA 6 of the right frontal lobe in the visual attention conditions. These conditions overlap with those found in the visual attention studies summarized by Chelazzi and Corbetta (2000), and with Bushara et al. (1999), and reinforce the importance of frontal and parietal brain regions for top-down attentional regulation of visual processing.

Unlike the Bushara et al. (1999) study discussed above, direct comparison of the visual and auditory conditions in our study did not reveal parietal regions that were differentially activated by auditory attention, and only one region in the right orbital frontal lobe (BA 11) that had higher rCBF during attention to dichotic than to visual stimuli. Directing attention to the right ear resulted in increased rCBF in left STG that was similar to that found in our previous studies. However, attend left instructions did not result in enhanced right STG flow. Instead, a region in the right precentral gyrus was activated, a finding similar to that found in a PET study reported by Tzourio et al. (1997), using directed attention instructions with left and right ear tone stimuli. In our study (O'Leary et al., 1997) subtraction of a resting baseline condition from the attend left and attend right dichotic conditions revealed activations in the right parietal lobe (BA 7), left frontal lobe (BA 4), right insula, and right cerebellum, but the network activated by auditory attention was much less extensive than that activated by visual attention.

Direct comparison of the two sensory modalities in O'Leary et al. (1997) suggested that the effects of directed attention were less spatially discrete for auditory than for visual attention. Attention to either ear resulted in increased rCBF in both left and right temporal lobe auditory cortices and little activation in frontal or parietal regions. Visually directed attention resulted in more localized activation in the occipital lobe contralateral to the direction of attention and widespread activation in other brain regions. We concluded that auditory attention might operate through brain stem mechanisms that have a more coarse and widespread effect on auditory processing than does the visual attention network. Bushara et al.'s finding that similar parietal and frontal mechanisms are involved in visual and auditory attention may have resulted from their use of auditory stimuli that were perceived to be localized in external space rather than dichotic stimuli that were perceived to be inside the head.

Hugdahl and colleagues (1999) have presented data from PET studies that include several dichotic paradigms that had not previously been assessed with functional imaging. They used dichotically presented CV and musical stimuli with "free report" instructions to the subjects (attend to both ears for a possible target). A baseline task involved pressing a response key each time a tone was heard. Behavioral data showed the expected perceptual asymmetry in the 12 right-handed subjects, with CV stimuli showing a significant REA and musical stimuli showing an LEA. The PET analysis showed blood flow asymmetries (regional normalized counts) that mirrored the behavioral findings. For both CV and musical stimuli there were significant bilateral activations in regions of the posterior STG that were very similar in location and extent to those found in studies from our laboratory. An important new finding was that in the absence of focused attention instructions, there were "stimulus-driven," bottom-up blood flow asymmetries, with greater activation in the left STG for CVs and in the right STG for musical stimuli.

Interpretation of the findings is complicated somewhat by the fact that correlations between perceptual asymmetry and brain activation measures were not significant. Thus, blood flow asymmetries were consistent with behavioral asymmetries for the group as a whole, but not on an individual basis. It is also the case that free-report instructions leave subjects free to choose a strategy to perform this difficult task. We have asked subjects how they perform in the free-report paradigm and have found considerable variability. Some subjects report that they attempt to divide attention, but others report biasing attention to the more difficult ear, or attending first to one ear and then attempting to quickly switch attention to the other ear (as in visual postexposural scanning), or other strategies. Thus, the free-report condition may have averaged across several different activation patterns resulting from differing strategies.

A second PET study (Hugdahl et al., 2000) assessed the effects of directed attention to dichotically presented CV and musical stimuli. In addition to the free report or "divided attention" instructions reported in Hugdahl et al. (1999), the 12 right-handed subjects were instructed to focus attention to the left or right ear to detect targets in streams of dichotically presented CV and musical stimuli. Behavioral data again showed the expected perceptual asymmetries, with better performance for CV stimuli when attention was focused right and better performance for musical stimuli when attention was focused left. The PET data showed an extremely interesting finding, with the divided attention conditions having higher flow in left and right STG than the focused attention conditions. Direct comparison of divided versus focused attention conditions revealed no regions in STG that were higher in the focused attention conditions. Instead, focusing attention to the left and right ears resulted in higher flow in the precuneus and inferior parietal lobes, with a trend toward higher activations in the parietal lobe contralateral to the direction of attention.

Hugdahl et al. (2000) interpreted these results as possible evidence that divided attention may result in greater rCBF because focused attention facilitates processing of stimuli from the attended ear. However, they also noted the possibility that dividing attention was a more difficult task than focusing attention, resulting in greater rCBF during divided attention conditions. This latter possibility seems unlikely, given evidence that more difficult perceptual tasks caused greater increases in rCBF in attention-related brain regions but reduced rCBF in sensory processing regions in comparison to easier tasks (Grady et al., 1995; Vandenberghe et al., 1995). Hugdahl et al.'s hypothesis that attention enhances processing seems a more likely explanation of their findings, particularly given evidence that attentional enhancement may involve suppression of processing of nonattended stimuli (e.g., Asbjørnsen and Hugdahl, 1995).

As noted above, we had previously found that binaural presentation of words and environmental sounds resulted in a similar pattern of bilateral STG when an RT baseline was subtracted from these conditions (O'Leary et al., 1996a). Dichotic presentation of the same stimuli with focused attention instructions and with the RT baseline subtracted resulted in an increase in rCBF in STG contralateral to the direction of attention and decreased rCBF in the STG ipsilateral to attention. We commented at that time:

In addition to increasing rCBF in the temporal lobe contralateral to the attended ear, attention also appears to decrease rCBF in auditory cortices processing stimuli from the non-attended ear. The evidence for this is less direct because comparisons must be made across stimulus type, and because attentional effects are confounded with binaural versus dichotic presentation. Inspection of Table 2, however, indicates that the right STG region showing increased flow (compared to baseline) for binaurally-presented words and environmental sounds was much less activated by dichotically-presented CVCs and words when attention was directed to the right ear. The decreased flow in right temporal lobe suggests that inhibition is occurring at a site in the auditory pathway prior to primary auditory cortex. Inhibition is an active process that increases metabolism and blood flow at the site at which it occurs. Therefore, the decrease in flow in right STG during dichotic, as compared to binaural, stimulation must result from inhibition occurring at least one synapse upstream from the right temporal lobe (p. 37).

We recently completed a reanalysis of data from our first dichotic study using the binaural condition as the comparison condition for the directed attention conditions (O'Leary et al., in preparation). Subtraction of the PET images for the binaurally presented words condition from the dichotically presented words attend-right condition provided very interesting findings. As expected, the dichotic condition had higher rCBF in the left STG (both Heschl's gyrus and the planum temporale), contralateral to the direction of attention, than did the binaural condition. In right STG there was a very focal decrease in rCBF in Heschl's gyrus in the dichotic compared to the binaural condition. Subtraction of the binaural environmental sounds condition from the dichotically presented environmental sounds condition revealed an opposite pattern of asymmetries. Although the activations did not reach the level of significance that we have traditionally used in our laboratory, there was higher rCBF in the right STG (t-max = 3.0) and lower rCBF in left STG (t-max = −2.7) in the dichotic environmental sounds attend-left condition in comparison to the binaural condition. Since the binaural condition did not involve spatially directed attention, this is strong evidence that focused attention acts to suppress activity in the nonattended ear in dichotic listening situations.

Summary

Functional imaging studies have added greatly to our knowledge of the brain mechanisms that result in perceptual asymmetries in the dichotic listening situation. Hugdahl and colleagues demonstrated that dichotic presentation of linguistic stimuli with free report instructions generated greater activation in left than in right auditory cortices (Hugdahl et al., 1999), whereas musical stimuli generated the opposite pattern of activation. This is an important finding because it gives insight into the brain mechanisms underlying the dichotic protocoll that is most frequently used in clinical and experimental studies of laterality. It generally supports the concept that bottom-up, stimulus-specific mechanisms contribute to perceptual asymmetries. Hugdahl et al. also found that focused attention conditions resulted in less activation in temporal lobes than did free report conditions, but found attention-related activation in other brain regions (precuneus, left and right parietal lobes).

The finding of greater activation during divided than focused attention appears to contrast with our finding that focused attention enhanced rCBF in auditory processing regions of the STG contralateral to the direction of attention. This was true whether the comparison condition was a simple task requiring a button press to an infrequent tone (O'Leary et al., 1996a; Hurtig et al., submitted) or involved target detection during binaural presentation of the same stimuli as used in the dichotic condition (O'Leary et al., in preparation). The differences in the pattern of the results from the two groups is most likely due to the comparison conditions used to assess the effects of focused attention. The divided attention instructions used in Hugdahl et al. (2000) may result in enhanced processing of stimuli from both ears, without the suppression effects seen with focused attention instructions in our studies (O'Leary et al., 1996a, in preparation). Thus, recent functional imaging studies generally support Asbjørnsen and Hugdahl's (1995) suggestion that attention acts both to enhance processing at the attended ear and to inhibit or suppress processing in the nonattended ear.

OVERALL SUMMARY

There has been a great deal of progress in understanding the cognitive/ brain mechanisms underlying dichotic perceptual asymmetries and attentional effects on these asymmetries. Findings from recent behavioral dichotic studies indicate that the REA for dichotically presented linguistic stimuli results at least partially from automatic, preattentional processing based upon the hardwired properties of the auditory system. But attention also clearly influences ear asymmetries, and a number of studies have attempted to assess whether attention acts to alter early (perceptual) or late (response selection) processes. Evidence from behavioral and electrophysiological studies reviewed above indicates that attention can act at both early and late stages to enhance processing of stimuli at attended locations. Recent models of attention that are based upon neurophysiological data concerning brain function indicate that spatially selective attention may influence processing at many different locations in the brain. These range from enhancement of attended stimuli in early sensory regions to attention-based selection of action-related systems. Functional imaging studies have provided support for the role of bottom-up, stimulus-specific mechanisms in the generation of perceptual asymmetries. PET studies also have indicated that attention may act to enhance processing of stimuli in the attended channel and to suppress processing of unattended stimuli.

REFERENCES

Alho, K., Medvedev, S. V., Pakhomov, S. V., Roudas, M. S., Tervaniemi, M., Reinikainen, K., Zeffiro, T., & Näätänen, R. (1999). Selective tuning of the left and right auditory cortices during spatially directed attention. *Cognitive Brain Research, 7*, 335–341.

Allport, A. (1992). Attention and control: Have we been asking the wrong questions? A Critical review of twenty-five years. In D. E. Meyer & S. Kornblum (Eds.), *Attention and performance XIV. Synergies in experimental psychology, artificial intelligence and cognitive neuroscience* (pp. 183–218). Cambridge, MA: MIT Press.

Andreasen, N. C., Cizadlo, T., Harris, G., Swayze, V. 2nd, O'Leary, D. S., Cohen, G., Ehrhardt, J., & Yuh, W. T. (1993). Voxel processing techniques for the antemortem study of neuroanatomy and neuropathology using magnetic resonance imaging. *Journal of Neuropsychiatry, 5*, 121–130.

Asbjørnsen, A. E., & Bryden, M. P. (1996). Biased attention and the fused dichotic word test. *Neuropsychologia, 34*, 407–411.

Asbjørnsen, A. E., & Hugdahl, K. (1995). Attentional effects in dichotic listening. *Brain and Language, 49*, 189–201.

Awh, E., Jonides, J., & Reuter-Lorenz, P. A. (1998). Rehearsal in spatial working memory. *Journal of Experimental Psychology: Human Perception and Performance, 24*, 780–790.

Berlin, C. I., Lowe-Bell, S. S., Cullen, J. K. Jr., & Thompson, C. L. (1973). Dichotic speech perception: An interpretation of right-ear advantage and temporal offset effects. *Journal of the Acoustical Society of America, 53*, 699–709.

Bryden, P. M. (1978). Strategy effects in the study of hemispheric asymmetry. In Underwood, G. (Ed.), *Strategies of information processing* (pp. 447–458). London: Academic Press.

Bryden, M. P., & Murray, J. E. (1985). Towards a model of dichotic listening performance. *Brain and Cognition, 4*, 241–257.

Bushara, K. O., Weeks, R. A., Ishii, K., Catalan, M. J., Tian, B., Rauschecker, J. P., & Hallett, M. (1999). Modality-specific frontal and parietal areas for auditory and visual spatial localization in humans. *Nature Neuroscience, 2*, 759–766.

Caplan, D. (1992). *Language: Structure, processing and disorders*. Cambridge MA: MIT Press.

Chelazzi, L., & Corbetta, M. (2000). Cortical mechanisms of visuospatial attention in the primate brain. In M. Gazziniga (Ed.), *The new cognitive neurosciences*. Second edition. Cambridge, MA: MIT Press.

Corbetta, M., Akbudak, E., Conturo, T. E., Snyder, A. Z., Ollinger, J. M., Drury, H. A., Linenweber, M. R., Petersen, S. E., Raichle, M. E., Van Essen, D. C., & Shulman, G. L. (1998). A common network of functional areas for attention and eye movements. *Neuron, 21*, 761–773.

Corbetta, M., Kincade, J. M., Ollinger, J. M., McAvoy, M. P., & Schulman, G. L. (2000). Voluntary orienting is dissociated from target detection in human posterior parietal cortex. *Nature Neuroscience, 3*, 292–297.

Corbetta, M., Miezin, F. M., Shulman, G. L., & Peterson, S. E. (1993). A PET study of visual spatial attention. *Journal of Neuroscience, 13*, 1202.

Crick, F. (1984). Function of the thalamic reticular complex: The searchlight hypothesis. *Proceedings of the National Academy of Sciences, USA, 81*, 4586–4590.

Desimone, R., & Duncan, J. (1995). Neural mechanisms of selective visual attention. *Annual Review of Neuroscience, 18*, 193–222.

Desimone, R., Wessinger, M., Thomas, L., & Scheider, W. (1990). Attentional control of visual perception: Cortical and subcortical mechanisms. *Cold Spring Harbor Symposia on Quantatative Biology, 55*, 963–971.

Grady, C. L., et al. (1995). The effect of increasing perceptual difficulty on cerebral blood flow activation. *Human Brain Mapping, 1* (Suppl. 1), 270.

Griffiths, T. D., Rees, G., Rees, A., Green, G. G., Witton, C., Rowe, D., Buchel, C., Turner, R., & Frackowiak, R. S. (1998). Right parietal cortex is involved in the perception of sound movement in humans. *Nature Neuroscience, 1*, 74–79.

Hansen, J. C., & Hillyard, S. A. (1980). Endogenous brain potentials associated with selective auditory attention. *Electroencephalography and Clinical Neurophysiology, 49*, 277–290.

Haxby, J. V., Horwitz, B., Ungerleider, L. G., Maisog, J. M., Pietrini, P., & Grady, C. L. (1994). The functional organization of human extrastriate cortex: A PET-rCBF study of selective attention to faces and locations. *Journal of Neuroscience, 14,* 6336–6353.

Heinze, H. J., Mangun, G. R., Burchert, W., Hinrichs, H., Scholz, M., Munte, T. F., Gos, A., Scherg, M., Johannes, S., Hundeshagen, H., et al. (1994). Combined spatial and temporal imaging of brain activity during visual selective attention in humans. *Nature, 372,* 543–546.

Hillyard, S. A., Hink, R. F., Schwent, V. I., & Picton, T. W. (1973). Electrical signs of selective attention in the human brain. *Science, 182,* 177–179.

Hiscock, M., & Beckie, J. L. (1993). Overcoming the right ear advantage: A study of focused attention in children. *Journal of Clinical and Experimental Neuropsychology, 15,* 754–772.

Hopfinger, J. B., Buonocore, M. H., & Mangun, G. R. (2000). The neural mechanisms of top-down attentional control. *Nature Neuroscience, 3,* 284–291.

Horwitz, B. (1991). Functional interactions in the brain: Use of correlations between regional metabolic rates. *Journal of Cerebral Blood Flow and Metabolism, 11,* A114–A120.

Howard, D., Patterson, K., Wise, R., Brown, W. D., Friston, K., Weiller, C., & Frackowiak, R. (1992). The cortical location of the lexicons. *Brain, 115,* 1769–1782.

Hugdahl, K. (1995). Dichotic listening: Probing temporal lobe functional integrity. In R. J. Davidson & K. Hugdahl (Eds.), *Brain asymmetry* (pp. 123–156). Cambridge MA: MIT Press.

Hugdahl, K., & Andersson, L. (1986). The "forced attention paradigm" in dichotic listening to CV-syllables: A comparison between adults and children. *Cortex, 22,* 417–432.

Hugdahl, K., Brønnick, K., Kyllingsbaek, S., Law, I., Gade, A., & Paulson, O. B. (1999). Brain activation during dichotic presentations of consonant-vowel and musical instrument stimuli: A 15O-PET study. *Neuropsychologia, 37*(4), 431–440.

Hugdahl, K., Carlsson, G., Uvebrant, P., & Lundervold, A. J. (1997). Dichotic listening performance and intracarotid amobarbitol injections in children and adolescents: Comparisons pre- and post-operatively. *Archives of Neurology, 54,* 1494–1500.

Hugdahl, K., Law, I., Kyllingsbaek, S., Bronnick, K., Gade, A., & Paulson, O. B. (2000). Effects of attention on dichotic listening: An 15O-PET study. *Human Brain Mapping 10*(2), 87–97.

Kesler, M. L. (1997). Correlations between brain regions during auditory selective attention: A positron emission tomography (PET) study. Ph.D. dissertation.

Kesler, M. L., O'Leary, D. S., Hurtig, R. R., & Andreasen, N. C. (1995). A positron emission tomography (PET) study of attention to auditory stimuli. *Society for Neuroscience Abstracts, 21*(2), 937.

Kimura, D. (1961). Cerebral dominance and the perception of verbal stimuli. *Canadian Journal of Psychology, 15,* 156–165.

Kinsbourne, M. (1970). The cerebral basis of lateral asymmetries in attention. *Acta Psychologia, 33*, 193–201.

Kinsbourne, M. (1973). The control of attention by interaction between the cerebral hemispheres. In S. Kornblum (Ed.), *Attention and performance IV*. (pp. 239–258). New York: Academic Press.

Liégeois-Chauvel, C., Musolino, A., & Chauvel, P. (1991). Localization of the primary auditory area in man. *Brain, 114*, 139–153.

Løberg, E. M., Hugdahl, K., & Green, M. F. (1999). Hemispheric asymmetry in schizophrenia: A "dual deficits" model. *Biological Psychiatry, 45*, 76–81.

Marr, D. (1992). *Vision*. San Francisco: W. H. Freeman.

Mesulam, M. M. (1990). Large-scale neurocognitive networks and distributed processing for attention, language, and memory. *Annals of Neurology, 28*(5), 597–613.

Mondor, T. A. (1994). Interaction between handedness and the attentional bias during tests of dichotic listening performance. *Journal of Clinical and Experimental Neuropsychology, 16*, 377–385.

Mondor, T. A., & Bryden, M. P. (1991). The influence of attention on the dichotic REA. *Neuropsychologia, 29*, 1179–1190.

Näätänen, R. (1992). *Attention and brain function*. Hillsdale, NJ: Lawrence Erlbaum Associates.

Näätänen, R., Gaillard, A. W. K., & Mantysalo, S. (1978). Early selective attention effect on evoked potential reinterpreted. *Acta Psychologia, 42*, 313–329.

Nobre, A. C., Sebestyen, G. N., Gitelman, D. R., Mesulam, M. M., Frackowiak, R. S., & Frith, C. D. (1997). Functional localization of the visuospatial attention system using positron-emission tomography. *Brain, 120*, 515–533.

O'Leary, D. S., Andreasen, N. C., Hurtig, R. R., Hichwa, R. D., Watkins, G. L., Boles Ponto, L. L., Rogers, M., & Kirchner, P. T. (1996a). A regional cerebral blood flow study of language and auditory attention. *Brain and Language, 53*, 20–39.

O'Leary, D. S., Andreasen, N. C., Hurtig, R. R., Kesler, M. L., Rogers, M., Arndt, S., Cizadlo, T., Watkins, G. L., Boles Ponto, L. L., Kirchner, P. T., & Hichwa, R. D. (1996b). Auditory attentional deficits in patients with schizophrenia: A positron emission tomography study. *Archives of General Psychiatry, 53*, 633–641.

O'Leary, D. S., Andreasen, N. C., Hichwa, R., Hurtig, R. R., Watkins, G. L., & Boles Ponto, L. L. (1997). Auditory and visual attention assessed with PET. *Human Brain Mapping, 5*, 422–436.

O'Leary, D. S., Andreasen, N. C., Hichwa, R., Watkins, G. L., & Boles Ponto, L. L. (in preparation). Surpression of blood flow in Heschl's gyrus ipsilateral to the direction of auditory attention.

O'Leary, D. S., Andreasen, N. C., Hichwa, R., Watkins, G. L., & Boles Ponto, L. L. (1999). The components of spatial working memory: A PET study assessing spatial attention and the maintenance and updating of location information. *NeuroImage, 9*, 961.

Pelizzari, C. A., Chen, G. T. Y., Spelbring, D. R., Weichselbaum, R. R., & Chen, C. T. (1989). Accurate three-dimensional registration of CT, PET, and/or MR images of the brain. *Journal of Computer Assisted Tomography, 13,* 20–26.

Posner, M. I., & Dhaene, S. (1994). Attentional networks. *Trends in Neuroscience, 17*(2), 75–79.

Posner, M. I., & Petersen, S. E. (1990). The attention system of the human brain. *Annual Review of Neuroscience, 13,* 25–42.

Posner, M. I., Snyder, C. R., & Davidson, B. J. (1980). Attention and the detection of signals. *Journal of Experimental Psychology: General, 109,* 160–174.

Rizzolatti, G., Riggio, L., & Shelige, B. B. (1994). Space and selective attention. In C. Umilata and M. Moscovitch (Eds.), *Attention and performance XV: Conscious and nonconscious information processing* (pp. 231–265). Cambridge MA: MIT Press.

Roudas, M. S. (1996). Direction of auditory attention affects hemispheric distribution of brain activity: A PET study. *Neuroimage, 3,* S196.

Schmahmann, J. D. (1998). Dysmetria of thought: Clinical consequences of cerebellar dysfunction on cognition and affect. *Trends in Cognitive Science, 2,* 362–371.

Spellacy, F., & Blumstein, S. (1970). The influence of language set on ear preference in phoneme recognition. *Cortex, 6,* 430–439.

Studdert-Kennedy, M., & Shankweiler, D. P. (1970). Hemispheric specialization for speech perception. *Journal of the Acoustic Society of America, 48,* 579–594.

Talairach, J., & Tournoux, P. (1988). *Co-planar stereotaxic atlas of the human brain. 3-D proportional system: An approach to cerebral imaging.* Stuttgart and New York: Georg Thieme Verlag.

Tzourio, N., Massioui, F. E., Crivello, F., Joliot, M., Renault, B., & Mazoyer, B. (1997). Functional anatomy of the human auditory system. *Neuroimage, 5,* 63–77.

Ungerleider, L. G., & Haxby, J. V. (1994). "What" and "where" in the human brain. *Current Opinions in Neurobiology, 4,* 157–165.

Vandenberghe, R., et al. (1995). Superior parietal blood flow depends on the number of attended attributes. In *Human brain mapping, Supplement 1, First International Conference on the Functional Mapping of the Human Brain* (p. 269). Paris: John Wiley & Sons.

Vandenberghe, R., Dupont, P., De Bruyn, B., Bormans, G., Michiels, J., Mortelmans, L., & Orban, G. A. (1996). The influence of stimulus location on the brain activation pattern in detection and orientation discrimination. A PET study of visual attention. *Brain, 119,* 1263–1276.

Wexler, B. E., & Hawles, T. (1983). Increasing the power of dichotic methods: The fused rhymed words test. *Neuropsychologia, 21,* 59–66.

Wexler, B. E., & Hawles, T. (1985). Dichotic listening tests in studying brain-behavior relationships. *Neuropsychologia, 23,* 545–559.

Wise, R., Chollet, F., Hadar, U., Friston, K., Hoffner, E., & Frackowiak, R. (1991). Distribution of cortical neural networks involved in word comprehension and word retrieval. *Brain, 114*, 1803–1817.

Woldorff, M. G. (1995). Selective listening at fast dichotic rates: So much to hear, so little time. In M. Karmos, V. Molnar, V. Csepc, & J. E. Desmedt (Eds.), *Perspectives of event-related potentials research* (EEG Suppl. 44) (pp. 32–51). Amsterdam: Elsevier Science.

Woldorff, M. G. (1996). Visual spatial attention: Integration of PET and ERP data. *Neuroimage, 3*, S242.

Woldorff, M. G., & Hillyard, S. A. (1991). Modulation of early auditory processing during selective listening to rapidly presented tones. *Electroencephalography and Clinical Neurophysiology, 79*, 170–190.

Woodruff, P. W. R., Benson, R. R., Talavage, T., Kwong, K. K., Bandettini, P. A., Goodman, J., Belliveau, J. W., & Rosen, B. R. (1995). Modulation of auditory cortical attention demonstrated with functional MRI. *Human Brain Mapping, 1*(Suppl. 1), 190.

Woods, R. P., Cherry, S. R., & Mazziotta, J. C. (1992). Rapid automated algorithm for aligning and reslicing PET images. *Journal of Computer Assisted Tomography, 16*(4), 620–633.

Woods, S., Hiscock, M., & Widrig, M. (2000). Selective attention fails to alter the dichotic lag effect: Evidence that the lag is preattentional. *Brain and Language, 71*, 373–390.

Worsley, K. J., Evans, A. C., Marrett, S., & Neelin, P. (1992). A three dimensional statistical analysis for CBF activation studies in human brain. *Journal of Cerebral Blood Flow and Metabolism, 12*, 900–918.

Zatorre, R. J., Mondor, T. A., & Evans, A. C. (1999). Auditory attention to space and frequency activates similar cortical regions. *Neuroimage, 10*(5), 544–554.

V   Emotional Laterality

14 The Functional Neuroimaging of Human Emotion: Asymmetric Contributions of Cortical and Subcortical Circuitry

Diego Pizzagalli, Alexander J. Shackman, and
Richard J. Davidson

Affective neuroscience is the subdiscipline of the biobehavioral sciences
that examines the underlying neural bases of mood and emotion. The
application of this body of theory and data to the study of normal
emotion, disorders of emotion, and affective style is helping to generate
a new understanding of the brain circuitry underlying these phenomena. Moreover, parsing the heterogeneity of both normal and abnormal
emotional processes on the basis of known circuits in the brain is providing a novel and potentially very fruitful approach to classification
and subtyping that does not rely on the descriptive nosology of personality theory and psychiatric diagnosis; rather, it is based upon more
objective characterization of specific affective processing deficits in normal individuals and in patients with mood disorders. At a more general level, this approach is helping to bridge the wide chasm between
the literatures that have focused on normal emotion and on the disorders of emotion. Historically, these research traditions have had
little to do with one another and have emerged completely independently. However, affective neuroscience has helped to integrate these
approaches into a more unified project that is focused upon the understanding of normal and pathological individual differences in affective style, the constituent components, and their neural bases (see, e.g.,
Davidson, Jackson, et al., 2000, Davidson, 2000).

Affective neuroscience takes as its overall aim a project which is similar to that pursued by its cognate discipline, cognitive neuroscience,
though it is focused instead on affective processes. The decomposition of cognitive processes into more elementary constituents that can
then be studied in neural terms has been remarkably successful. We no
longer query subjects about the contents of their cognitive processes

because many of the processes so central to important aspects of cognitive function are opaque to consciousness. Instead, modern cognitive scientists and neuroscientists have developed laboratory tasks to interrogate and reveal more elementary cognitive function. These more elementary processes can then be studied using imaging methods in humans, lesion methods in animals, and the study of human patients with focal brain damage. Affective neuroscience approaches emotion using the same strategy. Global constructs of emotion are giving way to more specific and elementary constituents that can be examined with objective laboratory measures. For example, the time course of emotional responding and the mechanisms that are brought into play during the regulation of emotion can now be probed using objective laboratory measures. These constructs may be particularly important for understanding mood disorders because patients with depression may suffer from abnormalities in emotion regulation and persistence of negative affect. Patients with such abnormalities may differ from those whose primary deficit may be in reactivity to positive incentives.

Previously constructs such as emotion regulation were mostly been gleaned from self-report measures whose validity has been seriously questioned (e.g., Kahneman, 1999). While the phenomenology of emotion provides critical information to the subject that helps guide behavior, it may not be a particularly good source for making inferences about the processes and mechanisms that underlie emotion and its regulation. Though it is still tempting and often important to obtain measures of subjects' conscious experience of the contents of their emotional states and traits, these no longer constitute the sole source of information about emotion.

This review will feature data that have mostly been derived from human neuroimaging studies. Neuroimaging methods provide unique in vivo data on human brain function that can be then be associated with behavioral and/or self-report measures. Since certain mechanisms of emotion may differ in humans compared with other species (e.g., subjective experiences of emotion or more developed capacity for emotion regulation), the opportunity to study these questions in humans with methods that allow for the interrogation of brain function throughout the brain volume is very significant. Some methods allow for the assessment of the time course of neural activation (e.g., event-related functional magnetic resonance imaging; fMRI) and other methods permit inferences to be drawn about connectivity among brain

D. Pizzagalli, A. J. Shackman, and R. J. Davidson

regions. Finally, positron emission tomography (PET) enables the investigator to probe the neurochemistry of the brain and evaluate how it may be affected by behavioral challenges.

The major limitation of the evidence derived from neuroimaging studies is that the data are correlative in nature, and it is therefore difficult to make causal inferences about the role of specific circuits in behavior. However, when neuroimaging data in humans are combined with more invasive studies in animals where the same circuitry can be directly manipulated, powerful strategies become available for making causal inferences.

This review will focus on selected fMRI and PET studies published between 1993 and 2001 that specifically manipulated affect or investigated emotional processing, and that bear on our understanding of asymmetries in the underlying neural circuitry. We will not treat studies that primarily involve the perception of emotional information, such as facial expressions. While interesting and important, and clearly relevant to the perception of emotional information, these findings may not directly bear on our understanding of the neural substrates of emotion per se, despite the fact that such data are often casually interpreted as if the perception and production of emotion were necessarily utilizing the identical circuitry. We will also focus primarily upon studies in normal subjects because we have recently published several reviews of similar questions in psychiatric patients (Davidson, Putnam, et al., 2000; Davidson et al., 2002). However, when pertinent, data from patient studies as well as from animal studies will be briefly mentioned.

CONCEPTUAL AND METHODOLOGICAL CONSIDERATIONS IN NEUROIMAGING STUDIES OF EMOTION AND AFFECTIVE STYLE

PET and fMRI provide powerful and complementary information that has not been possible to acquire with other methods. These techniques enable scientists to examine regional patterns of activation in normal, intact humans with considerable spatial precision and, in the case of fMRI, with temporal resolution on the order of seconds. With PET, in addition to its use as a measure of hemodynamic or metabolic activity, it can also be used to probe components of neurotransmission in vivo in relation to behavioral performance (e.g., Koepp et al., 1998). The application of these methods to the study of emotion has burgeoned over the past several years and has generated a new corpus of literature on the circuitry associated with selective features of emotional responding and affective traits. There are a number of critical conceptual and methodological issues that are fundamental to neuroimaging studies of emotion that are highlighted below.

1. *The perception of emotional information must be carefully distinguished from the production of emotion.* There are many studies that present facial expressions of emotion as stimuli to subjects. The presentation of facial expressions of emotion does not necessarily (nor even likely) elicit any emotion. Thus, when investigators use this procedure, it is important that it be described as a study of the perception of emotional faces and not a study about emotion per se.

2. *The control conditions against which emotion activation is compared crucially influence the nature of the data obtained.* When using subtractive methodology, it is helpful to control for as much of the stimulus content as possible in order to isolate the effects of emotion per se. Thus, for example, the comparison of a condition during which subjects were self-generating emotional imagery against a resting baseline would be problematic (e.g., Pardo et al., 1993) because any effects observed might not be a function of the particular emotion that was aroused, but rather the cognitive processes involved in retrieving information from memory and voluntarily generating visual imagery. It is good practice to include more than one emotion condition (e.g., both positive and negative) because any effect produced as a consequence of simply generating emotion per se should be common to the two emotions, while differences between conditions can be attributed to the specific nature of the emotional process elicited.

3. *Stimuli designed to elicit different emotions must be matched on arousal and physical characteristics.* Arousal can be inferred in several different ways, including self-report and skin conductance measures. Differences in patterns of activation observed between two emotion conditions that are not matched on intensity or arousal obviously can result from a failure to match appropriately, and might be more a function of the arousal differences rather than of the emotion differences between conditions (see Davidson et al., 1990 for more extended discussion). A related issue is the need to match stimuli across emotion and control conditions on physical properties such as color, the presence of faces,

D. Pizzagalli, A. J. Shackman, and R. J. Davidson

spatial frequency, and related variables. Some differences found between emotion conditions might conceivably be a function of physical differences between the stimuli that have nothing directly to do with emotion.

4. *Putatively asymmetric effects must be rigorously statistically interrogated.* Many investigators, using both PET and fMRI, have reported asymmetric changes associated with emotion. In most cases, claims about an activation being asymmetric were made on the basis of voxels in one hemisphere that exceeded statistical threshold whereas homologous voxels in the opposite hemisphere did not. However, such an analytic strategy, while typical, is only testing for main effects of condition. To demonstrate an actual difference between the two hemispheres, it is necessary to test the condition x hemisphere or group x hemisphere interaction. The fact that such tests are rarely performed is largely a function of the fact that while they are conceptually straightforward, their implementation is complex for a variety of reasons, including the lack of availability of commercial software for this purpose and, most important, the fact that brains are not anatomically symmetric and thus it would be hazardous to simply identify the homologous region of the brain to evaluate a putatively asymmetric effect. Having said this, it must be noted that such tests would still represent a considerable improvement over what is now standard practice. If the Hemisphere x Condition or Hemisphere x Condition interaction is not statistically significant, it is not legitimate to claim that an asymmetric finding is present, because the lack of a significant interaction means that the changes found in one hemisphere are not significantly different from those observed in the other, even if the effects are independently significant in one hemisphere but not in the other. Moreover, it is possible for significant interactions to arise in the absence of any significant main effects.

These methodological obstacles to making inferences about patterns of asymmetric activation can be further worsened if the signal-to-noise ratio (SNR) within regions of interest is inhomogeneous because of susceptibility artifacts with fMRI. This latter problem could especially pertain to subcortical regions, such as the amygdala. Recently, LaBar and colleagues (2001) explicitly tested the hypothesis that "asymmetrical" results in task-related amygdalar activation may be artificially caused by SNR dropouts due to susceptibility artifacts from the adjacent sinus. The authors used an algorithm to generate SNR maps thresholded at the minimum SNR required to observe reliable activation for a given fMRI protocol. The results showed that SNR was crucial for explaining variability in the pattern of amygdala activation across subjects: unilateral activation, bilateral activation, or no activation was highly dependent on the SNR in the amygdalar region. These findings underscore the care and caution required in the interpretation of asymmetric findings with neuroimaging methods such as fMRI.

5. *The processes of emotion regulation must ultimately be disentangled from those associated with the generation of emotion per se.* Mechanisms that regulate emotion—those processes which maintain, enhance, or suppress an emotion—are activated coterminously with the generation of emotion. This complicates the task of the scientist examining neuroimaging data and making inferences about the activations that are putatively associated with the elicited emotion. Some of the activations that have been observed could conceivably be a part of circuitry which serves to regulate emotion. While this topic is complex and has important conceptual and methodological implications, it cannot be treated extensively here other than to suggest at the outset that some of the inconsistencies which plague this literature may be associated with unintended variations in emotion regulation. Explicit manipulation of regulatory parameters may be one method for addressing this problem (see Davidson, Putnam, et al., 2000 for review).

REVIEW OF HUMAN NEUROIMAGING (FMRI/PET) STUDIES ON EMOTION AND AFFECTIVE STYLES

Classical Fear Conditioning

Classical or Pavlovian conditioning (Pavlov, 1927) is a form of associative learning involving a relationship between a neutral event and an event with biological significance, and thus contains elements of both memory and emotional processing (see Hugdahl, 1995 for review). In classical conditioning, the neutral stimulus becomes behaviorally significant by being contingently coupled with a salient unconditioned stimulus. Several neuroimaging studies have investigated the neural substrates of classical conditioning. In this paradigm, three experimental phases are usually distinguished. In a habituation or preconditioning phase, emotionally neutral stimuli are presented without additional

D. Pizzagalli, A. J. Shackman, and R. J. Davidson

intervening variables. During the acquisition or conditioning phase, initially neutral stimuli (conditioned stimuli, CS) become behaviorally salient (CS+) because of temporal pairing with an aversive unconditioned stimulus (US). In the extinction or postconditioning phase, the CS+ is presented without US.

In one of the first PET studies of classical fear conditioning, Hugdahl and coworkers (Hugdahl et al., 1995) scanned subjects during a habituation and an extinction phase, where auditory tones (CS) were presented alone. Between these two phases, the subjects were conditioned to the tones by pairing them with electric shocks (US). The results showed a pattern of right-lateralized activation involving the orbitofrontal cortex (OFC), dorsolateral prefrontal cortex (DLPFC), inferior and superior frontal cortices, and inferior and middle temporal cortices.

In a later PET study, Morris et al. (1997) employed a differential classical conditioning paradigm, using facial expressions as CS and an aversive burst of white noise as US. During the extinction phase, the CS^+ elicited stronger right-lateralized activation than the CS^- in the pulvinar nucleus of the thalamus, OFC (Brodmann area [BA]10; Brodmann, 1909), superior frontal gyrus (BA46), and anterolateral thalamus. Furthermore, activation in the right amygdala, the right basal forebrain, right hippocampal gyrus, and bilateral fusiform gyrus was significantly correlated with the CS^+-modulated activity in the right pulvinar.

In a follow-up study, Morris and coworkers (Morris, Friston, et al., 1998) investigated brain regions showing learning-related modulation in the auditory cortex as a consequence of conditioning. When auditory CS (tones, 200 Hz and 8000 Hz) previously paired with an aversive noise burst (US) were presented alone, learning-modulated activity was observed in the auditory cortex. Regression analyses indicated that conditioned activity within the auditory cortex (bilateral transverse temporal gyrus) covaried with activity in the amygdalae, basal forebrain, and right OFC (and to a lesser extent in the anterior insula and anterior cingulate cortex [ACC]).

In a later $H_2^{15}O$ PET study, Morris, Ohman, et al. (1998) used a backward masking procedure to present the CS^+ (an angry face previously paired with a burst of white noise) and CS^- (another angry face never paired with noise) below the level of conscious awareness. Whereas the left amygdala was activated when the CS^+ was presented above the level of awareness, right amygdalar activation was observed when the CS^+ was presented below the level of conscious awareness. Although the authors formally tested the masking x hemisphere interaction, the amygdalar activation for masked (medial and inferior) and unmasked (superior and posterior) stimuli was rather different. In fact, the voxels in the left ($x = -16$, $y = -8$, $z = -14$) and right ($x = 18$, $y = -2$, $z = -28$) amygdala were displaced by 15.36 mm (Euclidean distance).

Summary The data on conditioning implicate both PFC and amygdala in associative learning. First, it should be noted that the extant studies which have reported asymmetric effects have all been performed with aversive learning paradigms. It will be important in the future to examine appetitive learning to determine if the effects that have been reported for the aversive context are different during appetitive learning. Second, it is difficult to disentangle the active inhibitory processes that are presumably occurring during extinction from the CS-elicited emotional response prior to complete extinction. This makes the pattern of neural activity during extinction particularly difficult to interpret. Despite these caveats, several generalizations can be offered. During extinction in aversive conditioning, the CS+ has been found to elicit greater right-sided activation in several PFC regions, including the superior frontal gyrus and the OFC. In addition, some evidence indicates activation of the amygdala. The Morris, Ohman, et al. (1998) study reported asymmetric differences in amygdala activation in response to masked versus unmasked CS^+'s, with the former associated with greater right amygdala activation compared with the latter. However, these asymmetric effects in the amygdala were not in homologous regions.

With the sole exception of the Morris, Ohman, et al. (1998) study, the other studies of conditioning where asymmetric effects were reported did not rigorously evaluate the Condition x Hemisphere interactions. The lack of formal interaction testing precludes the drawing of definitive conclusions about asymmetric effects that distinguish between conditions. Finally, careful study of the differences between the acquisition and extinction phases is required before concluding that activations observed are associated with emotional effects of CS presentations versus the active inhibitory mechanisms of extinction.

D. Pizzagalli, A. J. Shackman, and R. J. Davidson

Reward and Punishment Processing

Reward and punishment are crucial variables for the regulation of behavior. Reward is associated with approach behavior, acts as positive reinforcer (i.e., increases and maintains the occurrence of behavior that leads to reward), and typically triggers pleasurable feelings. Animal studies have stressed the role of the basal ganglia (ventral striatum, particularly the nucleus accumbens and ventral pallidum), OFC, and DLPFC in reward processing. For example, in animals, neurons in the ventral striatum are activated before an expected reward, suggesting that they may encode reward representation (for a review, see Schultz et al., 2000). Human lesion and invasive animal data suggest that the ventral OFC is crucial for monitoring of response-outcome relations (for review, see Rolls 2000), especially when reversal learning and extinction are involved. Despite the extensive study of the neural substrates of reward processing in animals, it is only in recent years that the neural activation associated with reward and punishment processing has been studied in the human brain.

Thut and coworkers (1997) published the first human neuroimaging study aimed at investigating brain structures involved in reward processing. $H_2{}^{15}O$ PET scans were obtained while subjects performed a prelearned delayed go-no go task in which abstract shapes predicted the occurrence of a go (speeded key press) or no go trial (no key press). Abstract (the word "OK") or monetary reinforcement was given if their reaction time was under a given limit. Compared to the abstract reinforcement, monetary reinforcement elicited stronger activation in the lateral prefrontal cortex (BA10/44), OFC (BA47), thalamus, and midbrain, all in the left hemisphere. Thus, these results highlight a pivotal role for left-sided activation of the OFC and DLPFC in directing voluntary behavior toward appetitive goals.

Using ^{11}C-labeled raclopride and PET, Koepp et al. (1998) assessed changes in levels of extracellular dopamine while subjects were engaged in a goal-directed video game with monetary incentive. Compared to a control scan, playing the video game was associated with reduced raclopride binding in the striatum, reflecting increased release and binding of dopamine to its receptors. Highlighting the role of the striatum in goal-directed behavior, binding reduction in the striatum (especially left ventral) was positively correlated with task performance.

Since the ventral striatum receives important projections from the OFC, amygdala, and ACC, the association between ventral striatum and task performance may suggest that the dopamine changes were related to affective components of the task.

Using a computerized gambling task and $H_2{}^{15}O$ PET, Rogers and colleagues (1999) explored brain regions involved in deciding between a choice associated with unlikely, yet larger, reward as well as punishment and likely, yet smaller, rewards or punishments. Thus, in the former condition, despite the presence of large potential rewards, the opportunity for large potential punishments was also present. Results showed a strongly asymmetric pattern in frontal regions. Whereas increased regional cerebral blood flow (rCBF) during decision-making was observed in several regions of the right PFC (inferior and orbital PFC, BA11; medial frontal gyrus, BA10/11; orbital gyrus, BA11; and inferior frontal gyrus, BA47), -decreased rCBF was observed in, among other regions, the left medial frontal gyrus (BA10).

Delgado et al. (2000) also explored the neural substrates underlying feedback in a gambling task. Subjects were scanned while they were presented with a card with a hidden number that needed to be guessed ("smaller or greater than a given threshold?"). Using an event-related fMRI design, reward trials (win money), neutral trials, and punishment trials (lose money) were alternated. In agreement with prior animal work, this study confirmed a primary role of striatal regions in response to reward-related information: correct guesses elicited more sustained and slowly decaying bilateral activation in the dorsal striatum (caudate) and left medial temporal lobe compared to incorrect, and thus punished, guesses. The left-lateralized effect confirmed prior findings of greater involvement of left regions in reward-related information in similar tasks (Koepp et al., 1998; Thut et al., 1997; Zalla et al., 2000).

Employing fMRI and a simple reaction time embedded in a fictitious but engaging competitive tournament, Zalla et al. (2000) explored the role of the amygdala and other regions in processing "winning" or "losing" information. For the subjects, winning and losing depended on the response speed in a cued reaction time task (in reality, winning and losing were parametrically varied independently of performance). Results showed a laterality effect in the amygdalae: Whereas the left amygdala was associated with parametric increases in winning, the right amygdala was associated with parametric increases in losing.

D. Pizzagalli, A. J. Shackman, and R. J. Davidson

Further, winning was associated with increased activation in the left inferior frontal gyrus (BA44), left hippocampus, and right OFC (BA47). Conversely, losing elicited increased activation in three right hemispheric regions: PFC (BA9), putamen, and globus pallidum. Besides confirming a stronger involvement of left and right (especially frontal) regions in approach- and withdrawal-related states, respectively, this study showed, for the first time in the intact human brain, an involvement of the left amygdala in reward-related information.

Using a prelearned delayed pattern recognition task and $H_2^{15}O$ PET, Künig et al. (2000) compared brain activation in Parkinson's patients and control subjects. Subjects were engaged in a match-to-sample task involving three reinforcement conditions depending on subjects' performance: positive symbolic ("OK") reinforcement, monetary reinforcement, and no reinforcement (nonsense feedback). In controls, both positive reinforcements elicited bilateral activation in the ACC (BA24) and caudate, as well as activation in the left cerebellum and left medial frontal gyrus; monetary rewards additionally elicited bilateral striatal activation and left midbrain activation. Further, general processing of positive reinforcements involved additional left hemispheric regions, the inferior parietal gyrus (BA40) and medial temporal gyrus (BA21). These results confirm (a) an important role of dopaminergic mesostriatal/mesocorticolimbic and DLPFC regions in reward processing, and (b) a left hemispheric preponderance in such processes.

O'Doherty, Kringelbach, et al. (2001) further explored the role of the human OFC in abstract representations of reward and punishment. Subjects performed a visual reversal-learning task in which they attempted to determine by trial and error which of two stimuli was linked to (fictive) reward or punishment (stimulus-reinforcement contingencies were probabilistically determined). Results suggested a striking dissociation within the OFC with respect to reward or punishment: Whereas the medial (bilateral) OFC was involved in reward outcomes, the right lateral OFC (BA10/11) was implicated in punishment outcomes. Further, correlational analyses revealed an asymmetrical pattern in the OFC: the left medial and right lateral OFC were positively correlated with reward and punishment magnitude, respectively.

Summary The findings reviewed in this section are consistent with earlier electrophysiological findings that suggest asymmetric activation in regions of the PFC that differentiate between reward and punishment and approach- and withdrawal-related emotion (see Davidson, 2000; Davidson, Jackson, et al., 2000 for reviews). Moreover, the neuroimaging data permit more specific and differentiated anatomical specification, and indicate that asymmetries are observed in both orbital/ventral and dorsolateral regions of the PFC. Results from O'Doherty, Kringelbach, et al. (2001) suggest that medial territories in the OFC may crucially involved in reward outcomes, whereas lateral (possibly right) OFC (BA10/11) may be more involved in punishment outcomes. In addition, the neuroimaging data suggest that asymmetries may also be present in the amygdala. Although replication of this laterality effect is warranted, it is interesting to note that in rodents there is evidence suggesting a predominant role of the right amygdala rather than the left in memory consolidation for aversive experiences (Coleman-Mesches & McGaugh, 1995a, 1995b).

Two cautions require explicit mention in considering this literature. First, in addition to the asymmetric patterns of activation highlighted above, there were often other bilateral activations present in response to the incentive conditions that were studied. Thus, the asymmetry effects should be considered rather than a matter of degree and in any absolute fashion. Moreover, these findings should be placed within an overall circuit that may include both bilateral and asymmetric effects. Second, many of the studies did not formally test the condition x hemisphere interactions. Thus it is not always possible to know if the particular asymmetric finding that is reported is significantly greater for one hemisphere region than the other. The few studies where explicit tests for asymmetry were conducted have been noted.

Externally Elicited Affect

In 1996, our laboratory published the first report of amygdalar activation in response to complex aversive visual stimuli (Irwin et al., 1996). In this study, three coronal slices were acquired while female participants viewed alternating blocks of aversive and neutral complex pictures from the International Affective Picture Series (IAPS; Lang et al., 1995). When contrasting the BOLD (blood oxygen level-dependent) signal between neutral and negative pictures, bilateral amygdalar activation emerged during the latter condition.

In a series of influential PET studies, Lane, Reiman, and coworkers investigated several aspects of the functional neuroanatomy of affect,

D. Pizzagalli, A. J. Shackman, and R. J. Davidson

including the manner in which affect was elicited (internally generated versus elicited by external stimuli; Reiman et al., 1997) and the impact of differential attentional focus toward the affective state (Lane, Fink, et al., 1997). In a first study, Reiman et al. (1997) contrasted film- and recall-generated emotion without considering the valence or discrete emotion involved (happiness, sadness, disgust). Film-generated emotion elicited stronger activation in bilateral occipitotemporoparietal regions, lateral cerebellum, hypothalamus, anterior temporal cortex, amygdala, and hippocampus; recall-generated emotion induced stronger activation in the anterior insula. There were no pronounced asymmetric effects in these studies.

The main goal of the fMRI study by Canli et al. (1998) was to explicitly test the laterality-valence hypothesis. The task involved presentation of positively and negatively valenced pictures. For those subjects who rated the positive and negative pictures comparably in arousal, greater left hemispheric activity for positive than for negative affective pictures was observed in middle frontal (BA6/8) and middle/superior temporal (BA21/38) structures. Conversely, compared to positive, negative pictures elicited greater right hemispheric activation in inferior frontal PFC.

Using an fMRI protocol with coverage limited to occipital and occipitoparietal regions, Lang et al. (1998) explored the role of the visual cortex in processing emotional and neutral IAPS pictures. Both pleasant and unpleasant pictures elicited larger clusters of activation in bilateral occipitoparietal, and especially occipital, regions. Aversive pictures specifically activated right parietal regions and right BA18, whereas pleasant pictures were associated with larger activation in the left fusiform and right lingual gyri.

In a study that effectively exploited an ideographic approach to the elicitation of positive, approach-related emotion, Bartels and Zeki (2000) scanned 17 subjects while they observed photographs of their romantic partner and friends. Presentation of the partner's face was accompanied by positive affect and increased arousal, as assessed in separate psychophysiological sessions. The results showed a pattern of asymmetrical effects. Perception of the loved person was associated with activation in various subcortical and paralimbic regions in the left hemisphere (middle insula); head of the caudate nucleus; putamen), as well as bilateral activation in the ACC (BA24) and posterior hippocampus. *De*activations (friends > partner) were observed in several right-sided regions: PFC (BA9/46), parietal (BA39/19), middle temporal cortex (BA21/22), and posterior cingulate gyrus (BA23/29/30), as well as medial PFC (BA9) and left posterior amygdaloid region.

Kawasaki et al. (2001) recorded single-unit responses to aversive pictures in the right ventral PFC of a patient implanted for diagnostic purposes. Results showed selective responses to aversive stimuli in the right PFC between 120 and 160 ms, suggesting that the PFC can provide rapid (and likely coarse) categorization of emotional information.

A number of studies have used auditory stimuli to elicit emotion while measures of brain function were examined with PET or fMRI. Lorberbaum et al. (1999) scanned mothers while they heard cries of unfamiliar infants, which elicited more sadness and urge to help than a control sound (white noise). Based on prior animal work postulating the cingulate cortex in maternal behavior (MacLean, 1990; Devinsky et al., 1995), the authors hypothesized a primary role of this brain region during exposure to infant cries. Compared to the control sounds, infant cries were indeed associated with increased fMRI signal in the subgenual ACC, extending to the medial PFC and superior frontal gyrus, all in the right hemisphere. Right PFC involvement in this mildly distressing situation is consistent with the approach-withdrawal model (Davidson, 2000). However, since no control emotional condition was used, it is unclear whether right ACC and PFC activation was linked to valence per se, unspecific arousal, or attention-engaging mechanisms present in the infant cry condition.

Based on the observation that music can be a potent emotional elicitor, Blood et al. (1999) used unfamiliar music passages manipulated in their degree of dissonance to study the neural correlates of affective responses to music. Increasing dissonance was positively correlated with rCBF in the right parahippocampal gyrus (BA28/36) and right precuneus (BA7), and negatively correlated with rCBF in the OFC (bilateral, BA13/14), subcallosal ACC (BA25), and right frontal polar cortex (BA10). Similarly, unpleasantness ratings were positively correlated with activity in the right parahippocampal region as well as in the posterior cingulate cortex (BA-23/31), and negatively correlated with rCBF in the right OFC and medial subcallosal ACC.

In an event-related fMRI study, Goel and Dolan (2001) explored the brain substrates of humor by presenting semantic and phonological jokes. When comparing funny to nonfunny jokes (both semantic and phonological), the former were associated with stronger activation in the medial ventral PFC (BA10/11). In this region, pleasantness ratings of the jokes were positively correlated with the BOLD signal. Thus, these results suggest that positively valenced, auditorily presented affective information activates regions associated with reward representation (Rolls, 2000).

Olfactory stimuli involve a strong hedonic component (pleasant vs. unpleasant), and are thus ideal for eliciting approach and withdrawal tendencies in both animals and humans. In one of the first neuro-imaging studies using emotionally charged olfactory stimuli, Zatorre et al. (1992) reported right OFC activation during exposure to pleasant, neutral, and aversive olfactory stimuli. A series of subsequent PET and fMRI studies have been conducted to examine patterns of regional brain activity during pleasant and unpleasant odorant stimulation (e.g., Zald & Pardo, 1997; Zatorre et al., 2000; O'Doherty et al., 2000). These studies have not found systematic variations in the asymmetry of activation produced by stimuli of different valences. What does appear to be similar across all of these studies is activation of regions of OFC. This common focus of activation is likely a consequence of two factors. First is the suggestion that OFC represents a brain region for primary olfactory processing (see Rolls, 1999 for review). And second, OFC activation has been hypothesized to occur during reversal learning (e.g., Rolls, 2000). In response to olfactory stimuli, it is frequently observed that the hedonic valence of the stimulus to which an individual is exposed changes rapidly over time. Thus, the OFC is likely to be activated in such circumstances. The rapidly changing hedonic nature of olfactory stimuli also may account for some of the variability in the findings of studies that have attempted to contrast pleasant and unpleasant odors.

In an fMRI study, O'Doherty, Rolls, et al. (2001) investigated the role of the OFC and amygdala during presentation of both pleasant (glucose) and aversive (salt) tastes. Compared to neutral, both pleasant and aversive tastes elicited stronger bilateral activation in the amygdala, OFC, and insula/frontal operculum. Within the OFC there were both overlapping and unique regions of activation for the two valences (the aversive condition elicited slightly more medial OFC activation). Whereas these results confirmed that both pleasant and unpleasant tastes are represented in the OFC, amygdalar activation in response to the glucose condition implies that the amygdala activates to both aversive and appetitive stimuli. Direct contrasts between the pleasant and unpleasant taste conditions were not performed, and thus we cannot evaluate whether activation in the amygdala was greater for unpleasant compared with pleasant stimuli.

In an event-related fMRI study, Critchley et al. (2001) investigated brain activation during outcome anticipation in a two-choice decision-making task associated with monetary reward or punishment. The independent variables of interest were the degree of uncertainty (parametrically varied) and autonomic arousal (indexed via on-line skin conductance response recording). During the anticipatory period (prefeedback), the strongest foci of activation were in the right OFC and anterior insula. What was of particular interest in this report was the association observed between activation of the right DLPFC and right ACC, and electrodermal activity.

Summary Most of the studies reviewed in this section involved the presentation of visual emotional stimuli, typically film clips or pictures. One of the methodological conundrums of laboratory research on emotion is that laboratory environments are typically not places where strong emotions are expected to occur, and thus efforts to elicit such emotion in subjects may be thwarted by regulatory strategies invoked by subjects to attenuate the magnitude of the elicited affect. Often these regulatory maneuvers are generated nonconsciously. Thus, the activations that are observed during such experiments may reflect an unknown mixture of processes associated with the generation of emotion as well as with the regulation of that emotion.

Some of the studies reviewed in this section did not find reliable asymmetric effects in response to externally elicited emotion. In the experiments of the Arizona group (Reiman et al., 1997; Lane, Reiman, et al., 1997b), both cortical and limbic regions were activated, but not asymmetrically. The relatively diffuse pattern of activation found in these studies may reflect the complex nature of the emotions that were produced by the film clips used by these investigators to provoke emotion. These are complex film clips that produce a differentiated range of emotional changes over their courses. In earlier work conducted in our laboratory using film clips as elicitors and brain electrical activity measures to make inferences about regional brain activation, we, too, found that examining the data across the entire length of a short film clip (i.e., 2 min), no reliable asymmetries were observed (Davidson et al., 1990).

D. Pizzagalli, A. J. Shackman, and R. J. Davidson

It was only when we extracted very short epochs (on the order of a few seconds) of brain electrical activity that were coincident with objectively coded facial expressions of emotion that systematic asymmetrical effects were observed. Unfortunately, this was not possible using PET, since the data were averaged across approximately 2 min of the film clip. Using event-related fMRI and objective peripheral measures of emotion induction (e.g., skin conductance measures), other investigators have reported robust asymmetric effects (e.g., Critchley et al., 2001). Canli et al. (1998) also found that for subjects who rated positive and negative pictures comparably in arousal, asymmetric fMRI signal changes were observed, with greater right-sided activation in the inferior frontal PFC in response to negative than to positive pictures.

The use of briefer stimuli in the visual modality, including ideographically chosen stimuli (as in Bartels & Zeki, 2000), was associated with more consistent asymmetric effects compared with longer duration film clips, with the exception of stimuli whose repetitive presentation changes their hedonic value. Olfactory and gustatory stimuli are an example of this latter type, where rapid changes in hedonic effects over time may produce complex and difficult to interpret patterns of activation. Affective acoustic stimuli such as infant cries have been found to produce strong right-lateralized changes. It may be easier to elicit stronger emotion in the auditory modality than in the visual modality. Finally, the use of reward and punishment contingencies, as described earlier, may be particularly promising, and can be usefully be exploited using event-related fMRI paradigms. The strong associations reported between the magnitude of electrodermal changes and right PFC activations in Critchley et al. (2001) needs to be replicated and examined further. These findings also suggest that it is particularly for subjects showing strong autonomic changes that these right-sided activations are apparent. These data indicate that the mere presentation of particular incentives is insufficient to guarantee an emotional response. It may be only for that subset of subjects showing objective signs of emotion that lateralized activations of the type described are found.

CONCLUSION

This chapter presented a selective review of recent PET and fMRI studies on human emotion that have reported lateralized activations. In general, where such lateralized changes have been reported, they are most often supportive of the approach-withdrawal framework articulated in a series of publications by Davidson and his colleagues (e.g., Davidson, 1998, 2000; Davidson, Jackson, et al., 2000). However, it is also apparent that lateralized PFC changes associated with approach and withdrawal-related emotion are not consistently obtained. The inconsistencies in the literature are likely a function of a multitude of causes, including methodological issues in the statistical assessment of asymmetry, variability in affective responses that are elicited by particular stimulus conditions, and the failure to utilize proper control conditions in the experiments. Having said this, it must also be noted that when asymmetries are observed, they are a matter of degree and are by no means absolute. Moreover, the PFC is part of a more complex circuit that includes other cortical and subcortical zones interconnected with the PFC. It is conceivable that similar emotional states can arise as a consequence of somewhat different patterns of activation within this circuitry, and that the differences among these emotional states may be discovered only with more precise and detailed probing of the cognitive, attentional, memory, and motor changes associated with these emotional variants. For a detailed discussion of the functional and evolutionary significance and origins of these asymmetries associated with emotion, the interested reader can consult reviews by Davidson (Davidson, 2000; Davidson, Jackson, et al., 2000).

The data on amygdala asymmetries are complex and also not entirely consistent. Where studies have examined relations between activation in the left and right amygdala and measures of negative affect, they report stronger associations with the right amygdala than with the left amygdala more often than would be expected by chance. The Morris, Ohman, et al. (1998) study is the only one to suggest that the right amygdala is preferentially involved in the processing of nonconscious information, whereas the left amygdala is involved in the processing of conscious emotional information. Zalla et al. (2000) suggest that the left amygdala is involved in reward and appetitive processing, while the right amygdala is more involved in punishment and aversive processing. These claims all require systematic replication.

It is clear that research on asymmetrical activations in hemodynamic neuroimaging research is still very much in its infancy, and there are many methodological and conceptual problems to resolve in the future. The availability of these methods will enable investigators to systemically examine both cortical and subcortical asymmetries with a level of spatial and temporal precision not previously available. This bodes well for resolving some of these problems in the future.

ACKNOWLEDGMENTS

The research from the Laboratory for Affective Neuroscience was supported by NIMH grants (MH40747, P50-MH52354, MH43454) and by an NIMH Research Scientist Award (K05-MH00875) to Richard J. Davidson. Diego Pizzagalli was supported by grants from the Swiss National Research Foundation (81ZH-52864) and "Holderbank"-Stiftung zur Förderung der Wissenschaftlichen Fortbildung. AJS was supported by fellowships from NSF and the NIMH training program in emotion research.

REFERENCES

Bartels, A., & Zeki, S. (2000). The neural basis of romantic love. *Neuroreport, 11*, 3829–3834.

Blood, A. J., Zatorre, R. J., Bermudez, P., & Evans, A. C. (1999). Emotional responses to pleasant and unpleasant music correlate with activity in paralimbic brain regions. *Nature Neuroscience, 2*, 382–387.

Brodmann, K. (1909/1994). *Localisation in the cerebral cortex*. London: Smith-Gordon.

Canli, T., Desmond, J. E., Zhao, Z., Glover, G., & Gabrieli, J. D. (1998). Hemispheric asymmetry for emotional stimuli detected with fMRI. *NeuroReport, 9*, 3233–3239.

Coleman-Mesches, K., & McGaugh, J. L. (1995a). Differential effects of pretraining inactivation of the right or left amygdala on retention of inhibitory avoidance training. *Behavioral Neuroscience, 109*, 642–647.

Coleman-Mesches, K., & McGaugh, J. L. (1995b). Differential involvement of the right and left amygdala in expression of memory for aversively motivated training. *Brain Research, 670*, 75–81.

Critchley, H. D., Mathias, C. J., & Dolan, R. J. (2001). Neural activity in the human brain relating to uncertainty and arousal during anticipation. *Neuron, 29*, 537–545.

Davidson, R. J. (1998). Affective style and affective disorders: Perspectives from affective neuroscience. *Cognition and Emotion, 12*, 307–320.

Davidson, R. J. (2000). Affective style, psychopathology and resilance: Brain mechanisms and plasticity. *American Psychologist, 55*, 1193–1214.

Davidson, R. J., Ekman, P., Saron, C., Senulis, J., & Friesen, W. V. (1990). Approach/withdrawal and cerebral asymmetry: Emotional expression and brain physiology. *Journal of Personality and Social Psychology, 58*, 330–341.

Davidson, R. J., Jackson, D. C., & Kalin, N. H. (2000). Emotion, plasticity, context and regulation. *Psychological Bulletin, 126,* 890–906.

Davidson, R. J., Pizzagalli, D., Nitschke, J. B., & Putman, K. (2002). Depression: Perspectives from affective neuroscience. *Annual Review of Psychology, 53,* 545–574.

Davidson, R. J., Putnam, K. M., & Larson, C. L. (2000). Dysfunction in the neural circuitry of emotion egulation: A possible prelude to violence. *Science, 289,* 591–594.

Delgado, M. R., Nystrom, L. E., Fissell, C., Noll, D. C., & Fiez, J. A. (2000). Tracking the hemodynamic responses to reward and punishment in the striatum. *Journal of Neurophysiology, 84,* 3072–3077.

Devinsky, O., Morrell, M. J., & Vogt, B. A. (1995). Contributions of anterior cingulate cortex to behaviour. *Brain, 118,* 279–306.

Goel, V., & Dolan, R. J. (2001). The functional anatomy of humor: Segregating cognitive and affective components. *Nature Neuroscience, 4,* 237–238.

Hugdahl, K. (1995). Classical conditioning and implicit learning: The right hemisphere hypothesis. In R. J. Davidson & K. Hugdahl (Eds.), *Brain Asymmetry* (pp. 235–267). Cambridge, MA: MIT Press.

Hugdahl, K., Beradi, A., Thompson, W. L., Kosslyn, S. M., Macy, R., Baker, D. P., Alpert, N. M., & LeDoux, J. E. (1995). Brain mechanisms in human classical conditioning: A PET blood flow study. *NeuroReport, 6,* 1723–1728.

Irwin, W., Davidson, R. J., Lowe, M. J., Mock, B. J., Sorenson, J. A., & Turski, P. A. (1996). Human amygdala activation detected with echo-planar functional magnetic resonance imaging. *NeuroReport, 7,* 1765–1769.

Kahneman, D. (1999). Objective happiness. In E. Kahneman, E. Diener, & N. Schwartz (Eds.), *Well-being: The foundations of hedonic psychology* (pp. 3–25). New York: Russell Sage Foundation.

Kawasaki, H., Adolphs, R., Kaufman, O., Damasio, H., Damasio, A. R., Granner, M., Bakken, H., Hori, T., & Howard, M. A. III. (2001). Single-neuron responses to emotional visual stimuli recorded in human ventral prefrontal cortex. *Nature Neuroscience, 4,* 15–16.

Koepp, M. J., Gunn, R. N., Lawrence, A. D., Cunningham, V. J., Dagher, A., Jones, T., Brooks, D. J., Bench, C. J., & Grasby, P. M. (1998). Evidence for striatal dopamine release during a video game. *Nature, 393,* 266–268.

Künig, G., Leenders, K. L., Martin-Solch, C., Missimer, J., Magyar, S., & Schultz, W. (2000). Reduced reward processing in the brains of Parkinsonian patients. *NeuroReport, 11,* 3681–3687.

LaBar, K. S., Parrish, T. B., Gitelman, D. R., & Mesulam, M.-M. (2000). Impact of signal-to-noise on functional MRI of the amygdala during emotional picture encoding. *NeuroReport, 12,* 3461–3464.

Lane, R. D., Fink, G. R., Chau, P. M.-L., & Dolan, R. J. (1997). Neural activation during selective attention to subjective emotional responses. *NeuroReport, 8,* 3969–3972.

Lane, R. D., Reiman, E. M., Ahern, G. L., Schwartz, G. E., & Davidson, R. J. (1997). Neuroanatomical correlates of happiness, sadness, and disgust. *American Journal of Psychiatry*, *154*, 926–933.

Lang, P. J., Bradley, M. M., & Cuthbert, B. N. (1995). *International Affective Picture System (IAPS): Technical manual and affective ratings*. Gainsville: Center for Research in Psychophysiology, University of Florida.

Lang, P. J., Bradley, M. M., Fitzsimmons, J. R., Cuthbert, B. N., Scott, J. D., Moulder, B., & Nangia, V. (1998). Emotional arousal and activation of the visual cortex: An fMRI analysis. *Psychophysiology*, *35*, 199–210.

Lorberbaum, J. P., Newman, J. D., Dubno, J. R., Horwitz, A. R., Nahas, Z., Teneback, C. C., Bloomer, C. W., Bohning, D. E., Vincent, D., Johnson, M. R., Emmanuel, N., Brawman-Mintzer, O., Book, S. W., Lydiard, R. B., Ballenger, J. C., & George, M. S. (1999). Feasibility of using fMRI to study mothers responding to infant cries. *Depression & Anxiety*, *10*, 99–104.

MacLean, P. D. (1990). *The triune brain in evolution: Role in paleocerebral functions*. New York: Plenum Press.

Morris, J. S., Friston, K. J., & Dolan, R. J. (1997). Neural responses to salient visual stimuli. *Proceedings of the Royal Society of London*, *B264*, 769–775.

Morris, J. S., Friston, K. J., & Dolan, R. J. (1998). Experience-dependent modulation of tonotopic neural responses in human auditory cortex. *Proceedings of the Royal Society of London*, *B265*, 649–657.

Morris, J. S., Ohman, A., & Dolan, R. J. (1998). Conscious and unconscious emotional learning in the human amygdala. *Nature*, *393*, 467–470.

O'Doherty, J., Kringelbach, M. L., Rolls, E. T., Hornak, J., & Andrews, C. (2001). Abstract reward and punishment representations in the human orbitofrontal cortex. *Nature Neuroscience*, *4*, 95–102.

O'Doherty, J., Rolls, E. T., Francis, S., Bowtell, R., & McGlone, F. (2001). Representation of pleasant and aversive taste in the human brain. *Journal of Neurophysiology*, *85*, 1315–1321.

O'Doherty, J., Rolls, E. T., Francis, S., Bowtell, R., McGlone, F., Kobal, G., Renner, B., & Ahne, G. (2000). Sensory-specific satiety-related olfactory activation of the human orbitofrontal cortex. *NeuroReport*, *11*, 893–897.

Pardo, J. V., Pardo, P. J., & Raichle, M. E. (1993). Neural correlates of self-induced dysphoria. *American Journal of Psychiatry*, *150*, 713–719.

Pavlov, I. P. (1927). *Conditioned reflexes*. Oxford: Oxford University Press.

Reiman, E. M., Lane, R. D., Ahern, G. L., Schwartz, G. E., Davidson, R. J., Friston, K. J., Yun, L. S., & Chen, K. (1997). Neuroanatomical correlates of externally and internally generated human emotion. *American Journal of Psychiatry*, *54*, 918–925.

Rogers, R. D., Owen, A. M., Middleton, H. C., Williams, E. J., Pickens, J., Sahakian, B. J., & Robbins, T. W. (1999). Choosing between small, likely rewards and large, unlikely rewards activates inferior and orbital prefrontal cortex. *Journal of Neuroscience, 20,* 9029–9038.

Rolls, E. T. (1999). *The brain and emotion.* New York: Oxford University Press.

Rolls, E. T. (2000). The orbitofrontal cortex and reward. *Cerebral Cortex, 10,* 284–294.

Schultz, W., Tremblay, L., & Hollerman, J. R. (2000). Reward processing in primate orbitofrontal cortex and basal ganglia. *Cerebral Cortex, 10,* 272–283.

Thut, G., Schultz, W., Roelcke, U., Nienhusmeier, M., Missimer, J., Maguire, R. P., & Leenders, K. L. (1997). Activation of the human brain by monetary reward. *NeuroReport, 8,* 1225–1228.

Zald, D. H., & Pardo, J. V. (1997). Emotion, olfaction, and the human amygdala: Amygdala activation during aversive olfactory stimulation. *Proceedings of the National Academy of Sciences, USA, 94,* 4119–4124.

Zalla, T., Koechlin, E., Pietrini, P., Basso, G., Aquino, P., Sirigu, A., & Grafman, J. (2000). Differential amygdala responses to winning and losing: A functional magnetic resonance imaging study in humans. *European Journal of Neuroscience, 12,* 1764–1770.

Zatorre, R. J., Jones-Gotman, M., Evans, A. C., & Meyer, E. (1992). Functional localization and lateralization of human olfactory cortex. *Nature, 360,* 339–340.

Zatorre, R. J., Jones-Gotman, M., & Rouby, C. (2000). Neural mechanisms involved in odor pleasantness and intensity judgments. *NeuroReport, 11,* 2711–2716.

15 Regional Brain Activity in Anxiety and Depression, Cognition/Emotion Interaction, and Emotion Regulation

Wendy Heller, Nancy S. Koven, and Gregory A. Miller

THE CONTEXT: CONCEPTUALIZING EMOTION

Anxious and depressed moods encapsulate many aspects of emotional functioning, and hence are superb targets for research aimed at understanding the neural implementation of emotion and emotional disorders. Each involves emotional experiences and physiological events that are associated with distinct cognitive characteristics which are observable in the domains of attention, memory, perception, and information processing. Each can be present to some degree in routine daily life, and each is regulated by individuals with varying degrees of efficiency. Each can foster adaptive engagement with the environment, a dysfunctional engagement that seriously interferes with adaptive living, or a complex combination of both.

Human emotion can be conceptualized as a set of processes that includes attention, appraisal, subjective feelings, and visceral and motor responses (e.g., Ellsworth, 1994). External stimuli are perceived and interpreted in the context of a personal history of experiences, involving perception in multiple channels, memory of multiple antecedents, appraisal, and evaluation. Actions are taken, including communication or suppression of information about one's responses; physiological preparation for action, involving autonomic and endocrine modulation; and attentional orientation. Potential and recently executed actions are evaluated with regard to their consequences, and feelings, experiences, and thoughts are generated and monitored on an ongoing basis with reference to both the present and the past for information about one's relationship to the environment.

Each of these processes has a time course of its own, and interactions between them are constant, fluid, and nonlinear. Research in psychophysiology has made it abundantly clear that the various systems engaged by emotional stimulation do not covary linearly or synchronously. Verbal report does not necessarily mirror activity in various autonomic systems; conversely, activity in these systems does not necessarily correlate with verbal report or overt action. Furthermore, none of these publicly available manifestations of emotion need closely track subjective experience. These observations have led to models of emotion that argue for loosely coupled components that can be dissociated from each other and from subjective experience (Ohman et al., 2000; Lang, 1968, 1993; Miller & Kozak, 1993). Such an emphasis on separable components that do not all reflect a unitary "feeling" state challenges the commonsense view that subjective experience is the fundamental manifestation of an emotion (Ohman et al., 2000). Indeed, recent theoretical and empirical research questions the wisdom of basing our definition of emotion on any one component or dimension (see Ellsworth, 1994; Russell & Feldman Barrett, 1999; Lerner & Keltner, 2000).

IMPLEMENTING EMOTION: CONCEPTUALIZING BRAIN MECHANISMS

The functioning of all these components must recruit neural circuitry that implements their activity, and the relevant circuitry is likely to involve multiple brain regions. However, much recent research in cognitive and affective neuroscience has focused on the neural circuits associated with fear (for review, see LeDoux, 1995), with motivational aspects of emotion (approach vs. withdrawal; e.g., Davidson, 1995), or with valence (pleasant vs. unpleasant; e.g., Heller & Nitschke, 1998). This emphasis has highlighted the anterior regions of the brain—dorsolateral, medial, and orbital prefrontal areas in particular—as well as the amygdala (e.g., Elliott et al., 2000; London et al., 2000; Volkow & Fowler, 2000). Such primary conceptual dimensions surely capture fundamental aspects of emotion that span human and animal engagement of the environment. Yet those regions and functions are nonetheless only a portion of the many phenomena involved in integrated emotional behavior. Our work and that of others has identified a broader network of brain regions involved in emotion that reflects other important processes, such as arousal, appraisal, attention, and memory. These findings suggest that a variety of cortical regions are involved in emotion, including, in addition to prefrontal regions, posterior cingulate, parietal, temporal, and occipital areas (e.g., Damasio et al., 2000). Subcortical regions have also been implicated in emotional responses, including thalamus, hypothalamus, cerebellum, and brain stem (e.g., Damasio et al., 2000) in addition to the amygdala.

Ultimately, all of these regions will need to be understood in terms of their role in implementing the various components of emotional activity. Furthermore, how these regions interact and the mechanisms by which they influence and modulate each other are essential, pressing questions, not only for the sake of basic science but also because these interactions are fundamental to understanding changes in cognition/emotion relationships in biochemical and behavioral domains, often the focus of clinical intervention.

NARROWING THE FOCUS: DECOMPOSING EMOTION AS AN INVESTIGATIVE STRATEGY

Such a comprehensive goal notwithstanding, pragmatically it is essential to parse the processes involved in emotion in some way that allows research an entry into the system. Various strategies have been adopted to this end. Emotions can be treated categorically (e.g., as discrete phenomena, such as anger, fear, and sadness; see Damasio et al., 2000) or dimensionally, extracting a small number of common factors that vary quantitatively across emotions.

Our approach to research on brain mechanisms of emotion has relied primarily on the latter strategy, resting in part on a neuropsychological model proposed by Heller (1986, 1990, 1993), and subsequently refined (e.g., Heller, Nitschke, Etienne, et al., 1997; Keller et al., 2000; Nitschke et al., 2000; Nitschke et al., 2001; Nitschke et al., 1999), in which psychological theories of emotion were used to decompose emotional states into two components, valence and arousal. Our approach integrated the dimensional circumplex model of emotion (based primarily on self-report measures; for review, see Larsen & Diener, 1992) with neuropsychological data on cognitive, emotional, and autonomic functioning during different affective states (figure 15.1). Based on evidence from EEG, hemodynamic, and lesion studies, our model posited that the valence dimension (pleasant, unpleasant) is dependent on functions of the

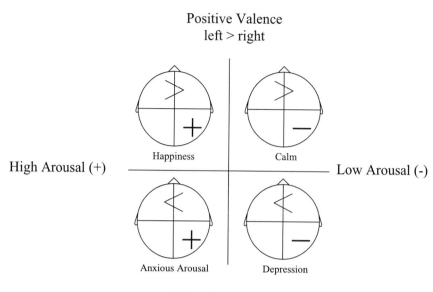

Positive Valence
left > right

High Arousal (+)

Happiness

Calm

Low Arousal (-)

Anxious Arousal

Depression

Negative Valence
right > left

Figure 15.1 A neuropsychological model of emotion that superimposes the two dimensions, valence and arousal, of the emotion circumplex onto asymmetric patterns of activity associated with specific regions of the brain. According to this model, valence (positive, negative) is dependent on functions of the anterior brain regions, while arousal (high, low) is dependent on right posterior brain regions.

anterior regions. Bias toward a particular valence pole is associated with the relative activity level of the left and right hemispheres. When the left frontal region is active relative to the right, affective valence is pleasant, whereas when the right frontal region is active relative to the left, affective valence is unpleasant. The association of valence with asymmetric activity of the anterior regions has been extensively studied (for reviews, see Davidson, 1992; Heller, 1990).

In contrast to valence, our model posited that the arousal dimension (or activation dimension; Larsen & Diener, 1992) depends on right posterior regions of the brain. More activity in this region is associated with higher self-reported arousal. This aspect of the model was based on theoretical and empirical work by numerous authors (e.g., Heilman et al., 1985; Hugdahl, 1995; Levy et al., 1983b; Tucker, 1981; Wittling, 1995) suggesting a special role for the right hemisphere in emotion-

W. Heller, N. S. Koven, and G. A. Miller

related arousal functions. The arousal component of our model derived empirical support from studies examining patients with brain damage compared to people without brain damage (for reviews, see Gainotti et al., 1993; Heller, Nitschke, & Lindsay, 1997; Wittling, 1995) and from research on conditioning and emotional responding in people without brain damage (e.g., Wittling, 1995).

We have used our emotion-processing model to predict patterns of brain activity during depression and anxiety, employing behavioral performance, autonomic activity, EEG, and fMRI measures. Since depression and anxiety both involve unpleasant valence, a similar pattern of brain activity was predicted for the anterior regions. However, self-reported depression and anxiety typically fall on opposite sides of the arousal dimension. Therefore, we expected them to be differentiated by opposing patterns of brain activity in right posterior regions. Anxiety should be associated with increased activity and depression with decreased activity.

However, this straightforward pair of predictions is greatly complicated by the substantial comorbidity often seen in clinical and non-clinical anxiety and depression. It is not yet clear whether it is best to consider anxiety and depression as largely distinct but often co-occurring rather than largely overlapping, each with some distinct characteristics, and if so, what those distinct characteristics are. In any case, research designs must address the comorbidity systematically, and this often has not been done.

We investigated our model of regional brain specificity in emotion and psychopathology using a variety of paradigms. In behavioral studies we examined performance on the Chimeric Faces Task (CFT; Levy et al., 1983a, 1983b), a free-vision test of face processing that elicits a strong attentional bias in right-handers toward the left side of space (see figure 15.2). Numerous studies have confirmed that individual differences in the magnitude of the hemispatial bias on the CFT reflect meaningful variations in the degree to which one hemisphere is engaged relative to the other (for review, see Heller et al., 1995).

Based on our hypothesis that anxiety and depression would be associated with opposing patterns of posterior right hemisphere activity, we predicted that hemispatial biases on the CFT would reflect this divergence. In an initial study (Heller et al., 1995), we looked at CFT scores in undergraduates selected to form extreme groups on the basis of questionnaires of anxiety and depression. As predicted, there

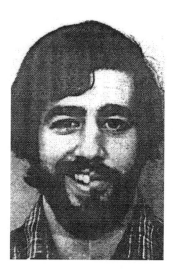

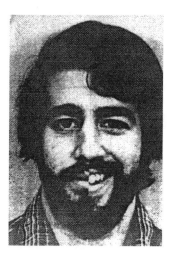

Figure 15.2 Example of a chimeric face used in the CFT, a free-vision test of face processing that elicits a strong attentional bias in right-handers toward the left side of space, indicating engagement of the contralateral right hemisphere. (Levy et al., 1983a.) Respondents are directed to look at the pair of faces for five seconds and then to indicate which of the two images, top or bottom, looks happier to them.

W. Heller, N. S. Koven, and G. A. Miller

were significant main effects for both anxiety and depression: high-anxious subjects showed a larger right-hemisphere bias than did low-anxious subjects, whereas high-depressed subjects showed a smaller right-hemisphere bias than did low-depressed subjects. The effect of comorbidity on hemispatial bias on the CFT in this study was very clear. High-anxious subjects who were not depressed had the largest right-hemisphere bias (significantly different from zero), whereas high-depressed subjects who were not anxious had the smallest right-hemisphere bias (not different from zero). Subjects who were both depressed and anxious were intermediate and very similar to controls. This study thus supported our prediction that anxiety and depression would be associated with distinct levels of right-hemisphere activity. Furthermore, that the comorbid group fell in between, with the effects of anxiety and depression essentially canceling out, is precisely what our model would predict in the face of comorbidity.

We obtained converging evidence for opposing posterior asymmetries in anxiety and depression in a subsequent study using a conventional clinical sample (Keller et al., 2000). Participants were adults diagnosed with major depression and community controls. In this sample, higher scores on an anxiety measure were associated with a larger right hemisphere bias, whereas higher scores on a depression measure were associated with a smaller right hemisphere bias. Importantly, these patterns emerged only when the variance associated with the other measure was partialed out. The findings were replicated in a third sample involving a large group of undergraduates selected on the basis of questionnaire scores for anxiety and depression subtypes (Keller et al., 2000). Taken together, the results of these studies confirmed our prediction that anxiety and depression are associated with opposing patterns of brain activity for the right posterior region, and further convinced us of the need to distinguish anxiety and depression in experimental designs.

The predictions of our model were subsequently examined in an EEG study of brain activity in anxiety and depression in questionnaire-selected college students. The EEG findings, however, were not consistent with our predictions (Heller, Nitschke, Etienne, et al., 1997). Based on resting EEG alpha activity (inversely related to regional brain activity), anxious subjects showed greater left hemisphere brain activity than did controls, the opposite of what our model would predict. The scores for depressed-only and depressed-plus-anxious subjects were similiar to those of controls, and both groups tended to show less lateralization than anxious-only subjects.

These EEG findings are consistent with a subset of studies in the literature on anxiety that report increased activity in left hemisphere regions. On the other hand, our aforementioned CFT results were consistent with studies reporting increased activity in right hemisphere regions in anxiety. In hopes of resolving the discrepancy, we turned to psychological models of anxiety for possible explanations. Indeed, various authors have argued for different types of anxiety. Clark, Watson, and colleagues (e.g., Clark & Watson, 1991) have emphasized anxious arousal in their tripartite model of depression and anxiety. Other authors, notably Barlow (1988, 1991), have discussed anxious apprehension as distinct from panic.

Developing such a differentiation of types of anxiety, we argued that panic, state anxiety, and sympathetic nervous system hyperactivity in response to immediate threat could be subsumed under the construct of anxious arousal (Heller et al., 1995; Heller & Nitschke, 1998; Heller, Nitschke, Etienne, et al., 1997; Miller, 2000; Nitschke et al., 2000). In contrast, worry, trait anxiety, and anticipation of future threat could be subsumed under the construct of anxious apprehension. Indeed, when we reconsidered the literature on brain activity in anxiety, we saw that studies which reported relative left hemisphere activity were more likely to have examined subjects who could be classified as anxious apprehensive, whereas those finding more right hemisphere activity were more likely to have investigated subjects experiencing anxious arousal (for review, see Nitschke et al., 2000).

This analysis of the literature needed systematic confirmation. As with the problem of comorbidity between anxiety and depression, however, studies comparing types of anxiety would have to deal with the likely but variable co-occurrence of anxious apprehension and anxious arousal. This could depend greatly on the particular sample recruited.

We tested the hypothesis of opposing patterns of asymmetry for anxious apprehension and anxious arousal by examining both types of anxiety in a single study (Heller et al., 1997a). Participants were selected on the basis of self-reported trait anxiety. We then manipulated anxious arousal on a within-subjects basis and contrasted regional brain activity (measured by EEG alpha) during rest periods with brain activity during a task in which participants listened to emotional narratives designed to elicit anxious arousal (e.g., fear and sad narratives that had previously received unpleasant valence and high arousal ratings). For frontal activity, group differences were unaffected by the narratives, with anxious participants showing a larger asymmetry in favor of left hemisphere activity than controls across both rest and listen periods. In contrast, group differences in right parietal activity varied with emotional content; for fear and sad narratives, anxious participants showed a selective increase in right parietal activity that was not demonstrated by controls. This effect was not seen for neutral and happy narratives. These results provided support for our view that anxious apprehension and anxious arousal are conceptually and topographically separable types of anxiety.

To replicate and extend the results of this within-subject manipulation of anxious arousal, we carried out a between-subjects manipulation (Nitschke et al., 1999). Subjects were selected using specific questionnaires of anxious apprehension and anxious arousal, and EEG activity was measured at rest. As predicted, the two groups differed significantly in their hemispheric asymmetries, with the anxious arousal group showing more right lateralization of brain activity than the anxious apprehension group. The fact that these two types of anxiety are distinguished electrophysiologically extends the psychological and physiological evidence suggesting that they are distinct constructs, and highlights the need to consider the presence of both in diagnostic, treatment, and research procedures.

The refinement of our model to include the distinction between types of anxiety allowed it to account better for the existing literature and produced testable new predictions that we were able to support. This refinement, however, complicated the simple two-dimensional model based on the circumplex. Frontal asymmetry depended not only on emotional valence but also on the nature of the cognitive processing that characterizes each type of anxiety. Anxious apprehension involves negative affect (which should be associated with increased right frontal activity), but it also involves considerable linguistic processing (and thus left frontal activity). Thus, a model that does not take into account the fact that rumination is part of anxious apprehension would not necessarily predict left frontal activity; it would only predict right frontal activity. Recent research on regional brain activity in anger provides another example of left frontal enhancement associated with emotionally negative contexts (Harmon-Jones & Allen, 1998). Some of these data favor an interpretation of the frontal asymmetry in emotion as reflecting the approach dimension of an approach-withdrawal dichotomy rather a valence dimension. More broadly, however, the evolution of this conceptualization of brain and emotion highlights the importance of examining the quality of the processing involved in a given context.

THE RETICULATION OF EMOTION AND COGNITION

In the work reviewed so far, pursuing hypotheses generated by a model based on the dimensions identified in the emotion circumplex enabled us to show that brain activity in anterior and right posterior regions differentiated depression from two types of anxiety, anxious apprehension and anxious arousal. Furthermore, our findings led us to argue that an understanding of these patterns of activity provides a powerful tool for understanding the cognitive characteristics of these disorders. Numerous studies, including electroencephalographic (EEG), event-related brain potential (ERP), and hemodynamic paradigms for measuring brain activity, have shown that activity in regions of the cortex specialized for particular modes of information processing covaries with performance on tasks that benefit from that type of computation. In the majority of studies, increased activity is associated with better performance (for review, see Heller & Nitschke, 1997), whereas deficient activity is associated with decrements in performance. In studies in which activity was not positively correlated with performance (e.g., Haier et al., 1992), the effects have been attributed to decreases in the use of nonessential brain areas with practice, changes in cognitive strategies, and changes in task demands. Based on these data, we have argued that the cognitive characteristics of depression and anxiety can in large part be anchored to corresponding levels of activity in critical regions of cortex (Heller & Nitschke, 1997; Nitschke et al., 2000).

Both types of anxiety, as well as depression, are characterized by specific cognitive biases and impairments (for reviews, see Eysenck, 1992; Heller & Nitschke, 1997; McNally, 1998; Nitschke et al., 2000; Nitschke & Heller, in press). Anxiety in general has been strongly associated with an attentional bias to threatening stimuli (for reviews, see Compton et al., 2000; McNally, 1998). In various paradigms, attention is captured by ambiguous, emotional, or threatening information; this phenomenon has been documented in trait and state anxiety and in

W. Heller, N. S. Koven, and G. A. Miller

every anxiety disorder category in the DSM-IV, including generalized anxiety disorder (e.g., Mathews & MacLeod, 1985), panic disorder (e.g., Ehlers et al., 1988), specific phobia (e.g., Watts et al., 1986), post-traumatic stress disorder (e.g., McNally et al., 1990), social phobia (e.g., Hope et al., 1990), and obsessive-compulsive disorder (e.g., Foa et al., 1993).

As reviewed above, we have suggested that anxious arousal and anxious apprehension are associated with distinct neural networks (Nitschke et al., 1999, 2000). Our EEG research suggested a special role for the right hemisphere in anxious arousal, as predicted by converging evidence from a variety of paradigms, including lesion studies of visual and spatial attention. Subsequent EEG, behavioral, and neuroimaging studies have supported and extended our understanding of a right hemisphere network involved in vigilance, alertness, and sustained (as opposed to selective) attention (Hager et al., 1998; Sturm et al., 1999). Attentional biases toward threat-related stimuli dovetail well with specializations of the right hemisphere for visual and spatial attention, vigilance, and autonomic arousal, and may be seen as reflecting the activity of a system engaged in "emotional surveillance," a term coined originally by David Bear (Nitschke et al., 2000). Thus, anxious arousal can be hypothesized to produce a set of behaviors that include attentional and other cognitive and physiological responses designed to evaluate and respond to the presence of a threat.

Anxiety is also reported to impair performance on many cognitive tasks, particularly when they are difficult or the conditions are stressful. Some of these deficits could reflect an emphasis on arousal-related cognitive processes, such as sustained attention or vigilance, that are not compatible with other cognitive processes, such as selective attention (as suggested by recent neuroimaging data, reviewed below). It is also possible that these deficits may reflect anxious apprehension, which could interfere with performance on attentionally demanding tasks due to the impact of worrisome thoughts on attention to task-relevant information. The neural mechanisms involved in anxious apprehension are likely to include areas involved in working memory, such as dorsolateral prefrontal cortex, Broca's area in left anterior cortex, and left posterior areas around the angular gyrus and supramarginal gyrus (Nitschke et al., 2000).

In depression, deficits have been described for explicit memory, a variety of executive functions, and visuospatial skills (for reviews, see

Heller & Nitschke, 1997, 1998). DSM-IV identifies difficulties in thinking and concentrating as fundamental components of major depressive episodes and dysthymia. Depression has been associated with abnormal metabolic activity in a variety of prefrontal regions, including decreased activity in medial prefrontal and anterior cingulate cortex (e.g., George et al., 1993; Dolan et al., 1994), dorsolateral prefrontal cortex (Elliott et al., 1997), and orbitofrontal cortex (Elliott et al., 1998). Decreased activity in these prefrontal brain regions can account for many of the cognitive impairments in depression, including memory for material on tasks that require or benefit from information-organizing strategies, the ability to access errors accurately, planning, problem-solving, and cognitive flexibility. Some of these cognitive functions have been linked to particular prefrontal regions (e.g., planning to the anterior cingulate and dorsolateral prefrontal regions; Elliott et al., 1997) but more work needs to be done to specify which regions are involved in different aspects of executive function (e.g., Miyake et al., 2000). Increased activity in some prefrontal regions has also been reported in depression (Drevets & Raichle, 1998), but it may be attributable to ruminative cognitions in the depressed sample. In future research, it will be important not only to examine the specific cognitive processes that are associated with activity in specific brain regions, but also essential to separate the contributions of anxious apprehension and anxious arousal to patterns of brain activity observed in depression, and vice versa.

Biases in attention, memory, and judgment have also been documented, with depressed people more likely to attend to unpleasant than pleasant stimuli, show better recall of unpleasant than pleasant information, and make more negative judgments about hypothetical and actual life events (for review, see Heller & Nitschke, 1997). These cognitive biases may be related to asymmetries in activity of prefrontal regions, with relatively higher right than left hemisphere activity associated with an increase in unpleasant valence.

A large neuropsychological literature has consistently associated depression with impairments on tasks associated with right posterior regions of the brain (e.g., Deldin et al., 2001; Keller et al., 2000; for review, see Heller & Nitschke, 1997). These findings are consistent with behavioral (Banich et al., 1992; Liotti & Tucker, 1992; Otto et al., 1987) and hemodynamic (Elliott et al., 1997) evidence that there is decreased activity in these brain regions as well. Bilateral deactivations in parietal, posterior cingulate, and retrosplenial cortex have also been reported (Mayberg et al., 1999; Pizzagalli et al., 2000), and it will be important in future research to identify the specific cognitive and behavioral functions of these areas and the ways in which they are affected by depression.

Based on these data and our theoretical perspectives, it is our view that cognition and emotion are integral, with regard not only to their effects on performance but also in terms of the neural structures involved. A contrasting viewpoint regarding the cortical structures supporting cognition and emotion was provided by Drevets and Raichle (1998), among others, who proposed that emotion and cognition are supported by separate systems. Drevets and Raichle argued that activity in areas associated with cognition is reciprocal to activity in areas associated with emotional processing. They make a distinction, therefore, between regions of the brain that process nonemotional thoughts and regions that process emotional thoughts. The hypothesis is supported by anatomical and behavioral data that the dorsolateral prefrontal cortex is implicated in executive control and working memory (Banich, 1997), whereas orbitofrontal cortex has been associated with emotional and affective processing (Damasio, 1995). Compatible with the Drevets and Raichle view, the anterior cingulate cortex appears to be divided into two main regions, a caudal portion that is more involved in cognitive functions and a rostral section that is more involved in affective processes (Devinsky et al., 1995). For example, Derbyshire et al. (1998) found that when PET data from individual subjects were examined, nonoverlapping regions of anterior cingulate were activated by painful heat stimulation compared to a color-word Stroop task.

Regardless of whether there are systems dedicated exclusively to cognition or to emotion in addition to systems contributing to both, it seems inescapable that emotion and cognition are extensively reticulated in both their neural circuitry and their behavioral manifestations (Miller, 1996; Miller & Keller, 2000). The hard distinctions sometimes drawn between emotion and cognition look less tenable as cognitive and affective neuroscience data and theory converge on shared concepts, such as a network view of emotion and its physiological implementation (e.g., Lang, 1979). Our recent studies of brain activity related to emotional self-regulation support this convergence as well.

WIDENING THE FOCUS: INVESTIGATING COGNITION IN EMOTION

An explication of the degree to which specific brain regions are active during cognitive or emotional processing or both has broad implications not only for our understanding of cognitive and emotional function in psychopathology but also for our understanding of the way in which the brain is organized. To examine further the neural networks involved in the cognitive components of anxiety and depression, we used a paradigm that involves attentional capture by emotional information. We have employed this paradigm in a recent series of fMRI experiments.

In the classic color-word Stroop task, nonemotional words are presented in a variety of colors, and the individual is asked to identify the ink color while ignoring the color content of the word (e.g., the word "blue" printed in red ink). Attentional selection is required, because the ink color must be attended regardless of the meaning of the word or the response to which it leads. Compared to a neutral baseline word, which has no intrinsic relationship to color (e.g., "table"), responses are facilitated if the word is the same as the ink color (e.g., the word "red" in red ink), and responses are slowed if the word name is in a different ink color (e.g., the word "blue" in red ink). The slowing of responses on incongruent trials is thought to result because word reading is relatively automatic compared to naming the ink color, and hence it is difficult to direct attention to the ink color over the word. The neural network involved in the color-word Stroop has been elucidated by a variety of researchers using hemodynamic brain-imaging techniques (e.g., Banich et al., 1998, 1999a, 1999b; Bench et al., 1993; Carter et al., 1995; Milham, Banich, Webb, Barad, et al., 1999; Milham, Banich, Webb, Wszalek, et al., 1999; Pardo et al., 1990) implicating a network of brain structures including prefrontal, anterior cingulate, parietal, and extrastriate cortex.

In a variant known as the emotional Stroop task, the content of the distractor words is either neutral ("sum"), negative ("die"), or positive ("joy"). A large body of evidence (reviewed by Williams et al., 1996) demonstrates that color naming is slowed in anxious subjects when the meaning of the distractor word is negative (e.g., "pain" in red ink). This finding has been taken as evidence that anxious subjects have particular difficulty filtering out threatening information, even when it is task-

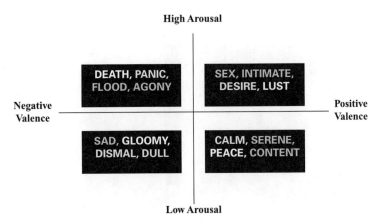

Figure 15.3 Examples of high- and low-arousal negative and high- and low-arousal positive words used in the emotional Stroop task. Participants are shown words, one at a time, and instructed to respond to the word's ink color (red, yellow, green, or blue) as quickly as possible and to ignore the meaning or content of the word.

irrelevant. We have recently found that with a carefully selected group of words such an effect can also be obtained in unselected individuals (Compton et al., 2000; Heller et al., 2000).

To investigate the predictions of our model of regional brain activity in emotion and psychopathology, as well as to examine the extent to which distinct and overlapping regions are involved in the classic color-word Stroop (a purely cognitive task) versus the emotional Stroop task, we compared regional hemodynamic responses on color-word versus emotional Stroop tasks. Emotional words were distinguished according to valence and arousal, producing four sets of stimuli: high-arousal negative, or threat (e.g., death, panic); low-arousal negative, or depressed (e.g., sad, gloomy); high-arousal appetitive (e.g., sex, lust), and low-arousal appetitive (e.g., calm, peace) (figure 15.3).

Both color-conflicting and high-arousal emotional words activated dorsolateral and prefrontal regions, indicating a common network for attentional selection (see figure 15.4 for areas activated by color-conflicting and threat words). High-arousal emotional words also activated left lateral orbitofrontal regions that were not significantly activated by color-conflicting words (figure 15.5). Low-arousal words of either valence did not produce reliable activation relative to neutral words.

A. Incongruent Color

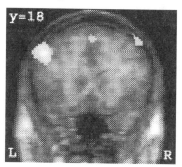

B. Negative High Arousal

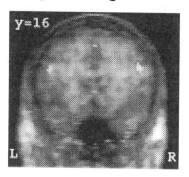

Figure 15.4 Both color-conflicting (*A*) and high-arousal threat words (*B*) activated inferior frontal, medial frontal, and parietal areas, indicating an extensive network for attention selection. In both examples, light areas indicate activation.

Although both positive and negative high-arousal words produced robust activation in comparison to low-arousal words, the pattern of activation varied with valence. Threat words uniquely activated temporal, parietal, and occipital regions of the right hemisphere, as well as a region in the left inferior frontal gyrus (see figure 15.6 for activated right hemisphere regions). High-arousal appetitive words activated bilateral inferior frontal regions.

Across all Stroop conditions, only threat words activated posterior regions of the right hemisphere. These findings for right posterior cortex support previous theorizing that these regions may be specialized

W. Heller, N. S. Koven, and G. A. Miller

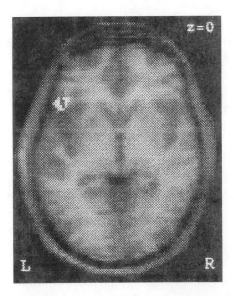

Figure 15.5 Unlike color-conflicting words, the high-arousal emotional words activated a left lateral orbitofrontal region. The light area indicates activation.

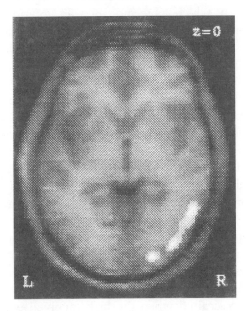

Figure 15.6 High-arousal threat words showed a unique pattern of activity in temporal, parietal, and occipital regions of the right hemisphere. Light areas indicate activation.

Regional Brain Activity in Anxiety and Depression

for "threat monitoring" or emotional surveillance (Nitschke et al., 2000). That is, right posterior regions may be especially responsive to stimuli with threatening meaning, such as threat words, and may play a crucial role in directing attention toward potential danger.

The asymmetry in left inferior frontal activation for threat words is inconsistent with some previous research indicating increased right anterior activation for negatively valenced stimuli (e.g., Davidson, 1995). One factor that may account for this difference is the nature of the task involved. In this study, the emotional words in the Stroop task were not designed to induce negative mood, and therefore may not be comparable to the negative stimuli used in prior studies of anterior asymmetry. However, the increased left inferior activation in response to threatening words is consistent with prior research suggesting increased left anterior involvement in anxious apprehension (Nitschke et al., 2000). The high-arousal threat words may elicit a network of associations to threatening information, a function proposed by Damasio (1995) to be mediated by "convergence zones" in ventral frontal regions. Further research is needed to address this possibility.

The findings for high-arousal appetitive words complement previous findings in depression, which have indicated an anterior asymmetry favoring the right hemisphere superimposed on a bilateral *decrease* in activity (for review, see Heller & Nitschke, 1997). In the present data, a bilateral *increase* in activity was observed for high-arousal appetitive words. Although numerous previous studies have shown greater left than right asymmetries in response to positive stimuli, to our knowledge this is the first time a bilateral increase in activity for positive emotion has been observed. These findings are highly consistent with data that positive affect is associated with better performance on a broad range of executive tasks (for review, see Ashby et al., 1999).

The findings of this study support three main conclusions regarding the neural regions involved in cognitive processes in emotion. First, the regions identified in the emotional Stroop task have much in common with those involved in closely related, but nonemotional, selective attention tasks, supporting a neural-overlap model of the relationship between emotion and cognition. In conjunction, however, additional neural regions, including orbitofrontal, inferior frontal, and right posterior regions, were recruited when the task involved emotional distractors. Thus, additional, distinct regions of the brain were active when emotion was involved. Finally, the neural regions activated in the

W. Heller, N. S. Koven, and G. A. Miller

emotional Stroop task differ depending on the valence and arousal characteristics of the emotional stimuli, consistent with Heller's original model emphasizing the importance of emotional dimensions and its subsequent refinement (based on our EEG work) with regard to types of anxiety.

EMOTION REGULATION: AT THE INTERFACE OF COGNITION AND EMOTION

As noted above, anxiety and depression interfere with cognitive performance and adaptive function in a variety of domains. Although there are various ways in which people regulate negative (and positive) emotion using externally directed behaviors (such as exercising, seeking social support, and using drugs), several internally directed cognitive strategies have been identified as extremely important for managing anxious and depressed moods (Gross, 1999). Prominent among these cognitive strategies is the inhibition or suppression of negative emotion (Gross & Levenson, 1997). There are notable individual differences in the ability to inhibit negative emotion. Some people appear to be simply indisposed to negative emotion and, unless confronted with a significant immediate threat, in general do not react with anxiety or depression to emotional events. Others are characterized by strong reactions to a variety of emotional challenges. A third style, termed repression, characterizes people who tend to respond to situations with anxiety but who avoid or suppress the affect in such a way as to diminish the impact of the emotional challenge (for review see Bonanno & Siddique, 1999).

The emotional Stroop task provides a useful paradigm for the investigation of individual differences in the degree to which people are able to ignore emotional information. The degree to which the meaning of an emotional word differentially influences reaction time reflects the process by which the individual regulates his or her emotional response to the word. Research has suggested that the bias toward threat words is associated with an engage/disengage mechanism reflecting attentional systems in posterior parietal regions of the brain (e.g., Posner & Petersen, 1990; Stormark et al., 1995).

Employing the emotional Stroop task described above in a subsequent fMRI study, we investigated individual differences in brain activation and deactivation associated with different patterns of reaction

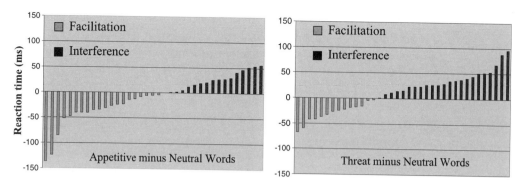

Figure 15.7 Two separate analyses were performed on the fMRI data, one that used groups divided on the basis of their appetitive Stroop effect (i.e., average reaction time to appetitive words minus the average reaction time to neutral words) and one that used groups divided on the basis of their threat Stroop effect (i.e., average reaction time to threat words minus average reaction time to neutral words). The first comparison involved one group showing appetitive facilitation (N = 22) and another group showing appetitive interference (N = 15). The second comparison involved one group showing threat facilitation (N = 14) and another group showing threat interference (N = 23). In all cases, an interference effect is characterized by a reaction time with a positive value, and a facilitation effect is characterized by a reaction time with a negative value.

time to threat and high-arousal appetitive words. The 37 participants showed a wide range of reaction time differences between neutral and emotional words, from facilitation (faster on emotional than neutral words) to interference (slower on emotional than neutral words). Based on this variability, we carried out two analyses, in each of which the sample was divided into two groups: one on the basis of reaction time to threat words, and one on the basis of reaction time to appetitive words (see figure 15.7). In addition, participants were given a number of questionnaires designed to measure traits, states, and symptoms of relevance to psychopathology. Choice of questionnaires was driven by previous research in which we demonstrated that the constructs involved were robust, relatively independent, and associated with unique patterns of brain activity. Questionnaires included the Mood and Anxiety Symptom Questionnaire (Watson et al., 1995), to assess anxious arousal and anhedonic depression; the Penn State Worry Questionnaire (Meyer et al., 1990), to assess anxious apprehension; and the Positive and Negative Affect Scale to assess for positive and negative affect.

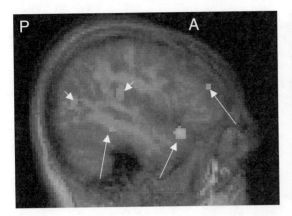
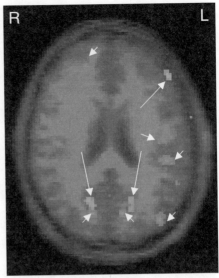

Figure 15.8 Pattern of brain activation during trials of threat words. The threat facilitation group (long arrows) shows activity in left anterior temporal (BA 38), left dorsolateral prefrontal (BA 46), and bilateral precuneus (BA 31) regions. The threat interference group (short arrows) shows activity in posterior left superior frontal (BA 22), right medial frontal (BA 9), bilateral precuneus (BA 18), and left middle occipital (BA 19) regions.

These different patterns of reaction time were associated with differences in asymmetric activation in prefrontal, temporal, parietal, and occipital regions of the brain. In the first analysis, subjects showing response facilitation by threat words exhibited a pattern of left dorsolateral prefrontal, left anterior temporal, and bilateral precuneus activation (see figure 15.8). Furthermore, this pattern was predicted by higher scores on positive affect. These results suggest that individuals biased toward positive affect, and hence approach behavior, activate brain circuits involved in approach (e.g., left prefrontal and temporal regions) that overlap with regions engaged by selective attention tasks (left hemisphere frontal and parietal regions; Corbetta et al., 1990; Coull & Nobre, 1998; Sturm et al., 1999). In contrast, people who showed interference to threat words demonstrated a pattern of activation in right medial frontal, posterior left superior temporal, and bilateral occipital cortex (see figure 15.8) and bilateral deactivation of parietal cortex (see figure 15.9). This pattern was predicted by higher scores on anxious arousal. These results suggest that for individuals prone to anxious

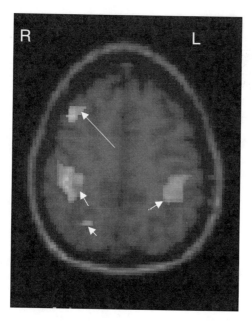

Figure 15.9 Pattern of brain deactivations during trials of threat words. The threat facilitation group (short arrows) shows right middle frontal (BA 8) deactivation, whereas the threat interference (long arrow) group shows bilateral superior (BA 7) and inferior parietal (BA 40) deactivation.

arousal, threat words activate brain circuits associated with withdrawal and negative valence (right frontal) and panic (occipital; for review, see Nitschke et al., 2000; Nitschke & Heller, in press). Bilateral deactivation of the parietal cortex may reflect the active attempt to suppress the attentional orientation or shift toward the threatening, but task-irrelevant, information (see Posner & Petersen, 1990).

The second analysis compared people showing facilitation to appetitive words to people showing interference to appetitive words. Those with facilitation had left prefrontal, left temporal, and bilateral parietal activation (see figure 15.10). These findings suggest that similar brain circuits are involved in appetitive facilitation as are involved in facilitation to threat words. In contrast, those with interference had right superior frontal, right middle temporal, and retrosplenial cortex activation (see figure 15.10), and this pattern was predicted by higher scores on anhedonic depression and anxious apprehension. These results suggest that people prone to depression and anxious apprehen-

W. Heller, N. S. Koven, and G. A. Miller

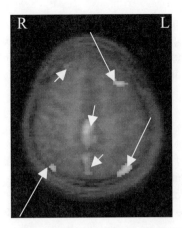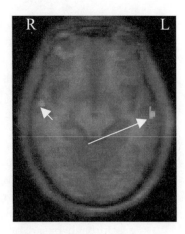

Figure 15.10 Patterns of brain activation during trials of appetitive words. The appetitive facilitation group (long arrows) shows activation in left middle frontal (BA 8/9; *left panel*), bilateral parietal (BA 39; *left panel*), and left anterior middle temporal (BA 21; *right panel*) regions. The appetitive interference group (short arrows) shows a pattern of right superior frontal (BA 8; *left panel*), posterior cingulate (BA 31; *left panel*), and right anterior middle temporal (BA 21; *right panel*) activation.

sion reacted with withdrawal and negative valence toward appetitive words (perhaps because they were all sex-related), and hence engaged the relevant brain circuits. Activation in retrosplenial cortex is consistent with other findings that this region is involved in emotionally arousing information processing, as well as in episodic memory (see Maddock & Buonocore, 1997, for a discussion of similar findings for threat words).

These findings extend our previous research on anxiety and depressed mood by addressing brain mechanisms involved in cognitive processes fostered by both negative and positive emotions. The data are consistent with hypotheses that we and others have put forth regarding the importance of a right hemisphere system that plays an executive role in modulating attention and vigilance in anxiety, especially in anxious arousal (i.e., panic or fear). This right hemisphere system promotes sympathetic nervous system activity, spatial attention, visual scanning of the environment, and sensitivity to meaningful nonverbal cues. These characteristics are very adaptive in the context of a threatening situation. However, when threat is not present or when an individual is prone to perceive, falsely, a threat to be present (as is the case in many anxiety disorders), the activity of this emotional surveillance system interferes with adaptive selective attention and with accurate and quick responses to the task at hand. A predisposition to be anxiously aroused seems to engage this right hemisphere system; positive affect, on the other hand, is associated with activity in left hemisphere neural circuits thought to be involved in approach behavior and in selective attention.

IN CONCLUSION: BEYOND VALENCE AND AROUSAL

By focusing on dimensions of emotional experience that emerge when self-reports of feeling are examined, the circumplex model of emotion provided a useful method for distilling certain aspects of emotional responses that could then be related to brain function. However, an approach based on the circumplex model limits the degree to which one can link aspects of emotion that are not readily represented by valence and arousal to brain function. For example, a variety of cognitive processes associated with emotion, including memory, attention, and information processing (e.g., verbal rumination in anxious apprehension), are likely to involve specific brain regions and interactions between them that do not map onto the relationships described by our neuropsychological model of emotion based on the circumplex.

Furthermore, dimensional models like the circumplex and dimensional concepts like approach-withdrawal are limited by their lack of specificity. Fear and anger cannot be differentiated by the circumplex model, since each involves unpleasant valence. They can be differentiated by approach-withdrawal motivation. In contrast, anger and happiness can be differentiated by the circumplex, since one involves unpleasant, and the other pleasant, valence, but both involve approach motivation. Similarly, negative affect draws on aspects of both valence and arousal. Although clearly of great interest in understanding anxiety, depression, and their shared and distinct aspects, negative affect has yet to be mapped successfully onto regional brain activity. It may be that adding dimensions to the model would preserve it, but in decades of work on dimensions of emotion, no consensus has emerged on the nature of the third dimension, if any.

As noted above, recent research has indicated increased left anterior activity in anger, which is consistent with approach motivation but not with positive valence (Harmon-Jones & Allen, 1998). If fear and anger are distinguished from each other by their patterns of left anterior brain activity, anger and happiness are not (at least not to date with scalp-recorded EEG; an appropriate fMRI study would be valuable). The possibility that motivational disposition generates, produces, or is essentially identical to or synonymous with affective valence (Davidson, 1998; Lang, 1995) is called into question. If motivational disposition can be dissociated from valence (whether orthogonal to it or not), and if asymmetric patterns of brain activity reflect motivational disposition and not valence, then what brain regions are involved in distinguishing pleasant from unpleasant experience? How is the difference between anger and happiness coded in the brain?

To accurately describe the neural circuitry that implements the full range of emotional responses, it will be necessary to go beyond the circumplex model and other dichotomous dimensions and to focus not simply on the isolated activity of a few brain regions, but on the interactions of numerous brain regions. The circumplex model can be greatly enhanced by incorporating a functional connectivity approach; when we begin to understand how activity in one brain region modulates activity in other regions both simultaneously and sequentially, we will achieve a more global picture of brain modulation of emotional functioning.

Current research in emotion emphasizes the need to refine theories and to better characterize the components involved. For example, Russell and Feldman Barrett (1999) distinguish core affect from evaluation as subclasses of emotion that will be best represented by different descriptive structures (e.g., categorical, dimensional, hierarchical). The more we can clarify the psychological structures, the more we can enhance the precision of our neuroanatomical and neurophysiological probes.

REFERENCES

American Psychiatric Association. (1994). *The diagnostic and statistical manual of mental disorders*. Fourth edition. Washington, DC: American Psychiatric Association.

Ashby, F. G., Isen, A. M., & Turken, A. U. (1999). A neuropsychological theory of positive affect and its influence on cognition. *Psychological Review, 106*, 529–550.

Banich, M., Milham, M., Atchley, R., Cohen, N., Webb, A., Wszalek, T., Kramer, A., Liang, Z. P., Wright, A., Shenker, J., & Magin, R. (1998). fMRI activation of cingulate regions by both spatial and color Stroop tasks. *Society for Neuroscience Abstracts, 24*, 1179.

Banich, M. T. (1997). *Neuropsychology: The neural bases of mental function*. Boston: Houghton-Mifflin.

Banich, M. T., Milham, M., Atchley, R., Cohen, N., Webb, A., Wszalek, T., Kramer, A., Liang, Z. P., Barad, V., Gullett, D., Shah, C., & Brown, C. (1999a). fMRI activations due to attentional selection can be dependent upon nature of information to be ignored. Paper presented at Annual Meeting of the Cognitive Neuroscience Society, Washington, DC.

Banich, M. T., Milham, M. P., Atchley, R., Cohen, N. J., Webb, A., Wszalek, T., Kramer, A., Liang, Z. P., Barad, V., Gullet, D., Shah, C., & Brown, C. (1999b). Dissociation of frontal and cingulate activity in attentional control. Paper presented at 5th International Conference on Functional Mapping of the Human Brain, Düsseldorf, Germany.

Banich, M. T., Stolar, N., Heller, W., & Goldman, R. B. (1992). A deficit in right-hemisphere performance after induction of a depressed mood. *Neuropsychiatry, Neuropsychology & Behavioral Neurology, 5*, 20–27.

Barlow, D. H. (1988). *Anxiety and its disorders: The nature and treatment of anxiety and panic*. New York: Guilford.

Barlow, D. H. (1991). Disorders of emotion. *Psychological Inquiry, 2*, 58–71.

Bench, C. J., Frith, C. D., Grasby, P. M., Friston, K. J., Paulesu, E., Frackowiak, R. S. J., & Dolan, R. J. (1993). Investigations of the functional anatomy of attention using the Stroop test. *Neuropsychologia, 31*, 907–922.

Bonanno, G. A., & Siddique, H. I. (1999). Emotional dissociation, self-deception, and psychotherapy. In J. L. Singer & P. Salovey (Eds.), *At play in the fields of consciousness: Essays in honor of Jerome L. Singer* (pp. 249–270). Hillsdale, NJ: Lawrence Erlbaum Associates.

Carter, C. S., Mintun, M., & Cohen, J. D. (1995). Interference and facilitation effects during selective attention: An H-2-15-O PET study of Stroop task performance. *Neuroimage, 2*, 264–272.

Clark, L. A., & Watson, D. (1991). Tripartite model of anxiety and depression: Psychometric evidence and taxonomic implications. *Journal of Abnormal Psychology, 100*, 316–336.

Compton, R. J., Banich, M. T., Mohanty, M. P., Milham, M. P., Miller, G. A., Scalf, P. E., & Heller, W. (submitted). Paying attention to emotion: An fMRI investigation of cognitive and emotional Stroop tasks.

Compton, R. J., Heller, W., Banich, M. T., Palmieri, P. A., & Miller, G. A. (2000). Responding to threat: Hemispheric asymmetries and interhemispheric division of input. *Neuropsychology, 14*, 254–264.

Corbetta, M., Miezin, F. M., Dobmeyer, S., Shulman, G. L., & Peterson, A. (1990). Attentional modulation of neural processing of shape, color, and velocity in humans. *Science, 248*, 1556–1559.

Coull, J. T., & Nobre, A. C. (1998). Where and when to pay attention: The neural systems for directing attention to spatial locations and to time intervals as revealed by both PET and fMRI. *Journal of Neuroscience, 18*, 7426–7435.

Damasio, A. R. (1995). On some functions of the human prefrontal cortex. In J. Grafman & K. J. Holyoak (Eds.), *Structure and functions of the human prefrontal cortex. Annals of the New York Academy of Sciences, 769*, 241–251.

Damasio, A. R., Grabowski, T. J., Bechara, A., Damasio, H., Ponto, L. L. B., Parvizi, J., & Hichwa, R. D. (2000). Subcortical and cortical brain activity during the feeling of self-generated emotions. *Nature Neuroscience, 3*, 1049–1056.

Davidson, R. J. (1992). Prolegomenon to the structure of emotion: Gleanings from neuropsychology. *Cognition & Emotion, 6*, 245–268.

Davidson, R. J. (1995). Cerebral asymmetry, emotion, and affective style. In R. J. Davidson & K. Hugdahl (Eds.), *Brain asymmetry* (pp. 361–387). Cambridge, MA: MIT Press.

Davidson, R. J. (1998). Affective style and affective disorders: Perspectives from affective neuroscience. *Cognition & Emotion, 12*, 307–330.

Deldin, P. J., Keller, J., Gergen, J. A., & Miller, G. A. (2001). Cognitive bias and emotion in neuropsychological models of depression. *Cognition & Emotion, 15*, 787–802.

Derbyshire, S. W. G., Vogt, B. A., & Jones, A. K. P. (1998). Pain and Stroop interference tasks activate separate processing modules in anterior cingulate cortex. *Experimental Brain Research, 188*, 52–60.

Devinsky, O., Morrell, M. J., & Vogt, B. A. (1995). Contributions of anterior cingulate cortex to behaviour. *Brain, 118*, 279–306.

Dolan, R. J., Bench, C. J., Brown, R. G., Scott, L. C., & Frackowiak, R. S. J. (1994). Neuropsychological dysfunction in depression: The relationship to regional cerebral blood flow. *Psychological Medicine, 24*, 849–857.

Drevets, W. C., & Raichle, M. E. (1998). Reciprocal suppression of regional cerebral blood flow during emotional vesus higher cognitive processes: Implications for interactions between emotion and cognition. *Cognition & Emotion, 12*, 353–385.

Ehlers, A., Margraf, J., Davies, S., & Roth, W. T. (1988). Selective processing of threat cues in subjects with panic attacks. *Cognition & Emotion, 2*, 201–219.

Elliott, R., Baker, S. C., Rogers, R. D., O'Leary, D. A., Paykel, E. S., Frith, C. D., Dolan, R. J., & Sahakian, B. J. (1997). Prefrontal dysfunction in depressed patients performing a complex planning task: A study using positron emission tomography. *Psychological Medicine, 27*, 931–942.

Elliott, R., Dolan, R. J., & Frith, C. D. (2000). Dissociable functions in the medial and lateral orbitfrontal cortex: Evidence from human neuroimaging studies. *Cerebral Cortex, 10*, 308–317.

Elliott, R., Sahakian, B. J., Michael, A., Paykel, E. S., & Dolan, R. J. (1998). Abnormal neural response to feedback on planning and guessing tasks in patients with unipolar depression. *Psychological Medicine, 28*, 559–571.

Ellsworth, P. C. (1994). William James and emotion: Is a century of fame worth a century of misunderstanding? *Psychological Review, 101*, 222–229.

Eysenck, M. W. (1992). *Anxiety: The cognitive perspective*. Hove, UK: Lawrence Erlbaum Associates.

Foa, E. B., Ilai, D., McCarthy, P. R., Shoyer, B., & Murdock, T. B. (1993). Information processing in obsessive-compulsive disorder. *Cognitive Therapy and Research, 17,* 173–189.

Gainotti, G., Caltagirone, C., & Zoccolotti, P. (1993). Left/right and cortical/subcortical dichotomies in the neuropsychological study of human emotions. *Cognition & Emotion, 7,* 71–93.

George, M. S., Ketter, T. A., & Post, R. M. (1993). SPECT and PET imaging in mood disorders. *Journal of Clinical Psychiatry, 54,* 6–13.

Gross, J. (1999). Emotion regulation: Past, present, future. *Cognition & Emotion, 13,* 551–573.

Gross, J., & Levenson, R. W. (1997). Hiding feelings: The acute effects of inhibiting positive and negative emotion. *Journal of Abnormal Psychology, 106,* 95–103.

Hager, F., Volz, H. P., Gaser, C., Mentzel, H.-J., Kaiser, W. A., & Sauer, H. (1998). Challenging the anterior attentional system with a continuous performance task: A functional magnetic resonance imaging approach. *European Archives of Psychiatry and Clinical Neuroscience, 248,* 161–170.

Haier, R. J., Siegel, B. V., Jr., MacLachlan, A., Soderling, E., Lottenberg, S., & Buchsbaum, M. S. (1992). Regional glucose metabolic changes after learning a complex visuospatial/motor task: A positron emission tomography study. *Brain Research, 570,* 134–143.

Harmon-Jones, E., & Allen, J. B. (1998). Anger and frontal brain activity: EEG asymmetry consistent with approach motivation despite negative affective valence. *Journal of Personality & Social Psychology, 74,* 1310–1316.

Heilman, K. M., Watson, R. T., & Valenstein, E. (1985). Neglect and related disorders. In K. M. Heilman & E. Valenstein (Eds.), *Clinical neuropsychology* (pp. 243–293). New York: Oxford University Press.

Heller, W. (1986). Cerebral organization of emotional function in children. Ph.D. dissertation, University of Chicago.

Heller, W. (1990). The neuropsychology of emotion: Developmental patterns and implications for psychopathology. In N. Stein, B. L. Leventhal, & T. Trabasso (Eds.), *Psychological and biological approaches to emotion* (pp. 167–211). Hillsdale, NJ: Lawrence Erlbaum Associates.

Heller, W. (1993). Neuropsychological mechanisms of individual differences in emotion, personality, and arousal. *Neuropsychology, 7,* 476–489.

Heller, W., Banich, M. T., Herrington, J. D., Mohanty, A., Fisher, J. E., Jacobson, B. L., Scalf, P., Erickson, K. I., Koven, N. S., Compton, R. J., & Miller, G. A. (2000). Differential brain activation in response to positive and threat stimuli in an emotional Stroop paradigm. Paper presented at the Annual Meeting of the Society for Research in Psychopathology, Boulder, CO.

Heller, W., Etienne, M., & Miller, G. A. (1995). Patterns of perceptual asymmetry in depression and anxiety: Implications for neuropsychological models of emotion and psychopathology. *Journal of Abnormal Psychology, 104*, 327–333.

Heller, W., & Nitschke, J. B. (1997). Regional brain activity in emotion: A framework for understanding cognition in depression. *Cognition & Emotion, 11*, 637–661.

Heller, W., & Nitschke, J. B. (1998). The puzzle of regional brain activity in depression and anxiety: The importance of subtypes and comorbidity. *Cognition & Emotion, 12*, 421–447.

Heller, W., Nitschke, J. B., Etienne, M. A., & Miller, G. A. (1997a). Patterns of regional brain activity differentiate types of anxiety. *Journal of Abnormal Psychology, 106*, 376–385.

Heller, W., Nitschke, J. B., & Lindsay, D. L. (1997b). Neuropsychological correlates of arousal in self-reported emotion. *Cognition & Emotion, 11*, 383–402.

Hope, D. A., Rapee, R. M., Heimberg, R. G., & Dombeck, M. J. (1990). Representations of the self in social phobia: Vulnerability to social threat. *Cognitive Therapy and Research, 14*, 177–189.

Hugdahl, K. (1999). Classical conditioning and implicit learning: The right hemisphere hypothesis. In R. J. Davidson & K. Hugdahl (Eds.), *Brain asymmetry*. Cambridge, Mass.: MIT Press.

Keller, J., Nitschke, J. B., Bhargava, T., Deldin, P. J., Gergen, J. A., Miller, G. A., & Heller, W. (2000). Neuropsychological differentiation of depression and anxiety. *Journal of Abnormal Psychology, 109*, 3–10.

Lang, P. J. (1968). Fear reduction and fear behavior: Problems in treating a construct. In J. M. Shlien (Ed.), *Research in psychotherapy*. Vol. 3 (pp. 90–102). Washington, DC: American Psychological Association.

Lang, P. J. (1979). A bio-informational theory of emotional imagery. *Psychophysiology, 16*, 495–512.

Lang, P. J. (1993). The network model of emotion: Motivational connections. In R. S. Wyer, Jr., & T. K. Srull (Eds.), *Perspectives on anger and emotion: Advances in social cognition*. Vol. 6 (pp. 109–133). Hillsdale, NJ: Lawrence Erlbaum Associates.

Lang, P. J. (1995). The emotion probe: Studies of motivation and attention. *American Psychologist, 50*, 372–385.

Larsen, R. J., & Diener, E. (1992). Promises and problems with the circumplex model of emotion. In M. S. Clark (Ed.), *Review of Personality and Social Psychology* (pp. 25–59). Newbury Park, CA: Sage.

LeDoux, J. E. (1995). Emotion: Clues from the brain. *Annual Review of Psychology, 46*, 209–235.

Lerner, J. S., & Keltner, D. (2000). Beyond valence: Toward a model of emotion-specific influences on judgement and choice. *Cognition & Emotion, 14*, 473–493.

Levy, J., Heller, W., Banich, M. T., & Burton, L. A. (1983a). Are variations among right-handed individuals in perceptual asymmetries caused by characteristic arousal differences between hemispheres? *Journal of Experimental Psychology: Human Perception and Performance, 9,* 329–359.

Levy, J., Heller, W., Banich, M. T., & Burton, L. A. (1983b). Asymmetry of perception in free viewing of chimeric faces. *Brain & Cognition, 2,* 404–419.

Liotti, M., & Tucker, D. M. (1992). Right hemisphere sensitivity to arousal and depression. *Brain & Cognition, 18,* 138–151.

London, E. D., Ernst, M., Grant, S., Bonson, K., & Weinstein, A. (2000). Orbitofrontal cortex and human drug abuse: Functional imaging. *Cerebral Cortex, 10,* 334–342.

Maddock, R. J., & Buonocore, M. H. (1997). Activation of left posterior cingulate gyrus by the auditory presentation of threat-related words: An fMRI study. *Psychiatry Research: Neuroimaging Section, 75,* 1–14.

Mathews, A., & MacLeod, C. (1985). Selective processing of threat cues in anxiety states. *Behaviour Research and Therapy, 23,* 563–569.

Mayberg, H. S., Liotti, M., Brannan, S. K., McGinnis, S., Mahurin, R. K., Jerabek, P. A., Silva, J. A., Tekell, J. L., Martin, C. C., Lancaster, J. L., & Fox, P. T. (1999). Reciprocal limbic-cortical function and negative mood: Converging PET findings in depression and normal sadness. *American Journal of Psychiatry, 156,* 675–682.

McNally, R. J. (1998). Information-processing abnormalities in anxiety disorders: Implications for cognitive neuroscience. *Cognition & Emotion, 12,* 479–495.

McNally, R. J., Kaspi, S. P., Riemann, B. C., & Zeitlin, S. B. (1990). Selective processing of threat cues in posttraumatic stress disorder. *Journal of Abnormal Psychology, 99,* 398–402.

Milham, M. P., Banich, M. T., Webb, A., Barad, V., Cohen, N. J., Wszalek, T., Kramer, A., Liang, Z. P., Gullett, D., Shah, C., & Brown, C. (1999). Activity of cingulate based attentional system in Stroop task is dependent upon response eligibility: A hybrid blocked/event-related fMRI design. Paper presented at 5th International Conference on Functional Mapping of the Human Brain, Düsseldorf, Germany.

Milham, M., Banich, M., Webb, A., Wszalek, T., Gullet, D., Brown, C., Shah, C., DiGirolamo, G., Cohen, N., Kramer, A., & Liang, Z. P. (1999). fMRI study using trained associations in a Stroop-like task verifies the generality of the neural bases of selection attention. Paper presented at the Society for Neuroscience Meeting, Miami Beach, FL.

Miller, G. A. (1996). Presidential address: How we think about cognition, emotion, and biology in psychopathology. *Psychophysiology, 33,* 615–628.

Miller, G. A. (2000). Cognition/emotion: Integration and comorbidity. Invited presentation, NIMH conference "From Neurobiology to Psychopathology: Integrating Cognition and Emotion," Bethesda, MD.

Miller, G. A., & Keller, J. (2000). Psychology and neuroscience: Making peace. *Current Directions in Psychological Science, 9,* 212–215.

Miller, G. A., & Kozak, M. J. (1993). A philosophy for the study of emotion: Three-systems theory. In A. Ohman & N. Birbaumer (Eds.), *The organization of the emotions* (pp. 31–47). Toronto: Hogrefe International.

Miyake, A., Friedman, N. P., Emerson, M. J., Witzki, A. H., & Howerter, A. (2000). The unity and diversity of executive functions and their contributions to complex "frontal lobe" tasks: A latent variable analysis. *Cognitive Psychology, 41,* 49–100.

Nitschke, J. B., & Heller, W. (In press). The neuropsychology of anxiety disorders: Affect, cognition, and neural circuitry. In D'Haenen (Ed.), *Textbook of biological psychiatry.*

Nitschke, J. B., Heller, W., Imig, J., McDonald, R. P., & Miller, G. A. (2001). Distinguishing dimensions of anxiety and depression. *Cognitive Therapy and Research, 25,* 1–22.

Nitschke, J. B., Heller, W., & Miller, G. A. (2000). Anxiety, stress, and cortical brain function. In J. C. Borod (Ed.), *The neuropsychology of emotion* (pp. 298–319). New York: Oxford University Press.

Nitschke, J. B., Heller, W., Palmieri, P. A., & Miller, G. A. (1999). Contrasting patterns of brain activity in anxious apprehension and anxious arousal. *Psychophysiology, 36,* 628–637.

Öhman, A., Flykt, A., & Lundqvist, D. (2000). Unconscious emotion: Evolutionary perspectives, psychophysiological data and neuropsychological mechanisms. In R. D. Lane & L. Nadel (Eds.), *Cognitive neuroscience of emotion* (pp. 296–327). New York: Oxford University Press.

Otto, M. W., Yeo, R. A., & Dougher, M. J. (1987). Right hemisphere involvement in depression: Toward a neuropsychological theory of negative affective experiences. *Biological Psychiatry, 22,* 1201–1215.

Pardo, J. V., Pardo, P. J., Janer, K. W., & Raichle, M. E. (1990). The anterior cingulate cortex mediates processing selection in the Stroop attentional conflict paradigm. *Proceedings of the National Academy of Sciences, USA, 87,* 256–259.

Pizzagalli, D., Nitschke, J. B., Pascual-Marqui, R. D., Larson, C. L., Abercrombie, H. C., Schaefer, S. M., Oakes, T. R., Koger, J. V., Benca, R. M., & Davidson, R. J. (2000). Brain electrical correlates of depression derived from a new source localization method. Poster presented at the Society for Research in Psychopathology, Boulder, CO.

Posner, M. I., & Petersen, S. E. (1990). The attention system of the human brain. *Annual Review of Neuroscience, 13,* 25–42.

Russell, J. A., & Feldman Barrett, L. (1999). Core affect, prototypical emotional episodes, and other things called emotion: Dissecting the elephant. *Journal of Personality and Social Psychology, 76,* 805–819.

Stormark, K. M., Nordby, H., & Hugdahl, K. (1995). Attentional shifts to emotionally charged cues: Behavioural and ERP data. *Cognition & Emotion, 9,* 507–523.

Sturm, W., de Simone, A., Krause, B. J., Specht, K., Hesselmann, V., Radermacher, I., Herzog, H., Tellmann, L., Muller-Gartner, H. W., & Willmes, K. (1999). Functional anatomy of instrinsic alertness: Evidence for a fronto-parietal-thalamic-brainstem network in the right hemisphere. *Neuropsychologia, 37,* 797–805.

Tucker, D. M. (1981). Lateral brain function, emotion, and conceptualization. *Psychological Bulletin, 89,* 19–46.

Volkow, N. D., & Fowler, J. S. (2000). Addiction, a disease of compulsion and drive: Involvement of the orbitofrontal cortex. *Cerebral Cortex, 10,* 318–325.

Watson, D., Weber, K., Assenheimer, J. S., Clark, L. A., Strauss, M. E., & McCormick, R. A. (1995). Testing a tripartite model: I. Evaluating the convergent and discriminant validity of anxiety and depression symptom scales. *Journal of Abnormal Psychology, 104,* 3–14.

Watts, F. N., McKenna, F. P., Sharrock, R., & Trezise, L. (1986). Colour naming of phobia-related words. *British Journal of Psychology, 77,* 97–108.

Williams, J. M. G., Mathews, A., & MacLeod, C. (1996). The emotional Stroop task and psychopathology. *Psychological Bulletin, 120,* 3–24.

Wittling, W. (1995). Brain asymmetry in the control of autonomic-physiologic activity. In R. J. Davidson & K. Hugdahl (Eds.), *Brain asymmetry* (pp. 305–357). Cambridge: MIT Press.

16 The State and Trait Nature of Frontal EEG Asymmetry in Emotion

James A. Coan and John J. B. Allen

INTRODUCTION

Over 60 studies have now been published examining the relationship between asymmetrical electroencephalographic (EEG) activity over the frontal cortex and emotion or emotion-related constructs. Two research approaches typify this literature. The first involves correlating resting EEG activity with traitlike phenomena, such as temperament or psychopathology, or with state fluctuations in emotion. The second involves correlating state fluctuations in frontal EEG asymmetry with changes in emotional or motivational state. This chapter reviews this literature, highlighting the state or trait nature of these studies, and provides a framework for conceptualizing state- and trait-related EEG asymmetry as it relates to emotion and emotion-related processes.

Current Conceptualizations of Asymmetries in Cortical Activation

Frontal EEG asymmetries have most frequently been associated with motivational and affective traits and states, most notably fundamental approach and withdrawal orientations and actions (Davidson, 1993). According to the approach/withdrawal model of frontal EEG asymmetry, relatively greater left frontal activity should generally result in either an approach orientation or an approach-oriented action (Davidson, 1993). In contrast, relatively greater right frontal activation should generally result in either a withdrawal orientation or a withdrawal-oriented action (Davidson, 1993). This primarily motivational model of frontal EEG asymmetry overlaps substantially (Davidson, 1992) with more affective models, such as the valence model. According to the valence model, relatively greater left frontal activation is associated with positively valenced emotions, while relatively greater right frontal activation is associated with negatively valenced emotions (Davidson, 1992). In recent years, evidence associating relatively greater left frontal activation with trait and state anger (Harmon-Jones, 2000a; Harmon-Jones & Allen, 1998), as well as with general behavioral activation tendencies independent of valence (Harmon-Jones & Allen, 1997; Sutton & Davidson, 1997), suggests that the approach/withdrawal model is the most universal model of frontal EEG asymmetry. The valence model is, obviously, unable to accommodate these recent anger findings, since anger is a negatively valenced emotion characterized by relative left frontal activation. Within both the approach/withdrawal and the valence models, frontal EEG asymmetry has been associated with both traitlike and state-dependent processes.

The vast majority of work in this area focuses on frontal activation asymmetry as a trait measure. From this perspective, trait frontal asymmetries have most commonly been associated with other traits, such as sociability, behavioral activation, or aggression (Harmon-Jones & Allen, 1997; Harmon-Jones & Allen, 1998; Schmidt, 1999), or with various forms of psychopathology, such as depression and anxiety (Allen et al., 1993; Henriques & Davidson, 1991; Weidemann et al., 1999). To a lesser degree, trait levels of frontal EEG asymmetry have been used to predict the magnitude of state-dependent fluctuations in affective reports (Tomarken et al., 1990; Wheeler et al., 1993). By contrast, a smaller number of studies have examined state-dependent changes in EEG asymmetry, associating fluctuations in frontal EEG asymmetries with concomitant fluctuations in affective states (Coan et al., 2001; Ekman & Davidson, 1993).

Although traitlike frontal EEG asymmetry has been associated with state-dependent affective responses, usually in the form of self-report, little is known about how trait and state frontal EEG asymmetries are related. In fact, no published studies, and only the published abstract of one author (Hagemann, Naumann, Luerken, & Bartussek, 1999a) and a recent symposium (Coan & Allen, 2000b; Harmon-Jones, 2000b; Hagemann, 2000; Kline, 2000), were found that involved any investigation of the relationship between trait levels and state-related changes in frontal EEG asymmetry.

For the purposes of this chapter, trait frontal EEG asymmetry will refer to asymmetries that are intraindividually consistent across time, or asymmetries examined in research studies that make this assumption even though asymmetries may not be measured on multiple occasions. Research of this type would argue that frontal EEG asymmetries represent properties of the individuals possessing them—that is, that individuals possess certain frontal EEG asymmetries as relatively stable traits. These traits, it is further argued (and demonstrated with ample research—see, e.g., Davidson, 1998a), serve as diatheses that increase risk for psychopathology, and that predict other traits and behaviors. These traits modulate state measures such as emotional reactivity, usually in the form of a verbal report (Davidson, 1998a; Wheeler et al., 1993).

State frontal EEG asymmetries, by contrast, may be thought of as those which are responsive to specific environmental conditions (Cattell & Scheier, 1961). Examples of this would include person-independent differences in frontal EEG asymmetry resulting from different voluntary emotional facial expressions (Coan et al., 2001; Ekman & Davidson, 1993). For example, Ekman and Davidson (1993) found that smiles that included the activation of the orbicularis pars lateralis muscle (the Duchenne smile) resulted in an increase in left frontal activation relative to ("unfelt") smiles that did not include this movement. State-oriented inquiries such as this would argue that state-related changes in frontal EEG asymmetries represent properties of the states per se (in the case of the example, properties of Duchenne and unfelt smiles), and assume that such state-EEG relationships generalize across individuals. Thus trait studies of EEG asymmetry adopt an individual differences approach, while state studies of frontal EEG asymmetry assume a normative approach.

The Nature of Frontal EEG Asymmetry

Before reviewing the literature on frontal EEG asymmetry and emotion, several issues relevant to the interpretation of frontal EEG asymmetry (or, indeed, any hemispheric asymmetry in scalp-recorded EEG) are worth highlighting. The first concerns the dependent measure: alpha activity, typically in the 8–13 Hz range, is extracted at any given site. Alpha, however, is generally thought to be inversely related to brain activation, since blocking of or decreases in alpha are seen when underlying cortical systems engage in active processing (e.g., Davidson, Chapman, et al., 1990). The assumption underlying research examining frontal EEG asymmetries, therefore, is that an asymmetry in alpha represents an asymmetry in the *opposite* direction in terms of activation of cortical regions.[1] This alpha/activation inverse can make reading the literature challenging. For example, many reports discuss correlations between depression and relatively greater left frontal alpha, leaving the reader to remember that the sign attributed to the correlation will have to be reversed in order to correspond to relatively greater left frontal *activation*. In the present chapter, therefore, asymmetries will be reported in terms of activation, to relieve the reader of additional cognitive operations to interpret the findings.

A second set of issues concerns the problem of what actually produces the asymmetry effects. Many investigators, for example, report a hemispheric difference score between homologous sites. This common practice usually involves subtracting the natural log (ln) of the right hemisphere alpha from that of the left hemisphere (ln[Right] − ln[Left]). The resultant difference score provides a unidimensional scale, wherein higher scores indicate relatively greater left frontal activation and lower scores indicate relatively greater right frontal activation (keeping in mind the putative inverse relationship between alpha and activation). The difficulty with the use of such a difference metric[2] is in ascertaining whether one, the other, or both of the hemispheres are involved in producing the difference. Fortunately, many investigators compare left and right hemispheric alpha power in addition to or instead of computing the difference score. Nonetheless, regardless of whether results are expressed as difference scores or constituent scores, it can be challenging when reading the literature to determine what is actually changing relative to what. In depression studies, for example, one will variously encounter "greater right frontal activation" (e.g., Schaffer et al., 1983, p. 758) and "lower left frontal activation" (e.g., Gotlib et al., 1998, p. 449). It is not always clear whether a single hemisphere has a particular stake in certain effects, or whether the critical determinant is the relative difference between hemispheres, however obtained.

Related to the issue of whether left or right hemisphere changes are producing effects is the observation that the difference between hemispheres is relatively small compared to the overall magnitude of activity in each hemisphere. The correlation between homologous sites (e.g., F3 and F4, or F7 and F8) is substantial, ranging from .95 to .99 (e.g., Tomarken, Davidson, Wheeler, & Kinney, 1992). The asymmetry, then, accounts for little variance in overall EEG activity, but captures im-

James A. Coan and John J. B. Allen

portant variance related to motivation and emotion. In fact, when the impact of the homologous lead is statistically controlled prior to calculating the difference score (cf. Fox et al., 1995), the relationship of asymmetry to criterion measures appears to be enhanced.

About the Tables

The tables included in the forthcoming pages summarize the literature on EEG hemispheric asymmetries in emotion, confined to frontal regions only. They are intended to provide certain details of general interest as well as of interest to the study of EEG asymmetry in particular. Of general interest are various sample characteristics, along with a tabular summary of the results. In addition, information has been provided that is of particular interest to investigators who may intend to conduct studies of this nature. For example, as one peruses any of the tables, one will immediately recognize that most reports include only right-handed participants. This is generally attributed to evidence (e.g., Bryden, 1982) that hemispheric lateralization may be partially a function of handedness. These tables include the specification of handedness in the attempt to identify studies where handedness either is not addressed or is mixed (interindividually, not intraindividually). (To our knowledge, there are no published studies utilizing a left-handed-only sample.) Also, it is increasingly apparent that different references (e.g., vertex, linked mastoids, left ear, etc.) each contribute unique sources of variance and error to the analysis of asymmetries in scalp-recorded EEG (Henriques & Davidson, 1991; Reid et al., 1998). Because no reference has thus far unequivocally emerged as preferred, a column for the reference scheme used in each study has been included, in the hope that this may prove useful.

FRONTAL EEG ACTIVATION ASYMMETRY AS A TRAIT MEASURE

In his classic article, Allport (1966) proposed eight properties of traits. First, he asserted that traits must have more than nominal existence. Second, he argued that traits must be more generalized than habits. Third, he proposed that traits must be determinative of behavior. The remaining properties read like a checklist: fourth, traits should be established empirically; fifth, traits should be only relatively independent of other traits; sixth, traits should not be synonymous with moral or social judgments; seventh, traits can be studied idiomorphically or in terms of their distributions in the general population; and eighth, acts or habits that are inconsistent with a given trait do not necessarily constitute evidence of the nonexistence of that trait (Allport, 1966). His subsequent discussion, like so many discussions of personality traits, centers on how traits are to be measured and, to a lesser extent, whether traits can ever be considered "real" or only as hypothetical constructs. As a trait measure, frontal EEG asymmetry appears to satisfy each of Allport's criteria.

With regard to measurement, the primary issue in determining the traitlike qualities of frontal EEG asymmetry involves establishing the measure's stability. Because the asymmetry can be measured more or less directly, it is less vulnerable (though by no means invulnerable) to the myriad measurement errors surrounding other traitlike constructs. Addressing the issue of stability, Tomarken, Davidson, Wheeler, and Kinney (1992) assessed the psychometric properties of traitlike frontal EEG asymmetries and were able to determine that frontal EEG asymmetry showed high internal consistency (Cronbach's alphas ranging from .81 to .90) and acceptable test-retest stability (intraclass correlations ranging from .53 to .72 within single assessments, and from .69 to .84 across 3 weeks). In another study, Jones, Field, Davalos, and Pickens (1997) found that frontal EEG asymmetry recorded at 3 months of age was highly correlated with the same asymmetry at 3 yrs ($r = .66$, $p < .01$). Similar figures come from Hagemann (2000), who found that across four different measurement occasions, 60% of the variance of the asymmetry measures was due to individual differences of a temporally stable latent trait, and 40% of the variance of the asymmetry scores was due to occasion-specific fluctuations. On the other hand, some studies have specifically examined subjects who show the greatest cross-session consistency (e.g., Wheeler et al., 1993), reasoning that the strongest relationships to other traits should be shown by those who are consistent on the measure of trait EEG asymmetry (cf. Bem & Allen, 1974).

Apart from its psychometric properties, trait frontal EEG asymmetry has been associated with other relatively stable traits (e.g., Harmon-Jones & Allen, 1997) and risk for psychopathology (e.g., Henriques & Davidson, 1990), and has been found to change little despite changes in clinical status in depression (Allen et al., 1993; Urry et al., 1999; although see Debener et al., 2000). Trait frontal EEG asymmetry has been used to predict the intensity of emotion in response to emotionally evocative films (Wheeler et al., 1993), and has predicted basal natural killer cell immune function (Davidson et al., 1999). In children, it has predicted internalizing and externalizing difficulties (Fox et al., 1996), and, in infants, crying behavior in response to maternal separation (Davidson & Fox, 1989). Traitlike frontal EEG asymmetry has, in part, characterized the infants of depressed mothers (e.g., Dawson, Frey, Panagiotides, et al., 1997). Given the very wide range of relationships that trait frontal EEG asymmetry appears to have, it will be useful to review the entire literature in some detail, categorizing the literature on traitlike asymmetry into manageable subsections, specifically trait frontal EEG and its relationship to other traitlike measures, trait frontal EEG asymmetry and psychopathology, and trait frontal EEG asymmetry as a predictor of state-dependent changes in emotion.

Trait Frontal EEG Asymmetry and other Traitlike Measures

A comprehensive tabular summary of this literature can be found in table 16.1. Although no attempt will be made to review every report within this chapter, a number of particularly influential and interesting studies should be highlighted.

Frontal EEG asymmetry is thought to relate to various personality traits. Following from the approach/withdrawal model of asymmetry, trait patterns of propensities to approach or engage with the environment or to withdraw from the environment should be associated with this EEG measure. A clear example of this can be found with Carver and White's (1994) BIS/BAS scales, which are intended to measure Gray's (1972, 1987) behavioral inhibition and activation systems (BIS and BAS, respectively) as traits. According to Gray, the BIS initially inhibits action and subsequently guides behavior toward removing or avoiding an undesirable stimulus. The BAS essentially functions in the opposite manner, responding to incentives and guiding organisms toward attaining a desirable stimulus. Several researchers have identified a relationship between these systems and frontal EEG asymmetry (Coan & Allen, 2000a; Harmon-Jones & Allen, 1997; Sutton & Davidson, 1997). Sutton and Davidson (1997) proposed that the BIS and BAS should map closely onto withdrawal and approach tendencies, respectively, and indeed found that relatively greater left frontal activation was

Table 16.1 Trait frontal EEG asymmetry and other traitlike measures

Citation	Sample number	Age info	Sex	Handedness	Reference scheme
Davidson et al., 1999	24	17–21 yrs.	F/M	R	LM
Fox et al., 1995	48	49–62 months	F/M	No info	Cz
Hagemann et al., 1999b	36	Mean = 24.7	F/M	R	Cz
Harmon-Jones, 2000a	97	Mean = 19 yrs.	F/M	R	Linked ears
Harmon-Jones & Allen, 1997	37	No info	F	R	Cz
Jacobs & Snyder, 1996	40	18–53 yrs.	M	R	LM
Jones et al., 1997c	87 (infants)	No info	F/M	No info	Cz
Kang et al., 1991	20	17–20 yrs.	F	R	Cz, LM
Kalin et al., 2000	17 (rhesus monkeys)	Longitudinal data @ 4, 8, 14, 40, & 52 months	F/M	No info	No info
Kline et al., 1998	60 women 25 men	17–33 yrs.	F/M	R	Linked ears
Kline et al., in press	141 women 94 men	Mean = 20.4	F/M	R	No info
Moss et al., 1985	12 (Japanese) 12 (Westerners)	J Mean = 32.6 yrs. W Mean = 29.1 yrs.	F	R	Cz
Merckelbach et al., 1996	29	22–38 yrs.	F	No info	A1
Schmidt, 1999	40 (extreme scorers selected from among 271)	Mean = 20.97 yrs.	F	R	Cz

James A. Coan and John J. B. Allen

Independent variable	Dependent variable	Results summary
EEG @ F3/4, F7/8 & T3/4	Natural killer (NK) cell activity at rest, before exam, and following pos and neg film clips	↑ RFA, ↓ NK (rest) ↑ RFA, ↓ NK (exam) ↑ LFA, ↑ NK (pos film clip)
EEG @ F3/4, P3/4 & O1/2	Social competence (SC)	↑ RFA, ↓ SC ↑ LFA, ↑ SC
Positive affectivity (PA), negative affectivity (NA), extroversion (E), and neuroticism (N).	EEG @ F3/4, T3/4, C3/4, P3/4 A1/2	↑ NA, ↑ LATA
EEG @ F7/8, F3/4 & P3/4	Trait anger (A), anger attitudes (AA)	↑ A, ↑ LFA ↑ A*AA, ↑ LFA ↑ A, ↓ RFA
EEG @ F3/4 & P3/4	BIS/BAS	↑ LFA, ↑ BAS
EEG @ F3/4, P3/4	PANAS (PA & NA); BDI	↑ LFA, ↓ NA score ↑ LFA, ↓ BDI score
Baby groups: Overstimulating (O) vs. Understimulating (U) mothers.	EEG @ F3/4 & P3/4, various physio and beh. measures	O babies, ↑ LFA U babies, ↑ RFA (Mothers showed the same pattern as infants)
Extreme LFA and RFA groups	Natural killer (NK) cell, lymphocyte and T-cell activity	RFA group, ↓ NK activity
Extreme LFA and RFA groups in monkeys	Cerebrospinal fluid CRH	↑ RFA, ↑ CRH
Defensive Coping (EPQ-L scale)	EEG @ F3/4, FP1/2, F7/8, C3/4, T3/4, T5/6, P3/4, O1/2	For women, ↑ LFA ↑ defensiveness For men, ↑ LFA ↓ defensiveness
High (HD) vs. low (LD) defensiveness groups. Experimenter gender: same vs. opposite.	EEG @ F3/4, FP1/2, F7/8, C3/4, T3/4, T5/6, P3/4, O1/2	HD, ↑ LFA in presence of opposite sex.
Cultural group (J vs. W)	EEG @ T3/4 & P3/4	W = ↑ LPA
L vs. R hemisphere preference (questionnaire)	EEG @ F3/4 & P3/4	↑ LHP, ↑ LFA
Low shy vs. High shy Low soc vs. High soc	EEG @ F3/4, P3/4 & O1/2	↑ shyness, ↑ RFA ↑ soc, ↑ LFA high shy, high soc had ↑ LFA than high shy, low soc

Table 16.1 (continued)

Citation	Sample number	Age info	Sex	Handedness	Reference scheme
Schmidt & Fox, 1994	40 (extreme scorers selected from among 282)	No info	F	R	Cz
Sutton & Davidson, 1997	46	18–22 yrs.	F/M	R	LM
Tomarken & Davidson, 1994	90	No info	F	R	Cz
Tomarken et al., 1992a	90	17–21 yrs.	F	R	Cz, LM

RFA, right frontal activation, LFA, left frontal activation, RATA, right anterior temporal activation, LATA, left anterior temporal activation, RPA, right parietal activation, LPA, left parietal activation.

associated with both higher BAS scores and greater BAS-BIS differences scores. Relatively greater right frontal activation was associated with higher BIS scores (Sutton & Davidson, 1997). Work by Harmon-Jones and Allen (1997) and Coan and Allen (2000a), however, suggests that the relationship is robust for BAS, but not so robust for BIS.

While both of these reports found associations between relative left frontal activation and higher BAS scores, neither was able to detect an association between relative right frontal activation and BIS scores, suggesting that the theoretical association between withdrawal motivations and the BIS is more complex than that between approach motivations and the BAS (Coan & Allen, 2000a; Harmon-Jones and Allen, 1997). In part, this is suggested by the fact that, theoretically, Davidson's (1998a) withdrawal construct is potentially more heterogeneous than that of the BIS, whereas Davidson's approach and Carver and White's BAS constructs have more in common. For example, Davidson's withdrawal construct references movement, or tendencies toward movement, *away* from a stimulus. The BIS, on the other hand, may tap only one event in a chain of events that may lead to withdrawal behaviors; it is thought primarily to motivate behavioral inhibition in response to an aversive stimulus.

Thus, variance due to withdrawal orientations or actions may overlap only slightly with the BIS, with other withdrawal variance distrib-

Independent variable	Dependent variable	Results summary
Low shy vs. High shy Low soc vs. High soc	EEG @ F3/4, P3/4, A1/2 & O1/2	↓ soc, ↑ RFA low shy, high soc = ↑ RPA low shy, low soc = ↑ LPA
EEG @ F3/4 & P3/4	BIS/BAS, BAS-BIS diff score	↑ LFA, ↑ BAS ↑ RFA, ↑ BIS ↑ LFA, ↑ BAS-BIS diff
High Defensive (HD) vs. Low Defensive (LD)	EEG @ F3/4, F7/8, T3/4, C3/4 & P3/4	HD = ↑ LFA in F3/4 & F7/8
EEG @ F3/4, F7/8, T3/4, P3/4, C3/4	General positive and negative affect (PA and NA)	↑ LFA, ↑ PA ↑ LFA, ↓ NA

uted across Gray's (1972, 1987) fight/flight system (FFS), and even the BAS, which is to a lesser extent thought to motivate individuals to avoid punishing situations. Analogously, some individuals are motivated to avoid negative affect associated with certain situations; Tomarken and Davidson (1994) demonstrated a relationship between defensive coping style and frontal EEG asymmetry (see also Kline et al., 1998 for a replication with women but not men). In their analysis, high-defensive subjects, who presumably are motivated to avoid negative affect (Schwartz, 1990), showed higher levels of left frontal activation than low-defensive subjects.

The relationship between frontal EEG asymmetry and the BAS has highlighted the relative independence of the approach/withdrawal and valence continuums, but a more dramatic demonstration of this independence is found in the work of Harmon-Jones and Allen (1998) and, more recently, Harmon-Jones (2000a). In both of these studies, left frontal activation was associated with trait anger, a negatively valenced but approach-related emotion. That is, individuals who score more highly on measures of trait anger show relatively greater left frontal activation at rest. Harmon-Jones (2000a) found that trait anger is associated with both increased left frontal activity and decreased right frontal activity.

Trait approach and withdrawal dispositions indexed by frontal EEG asymmetry are likely to hold consequences for traits associated with social behavior. Fox et al. (1995) found evidence for this in children. In their analysis, children with greater right frontal activation generally were more inhibited socially, and scored lower on measures of social competency (Fox et al., 1995). In addition, children with greater left frontal activation were both more sociable and more socially competent. These results fit well with those of Schmidt and colleagues (Schmidt, 1999; Schmidt & Fox, 1994), who investigated the relationship between EEG asymmetry and similar traits in adults. Schmidt and Fox (1994) found that individuals scoring low on measures of sociability evidenced relatively greater right frontal activation. Schmidt (1999) subsequently determined that frontal EEG asymmetry was related to measures of sociability and shyness. Shyness was positively associated with relatively greater right frontal activation, while sociability was positively related to relatively greater left frontal activation (Schmidt, 1999). Interestingly, Schmidt also found that shy individuals who nevertheless scored high on measures of sociability possessed greater left frontal activation than other shy individuals with low sociability scores.

In recent work, Kalin and colleagues (2000) have begun to investigate other physiological traits that may underlie processes related to those reviewed above. In rhesus monkeys, they have found a positive relationship between extreme right frontal activation asymmetry at rest and high cerebrospinal fluid concentrations of corticotrophin-releasing hormone (CRH). CRH has been identified as a mediator of stress responses, as well as responses to fear, anxiety, and depression, with higher CRH levels associated with higher levels of stress (De Souza, 1995; Kalin et al., 2000).

Trait Frontal EEG Asymmetry and Psychopathology

Consistent with its relationships to other personality traits, frontal EEG asymmetry appears to be related to emotion-related psychopathology, and may tap a diathesis toward depression in particular, in that relative right frontal activation characterizes depressed individuals both when depressed and when in remission as well (table 16.2).

Links have been established between lower left frontal activation—or relatively more right frontal activation—and depression (e.g., Henriques & Davidson, 1990, 1991; Schaffer et al., 1983) and seasonal depression (Allen et al., 1993). In the first report in this domain, Schaffer et al. (1983), using the Beck Depression Inventory (BDI) as their measure of depression, found that high scorers on the BDI showed relatively greater right frontal activation, and subsequent studies found the same relationship among clinically diagnosed subjects (Allen et al., 1993; Gotlib et al., 1998; Henriques & Davidson, 1991). These results have, in some studies, included not only depressed individuals but also euthymic individuals who have suffered previous bouts of depression (Gotlib et al., 1998; Henriques & Davidson, 1990). This general relationship has been replicated and extended (e.g., Allen et al., 1993; Baehr et al., 1998; Debener et al., 2000), but not without some conflicting results (Reid et al., 1998). For example, Reid et al., in two separate and reasonably large samples, did not find frontal EEG asymmetry to discriminate depressed from nondepressed subjects. They highlighted the heterogeneous nature of depression, and suggested that frontal EEG asymmetry may tap one of several possible risk trajectories associated with the disorder. In addition, they emphasized the fact that traits will interact with the particular experimental environment, and that as yet unidentified aspects of the experimental environment may have masked, or interacted with, asymmetries that may have existed prior to measurement.

Further evidence of an association between frontal EEG asymmetry and depression can be found in studies finding relative right frontal activation in infants of depressed mothers (e.g., Dawson, Frey, Panagiotides, et al., 1999; Field et al., 1995). Dawson et al. (1997a) discovered that infants of depressed mothers showed less left frontal activity than those of nondepressed mothers. Further, left frontal activity discriminated infants whose mothers were diagnosed with major depression from those whose mothers were considered to be subthreshold. In other studies, Dawson and colleagues have demonstrated that infants of depressed mothers who show concomitant left frontal hypoactivation are less affectionate with their mothers (Dawson, Frey, et al., 1999a), and that infants of depressed mothers show evidence of left hypoactivation while at rest, while interacting with their mothers, and while interacting with familiar strangers. Field et al. (1995) independently achieved similar effects, reporting more right frontal activation (not less left frontal activation) in depressed versus nondepressed mothers, and highly similar differences in their respective infants.

These infant studies are important in their own right, but they also address, or hold the potential for addressing, the question of how trait frontal EEG asymmetry patterns originate. Because the infants studied

Table 16.2 Trait frontal EEG asymmetry and measures of psychopathology

Citation	Sample number	Age info	Sex	Handedness	
Allen et al., 1993	8 (4 with seasonal affective disorder; SAD)	No info	F	R	Cz
Baehr et al., 1998	24 (13 depressed)	43–57 yrs.	F/M	No info	Cz
Bruder et al., 2001	53	18–65	F/M	No info	Nose
Davidson et al., 2000	28	19–68 yrs.	F/M	R	LM
Davidson et al., 1985	20 (10 depressed)	18–23 yrs.	F/M	R	Cz
Dawson et al., 1997a	117 infants (54 with depressed mothers)	13–15 months	F/M	No info	LM
Dawson, Frey, Panagiotides, et al., 1999	99 infants (59 with depressed mothers)	13–15 months	F/M	R/L	LM
Dawson, Frey, Self, et al., 1999	117 infants (54 with depressed mothers)	13–15 months	F/M	No info	LM
Dawson et al., 1997b	30 infants	11–17 months	F/M	No info	Cz
Dawson, Klinger, et al., 1992	26 infants	11–17 months	F/M	No info	Cz
Debener et al., 2000	37 (15 depressed)	23–64 yrs.	F/M	L/R (most R)	Linked earlobes

Independent variable	Dependent variable	Results summary
SAD (S) vs. control (C) groups. Pre-post bright light treatment	EEG @ F3/4, P3/4 (alpha power reviewed here)	S ↓ LFA Unchanged by treatment
Depressed (D) and nondepressed (ND) groups (BDI median split)	Percent time spent with RFA vs. LFA in F3/4	D, ↑ pct time with RFA
Resting EEG @ F3/4, FP1/2, F7/8, FC5/6, FT9/10, C3/4, T7/8, CP5/6, TP9/10, P3/4, P7/8, P9/10, O1/2	Recovery vs. nonrecovery from depression following SSRI (Fluoxetine) treatment	In women: nonresponders, ↑ RA, but not specific to frontal region
Social phobics vs. controls anticipating public speech	EEG @ AF1/2, F3/4, F7/8, T3/4, P3/4, C3/4, Cz, and Fz in alpha 1 (8–10 Hz); and alpha 2 (10–13 Hz)	Alpha 1: phobics, ↑ RFA/RATA
Happy, sad, & neutral face pictures, depressed vs. non-depressed, left visual field (LVF) vs. right visual field (RVF)	EEG @ F3/4, P3/4	Group differences in frontal asymmetry between RVF and LVF presentations appears to account for group differences in self-report ratings of happiness in response to lateralized picture presentations
Depressed (D) vs. nondepressed (ND) mothers; major depression (MD) vs. subdepression (SD)	Infant EEG @ F3/4 & P3/4	D, ↓ LFA MD, ↓ LFA compared to SD
Depressed (D) vs. nondepressed (ND) mothers; interaction with mother vs. familiar adult	Infant EEG @ F3/4 & P3/4	D, ↓ LFA (across other conditions)
Depressed (D) vs. nondepressed (ND) mothers	Infant EEG @ F3/4 & P3/4; affection behaviors (AB)	D, ↓ AB (D & ↓ AB), ↓ LFA
Emotional faces during emotional stimuli; depressed (D) vs. nondepressed (ND) mothers	Infant EEG @ F3/4 & P3/4	Bilateral decrease in activation during negative faces in D group
Emotion conditions: play w/mother (P), stranger approach (SA), maternal separation (MS); depressed (D) vs. nondepressed (ND) mothers; secure (S) vs. insecure (IS) attachment	Infant EEG @ F3/4 & P3/4	S: If D, ↓ LFA during P D, ↓ RFA
Depressed (D) vs. nondepressed (ND) groups	EEG @ Fp1/2, F3/4, F7/8, C3/4, T3/4, T5/6, P3/4, O1/2	D, ↓ LFA, but not stable over time C, ↑ temporal stability in asymmetry

Table 16.2 (continued)

Citation	Sample number	Age info	Sex	Handedness	
Earnest, 1999	1 (case study)	14 yrs.	F	No info	Cz
Field et al., 1995	32	3–6 months	F/M	R (mothers)	Cz
Field et al., 2000	160 depressed, 100 nondepressed women, and 260 infants of these mothers	Mean = 17.8	F	No info	Cz
Fox et al., 1996	96	46–62 months	F/M	No info	Cz
Gotlib et al., 1998	Study 1: 77 Study 2: 59	No info	F	R	Cz
Henriques & Davidson, 1990	14 (6 previously depressed)	D mean: 37.4 yrs. C mean: 34.7 yrs.	F/M	R	Cz, LM
Henriques & Davidson, 1991	28 (15 depressed)	31–57 yrs.	F/M	R	Cz, LM, AR
Heller et al., 1997	40 (24 anxious)	No info	F/M	R	LM
Jones & Field, 1999	30	Mean = 18.8 yrs.	No info	No info	Cz
Jones, Field, & Davalos, 1998	25 infants of depressed mothers	1 month	F/M	No info	Cz
Jones, Field, Fox, et al., 1998	63 infants (35 with depressed mothers)	1 week	F/M	No info	Cz
Jones et al., 1997b	44 infants (23 with depressed mothers)	1 month, 3 months (longitudinal)	F/M	No info	Cz
Nitschke et al., 1999	67	17–20 yrs.	F/M	R	LM

James A. Coan and John J. B. Allen

Independent variable	Dependent variable	Results summary
Pre and post biofeedback treatment to ↑ LFA	BDI score	Lower BDI score post treatment
Depressed (D) vs. nondepressed (ND) mothers	Infant and mother EEG @ F3/4 & P3/4	D, ↑ RFA (mothers and infants)
Depressed (D) vs. nondepressed (ND) mothers and their respective infants	Infant and mother EEG @ F3/4 & P3/4	D, ↑ RFA (mothers and infants)
EEG @ F3/4, P3/4 & O1/2	Sociability (S), externalizing (E) and internalizing (I)	(↑ S & ↑ RFA), ↑ E (↓ S & ↑ RFA), ↑ I
Previously depressed (PD), depressed (D) & never depressed (Nev) groups	EEG @ F3/4, mood/cognitive measures	PD, D, ↓ LFA No other effects, suggesting no cognitive mediation
Never depressed (Nev) & previously depressed (PD) groups	EEG @ F3/4, F7/8, T3/4, T5/6, P3/4, C3/4	D, ↓ LFA D, ↑ RPA
Depressed (D) vs. nondepressed (ND) groups	EEG @ F3/4, F7/8, T3/4, T5/6, P3/4, C3/4	Cz: D, ↑ RFA AR: D, ↑ RFA LM: no effects
Anxious (A) & control (C) groups; panic (P) vs. worry (W) tasks	EEG @ F3/4, A1/2, P3/4	A, ↑ LFA (A & P), ↑ RFA
Music (Mu) vs. massage (Ma) therapy; pre, during, & post tests	Depression measures & EEG @ F3/4, P3/4	LFA increased from pre to during, and from during to post in both Mu and Ma
Pre, during, and post massage	Infant EEG @ F3/4 & P3/4	↓ RFA from pre to during and from during to post
Depressed (D) vs. nondepressed (ND) mothers	Infant EEG @ F3/4 & P3/4, vagal tone	D, ↓ LFA D, ↓ Vagal tone
Depressed (D) vs. nondepressed (ND) mothers	Infant EEG @ F3/4 & P3/4	D, ↑ RFA ↑ RFA, ↑ Neg affect pattern stable
Anxious apprehension (AAp), anxious arousal (AAr), depressed (D), comorbid (CM), & control groups (C)	EEG @ F3/4, F7/8, T3/4, T5/6, P3/4	AAr, ↓ LFA Aap no ↓ LFA

Table 16.2 (continued)

Citation	Sample number	Age info	Sex	Handedness	
Papousek et al., 2001	Study 1: 25 men 25 women Study 2: 47 men 43 women	No info	F/M	R	Nose
Petruzzello & Landers, 1994	19	Mean = 22.7 yrs.	M	R	LM
Reid et al., 1998	Study1: 36 (17 depressed); Study 2: 27 (13 depressed)	1 mean = 18.5 yrs. 2 mean = 27.5 yrs.	F	R	Cz, LM, AR
Rosenfeld et al., 1996	5	No info	F/M	R	Cz
Urry et al., 1999	23 Depressed	18–45	F	R	Cz, LM, AR
Schaffer et al., 1983	15 (6 depressed)	No info	F/M	R	Cz
Weidemann et al., 1999	48 (23 with panic disorder)	Mean = 36.6 yrs.	F/M	R	Cz

RFA, right frontal activation, LFA, left frontal activation, RATA, right anterior temporal activation, LATA, left anterior temporal activation, RPA, right parietal activation, LPA, left parietal activation.

in these reports were being raised by their biological mothers, it would be difficult to tease apart the influence of genes versus environment in producing relatively greater right/lower left activation in the children of depressed mothers. On the other hand, EEG spectra are modestly heritable (Lykken et al., 1982), and a conference report suggests that frontal EEG asymmetry shows greater similarity in monozygytic twins than dizygotic twins (MacDhomhail et al., 1999). An important next

James A. Coan and John J. B. Allen

Independent variable	Dependent variable	Results summary
Resting EEG and electrodermal activity (EDA) at two time points (T1 and T2). Depression (D) and anxiety (A) measured.	EEG @ FP1/2, F3/4, P3/4	Studies 1 and 2: If ↑ RFA AND ↑ anxiety, ↑ EDA Assorted findings in beta band.
Pre and post rigorous exercise conditions	EEG @ F3/4, T3/4; state measures of anxiety level	Anxiety decreased post exercise. LFA increased post exercise.
(1) Depressed (D) vs. non-depressed (ND) groups (BDI); (2) Depressed (D) vs. non-depressed (ND) groups (SCID)	EEG @ Fp1/2, F3/4, F7/8, T3/4, T5/6, P3/4, C3/4, O1/2, A1/2, FTC1/2, TCP1/2, PO1/2	D & ND not different (both studies) ↑ left anterior temporal activation in depressed (Study 2, in LM reference, trend in AR reference)
EEG @ F3/4	Pre and post therapy session reports of affect; affect change (AC) score	Subjects with ↑ LFA at beginning of session show ↑ change from neg to pos affect
Time of assessment—to examine stability of asymmetry over time in depression	EEG @ F3/4, F7/8, T3/4, others not reported	Asymmetry stable across 3–5 monthly assessments, median intraclass correlation = .63
High vs. low BDI scores	EEG @ F3/4, P3/4	↑ BDI, ↑ RFA
Panic (P) vs. control groups (C); conditions: rest (R), neutral stim (N), panic stim (Pn), anxiety stim (A), emotional stim (E), motor task (M)	EEG @ F3/4, P3/4	Rest: P, ↑ RFA A: P, ↑ RFA P, ↓ LFA when shown erotic pictures

step would be to assess the infants of depressed versus nondepressed adoptive mothers.

If frontal EEG asymmetry is a trait related to risk, and perhaps to genetic risk, then one would expect that there would be relatively little change in asymmetry as episodes of depression or other psychopathology wax and wane. To date, the data are somewhat mixed, suggesting some traitlike stability in the face of changes that may or may not track the severity of symptomatology. Jones and Field (1999) found in depressed adolescents that change in resting frontal EEG asymmetry could be accomplished in the course of a music or massage therapy session. While the asymmetries in their participants continued (at the group level) to demonstrate relative right activation, the magnitude of this asymmetry was attenuated during and after the session relative to a presession baseline. In applying their efforts toward infants, Jones and colleagues used massage therapy to alter resting frontal EEG asymmetry (Jones, Field, & Davalos, 1998). In their sample of 25 one-month-old infants, they were able to reduce frontal EEG lateralization favoring the right with massage, demonstrating changes from the pretest to the midtreatment measure, as well as from midtreatment to the posttest.

Two studies have specifically examined the stability of asymmetry across time in individuals undergoing treatment for depression. Debener et al. (2000) examined 15 medicated depressed patients on two occasions separated by 2 weeks. These investigators found, as expected, relatively greater left frontal activation in control than in depressed subjects, and found adequate test-retest stability of EEG asymmetry only in control but not depressed subjects. No systematic change in asymmetry across sessions was observed in the depressed patients, however, and asymmetry was not related to measures of daily mood; the asymmetry was simply variable across sessions in these patients. By contrast, Urry et al. (1999) found evidence of better stability in EEG asymmetry in a sample of women receiving a nonpharmacological intervention (Allen et al., 1998). Across three assessments in 3 months for all 23 subjects, and across five assessments in 5 months for 12 of the subjects, the median intraclass correlations of stability was .63, which is very similar to the test-retest values observed for control subjects in Debener et al.'s study. Also similar between the two studies was that the instability in the depressed subjects in Urry et al. (1999) was not related to clinical status or mood state. Thus the majority of findings with depressed patients suggest some underlying stability across time (with the excpeption of the Debener et al. study), with variations across occasions of assessment that have yet to be explained fully.

Although the vast majority of clinically relevant frontal EEG studies concern depression, anxiety disorders have also been examined. These studies have produced a pattern of results that the approach/withdrawal model cannot fully accommodate. Some, for example, have found that anxious individuals show relatively greater left frontal activation (Heller et al., 1997). Others have associated panic disorder (Wiedemann et al., 1999) and social phobia (Davidson et al., 2000)

James A. Coan and John J. B. Allen

with relatively greater right frontal activation. Heller and Nitschke (1997) have proposed a revised valence model, suggesting that anxious apprehension, a symptom that cuts across both the anxiety and depressive disorder spectra, may account for cases where anxiety or depression is not associated with the typical frontal asymmetry pattern. The anxious apprehension aspect of the model has intuitive appeal, since it is reasonable to suppose that subvocal apprehensive ruminations may activate left anterior systems (Reid et al., 1998, p. 402). Some support for the model comes from Nitschke et al. (1999), who found that the expected pattern of relatively greater right frontal activation was present for subjects high in anxious arousal, but not those high in their measure of anxious apprehension. Other findings in that study were not consistent with their model, however, and may reflect the relatively small sample size in each subgroup, or may suggest a need for further theoretical revisions of both the approach/withdrawal and the revised valence model of Heller and Nitschke (1997).

Trait Frontal Asymmetry as a Predictor of State-Dependent Changes in Emotion

Whereas the previous section reviewed research suggesting that frontal EEG asymmetry may tap a diathesis to develop emotion-related psychopathology, analogous research has found that trait frontal EEG asymmetry predicts state-dependent emotional responses in the nonclinical range. Davidson (1998a) has proposed that trait EEG asymmetries index propensities for reacting in predictable ways to evocative stimuli. In this way, frontal EEG activation indexes what Davidson has called "affective style." Some affective styles, he argues, put people at risk for depression and anxiety as part of a diathesis-stress process. This section reviews a handful of reports detailing ways in which people possessing different traitlike patterns of frontal EEG asymmetry respond to evocative stimuli (table 16.3).

Some of the earliest work of this sort investigated individual differences in state reactions in infants. Davidson and Fox (1989) found that infants who cried in response to maternal separation had greater right frontal activation at rest than those who did not, a result subsequently replicated by Fox et al. (1992). They added a longitudinal component to their investigation and determined that this effect was modestly stable over 5 months.

Table 16.3 Trait frontal asymmetry as a predictor of state-dependent changes in emotion

Citation	Sample number	Age info	Sex	Handedness	
Allen et al., 2001	18	18–38	F	R	Cz
Davidson & Fox, 1989	13 infants	10 months	F	R (Parents)	Cz
Fox et al., 1992	(1) 33 infants (2) 13 infants	(1) 14–24 months (cross-sectional); (2) 7–12 months (longitudinal)	F/M	R/L	Cz
Hagemann et al., 1998	37	19–44 yrs.	F/M	R	Cz, LM
Tomarken et al., 1990	32	17–41 yrs.	F	R	Cz
Wheeler et al., 1993	90, but most analyses based on 26 with stable asymmetry across sessions	17–21 yrs.	F	R	Cz

RFA, right frontal activation, LFA, left frontal activation, RATA, right anterior temporal activation, LATA, left anterior temporal activation, RPA, right parietal activation, LPA, left parietal activation.

In the adult literature, frontal EEG asymmetries have typically been related to global positive and negative affect in response to emotionally evocative films or slides (e.g., Wheeler et al., 1993). Tomarken et al. (1990) asked participants to report affective responses to emotional film clips after taking EEG recordings at rest. Participants reported the intensity of their specific affects (e.g., fear, sadness) in reaction to the films. These specific affects were grouped into global ratings of positive and negative, and results indicated that individuals with greater right frontal activation at rest responded with more intense levels of negative affect to negatively valenced film clips, particularly those involving fear. Wheeler et al. (1993) replicated and extended this work. With ap-

James A. Coan and John J. B. Allen

Independent variable	Dependent variable	Results summary
Biofeedback training to move asymmetry toward left or right activation	Self-Report Emotion, Facial EMG	↑ RFA caused ↓ positive affect, ↓ zygomatic, and ↑ corrugator activity
EEG @ F3/4, P3/4	Infant response to maternal separation (crying vs. not-crying)	Criers, ↑ RFA Noncriers, ↑ LFA
EEG @ F3/4, P3/4	Infant response to maternal separation (crying vs. not-crying)	Criers, ↑ RFA Effects consistent over time.
EEG @ F3/4, T3/4, C3/4, P3/4, A1/2	Positive affect (PA), negative affect (NA), affective bias (AB), and generalized reactivity (GR), all in response to affective slides.	Cz, 8 min resting: ↑ LFA, ↑ PA Cz, 4 min eyes clsd: ↑ LFA, ↑ PA LM reference: No effects ↑ R T3/4, ↑ NA note: overall results equivocal with regard to A/W model
EEG @ F3/4, T3/4, P3/4, C3/4	Reported positive affect (PA) and negative affect (NA) following film clips	↑ RFA, ↑ NA ↑ RFA, ↑ PA-NA difference ↑ RFA, ↑ Fear report
EEG @ F3/4, T3/4, P3/4, C3/4	Reported positive affect (PA) and negative affect (NA) following film clips	↑ LFA, ↑ PA ↑ RFA, ↑ NA

proximately the same design, but with a sample that had consistent asymmetries across multiple resting assessment occasions, they found not only that individuals with greater right frontal activation exhibited more intense negative affect in response to negatively valenced films, but also that individuals with greater left frontal activation exhibited more intense positive affect to positively valenced films. Together, these studies suggest that there are individual differences in the propensity to respond emotionally, given emotionally evocative situations. These studies, considered jointly with those reviewed previously showing trait asymmetry may serve as a diathesis for emotion-related psychopathology, suggest a process by which an individual's affective style might put him or her at risk for certain affective disorders such as depression and anxiety (i.e., certain affective styles may predispose people to emotion-specific, or valence-specific, biased reactivity; Davidson, 1998a).

It is important to note that at least one attempt to replicate these findings has not been entirely successful (Hagemann et al., 1998). Hagemann et al. (1998) opted to use normed emotion-eliciting slides to evoke emotional reactions instead of using evocative films. As in Wheeler et al. (1993), resting frontal EEG was recorded prior to emotion-evoking stimuli, and the former was used to predict responses to the latter (Hagemann et al., 1998). Their results were inconsistent. For example, using the Cz reference montage, and eight minutes of eyes-opened and eyes-closed resting EEG data, Hagemann et al. (1998) did indeed find that individuals with greater left frontal activation at rest responded with more positive affect to positively valenced films. However, this effect did not generalize to frontal EEG recorded using a linked mastoids reference montage. To the extent that other significant results emerged, they were inconsistent with the approach/withdrawal model posited by Davidson (1998b). For example, when Hagemann et al. (1998) discovered a relationship between anterior temporal EEG asymmetry and negative affect, it was in the direction opposite the prediction of the approach/withdrawal model, that is, it was related to relatively greater left hemisphere activation at rest. Davidson (1998b) has argued that Hagemann et al.'s (1998) results were due to methodological inconsistencies with earlier studies. For example, Davidson (1998b) points out that in Wheeler et al.'s (1993) study, relationships were based on study participants with a demonstrated consistency in their frontal EEG pattern across 3 weeks. Further research is clearly required to resolve these inconsistencies.

FRONTAL EEG ACTIVATION ASYMMETRY AS A STATE MEASURE

Cattell and Scheier (1961) distinguished states from traits in the following way: traits, they argued, are predispositions to respond in particular ways over a variety of environmental conditions. States, on the other hand, are patterns of responses that are specific to certain environmental conditions (Cattell & Scheier, 1961). Here, the literature highlighting fluctuations in frontal EEG asymmetry that are condition specific is reviewed (table 16.4).

The approach/withdrawal model of frontal EEG asymmetry pertains to individual differences in trait levels, but also accommodates state changes. That is, environmental stimuli that encourage approach responses should result in relatively greater left frontal activation while environmental stimuli that encourage withdrawal responses should result in relatively greater right frontal activation. Indeed, there is evidence to support this prediction (e.g., Coan et al., 2001; Ekman et al., 1990; Davidson & Fox, 1982).

In early work, Davidson and Fox (1982)[3] showed films of an actress performing happy and sad faces to infants aged 10 to 12 months old while recording EEG in the frontal and parietal regions. They found that these infants showed evidence of increased left frontal activation while viewing the happy films, though no effect of the sad films was detected. In subsequent years, Fox and Davidson (1986, 1987, 1988) uncovered similar effects with both positive and negative affects. Using differently flavored drops, Fox and Davidson (1986) showed that infants as young as 2 to 3 days exhibited an increase in left frontal activation in response to a desirable flavor (sucrose), while exhibiting more right frontal activation in response to the neutral flavor (water). Later Fox and Davidson (1987) showed that 10-month-old infants who reached for their mothers during a mother approach task showed more concomitant left frontal activation than infants who did not. Further, they found that babies who cried in response to maternal separation showed an increase in right frontal activation. In a study that generally supported the approach/withdrawal over the valence model, Fox and Davidson (1988) later found that both anger and sadness in response to maternal separation resulted in relatively greater left frontal activation *unless* the baby was crying concomitantly, in which case anger and sadness appeared to result in relatively greater right frontal activation.

Although in most studies of EEG asymmetry sadness is associated with relative right frontal activation, sadness in the absence of crying was associated with relative left frontal activation in these infants. The authors reasoned that approach motivation may be involved in some sad states, and in this case may reflect the infants' attempt to regain the caregiver's presence. Davidson, Ekman, et al. (1990) used emotional films to investigate the relationship between emotional experience and frontal EEG asymmetry in adults. Interestingly, and in a way that would hold implications for emotion theory more generally, these researchers discovered that frontal EEG recordings averaged across the entire period of viewing the emotional films did not show evidence of differences in hemispheric activation. Rather, it was only during moments

Table 16.4 Frontal EEG activation asymmetry as a state measure

Citation	Sample number	Age info	Sex	Handedness	
Benca et al., 1999	17	35–63 yrs.	F/M	R	LM
Blackhart et al., 2002	36 men, 41 women	16–39 yrs.	F/M	R	LM
Coan et al., 2001	36	17–24 yrs.	F/M	R	Cz, LM, AR
Collet & Duclaux, 1986	24	18–45 yrs.	F/M	R	AR
Davidson, Ekman et al., 1990	11 from among 37	17–41 yrs.	F	R	Cz
Davidson & Fox, 1982	24 infants	~10 months	F	No info	Cz
Davidson et al., 1992	9 rhesus monkeys	~12 months	F/M	No info	LM
Davidson et al., 1993	9 rhesus monkeys	~12 months	F/M	No info	LM
Dawson, Panagiotides, et al., 1992b	21 infants	21 months	F/M	No info	Cz
Ekman & Davidson, 1993	14	No info	F/M	No info	LM
Ekman et al., 1990	31	17–41 yrs.	F	R	Cz
Fox & Davidson, 1987	35 infants	~10 months	F	R (parents)	Cz
Fox & Davidson, 1988	35 infants	~10 months	F	R (parents)	Cz
Fox & Davidson, 1986	16 infants	2–3 days	F/M	R (parents)	Cz

Independent variable	Dependent variable	Results summary
Wakefulness vs. various sleep stages (REM, Stg II, SWS)	EEG @ F3/4, F7/8, T3/4, T5/6, P3/4, O1/2	Waking EEG correlated with sleep (notably REM) in frontal and temporal regions
Pre and post EEG hookup mood ratings	EEG @ F3/4, FP1/2, F7/8, T3/4, T5/6, C3/4, P3/4, O1/2	Women: ↓ post mood, ↑ LFA Men: ↓ post mood, ↑ RFA
Voluntary emotional facial expressions grouped according to approach (A), withdrawal (W), and control (C) conditions	EEG @ F3/4, F7/8, FTC1/2, P3/4	W, ↓ LFA A = C
Emotional expression during emotional films; happy (H), sad (S), and neutral (N)	EEG @ F3/4, T1/2, T3/4, T5/6, C3/4, P3/4, O1/2	No effects
Emotional facial expressions during emotional film clips	EEG @ F3/4, C3/4, T3/4, P3/4	No effect of films per se Disgust (face), ↑ RATA Joy (face), ↑ LATA
Films of an actress performing happy vs. sad faces	EEG @ F3/4, P3/4	Happy, ↑ LFA Sad, no effect
Diazepam shot vs. vehicle	EEG @ F3/4, P3/4	Diazepam, ↑ LFA
Diazepam shot vs. vehicle	EEG @ F3/4, P3/4, freezing time in response to challenge	Those with most ↑ LFA to Diazepam showed longest duration freezing behavior
Baseline (B) vs. "mother out" (MO) conditions	EEG @ F3/4, P3/4	↑ overall frontal activation during MO
Duchenne (D) vs. unfelt smiles (U) vs. anger face (A)	EEG @ F3/4, F7/8, C3/4, T3/4, T5/6, P3/4, O1/2	D, ↑ LFA, LATA D, ↑ LFA than A
Emotional facial expressions during emotional film clips; Duchenne (D) vs. unfelt (U) smiles	EEG @ F3/4, C3/4, T3/4, P3/4	D, ↑ LATA U, ↑ RATA
Stranger approach (SA), mother approach (MA), maternal separation (MS) condition	EEG @ F3/4, P3/4	MA, ↑ LFA (mother reach sub-condition); (↑ LFA if vocalizing) MS + crying, ↑ RFA (↑ LFA if vocalizing)
Stranger approach (SA) vs. mother approach (MA); Facial expressions of joy (J), anger (A), sadness (S); Duchenne (D) vs. unfelt (U) smiles	EEG @ F3/4, P3/4	D, ↑ LFA than U A & S (no crying), ↑ LFA A & S (crying), ↑ RFA
Emotional facial expressions during taste conditions (sucrose [S], citric acid [CA], H_2O).	EEG @ F3/4, P3/4	1–3 Hz band: H_2O, ↑ RFA S, ↑ LFA 6–12 Hz band: H_2O, ↑ RFA S, ↑ LFA

Table 16.4 (continued)

Citation	Sample number	Age info	Sex	Handedness	
Gilbert et al., 1994	16	21–35 yrs.	F/M	R	No info
Hagemann & Naumann, 2001	31	19–36 yrs.	F/M	No info	Cz
Harmon-Jones & Sigelman, 2001	42	No info	M	R	LM
Jones & Fox, 1992	23	18–22 yrs.	F	R	Cz
Kline et al., 2000	49	Mean = 64.2 yrs.	F	No info	No info
Miller & Tomarken, 2001	30 men 30 women	Mean = 19 yrs.	F/M	L/R	Cz
Reeves et al., 1989	16	20–50 yrs.	F/M	R	LM
Sabotka et al., 1992	15	18–25 yrs.	F/M	R	LM
Tucker & Dawson, 1984	14 method actors	No info	F/M	R	LM
Waldstein et al., 2000	30	Mean = 24 years	F/M	R	Cz
Zinser et al., 1999	72	Mean = 26.3	F/M	R	Cz

RFA, right frontal activation, LFA, left frontal activation, RATA, right anterior temporal activation, LATA, left anterior temporal activation, RPA, right parietal activation, LPA, left parietal activation.

Independent variable	Dependent variable	Results summary
Various self-report measures	EEG @ F3/4, T3/4, P3/4 (others)	↑ BDI, ↑ RFA (in normals)
Ocular artifacts vs. no ocular artifacts in EEG recordings.	EEG @ FP1/2, F3/4, F7/8, T3/4, C3/4, T5/6, P3/4, O1/2	No significant effects of ocular artifact in the alpha range.
Baseline (B), insult (I), no-insult (NI) conditions	Self-reported anger (A) and aggression (AG); EEG @ F3/4, F7/8, P3/4	I produced, ↑ A, ↑ AG, ↑ LFA LFA correlated with Anger in I, not NI LFA correlated with Aggression in I, not NI
Emotional facial expressions during videos of anger (A), happiness (H), disgust (D), and sadness (S); positive (P) vs. negative (N) affectivity groups	EEG @ F3/4, T3/4, P3/4	H, ↑ LFA S, ↑ RFA D, ↑ RFA P, ↑ LFA during H N, ↑ RFA during H
Odor conditions; vanilla (V), neutral (N), valarian (VN).	EEG @ Fp1/2, F3/4, F7/8, O1/2, P3/4, T5/6	V, ↑ LFA
Incentive levels: Large reward (LR), reward (R), no reward (NR), punish (P), large punish (LP). Expectancy levels: high (HE), medium (ME), and low (LE). Response levels: active (A) and passive (PS). Hand response levels: left (LT) and right (RT).	EEG @ F3/4, C3/4, P3/4, AF3/4	↑ R, ↑ LFA Men: HE, ↑ LFA Women: LE, ↑ LFA LT, ↑ RFA RT, ↑ LFA
TV segments depicting positive (P) and negative (N) scenes	EEG @ F3/4, O1/2	P, ↑ LFA N, ↑ RFA
Reward (R) vs. punishment (P) conditions	Ratings of happiness (H) vs. sadness (S) during conditions; EEG @ F3/4, F7/8, T3/4, C3/4, O1/2, TP3/4; approach (finger press; FP) vs. withdrawal (finger lift; FL) responses	R, ↑ LFA P, ↑ RFA
Imagination condition; depressed (D) vs. sexually aroused (S)	EEG @ F3/4, C3/4, P3/4, O1/2	S, ↑ RFA compared to D
Imagination and film conditions; happiness (H) vs. anger (A)	EEG @ F3/4, C3/4, P3/4, O1/2 blood pressure (BP)	H, ↑ LFA compared to A ↑ RFA during anger, greater BP reactivity
Cigarette deprivation (D) and control (C) groups by 1 cigarette "anticipation" (A) and 2 cigarette "no wait" (N) groups (2 × 2 factorial)	EEG @ F3/4	D, A ↑ LFA Smoking itself, ↓ LFA

where participants showed emotional facial expressions that effects emerged. Even then, their effects were mainly in the anterior temporal rather than the frontal region, with disgust films eliciting more right anterior temporal activation and happy films eliciting more left anterior temporal activation (Davidson, Ekman, et al., 1990). Following up with the same data set, Ekman et al. (1990) investigated the difference between Duchenne smiles (those involving activation of the obicularis pars lateralis muscle) and "unfelt" smiles, finding that Duchenne smiles resulted in more left anterior temporal activation than unfelt smiles, a finding that replicated what had been found in infants several years before (Fox & Davidson, 1988). A subsequent test of the effects of voluntarily performed Duchenne versus unfelt smiles (Ekman & Davidson, 1993) also revealed that Duchenne smiles resulted in greater left activation in frontal and anterior temporal regions than did unfelt smiles.

Ekman, Davidson, and colleagues (Ekman et al., 1990; Davidson, Ekman, et al., 1990) have argued that the seeming dependence of state EEG asymmetry effects on moments during which participants are expressing emotions on their faces reflects the fact that emotional facial expressions are strongly tied to veridical emotional experiences. While this has theoretical appeal, a possible criticism is that the hemispheric differences identified in their work do not actually reflect differences in cortical activation, but rather muscle artifact in the alpha frequency band (8–13 Hz) resulting from asymmetrical facial expressions. This criticism is a legitimate concern in research of this type, although some have estimated that the effects of facial muscle alpha artifact are, if significant, small (Friedman & Thayer, 1991), and others have argued that facial muscle movement cannot alone account for cortical asymmetries, even when facial movement is pronounced (Coan et al., 2001).

This and other work (e.g., Harmon-Jones & Sigelman, 2001; Jones & Fox, 1992) suggests that lateralized frontal brain activity is an important element in the collection of properties that comprise what appear to be distinct emotions or emotional families (see Ekman, 1993). For example, consider five of the commonly hypothesized basic or modal emotions (e.g., Ekman, 1993; Scherer, 1994): anger, disgust, fear, joy, and sadness. The steadily accumulating work on emotion and lateralized frontal brain activation might lead one to predict that disgust, fear, and sadness would result in relatively greater right frontal activation, while anger and joy might result in relatively greater left frontal activation. This is because disgust, fear, and sadness, though most often thought of as negatively valenced, can be thought of as withdrawal emotions, while anger and joy can be thought of as approach emotions (Coan et al., 2001). It is this more general model that was tested by Coan et al. (2001) with voluntary facial expressions of these same five basic emotions, grouped and analyzed according the approach/ withdrawal motivational model. Coan et al. (2001) discovered that when EEG data resulting from voluntary facial expressions of these emotions were grouped according to the approach/withdrawal model, withdrawal-related emotions resulted in a dramatic decrease in left frontal activation compared to both approach and control conditions.

Although not designed to address the causal role of frontal EEG asymmetry, work by Rosenfeld et al. (1996) has shown that EEG asymmetry can covary with clinical state in the context of biofeedback training, further suggesting that EEG asymmetry is linked to emotional states. In a study designed to test specifically whether manipulating frontal EEG asymmetry would alter emotional responding, Allen et al. (2001) used biofeedback training and found that the direction of EEG change systematically biased affective reports, as well as affective EMG responses, in a manner consistent with the approach/withdrawal model.

The ability of state changes to predict subsequent emotion and behavior is further highlighted by a series of studies by Harmon-Jones and colleagues. In two separate anger-induction experiments (one reported in Harmon-Jones & Sigelman, 2001; one in Harmon-Jones et al., in press), the increase in left frontal activation following an insult predicted self-reports of anger. Also, in one experiment, the increase in left frontal activation predicted the extent of aggressive retaliatory behavior. Highlighting the state- and situation-specific nature of the relationship between state changes in EEG asymmetry and subsequent behavior, Harmon-Jones et al. (in press) found that only when coping responses were possible did left frontal activation occur in response to an anger-producing manipulation. They provided college students with a bogus radio broadcast indicating that an impending tuition increase was either certain or merely under consideration. Subjects who heard that the tuition increase was under consideration showed greater increases in left frontal activation than those who thought it was certain. Moreover, among those who thought that the increase was merely under consideration, the degree of state-related change in left frontal activation predicted coping actions (signing and collecting petitions). Collectively these studies support the motivational approach/ withdrawal model of frontal EEG asymmetry, highlighting not only that state-related changes in asymmetrical frontal activation occur in response to anger provoking situations, but also that such activation is seen when motivated behavior is likely to produce some resolution.

THE RELATIONSHIP BETWEEN TRAIT AND STATE FRONTAL EEG ASYMMETRY

We have seen that resting measures of frontal EEG asymmetry appear to tap trait approach versus withdrawal orientations that predict the intensity of certain affective responses and that may place individuals at risk for certain affective disorders. We have also seen that frontal EEG asymmetries vary with certain affective states, perhaps indicating that these affective states include a motivational dimension (e.g., fear has behavioral withdrawal properties while anger has behavioral approach properties).

When conceptualizing the relationship between trait and state frontal EEG asymmetry, there are three systematic sources of variation to consider:

1. Trait frontal asymmetry that is consistent across multiple sessions of measurement, derived from resting EEG assessments

2. Occasion-specific but reliable variations in frontal asymmetry that characterize the variation in resting EEG assessments across multiple sessions of measurement

3. State-specific changes in frontal asymmetry that characterize the difference between two conditions or between baseline resting levels and some condition.

The primary differences between sources 2 and 3 are that occasion-specific fluctuations are assumed to be characteristic of the individual,[4] independent of the intended experimental manipulations, whereas state-specific changes are thought to reflect changes in response to specific experimental manipulations. Occasion-specific fluctuations are assumed to characterize the individual throughout the evaluation session, whereas state-specific changes will by definition change with state manipulations. Most studies of trait frontal asymmetry are not designed to allow for the separation of sources 1 and 2, since most studies entail solely a single occasion of measurement of resting frontal asym-

James A. Coan and John J. B. Allen

metry. If occasion-specific fluctuations were not sizable, then a single assessment of trait levels would prove sufficient. This may not be the case. Recent evidence (Hagemann, 2000) suggests that reliable occasion-specific fluctuations account for approximately 40% of overall explained variance in resting frontal asymmetry, while the consistency across multiple sessions, presumably reflecting a stable trait, accounts for approximately 60%. Further, there may be individual differences in the magnitude of occasion-specific fluctuations. For example, Wheeler et al. (1993) selected a subset of 26 from among 81 women (i.e., 32% of the sample) who were classified as possessing stable asymmetry, meaning that 68% of the sample was classified as having unstable asymmetry.

In the remainder of this discussion, the distinction between trait levels and occasion-specific fluctuations will be collapsed, with both being subsumed under the rubric of trait levels. This is not because this distinction is unimportant; in fact, the limited data bearing on this distinction suggest it is relevant and will account for a sizable proportion of variance. Both sources of variation, however, are related to individual differences assessed with resting EEG, and can be considered jointly as trait variance in raising the question of how trait and state asymmetry may interact.

Because trait resting frontal EEG asymmetries predict affective responses, and because affective responses are associated with certain state-dependent changes in frontal EEG asymmetry, it is reasonable to hypothesize that resting frontal asymmetry will predict the magnitude of state-dependent change in frontal asymmetry associated with certain affective states. To date, there are no published studies that examine this relationship, although several works suggest there may be such a relationship (Coan & Allen, 2000b; Hagemann, 2000).

Conceptual Models for Understanding Trait-State Asymmetry Relationships

When considering the nature of the relationship between trait levels of frontal asymmetry and state-related changes in frontal asymmetry, there are at least four conceptual models that may prove useful in guiding and interpreting investigations: (1) the artifact model; (2) the correlated model; (3) the interactive model; and (4) the orthogonal model. The *artifact* model proposes that the level of the trait variable places artifactual constraints on the degree of state-related change possible. This could take the form of a simple floor or ceiling effect, but also might include the possibility that there are certain ranges of asymmetry in which change may be more or less likely. This artifact model would also subsume the possibility that there are artifactual constraints on the degree of change possible imposed by a curvilinear relationship between trait and state levels and the difference representing the change between them (cf. Chapman & Chapman, 1988).[5]

The second model for conceptualizing the relationship between trait levels and state changes in frontal asymmetry is the *correlated* model, in which simple linear correlations can express the degree of relationship. In the correlated model, trait and states are clearly related, but the correlated model remains agnostic about how or why.

The third model for conceptualizing the trait-state relationship is the *interactive* model. In this model, simple linear correlations would be insufficient to account for the relationship because different trait levels interact with situations to produce *nonlinear* effects in state changes. An analogue to this idea is the concept of *reaction range* in the field of behavioral genetics. A reaction range refers to the upper and lower limits for the phenotypic expression of a given genotype. These limits are constrained by an individual's genotypes, with certain genotypes showing much more or much less change as a function of environmental variations. Analogously, different levels of trait frontal EEG asymmetry may determine the "reaction ranges" of individuals' state asymmetry responses, although the ultimate determinant of such responses will be an amalgam of trait potentials and contextual constraints. For example, one might speculate that subjects with consistent extreme asymmetry across sessions (e.g., Wheeler et al., 1993) might be thought to have less potential for state-related change than subjects who are inconsistently trait-lateralized or who have approximately symmetrical activity.

The final model for conceptualizing the trait-state relationship is the *orthogonal* model, which asserts that state changes are unrelated to trait levels. This is of course a null hypothesis, and would be deemed likely only if many adequately powered tests failed to find a relationship between state change and trait levels. Such a finding would not necessarily mean that the state and trait mechanisms are unrelated. The same brain circuitry might be evoked to produce trait and state effects, but the elicitors under state and trait situations could be orthogonal.

James A. Coan and John J. B. Allen

Data Bearing on the Trait-State Relationship

There are few data available at present to test the viability of these models of the trait-state relationship, but data from two studies are germane. The first of these studies has been mentioned already: the state-trait structural model proposed by Hagemann (2000; see also Steyer et al., 1992). As mentioned above, this model assumes that cortical asymmetries recorded on multiple occasions load first on occasion factors. These occasion factors then load on a single higher-order trait factor (Hagemann, 2000). This trait-occasion model resulted in reasonably good fits to the covariance matrices derived from various cortical regions (fit statistics were collapsed across multiple cortical regions; All $\chi^2(\mathrm{df}=33) \leq 44.71$, all $p \geq .084$, all CFI $\geq .85$, all RMSEA $\leq .08$, all $p_{\mathrm{RMSEA}} \geq .215$; Hagemann, 2000; see figure 16.1). Hagemann (2000) then computed coefficients of state and trait specificity, and concluded that occasion-specific factors accounted for approximately 40% of overall explained variance, while the trait-specific factor accounted for approximately 60%. These results imply that trait cortical EEG asymme-

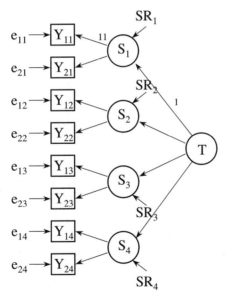

Figure 16.1 Trait-state interaction model. Findings here were summarized across eight scalp regions (Fp1/2, F7/8, F3/4, T3/4, C3/4, T5/6, P3/4, O1/2). All $\chi^2(\mathrm{df}=33) \leq 44.71$, all p $\geq .084$, all CFI $\geq .85$, all RMSEA $\leq .08$, all $p_{\mathrm{RMSEA}} \geq .215$. (From Hagemann, 2000.)

State and Trait of Frontal EEG Asymmetry in Emotion

tries are highly sensitive to day-to-day subject variations or variations in how the subjects react to the experimental context. Thus, Hagemann recommends constructing a model similar to his when conducting trait EEG asymmetry research, such that occasion variance can be accounted for and an optimally reliable trait-only factor can be extracted for subsequent analysis.

Missing from the Hagemann model, however, is how state-related changes would relate to either the trait or the occasion factors. In a related analysis to specifically address this issue, Coan and Allen (2000b) used trait measures of frontal EEG asymmetry to predict state change under experimentally manipulated conditions. Using a sample of data reported by Coan et al. (2001), Coan and Allen (2000b) used resting frontal EEG (trait) to predict the change in frontal EEG asymmetries evoked with a directed facial action (DFA) task where subjects were asked to perform voluntary emotional facial poses. The DFA manipulations resulted in state-dependent alterations in frontal EEG asymmetry. With three different reference schemes, Coan et al. (2001) found that the withdrawal condition resulted in significantly lower left frontal activation relative to approach and control conditions. In the same participants, a trait measure of frontal EEG asymmetry showed a predicted relationship to a trait variable: relatively greater left frontal EEG activation was associated with higher BAS scores (replicating earlier research by Sutton & Davidson, 1997 and Harmon-Jones & Allen, 1997).

With both trait and state-dependent EEG asymmetry showing predicted relationships with trait and state manipulations, respectively, the association between frontal asymmetries at rest with state-dependent changes was assessed using confirmatory structural equation modeling (SEM). Results using two of three reference schemes (average and Cz references) suggested that resting asymmetries were strongly related to the magnitude of change from resting baseline in approach state manipulations (model fit statistics for average and Cz reference schemes: $\chi^2 \leq 10.59$; $p \geq .23$; CFI $\geq .97$; RMSEA $\leq .11$; the structural model did not fit data derived using the linked mastoids reference scheme). Path coefficients between latent trait frontal and state-change frontal asymmetry variables were uniformly negative (-0.61 and -0.46 for average and Cz reference schemes, respectively; $p < .05$), suggesting that individuals who were more right frontally active at rest display a larger difference in the left-activation direction during the approach condition (figure 16.2). Alternatively, the results

James A. Coan and John J. B. Allen

Trait With Change During Approach State

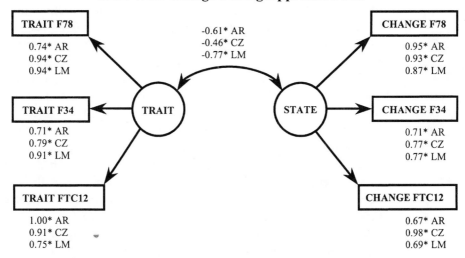

Trait With Change During Withdrawal State

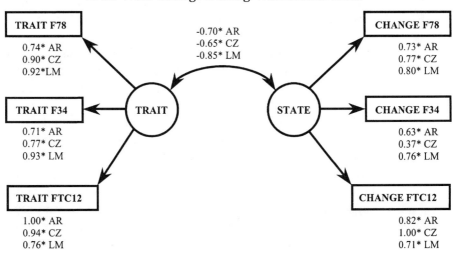

* = Path coefficient is statistically significant at the p < 0.05 level.

Figure 16.2 Trait/state-change confirmatory structural equation models. Fit statistics for models relating latent trait and approach state-change frontal asymmetry variables reveal good fits to data derived using the average and Cz reference schemes ($\chi^2 \leq 10.59$; $p \geq .23$; CFI $\geq .97$; RMSEA $\leq .11$), but not the linked mastoid scheme ($\chi^2 \leq 45.52$; $p \geq .00$; CFI $\geq .73$; RMSEA $\leq .40$). Fit statistics for models relating latent trait and withdrawal state-change frontal asymmetry variables reveal good fits to data derived using the average and Cz reference schemes ($\chi^2 \leq 7.61$; $p \geq .47$; CFI $= 1.00$; RMSEA $= .00$), but not the linked mastoid scheme ($\chi^2 = 48.94$; $p = .00$; CFI $= .71$; RMSEA $= .42$). Path coefficients for each reference scheme are listed in the diagram. (Coan & Allen, 2000b.)

suggest that individuals who are more left frontally active at rest display a smaller difference in the left-activation direction during the approach condition. While model fit was not achieved for the linked mastoid reference, path coefficients derived from this model mirror those of the other reference schemes exactly.

The results of an identical structural model applied to changes during the withdrawal condition also suggested that resting asymmetries were strongly related to the magnitude of change from resting baseline in *withdrawal* state manipulations in two of three reference schemes (fit statistics for average and Cz reference schemes: $\chi^2 \leq 7.61$; $p \geq .47$; CFI = 1.00; RMSEA = .00; the structural model again did not fit data derived using the linked mastoids reference scheme). Path coefficients between latent trait frontal and state-change frontal asymmetry variables were again uniformly negative ($-.70$ and $-.65$ for average and Cz reference schemes, respectively; $p < .05$), suggesting that individuals who were more right frontally active at rest displayed a smaller difference in the right-activation direction during the withdrawal condition. Alternatively, individuals who were more left frontally active at rest displayed a larger difference in the right-activation direction during the withdrawal condition.

These relationships between trait levels and state change were not some peculiar artifacts of the SEM analyses, but were almost invariably evident in the zero-order correlations between trait asymmetry at a given site and state changes at that same site, under both approach and withdrawal state manipulations. These findings are perhaps most consistent with the artifact model, which would suggest that individuals who are tonically most left frontally activated are constrained from moving in the left frontal direction, but have the greatest room to move in the right frontal direction. Alternatively, the correlated model would suggest an inverse relationship between trait levels and propensity for state-related change, an interpretation that is difficult to reconcile with any of the existing models of anterior asymmetry.

CONCLUSION

In this chapter we have attempted to review most of the literature on frontal cortical EEG activation asymmetries, emphasizing the differences and similarities between trait and state natures. Resting levels of cortical activation asymmetries are fairly stable and trait-like, showing high internal consistency and acceptable test-retest reliability (Tomarken, Davidson, Wheeler, et al., 1992). Resting levels of frontal activation asymmetry have been shown to predict other traitlike measures, such as shyness, sociability, levels of behavioral activation, trait anger, and even natural killer cell activity (Fox et al., 1995; Davidson et al., 1999; Harmon-Jones & Allen, 1997; Schmidt, 1999; Sutton & Davidson, 1997). Resting frontal asymmetry, as reviewed above, is associated with psychopathology in children and adults—most notably depression, but anxiety, and internalizing and externalizing problems as well (Dawson, Frey, Panagiotides, et al., 1999; Fox et al., 1996; Gotlib et al., 1998; Henriques & Davidson, 1991). Finally, it appears that frontal EEG asymmetry at rest predicts the magnitude of state-dependent affective responses (Davidson & Fox, 1989; Tomarken et al., 1990; Wheeler et al., 1993). State-related changes in frontal EEG asymmetry have also been shown to occur as a function of distinct affective states (Coan et al., 2001; Ekman et al., 1990; Davidson & Fox, 1982), with increases in relative left frontal activation being more associated with positively valenced, approach-oriented states and increases in relative right frontal activation being more associated with negatively valenced, withdrawal-oriented states.

This pattern of results has suggested a general framework for understanding frontal EEG asymmetries: the approach/withdrawal model (Davidson, 1992, 1998a, 1998b). This model asserts that EEG asymmetries over the frontal cortex—whether state-dependent or traitlike—index approach versus withdrawal tendencies and actions. According to the approach/withdrawal model, relatively greater left frontal activation is related to an approach orientation or action, while relatively greater right frontal activation is related to a withdrawal orientation or action.

An important question is whether, and to what extent, traitlike cortical activation asymmetries predict the magnitude of change in cortical asymmetries associated with specific affective states. Though preliminary, results reported by both Hagemann (2000) and Coan and Allen (2000b) suggest that superimposed on trait asymmetries are reliable and sizable variations across occasions of measurement, and that trait levels assessed at any given occasion are strongly, but in this instance negatively, related to state changes in response to experimental manipulations. Replication of the inverse trait-state relationship is obviously required before conclusive interpretations can be levied, but the limited findings to date suggest that trait levels can be sizable predictors of state-related changes in frontal asymmetry.

This chapter has proposed four models of trait/state associations: the artifact model, the correlated model, the interactive model, and the orthogonal model. Given recent findings cited here (Coan & Allen, 2000b; Hagemann, 2000), the orthogonal model is the only model at present that appears to be untenable. At present, the existing data can be interpreted in terms of either the artifact, correlated or interactive model. The limited data addressing these models to date is perhaps most strongly supportive of the artifact model. To adequately test the interactive model, other relevant variables that might modulate the re-lationship between trait levels and state change (e.g., the intensity of emotional experience) would need to be included explicitly in related analyses. A straightforward way of doing so initially would be to in-clude multiplicative terms in a structural model. Hagemann (2000) nor Coan and Allen (2000b) do not include multiplicative terms in their models. One can imagine a structural model based on Hagemann's data set wherein multiplicative terms representing the interaction of occasion and trait factors could be used to explain the observed vari-ance in cortical asymmetries. An improvement in the fit statistics of such a model would give credibility to the interactive model over and above evidence supportive of the artifact or correlated model. Theo-retically, the interactive model is more satisfying than the correlated model as well, since it is the more general of the two while not being so general as to ignore questions of how trait and state asymmetries may be related (as the correlated model does).

Future Directions

Apart from state/trait interactions, important questions about the nature of frontal EEG asymmetry remain. Although the approach/ withdrawal model appears to be the most parsimonious and best fit-ting account of the research to date, there remain inconsistencies that the model must explain or accommodate. Thus, although frontal EEG asymmetry appears to map well onto directional propensities to ap-proach or withdraw from environmental stimuli, the role of behavioral inhibition is at present unresolved. Frontal EEG asymmetry has incon-sistently correlated with one measure of behavioral inhibition. Further

James A. Coan and John J. B. Allen

work, using multiple measures of behavioral inhibition, will be necessary to clarify this relationship. It is also unknown whether behavioral inhibition attenuates or enhances changes in EEG asymmetry to approach and withdrawal related stimuli, or whether it has no effect at all.

Other future directions have been proposed by Davidson (1998a), who suggested that individual differences in the time course and in the magnitude of emotional responses are likely to be important for a deeper understanding of affective style. He called for the measurement of what he terms *affective chronometry*. Affective chronometry refers to changes in affective states in magnitude over time. It includes measures of what he has called *stimulus threshold, rise time to peak, peak response,* and *recovery time to baseline*. As applied to frontal asymmetry, the literature has just begun to address questions related to response thresholds and peak responses. Studies showing an increased likelihood to respond in certain affective directions given certain baseline asymmetry levels (e.g., right frontally activated babies being more likely to cry following maternal separation) provide compelling evidence of individual differences in stimulus thresholds.

As of this writing, no published reports chart response slopes or response recoveries with regard to fluctuations in frontal EEG asymmetry. The lack of such reports is due in part to constraints imposed by the measure; numerous EEG epochs across 30 seconds or much longer are collapsed to produce a reliable estimate of spectral power. On the other hand, EEG asymmetry is a dynamic process that may benefit from examination using real-time measures of asymmetry, or measures that are sensitive to short-lived perturbations from trait levels. Data that have examined the consistency of short (1 s) epochs of EEG asymmetry have found that nondepressed subjects produce asymmetry scores that reflect relative left activation on approximately 70% of epochs but relative right activation on the remainder (Allen et al., 2001; Baehr et al., 1998), and depressed subjects produce asymmetry scores indicative of relative left frontal activation on only 45% of epochs (Baehr et al., 1998). Thus even though reliable group differences in trait levels may exist between clinical populations and control subjects, there is substantial variability within any individual over relatively short periods of time. It is unknown whether similar variability will also be present in state-related epochs, or whether state-related changes will minimize the ongoing variability seen in the trait recordings.

In sum, frontal EEG asymmetry appears to be clearly related to affective processes—both stable and fleeting. While the underlying processes that drive frontal EEG asymmetry are not currently known, advances in the cognitive neuroscience of emotion will likely shed light on the structural and functional underpinnings of cortical asymmetry. Similarly, studies using behavioral genetics methods and studies specifically examining the effects of early environment will shed light on the genesis and malleability of trait levels of frontal EEG asymmetry. An important direction for this program of research will be to better understand how, and to what degree, state fluctuations in frontal EEG asymmetries can be controlled, as well as the degree to which trait asymmetries can be systematically altered. Research into state/trait frontal EEG asymmetry interactions will aid in these endeavors. The attempt to understand the relationship between frontal EEG asymmetry and various affective states and traits has resulted in a fruitful and multifaceted program of research. The future of research in this area promises to be no less so.

ACKNOWLEDGMENTS

This work was supported, in part, by a Young Investigator award from NARSAD (John Allen) and a graduate research fellowship from the National Science Foundation (James Coan).

NOTES

1. Other issues related to this assumption are beyond the scope of the current chapter, but include the assumption that reduced alpha is an adequate measure of activation (cf. Spydell & Sheer, 1982) and the assumption that the alpha recorded at a given scalp site is indicative of electrical activity generated in the underlying cortical regions.

2. Difference scores have been criticized for their greater unreliability than the constituent scores from which they are derived, but in most cases this criticism does not threaten the reliability of the results using an asymmetry difference score, since alpha values at any given site tend to be highly reliable, so that the difference score is also highly reliable (cf. Reid et al., 1998; Tomarken et al., 1992).

3. In this and many infant studies, the alpha band (8–13 Hz) is lower or expanded downward. Davidson and Fox (1982) recorded from 1 to 12 Hz. Other studies (e.g., Dawson et al., 1992) refer to alpha as being between 6 and 9 Hz in infants.

4. Such fluctuations might reflect individual difference variables (e.g., mood on the day of assessment) or, alternatively, the interaction of the individual with the experimental

milieu in a way that varies from session to session. Such effects would not be the result of the intended state-related experimental manipulations, but rather an interaction of subject characteristics with the general experimental milieu. These latter effects could result from unintended variations across experimenters or an interaction of subject and experimenter characteristics (Kline, 2000).

5. Chapman and Chapman (1988) present the case that mean difference scores will arti-factually be largest when total accuracy (the sum of the constituent scores) is near 50%. Although EEG asymmetry cannot be conceptualized in terms of accuracy, the factor that underlies the artifactual relationship, reliable variance, is relevant. Extrapolating from the derivations of Chapman and Chapman (1988), when trait levels have more variance than state levels, state-minus-trait asymmetry scores (i.e., state-related change) should be arti-factually negatively related to the sum of state and trait scores; when trait levels have less variance than state levels, the opposite artifactual relationship should obtain. Such an artifact could augment or nullify any valid relationships that might exist between trait levels and state change.

REFERENCES

Allen, J. J., Iacono, W. G., Depue, R. A., & Arbisi, P. (1993). Regional electroencephalo-graphic asymmetries in bipolar seasonal affective disorder before and after exposure to bright light. *Biological Psychiatry, 33*, 642–646.

Allen, J. J. B., Harmon-Jones, E., & Cavender, J. H. (2001). Manipulation of frontal EEG asymmetry through biofeedback alters self-reported emotional responses and facial EMG. *Psychophysiology, 38*, 685–693.

Allen, J. J. B., Schnyer, R. N., & Hitt, S. K. (1998). The efficacy of acupuncture in the treatment of major depression in women. *Psychological Science, 9*, 397–401.

Allport, G. W. (1966). Traits revisited. *American Psychologist, 21*, 1–10.

Baehr, E., Rosenfeld, J. P., Baehr, R., & Earnest, C. (1998). Comparison of two EEG asym-metry indices in depressed patients vs. normal controls. *International Journal of Psycho-physiology, 31*, 89–92.

Bem, D. J., & Allen, S. (1974). On predicting some of the people some of the time: The search for cross-situational consistencies in behavior. *Psychological Review, 81*, 506–520.

Benca, R. M., Obermeyer, W. H., Larson, C. L., Yun, B., Dolski, I., Kleist, K. D., Weber, S. M., & Davidson, R. J. (1999). EEG alpha power and alpha power asymmetry in sleep and wakefulness. *Psychophysiology, 36*, 430–436.

Blackhart, G. C., Kline, J. P., Donohue, K. F., LaRowe, S. D., & Joiner, T. E. (2002). Affec-tive responses to EEG preparation and their link to resting anterior EEG asymmetry. *Per-sonality and Individual Differences, 32*, 162–174.

Bruder, G. E., Stewart, J. W., Tenke, C. E., McGrath, P. J., Leite, P., Bhattacharya, N., & Quitkin, F. M. (2001). Electroencephalographic and perceptual asymmetry differences be-tween responders and nonresponders to an SSRI antidepressant. *Biological Psychiatry, 49*, 416–425.

Bryden, M. P. (1982). *Laterality: Functional asymmetry in the intact brain*. New York: Academic Press.

Carver, C. S., & White, T. L. (1994). Behavioral inhibition, behavioral activation, and affective responses to impending reward and punishment: The BIS/BAS scales. *Journal of Personality & Social Psychology, 67*, 319–333.

Cattell, R. B., & Scheier, I. H. (1961). *The meaning and measurement of neuroticism and anxiety*. New York: Ronald Press.

Chapman, L. J., & Chapman, J. P. (1988). Artifactual and genuine relationships of lateral difference scores to overall accuracy in studies of laterality. *Psychological Bulletin, 104*, 127–136.

Coan, J. A., & Allen, J. J. B. (2000a). *Trait frontal EEG asymmetry and its relationship behavioral activation system (BAS)*. Poster session presented at the annual meeting of the Society for Psychophysiological Research, San Diego, CA.

Coan, J. A., & Allen, J. J. B. (2000b). *Frontal EEG asymmetry in response to directed facial actions and its relationship to resting trait levels*. Paper presented at the annual meeting of the Society for Psychophysiological Research, San Diego, CA.

Coan, J. A., Allen, J. J. B., & Harmon-Jones, E. (2001). Voluntary facial expression and hemispheric asymmetry over the frontal cortex. *Psychophysiology, 38*, 912–925.

Collet, L., & Duclaux, R. (1986). Hemispheric lateralization of emotions: Absence of electrophysiological arguments. *Physiology and Behavior, 40*, 215–220.

Davidson, R. J. (1992). Anterior cerebral asymmetry and the nature of emotion. *Brain & Cognition, 20*, 125–151.

Davidson, R. J. (1993). Cerebral asymmetry and emotion: Conceptual and methodological conundrums. *Cognition & Emotion, 7*, 115–138.

Davidson, R. J. (1998a). Affective style and affective disorders: Perspectives from affective neuroscience. *Cognition & Emotion, 12*, 307–330.

Davidson, R. J. (1998b). Anterior electrophysiological asymmetries, emotion, and depression: Conceptual and methodological conundrums. *Psychophysiology, 35*, 607–614.

Davidson, R. J., Chapman, J. P., Chapman, L. J., & Henriques, J. B. (1990). Asymmetrical brain electrical activity discriminates between psychometrically-matched verbal and spatial cognitive tasks. *Psychophysiology, 27*, 528–543.

Davidson, R. J., Coe, C. C., Dolski, I., & Donzella, B. (1999). Individual differences in prefrontal activation asymmetry predict natural killer cell activity at rest and in response to challenge. *Brain, Behavior and Immunity, 13*, 93–108.

Davidson, R. J., Ekman, P., Saron, C. D., Senulis, J. A., & Friesen, W. V. (1990). Approach-withdrawal and cerebral asymmetry: Emotional expression and brain physiology I. *Journal of Personality and Social Psychology, 58*, 330–341.

Davidson, R. J., & Fox, N. A. (1982). Asymmetrical brain activity discriminates between positive and negative affective stimuli in human infants. *Science, 218*, 1235–1236.

Davidson, R. J., & Fox, N. A. (1989). Frontal brain asymmetry predicts infants' response to maternal separation. *Journal of Abnormal Psychology, 98*, 127–131.

Davidson, R. J., Kalin, N. H., & Shelton, S. E. (1992). Lateralized effects of diazepam on frontal brain electrical asymmetries in rhesus monkeys. *Biological Psychiatry, 32*, 438–451.

Davidson, R. J., Kalin, N. H., & Shelton, S. E. (1993). Lateralized response to diazepam predicts temperament style in rhesus monkeys. *Behavioral Neuroscience, 107*, 1106–1110.

Davidson, R. J., Marshall, J. R., Tomarken, A. J., & Henriques, J. B. (2000). While a phobic waits: Regional brain electrical and autonomic activity in social phobics during anticipation of public speaking. *Biological Psychiatry, 47*, 85–95.

Davidson, R. J., Schaffer, C. E., & Saron, C. (1985). Effects of lateralized presentations of faces on self-reports of emotion and EEG asymmetry in depressed and non-depressed subjects. *Psychophysiology, 22*, 353–364.

Dawson, G., Frey, K., Self, J., Panagiotides, H., Hessl, D., Yamada, E., & Rinaldi, J. (1999). Frontal brain electrical activity in infants of depressed and nondepressed mothers: Relation to variations in infant behavior. *Development & Psychopathology, 11*, 589–605.

Dawson, G., Klinger, L. G., Panagiotides, H., Hill, D., & Spieker, S. (1992). Infants of mothers with depressive symptoms: Electroencephalograhic and behavioral findings related to attachment status. *Child Development, 63*, 725–737.

Dawson, G., Panagiotides, H., Klinger, L. G., & Hill, D. (1992). The role of frontal lobe functioning in the development of infant self-regulatory behavior. *Brain and Cognition, 20*, 152–175.

Dawson, G., Panagiotides, H., Klinger, L. G., & Spieker, S. (1997b). Infants of depressed and non-depressed mothers exhibit differences in frontal brain electrical activity during expression of negative emotions. *Developmental Psychology, 33*, 650–656.

Dawson, G. D., Frey, K., Panagiotides, H., Osterling, J., & Hessl, D. (1997a). Infants of depressed mothers exhibit atypical frontal brain activity: A replication and extension of previous findings. *Journal of Child Psychology and Psychiatry, 38*, 179–186.

Dawson, G. D., Frey, K., Panagiotides, H., Yamada, E., Hessl, D., & Osterling, J. (1999). Infants of depressed mothers exhibit atypical frontal brain activity during interactions with mother and with familiar, non-depressed adults. *Child Development, 70*, 1058–1066.

Debener, S., Baeudecel, A., Nessler, D., Brocke, B., Heilemann, H., & Kayser, J. (2000). Is resting anterior EEG alpha asymmetry a trait marker for depression? *Neuropsychobiology, 41*, 31–37.

De Souza, E. B. (1995). Corticotropin-releasing factor receptors: Physiology, pharmacology, biochemistry and role in central nervous system and immune disorders. *Psychoneuroendocrinology, 20*, 789–819.

Earnest, C. (1999). Single case study of EEG biofeedback for depression: An independent replication in an adolescent. *Journal of Neurotherapy, 3*, 28–35.

Ekman, P. (1993). Facial expression and emotion. *American Psychologist, 48*, 384–392.

Ekman, P., & Davidson, R. J. (1993). Voluntary smiling changes regional brain activity. *Psychological Science, 4,* 342–345.

Ekman, P., Davidson, R. J., & Friesen, W. V. (1990). The Duchenne smile: Emotional expression and brain physiology II. *Journal of Personality and Social Psychology, 58,* 342–353.

Field, T., Fox, N. A., Pickens, J., & Nawrocki, T. (1995). Relative right frontal EEG activation in 3 to 6 month old infants of "depressed" mothers. *Developmental Psychology, 31,* 358–363.

Field, T., Pickens, J., Prodromidis, M., Malphurs, J., Fox, N. A., Bendell, D., Yando, R., Schanberg, S., & Kuhn, C. (2000). Targeting adolescent mothers with depressive symptoms for early intervention. *Adolescence, 35,* 381–414.

Fox, N. A., Bell, M. A., & Jones, N. A. (1992). Individual differences in response to stress and cerebral asymmetry. *Developmental Neuropsychology, 8,* 161–184.

Fox, N. A., & Davidson, R. J. (1986). Taste-elicited changes in facial signs of emotion and the asymmetry of brain electrical activity in human newborns. *Neuropsychologia, 24,* 417–422.

Fox, N. A., & Davidson, R. J. (1987). Electroencephalogram asymmetry in response to the approach of a stranger and maternal separation in 10 month old infants. *Develomental Psychology, 23,* 233–240.

Fox, N. A., & Davidson, R. J. (1988). Patterns of brain electrical activity during facial signs of emotion in 10 month-old infants. *Developmental Psychology, 24,* 230–246.

Fox, N. A., Rubin, K. H., Calkins, C. D., Marshall, T. R., Coplan, R. J., Porges, S. W., Long, J. M., & Shannon, S. (1995). Frontal activation asymmetry and social competence at four years of age. *Child Development, 66,* 1770–1784.

Fox, N. A., Schmidt, L. A., Calkins, C. D., Rubin, K. H., & Coplan, R. J. (1996). The role of frontal activation in the regulation and dysregulation of social behavior during the preschool years. *Development & Psychopathology, 8,* 89–102.

Friedman, B. H., & Thayer, J. F. (1991). Facial muscle activity and EEG recordings: Redundancy analysis. *Electroencephalography and Clinical Neurophysiology, 79,* 358–360.

Gilbert, D. G., Meliska, C. J., Wesler, R., & Estes, S. L. (1994). Depression, personality, and gender influence EEG, cortisol, beta-endorphin, heart rate, and subjective responses to smoking multiple cigarettes. *Personality and Individual Differences, 36,* 247–264.

Gotlib, I. H., Ranganath, C., & Rosenfeld, J. P. (1998). Frontal EEG asymmetry, depression, and cognitive functioning. *Cognition and Emotion, 12,* 449–478.

Gray, J. A. (1972). The psychophysiological basis of introversion-extraversion: A modification of Eysenck's theory. In V. D. Nebylitsyn & J. A. Gray (Eds.), *The biological bases of individual behavior* (pp. 182–205). San Diego: Academic Press.

Gray, J. A. (1987). *The psychology of fear and stress.* Cambridge: Cambridge University Press.

Hagemann, D. (2000). *State and trait properties of resting EEG asymmetry: Consequences for research strategies*. Paper presented at the annual meeting of the Society for Psychophysiological Research, San Diego, CA.

Hagemann, D., & Naumann, E. (2001). The effects of ocular artifacts on (lateralized) broadband power in EEG. *Clinical Neuropsychology, 112*, 215–231.

Hagemann, D., Naumann, E., Becker, G., Maier, S., & Bartussek, D. (1998). Frontal brain asymmetry and affective style: A conceptual replication. *Psychophysiology, 35*, 372–388.

Hagemann, D., Naumann, E., Luerken, A., & Bartussek, D. (1999a). EEG trait asymmetry and affective style I: Latent state and trait structure of resting asymmetry scores. Paper presented at the annual meeting of the Society for Psychophysiological Research, Grenada, Spain.

Hagemann, D., Naumann, E., Luerken, A., Becker, G., Maier, S., & Bartussek, D. (1999b). EEG asymmetry, dispositional mood and personality. *Personality & Individual Differences, 27*, 541–568.

Harmon-Jones, E. (2000a). Individual differences in anterior brain activity and anger: Examining the roles of attitude toward anger and depression. Unpublished manuscript, University of Wisconsin, WI.

Harmon-Jones, E. (2000b). Relationship between anger and asymmetrical frontal cortical activity. Paper presented at the annual meeting of the Society for Psychophysiological Research, San Diego, CA.

Harmon-Jones, E., & Allen, J. J. B. (1997). Behavioral activation sensitivity and resting frontal EEG asymmetry: Covariation of putative indicators related to risk for mood disorders. *Journal of Abnormal Psychology, 106*, 159–163.

Harmon-Jones, E., & Allen, J. J. B. (1998). Anger and frontal brain activity: EEG asymmetry consistent with approach motivation despite negative affective valence. *Journal of Personality & Social Psychology, 74*, 1310–1316.

Harmon-Jones, E., & Sigelman, J. (2001). State anger and prefrontal brain activity: Evidence that insult-related relative left prefrontal activation is associated with experienced anger and aggression. *Journal of Personality & Social Psychology, 80*, 797–803.

Harmon-Jones, E., Sigelman, J. D., bohlig, A., & Harmon-Jones, C. (in press). Anger, coping, and frontal cortical activity: The effect of coping potential on anger-induced left frontal activity. *Cognition and Emotion*.

Heller, W., & Nitschke, J. B. (1997). Regional brain activity in emotion: A framework for understanding cognition in depression. *Cognition and Emotion, 11*, 637–661.

Heller, W., Nitschke, J. B., Etienne, M. A., & Miller, G. A. (1997). Patterns of regional brain activity differentiate types of anxiety. *Journal of Abnormal Psychology, 106*, 376–385.

Heller, W., Nitschke, J. B., & Miller, G. A. (1998). Lateralization in emotion and emotional disorders. *Current Directions in Psychological Science, 7*, 26–32.

Henriques, J. B., & Davidson, R. J. (1990). Regional brain electrical asymmetries discriminate between previously depressed and healthy control subjects. *Journal of Abnormal Psychology, 99*, 22–31.

Henriques, J. B., & Davidson, R. J. (1991). Left frontal hypoactivation and depression. *Journal of Abnormal Psychology, 100*, 535–545.

Jacobs, G., & Snyder, D. (1996). Frontal brain asymmetry predicts affective style in men. *Behavioral Neuroscience, 110*, 3–6.

Jones, N. A., & Field, T. (1999). Massage and music therapies attenuate frontal EEG asymmetry in depressed adolescents. *Adolescence, 34*, 529–535.

Jones, N. A., Field, T., & Davalos, M. (1998). Massage therapy attenuates right frontal EEG asymmetry in one-month old infants of depressed mothers. *Infant Behavior and Development, 21*, 527–530.

Jones, N. A., Field, T., Davalos, M., & Pickens, J. (1997a). EEG stability in infants/children of depressed mothers. *Child Psychiatry and Human Development, 28*, 59–70.

Jones, N. A., Field, T., Fox, N. A., Davalos, M., Lundy, B., & Hart, S. (1998). Newborns of mothers with depressive symptoms are physiologically less developed. *Infant Behavior and Development, 21*, 537–541.

Jones, N. A., Field, T., Fox, N. A., Davalos, M., Malphurs, J., Carraway, K., Schanburg, S., & Kuhn, C. (1997c). Infants of intrusive and withdrawn mothers. *Infant Behavior and Development, 20*, 175–186.

Jones, N. A., Field, T., Fox, N. A., Lundy, B., & Davalos, M. (1997b). EEG activation in 1-month-old infants of depressed mothers. *Development & Psychopathology, 9*, 491–505.

Jones, N. A., & Fox, N. A. (1992). Electroencephalogram asymmetry during emotionally evocative films and its relation to positive and negative affectivity. *Brain and Cognition, 20*, 280–299.

Kalin, N. H., Shelton, S. E., & Davidson, R. J. (2000). Cerebrospinal fluid corticotropin-releasing hormone levels are elevated in monkeys with patterns of brain activity associated with fearful temperament. *Biological Psychiatry, 47*, 579–585.

Kang, D. H., Davidson, R. J., Coe, C. L., Wheeler, R. E., Tomarken, A. J., & Ershler, W. B. (1991). Frontal brain asymmetry and immune function. *Behavioral Neuroscience, 105*, 860–869.

Kline, J. P. (2000). State/trait interaction effects and anterior asymmetry: States, traits or straits? Paper presented at the annual meeting of the Society for Psychophysiological Research, San Diego, CA.

Kline, J. P., Allen, J. J. B., & Schwartz, G. E. (1998). Is left frontal brain activation in defensiveness gender specific? *Journal of Abnormal Psychology, 107*, 149–153.

Kline, J. P., Blackhart, G. C., & Joiner, T. E. (in press). Sex, lie scales and electrocaps: An interpersonal context for defensiveness and anterior electroencephalographic asymmetry. *Personality and Individual Differences*.

Kline, J. P., Blackhart, G. C., Woodward, K. M., Williams, S. R., & Schwartz, G. E. R. (2000). Anterior electroencephalographic asymmetry changes in elderly women in response to a pleasant and unpleasant odor. *Biological Psychology, 52*, 241–250.

Lambert, Z. V., Wildt, A. R., & Durand, R. M. (1988). Redundancy analysis: An alternative to canonical correlation and multivariate multiple regression in exploring interset associations. *Psychological Bulletin, 104*, 282–289.

Lykken, D. T., Tellegen, A., & Iacono, W. G. (1982). EEG spectra in twins: Evidence for a neglected mechanism of genetic determination. *Phsyiological Psychology, 10*, 60–65.

MacDhomhail, S., Allen, J. J. B., Katsanis, J., & Iacono, W. G. (1999). Heritability of frontal alpha asymmetry. Paper presented at the annual meeting of the Society for Psychophysiological Research, Grenada, Spain.

Merckelbach, H., Muris, P., Pool, K., DeJong, P., & Schouten, E. (1996). Reliability and validity of a paper and pencil test measuring hemisphere preference. *European Journal of Personality, 10*, 221–231.

Miller, A., & Tomarken, A. J. (2001). Task-dependent changes in frontal brain asymmetry: Effects of incentive cues, outcome expectencies, and motor responses. *Psychophysiology, 38*, 500–511.

Moss, E. M., Davidson, R. J., and Saron, C. (1985). Cross-cultural differences in hemisphericity: EEG asymmetry discriminates between Japanese and Westerners. *Neuropsychologia, 23*, 131–135.

Nitschke, J. B., Heller, W., Palmieri, P. A., & Miller, G. A. (1999). Contrasting patterns of brain activity in anxious apprehension and anxious arousal. *Psychophysiology, 36*, 628–637.

Papousek, I., & Schulter, G. (2001). Associations between EEG asymmetries and electrodermal lability in low vs. high depressive and anxious normal individuals. *International Journal of Psychophysiology, 41*, 105–117.

Petruzzello, S. J., & Landers, D. M. (1994). State anxiety reduction and exercise: Does hemispheric activation reflect such changes? *Medicine and Science in Sports and Exercise, 26*, 1028–1035.

Reeves, B., Lang, A., Thorson, E., & Rothschild, M. (1989). Emotional television scenes and hemispheric specialization. *Human Communication Research, 15*, 493–508.

Reid, S. A., Duke, L. M., & Allen, J. J. B. (1998). Resting frontal electroencephalographic asymmetry in depression: Inconsistencies suggest the need to identify mediating factors. *Psychophysiology, 35*, 389–404.

Rosenfeld, J. P., Baehr, E., Baehr, R., Gotlib, I. H., & Ranganath, C. (1996). Preliminary evidence that daily changes in frontal alpha asymmetry correlate with changes in affect in therapy sessions. *International Journal of Psychophysiology, 23*, 137–141.

Sabotka, S. S., Davidson, R. J., & Senulis, J. A. (1992). Anterior brain electrical asymmetries in response to reward and punishment. *Electroencephalography and Clinical Neurophysiology, 83*, 236–247.

Schaffer, C. E., Davidson, R. J., & Saron, C. (1983). Frontal and parietal electroencephalogram asymmetry in depressed and non-depressed subjects. *Biological Psychiatry, 18*, 753–762.

Scherer, K. R. (1994). Toward a concept of "modal emotions." In P. Ekman & R. J. Davidson (Eds.), *The nature of emotion: Fundemental questions* (pp. 25–31). New York: Oxford University Press.

Schmidt, L. A. (1999). Frontal brain electrical activity in shyness and sociability. *Psychological Science, 19*, 316–321.

Schmidt, L. A., & Fox, N. A. (1994). Patterns of cortical electrophysiology and autonomic activity in adults' shyness and sociability. *Biological Psychology, 38*, 183–198.

Schwartz, G. E. (1990). Psychobiology of repression and health: A systems approach. In J. L. Singer (Ed.), *Repression and dissociation: Implications for personality theory, psychopathology, and health* (pp. 405–434). Chicago: University of Chicago Press.

Spydell, J. D., & Sheer, D. E. (1982). Effect of problem solving on right and left hemisphere 40 Hertz activity. *Psychophysiology, 19*, 420–425.

Steyer, R., Ferring, D., & Schmitt, M. J. (1992). States and traits in psychological assessment. *European Journal of Psychological Assessment, 8*, 79–98.

Sutton, S. K., & Davidson, R. J. (1997). Prefrontal brain asymmetry: A biological substrate of the behavioral approach and inhibition systems. *Psychological Science, 8*, 204–210.

Tomarken, A. J., & Davidson, R. J. (1994). Frontal brain activation in repressors and non-repressors. *Journal of Abnormal Psychology, 103*, 339–349.

Tomarken, A. J., Davidson, R. J., & Henriques, J. B. (1990). Resting frontal brain asymmetry predicts affective responses to films. *Journal of Personality and Social Psychology, 59*, 791–801.

Tomarken, A. J., Davidson, R. J., Wheeler, R. E., & Doss, R. C. (1992a). Individual differences in anterior brain asymmetry and fundamental dimensions of emotion. *Journal of Personality and Social Psychology, 62*, 676–687.

Tomarken, A. J., Davidson, R. J., Wheeler, R. E., & Kinney, L. (1992b). Psychometric properties of resting anterior EEG asymmetry: Temporal stability and internal consistency. *Psychophysiology, 29*, 576–592.

Tucker, D. M., & Dawson, S. L. (1984). Asymmetric changes as method actors generated emotions. *Biological Psychiatry, 19*, 63–75.

Urry, H. L., Hitt, S. K., & Allen, J. J. B. (1999). Internal consistency and test-retest stability of resting EEG alpha symmetry in major depression. Paper presented at the annual meeting of the Society for Psychophysiological Research, Grenada, Spain.

Waldstein, S. R., Kop, W. J., Schmidt, L. A., Haufler, A. J., Krantz, D. S., & Fox, N. A. (2000). Frontal electrocortical and cardiovascular reactivity during happiness and anger. *Biological Psychology, 55*, 3–23.

Wheeler, R. E., Davidson, R. J., & Tomarken, A. J. (1993). Frontal brain asymmetry and emotional reactivity: A biological substrate of affective style. *Psychophysiology, 30*, 82–89.

Wiedemann, G., Pauli, P., Dengier, W., Lutzenberger, W., Birbaumer, N., & Buchkremer, G. (1999). Frontal brain asymmetry as a biological substrate of emotions in patients with panic disorders. *Archives of General Psychiatry, 56*, 78–84.

Zinser, M. C., Fiore, M. C., Davidson, R. J., & Baker, T. B. (1999). Manipulating smoking motivation impact on an electrophysiological index of approach motivation. *Journal of Abnormal Psychology, 108*, 240–252.

VI   Neurological Disorders

17 Agenesis of the Corpus Callosum

Maryse Lassonde and Hannelore C. Sauerwein

Agenesis of the corpus callosum (ACC) is a complex malformation of midline structures of the brain due to an axon migration disorder during early fetal development (Barkovitch et al., 1988). Most of the cases are sporadic, but genetic forms also exist both in humans and in animals (e.g., Andermann et al., 1972; Wahlsten, 1989).

Scientific interest in this brain defect, first described by Reil in 1812, was rekindled in the 1960s following the seminal work of Sperry (1961) and colleagues (Sperry et al., 1969) in split-brain animals and patients, and the subsequent finding by Sperry (1970) that individuals born without a corpus callosum do not display the typical disconnection deficits observed after surgical division of the cerebral commissures. ACC has since come to be regarded as a developmental model of the "split-brain" that, when compared with the surgically produced "split-brain," is uniquely suited for the study of the extent and limits of cerebral plasticity.

In the present chapter we describe the clinical and neuropsychological features of this complex malformation as well as the compensatory mechanisms that appear to be available to individuals born without the corpus callosum.

CLINICAL DESCRIPTION OF AGENESIS OF THE CORPUS CALLOSUM

Developmental Aspects

The development of the corpus callosum is preceded by that of the anterior commissure and the hippocampal commissure (Loeser & Alvord,

1968; Rakic & Yakovlev, 1968). All three forebrain commissures develop from a common primitive structure, the lamina terminalis. Depending on the time of insult, the anterior commissure may also be absent, whereas the hippocampal commissure is usually present (Loeser & Alvord, 1968).

The development of the corpus callosum begins in the seventh week of fetal life with the formation of the lamina reuniens, which serves as a precursor for both the anterior commissure and the corpus callosum. Callosal axon guidance toward and across the midline occurs around the 12th week of gestation (Gelot et al., 1998). Callosal fibers cross a preformed glial pathway. Arrested or delayed development of this structure results in failure of callosal fibers to bridge the interhemispheric fissure. The genu appears first, followed by the trunk and the splenium. The most anterior part, the rostrum, forms last (Rausch & Jinkins, 1994). By the 22nd week all parts of the corpus callosum are formed (Rakic & Yakovlev, 1968). Before this time, the presence or absence of the corpus callosum cannot be ascertained by prenatal sonographic examination (Bennet et al., 1996). The mature corpus callosum connects predominantly homologous areas in the association areas of all lobes, whereas primary sensory areas are largely devoid of callosal connections (Pandya & Seltzer, 1986).

Any noxious event interfering with fetal development may result in total or partial absence of the commissures, depending on the time of its occurrence. Thus, an insult occurring around the 7th week of gestation may prevent the formation of both the corpus callosum and the anterior commissure. An injury between the 7th and 12th weeks will result in total absence of the corpus callosum but presence of the anterior commissure, while a noxious event interrupting development between the 12th and the 20th week would produce various degrees of partial callosal agenesis (Rausch & Jinkins, 1994). Finally, arrest of development after the 20th week, at which time the corpus callosum is formed but has not yet achieved its full volume, will result in hypoplasia of the corpus callosum.

Clinical Features

Callosal agenesis is heterogeneous both in etiology and in presentation. It is often associated with other malformations of the brain, but it can also occur in isolation, in which case it is not necessarily accompanied

Maryse Lassonde and Hannelore C. Sauerwein

by clinical manifestations. More than 50 disorders have been described in association with this malformation (Geoffroy, 1994). ACC is part of five distinct syndromes: Aicardi syndrome (Aidardi & Chevrie, 1994), Menkes syndrome (see Geoffroy, 1994; Wiesniewski & Jeret, 1994), Andermann syndrome (Andermann et al., 1972), acrocallosal syndrome, and Shapiro syndrome (Geoffroy, 1994).

Aicardi syndrome occurs exclusively in females (or individuals with two X chromosomes) without familial recurrence. Clinically, it consists of a triad including agenesis of the corpus callosum (partial or complete), chorioretinal lacunae, and infantile spasms. Other abnormalities of the eyes, ribs, vertebrae, or heart may be present. The syndrome is always accompanied by severe mental retardation.

Menkes syndrome is transmitted through an X-linked inheritance but, in contrast to the Aicardi syndrome, affects only males. The syndrome occurs in infants with severe epileptogenic encephalopathy accompanied by ACC and profound mental retardation. Chemical analysis of brain tissue points to a reduction in lipids.

Andermann syndrome (Andermann et al., 1972; Andermann & Andermann, 1994) is a familial form of ACC that occurs in conjunction with sensorimotor neuropathy. The syndrome was first detected in the Saguenay-Lake St. Jean region of Quebec, an area with a high incidence of autosomal recessive disorders that can be traced back to early French settlers along the Saguenay River. The corpus callosum is missing in approximately 33 percent of the cases. The syndrome is characterized by progressive muscular atrophy of the upper and lower limbs, starting in childhood. By the age of 20, many of the afflicted patients are wheelchair-bound. Biopsy and postmortem studies reveal axon swelling and progressive demyelination in the nerve roots (Carpenter, 1994). Mental retardation is not a necessary feature of the syndrome, but many of the patients are mentally deficient.

The acrocallosal syndrome is another disorder that is transmitted through autosomal recessive inheritance. To date, 20 cases have been described in the literature (see Geoffroy, 1994). Characteristic features of the syndrome are macrocephaly, facial dysmorphism (epicanthus, hypertelorism, high-arched or cleft palate), polydactyly, ACC, and mental retardation. Less frequently, systemic malformations such as visceral abnormalities and congenital heart defects are present. In contrast to the Andermann syndrome, the structural abnormalities are not accompanied by neurological disease.

Shapiro syndrome, on the other hand, is a rare disorder of thermo-regulation of hitherto unknown origin. The syndrome consists of epi-sodic hyperhidrosis, hypothermia, and ACC (Geoffroy, 1994). A typical episode is characterized by lethargy, mutism, amnesia, and confusion. Neurological signs are ataxia, tremor, dysarthria, and hyperreflexia. Autopsy studies of one case showed neural loss and fibrillary gliosis in the hypothalamic infundibular nuclei. The association with the clinical and structural abnormalites and ACC remains to be explained.

Apart from these syndromes, ACC occurs infrequently in association with Chiari's syndrome, Dandy-Walker's syndrome, Apert syndrome, Zellweger syndrome, neurofibromatosis, facial cleft syndrome, fetal alcohol syndrome, postradiation encephalopathy, and midline tumors and cysts (Geoffroy, 1994; Jacobson & Jeeves, 1994). Many of these dis-orders seem to be genetically transmitted (e.g., Andermann & Ander-mann, 1994; Atlas et al., 1988; Baranzini et al., 1997; Donnenfeld et al., 1989; Inbar et al., 1997; Serur et al., 1988). Genetic factors have also been identified in strains of mice with ACC (Wahlsten & Bulman-Fleming, 1994).

Clinically, ACC may be accompanied by mental retardation, hydro-cephaly, epileptic seizures, hypo- or hyperreflexia, or ocular anomalies (Wisnewski & Jeret, 1994). Many of these patients show gyral abnor-malities (heterotopias, polymicrogyria, lissencephaly, etc.), which points to a migration disorder.

Radiological and Histopathological Findings

Agenesis of the corpus callosum is infrequently detected at autopsy (Loeser & Alvord, 1968). Antemortem diagnosis of this malformation was made earlier by pneumoencephalography (Davidoff & Dyke, 1934). More recently, less invasive imaging techniques such as CT scan, MRI, and sonography (Cioni et al., 1994; Rausch & Jinkins, 1994) are used to investigate cerebral abnormalities (figure 17.1). Functional MRI, assess-ing activation patterns of cortical areas, can provide additional infor-mation about structural defects.

All acallosal brains share certain structural modifications as a direct consequence of the absence of the interhemispheric commissure (Mel-anson & Salazar, 1994). Neuroradiological findings include exaggerated separation of the lateral ventricles, enlargement and anterior dis-placement of the third ventricle, enlargement and elongation of the

Maryse Lassonde and Hannelore C. Sauerwein

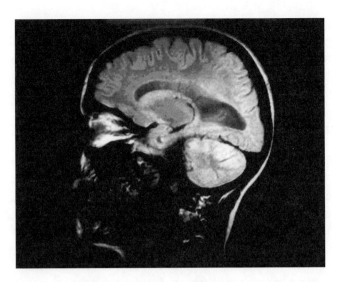

Figure 17.1 MRI, midsagittal plane, showing total agenesis of the corpus callosum.

interventricular foramen, and enlargement and continuity of the interhemispheric fissure with the third ventricle. Other characteristic features are "batwing" appearance of the frontal horns, dilatation of the posterior horns, and eversion of the cingulate gyrus (Melanson & Salazar, 1994; Meyer et al., 1998). In some cases, callosal axons that were prevented from crossing the midline during fetal development can be visualized as two parallel bands of white matter (the so-called Probst's bundle) running intrahemispherically on either side of the hemispheric fissure. The anterior commissure is present in most cases (Meyer et al., 1998; Rausch & Jinkins, 1994). However, it can also be absent or hypotrophied (Loeser & Alvord, 1968; Meyer & Röricht, 1998; Rausch & Jinkins, 1994). Furthermore, structural reorganization of cortical areas may be detected (Bittar et al., 2000). On the cellular level, histopathological studies in acallosal subjects have shown an important reduction of pyramidal cells in layer III of striate cortex, which is the target zone of callosal axons in the intact brain (Shoumura et al., 1975).

Incidence of ACC

ACC is found around the world but its incidence varies from country to country. It is estimated to be close to 1% in the general population

(Cioni et al., 1994) and between 2.2% and 2.4% among developmentally delayed children (see Wisniewski & Jeret, 1994). The number of newly diagnosed cases is highest in centers that routinely use prenatal sonographic examination. Overall, its occurrence is slightly higher in the male population (Wiesneski & Jeret, 1994).

NEUROPSYCHOLOGICAL FINDINGS IN ACC

Cognitive Abilities

Review studies of intellectual abilities of callosal agenesis patients without gross neuropathalogy (Chiarello, 1980; Sauerwein & Lassonde, 1994) have shown that individuals born without a corpus callosum can have normal intelligence, but most of the patients tested in a clinical setting tend to function at the low end of the normal range. Intellectual functioning may be still lower if other malformations of the nervous system coexist. However, a small proportion of the acallosals in each of these surveys (approximately 20%) fell in the high to superior range of mental abilities, among these a brilliant patient with a frontal cyst who was seen by our team. These findings indicate that agenesis of the corpus callosum per se is not the main cause of the cognitive impairments seen in many cases. It should also be kept in mind that acallosal individuals with normal intelligence rarely come to the attention of the clinician. If one adds the cases that are incidentally detected at autopsy and who reportedly lived normal, satisfying lives, the proportion of normally functioning individuals with ACC is even higher. In addition, routine use of prenatal sonography and imaging techniques has led to the detection of an increasing number of asymptomatic cases of callosal agenesis who do not display any cognitive or developmental disabilities.

Some authors have speculated that verbal and nonverbal functions may compete for resources in the acallosal brain, to the effect that verbal functions may develop at the expense of perceptual skills (Sperry, 1970) or vice versa (Saul & Sperry, 1968; Gazzaniga, 1970). In support of this hypothesis, Dennis (1977) found that half of the acallosal subjects had verbal deficits with well developed visuospatial functions, whereas the other half showed the reverse pattern. The author concluded that while the nature of the function which is disadvantaged is not predictable, lateralized functions appear to develop unevenly in the acallosal brain. However, an analysis of the intellectual quotient (IQ) obtained from 46 reviewed cases of the literature (Sauerwein & Lassonde, 1994) showed that this assumption does not hold true. When a discrepancy of one standard deviation was used to define a significant difference between verbal IQ and performance IQ, no imbalance was found between verbal and non-verbal functions.

Language Lateralization in ACC

Studies assessing language functions in ACC have shown deficits in syntactic-pragmatic functions in isolated cases of callosal agenesis (Dennis, 1981; Sanders, 1989), and it has been questioned whether such deficits may be related to anomalous lateralization of linguistic functions (Dennis, 1981). The question of how language is organized in the acallosal brain is of particular interest, since it has been postulated that the corpus callosum may be crucial for the development of hemispheric specialization (Corballis & Morgan, 1978; Doty et al., 1973; Moscovitch, 1977). According to this hypothesis, the hemisphere predisposed to treat linguistic information suppresses the development of verbal skills in its counterpart by way of the corpus callosum. Consequently, it was postulated that language might develop bilaterally in acallosal individuals. However, this hypothesis has not been supported by subsequent research (see Jeeves, 1986; Sauerwein & Lassonde, 1994).

To begin with, there is evidence that acallosal subjects are more efficient in identifying tachistoscopically presented stimuli in the right visual hemifield that projects to the left hemisphere (Ettlinger et al., 1972). Furthermore, dichotic listening studies have shown reliable ear preference in callosal agenesis subjects, although the side of the preferred ear seems to be less consistent in acallosals than in normal subjects (Chiarello, 1980). In neurologically intact subjects, simultaneous input to both ears results in a consistent right ear (left hemisphere) superiority for verbal material. This advantage is considered to be the result of the suppression of the weaker ipsilateral connections in favor of the stronger contralateral connections of the auditory pathway. In our own study (Lassonde et al., 1990), we observed the expected left hemisphere superiority for verbal stimuli in three out of four acallosal subjects. With regard to the magnitude of the asymmetry, the acallosal subjects showed smaller asymmetries than high IQ controls but larger asymmetries than low IQ subjects. This finding suggests that rather than enhancing hemispheric asymmetry, the corpus callosum, by allowing continuous information exchange between the hemispheres, may in some cases *reduce* the asymmetries. To carry this argument further, this would suggest that the absence of interhemispheric cross talk in the acallosal brain might favor a greater expression of such asymmetries.

Additional evidence against bilateral representation of language in the acallosal brain is derived from sodium amytal studies. This procedure is routinely used to determine language lateralization in epileptic patients slated for surgery. Injection of sodium amytal in the carotid artery temporarily anesthetizes the hemisphere ipsilateral to the site of injection. When the hemisphere that is dominant for speech is anesthetized, the patient becomes temporarily mute. Evidence of normal lateralization of speech in the left hemisphere has been found in all but two acallosal patients studied with this technique (see Sauerwein & Lassonde, 1994). Both individuals were left-handed. In fact, one documented case of unilateral representation of speech would suffice to weaken the hypothesis of bilateral organization of language in acallosals.

Finally, the surveys by Chiarello (1980) and Sauerwein and Lassonde (1994) have shown that the majority of acallosal subjects are right-handed, although there is a greater variability in this group, as would be expected in a clinical population. This would suggest that motor control also develops asymmetrically in the acallosal brain.

Interhemispheric Communication in ACC

Following the demonstration of specific disconnection deficits in patients with therapeutic section of the callosum by Sperry and collaborators (Sperry et al., 1969), the bulk of research in callosal agenesis has concentrated on the study of interhemispheric transfer of lateralized information in these individuals. Disconnection deficits in split-brain patients are demonstrable in the visual, tactile, and motor modalities in which sensory input and motor output are predominantly mediated by crossed connections. Thus, stimuli presented in the left visual field and to the left hand reach the right hemisphere, whereas information from the right side of perceptual space is conveyed to the left hemisphere. By the same token, motor output is principally controlled by the contralateral hemisphere.

Maryse Lassonde and Hannelore C. Sauerwein

Surgical section of the corpus callosum in adult patients results in a number of disconnection deficits (Sperry et al., 1969) that can be experimentally demonstrated when the subject has to compare sensory input that is channeled simultaneously to two different hemispheres or when one hemisphere is asked to respond to a stimulus received exclusively by the other hemisphere. Typically, these patients have difficulties carrying out bimanual comparisons of tactile stimuli placed in each hand out of their view. Furthermore, they are unable to compare visual stimuli presented in different visual hemifields. They also have difficulties transferring a light touch applied to the fingers of one hand to the other, nonstimulated hand. Finally, they are unable to name stimuli that are manipulated by the left hand or presented in the left visual field because the right hemisphere does not possess the mechanism for speech. Most of these deficits are permanent, although some recovery has been observed (Bogen & Vogel, 1975; Goldstein & Joynt, 1975), especially in younger patients (Lassonde et al., 1986, 1988, 1991).

In contrast, callosal agenesis patients tested with these paradigms do not show the typical disconnection deficits (e.g., Ettlinger et al., 1972; Berlucchi et al., 1995; Lassonde et al., 1991; Sauerwein et al., 1981; Saul & Sperry, 1968). Thus, acallosal subjects have no difficulties comparing objects or shapes placed in each hand out of view and making interfield comparisons of visual stimuli. Similarly, they are perfectly able to read letters in the left visual field and to name material presented unilaterally to the right hemisphere in the tactile or visual modality (e.g., Milner & Jeeves, 1979; Sauerwein et al., 1981; Sauerwein & Lassonde, 1983). Furthermore, they show continuity across the visual field when asked to read words that are split between the two visual fields (Corballis & Finlay, 2000).

Compensatory Mechanisms in ACC

The absence of disconnection deficits in acallosal subjects has been attributed to cerebral plasticity that would allow these individuals to develop compensatory mechanisms early in life which are not readily available to patients who undergo callosotomy at adulthood (see Jeeves, 1986, 1994).

One of the mechanisms that has been evoked to explain the ability of acallosal patients to name stimuli conveyed to the right hemisphere is the duplication of language functions in both hemispheres (Sperry,

1968a). However, while bilateral organization of language has been found in isolated cases, the studies discussed above indicate that this is not the norm.

With regard to visual transfer, the anterior commissure and/or subcortical commissures have been suggested as possible compensatory pathways when the callosal route is not available (Jeeves, 1965; Milner, 1994). The anterior commissure connects visual areas of the inferior temporal lobes. The fact that it is hypertrophied in some cases has given rise to the speculation that anterior callosal fibers which were prevented from crossing the midline may be rerouted through the anterior commissure, allowing for a wider interhemispheric distribution of this structure (Ettlinger et al., 1972; Rausch & Jinkins, 1994; Jeeves, 1994). However, magnetic resonance studies have shown that hypertrophy of this commissure, when present, is the exception rather than the rule (Rauch & Jinkins, 1994). Moreover, according to developmental studies in fetuses of acallosal mice (see Wahlsten & Ozaki, 1994), callosal axons that fail to cross the midline do not seem to reroute through the anterior commissure.

Nevertheless, the anterior commissure remains a likely compensatory pathway for interhemispheric transfer of certain kinds of visual information. This is evident from a study of two acallosal subjects, in one of whom the anterior commissure was also absent. The subject lacking the anterior commissure was impaired on a visual transfer task, whereas the other patient performed normally on these tasks (Fischer et al., 1992). Similarly, our team has described the case of an individual lacking the corpus callosum and the anterior commissure who could make interhemisperic comparisons of letters based on their shape, but was unable to compare the stimuli when the task required a lexical decision (Caillé et al., 1999). However, while the anterior commissure appears to be adequate to transfer visual pattern information, it seems to be less apt to transfer color (Corballis & Finlay, 2000) and visuospatial information (Martin, 1985).

The ability of acallosals to integrate tactile information from both hands has frequently been attributed to enhancement of ipsilateral connections of the somatosensory system, either through increased use of existing fibers or through recruitment of additional fibers as part of structural reorganization (Ettlinger et al., 1972; Dennis, 1976; Jeeves, 1986, 1994; Sauerwein et al., 1981; Lassonde et al., 1991). In the normal brain, crossed pathways of the sensory and motor systems take prece-

Maryse Lassonde and Hannelore C. Sauerwein

dence over uncrossed connections both in size and in function (Barr, 1972). There is some electrophysiological evidence for an enhancement of ipsilateral connections of the lemniscal pathway (Laget et al., 1977; Vanasse et al., 1994). In addition, uncrossed fibers of the ventral spino-thalamic pathway, a parallel somatosensory pathway that is is less lateralized, may be used by acallosals to achieve tactile transfer. These connections have been found to be sufficient to sustain the gradual reacquisition of size discrimination after the lemniscal pathways were severed (Mountcastle, 1984). The simultaneous use of crossed and uncrossed fibers would allow for integration of tactile input from both hands in a single hemisphere. In this case no interhemispheric transfer of information would be required.

Cross-cueing, as a behavioral mechanism of compensation, has occasionally been observed in commissurotomized patients and animals (Gazzaniga, 1970) and may also be used by acallosals. This strategy makes use of external cues (e.g., a movement, a sound, or an eye movement initiated by the stimulated hemisphere or elicited by the stimulus material) that can convey salient information to the nonstimulated hemisphere. Furthermore, given the fact that acallosal subjects have no difficulties verbally identifying stimuli channeled to either hemisphere, information that lends itself to verbal coding can be easily used by these subjects to cue the nonstimulated hemisphere. Again, no physiological transfer of information takes place in this case. As Sperry (1970) has pointed out, individuals without a corpus callosum may become so efficient at these strategies that they are not obvious to the naive observer. In experimental paradigms designed to investigate interhemispheric communication in these populations, great care is generally taken to control for these strategies.

Limitation of Compensatory Mechanisms

Given the size and the widespread distribution of the corpus callosum in normal cortex, the absence of this structure would be expected to affect the efficiency of interhemispheric transfer in some way, even in individuals who have had the opportunity early in life to develop other means of interhemispheric communication. Indeed, one of the major limitations of the compensatory mechanisms in acallosal subjects concerns the speed of transfer. Thus, response times for interhemispheric transfer in acallosal patients are consistently longer than those of controls (Jeeves, 1969; Lassonde et al., 1988; Sauerwein et al., 1981). Acallosal subjects have also been found to be limited with regard to the complexity of the material that is transferred (Gott & Saul, 1978; Karnath et al., 1991). Furthermore, they show poor motor integration on tasks requiring asynchronous, distal movements (e.g., Jeeves et al., 1988). In the tactile modality, deficits in cross-localization of touch (Geffen et al., 1994) and impaired transfer of tactuomotor learning (Ettlinger et al., 1972; Gott & Saul, 1978; Lassonde et al., 1995; Sauerwein et al., 1994) have been observed, which points to the limited capacity of the compensatory pathway(s) to mediate this type of information.

There is evidence that the absence of the corpus callosum also affects unilateral processing. This holds particularly true for functions that are more specialized in each hemisphere and that cannot be efficiently treated without input from the hemisphere which is more proficient in the processing of a given kind of information. These difficulties are discrete signs of interhemispheric disconnection in callosal agenesis. One example is the impaired performance of the right hand in the right hemispace reported by Temple & Ilsley (1994) in a visual neglect task that can be attributed to the dissociation between the left and the right hemisphere, the latter being more proficient in directing attention. Other examples are the right visual field impairments for judgment of stimulus location and word orientation observed by Martin (1985), and the right-hand deficits in spatial processing observed in the tactile part of the De Renzi rod test (Meerwaldt, 1983; Jeeves & Silver, 1988). In both cases the patient's left hemisphere is not as proficient as the right in analyzing the spatial information.

In addition, acallosal subjects display other problems that are more difficult to interpret in the context of interhemispheric disconnection. The visuoconstructive and perceptual deficits reported by Temple and Ilsley (1994) and Berlucchi et al. (1995) fall in this category. Similarly, the impairments in auditory verbal learning (Geffen et al., 1994a) and phonological processing Temple & Ilsley (1994), observed in some acallosal subjects, still need to be explained. Our own research indicates that acallosal subjects have difficulties judging the relative distance between objects (Lassonde, 1986). Their performance was at chance level in both the intra- and the interhemispheric condition.

Taken together, these observations have led us to postulate a facilitatory or modulating influence of the corpus callosum on the activity of

Maryse Lassonde and Hannelore C. Sauerwein

both hemispheres (Lassonde, 1986), a hypothesis that gains support from the electrophysiological studies of Bremer (1966, 1967) and, more recently, from research using transcranial magnetic stimulation to explore both inhibitory and excitatory interhemispheric interactions between the motor zones (Meyer et al., 1995) in normal subjects and in patients with callosal abnormalities (complete and partial agenesis, hyperplasia of the corpus callosum). In the latter study, patients with callosal pathology had higher thresholds at rest for excitatory contralateral motor responses than control subjects. The absence of transcallosal enhancement of cortical activity in individuals lacking the corpus callosum may explain, at least in part, the deficits in intrahemispheric processing described above.

Motor and Tactuomotor Functions in ACC

Studies in commissurotomzed patients have pointed to the important role of the corpus callosum in bilateral motor coordination and tactuomotor learning. These patients have difficulties performing fast, coordinated movements and learning new motor skills (Preilowski, 1972; Zaidel & Sperry, 1977). Acallosal individuals share a number of deficits that are observed in these patients. For example, they are clumsy and slow when performing bimanual coordination under speed stress (Chiarello, 1980; Jeeves, 1965; Sauerwein et al., 1981) and, like the surgical patients, they have been found to be impaired on tasks requiring continuous mutual monitoring of asymmetrical input from the two hands (Jeeves & Silver, 1988). Furthermore, recent studies carried out in our laboratory have shown that acallosal subjects have difficulties learning a complex visuomotor skill requiring the participation of both hemispheres (De Guise et al., 1999). This task involved procedural learning of unimanual and bimanual key-pressing responses to a fixed sequence of 10 visual stimuli. Although the acallosal subjects were able to learn this task unilaterally, they could not transfer the procedural skill to the untrained hemisphere. Furthermore, none of the subjects was able to learn the task in the bimanual condition.

Consistent deficits are further observed in interhemispheric transfer of tactile stimuli that do not lend themselves to verbal coding. As mentioned above, many acallosals have difficulties transferring the locus of a light touch on the fingertips from one hand to the other (Dennis, 1976; Geffen et al., 1994b).

Although section of the corpus callosum has been shown to abolish interhemispheric transfer of tactuomotor learning (Goldstein & Joynt, 1975), the results from acallosal subjects are equivocal. Some authors have reported impairments in intermanual transfer of formboard learning and pencil maze learning (Russell & Reitan, 1955; Ferris & Dorsen, 1975; Gott & Saul, 1978; Jeeves, 1979; Sauerwein & Lassonde, 1994), whereas others did not find any deficits on these tasks (Sauerwein et al., 1981, with a simpler formboard; Reynolds & Jeeves, 1977).

Subjects with callosal agenesis may also display other types of motor deficits that do not appear to be related to the lack of interhemispheric communication. These include defects in grip formation and in reaching toward a visual stimulus (Silver & Jeeves, 1994; Jakobson et al., 1994; Lassonde, 1994).

The impaired motor performance of acallosal subjects has been attributed to the increased use of ipsilateral or uncrossed motor projections in acallosals. Specifically, it has been postulated that in the absence of the corpus callosum, normal inhibition of the ipsilateral pathways may not take place, and as a result, output from uncrossed pathways competes with that of crossed pathways, thereby reducing the overall level of performance (Dennis, 1976; Jeeves, 1986; Jeeves & Silver, 1988). By the same token, it has been argued that an enhanced ipsilateral somotosensory pathway allows for intermanual integration of tactile information in the same hemisphere at the expense of sensory acuity (Dennis, 1976).

However, the hypothesis of an inhibitory role of the corpus callosum on uncrossed pathways is still open to debate, at least with respect to motor functions. Meyer et al. (1995) demonstrated an inhibitory action of the corpus callosum by showing that transcranial magnetic stimulation over the motor cortex of normal subjects suppressed voluntary activity in the ipsilateral hand, a response that was absent or delayed in patients with callosal pathology. In further support of an inhibitory action of the corpus callosum, Allison et al. (2000), using functional MRI in normal subjects, observed significant ipsilateral deactivation in a finger-thumb opposition task. In contrast, five acallosal subjects studied by our team with the same technique did not differ from normal controls with respect to ipsilateral deactivation (Reddy, Lassonde, & Matthews, 2000; Reddy, Lassonde, Bemasconi, et al., 2000). In fact, simple unilateral finger movements did not yield any differences between acallosals and normal controls with respect to the localization of the cortical motor regions activated by the task, the volumes of activation, or the relative hemispheric lateralization of activation. The results are not in favor of enhanced ipsilateral activation during motor performance in acallosal subjects. Furthermore, there is evidence that not all acallosal subjects show the bimanual coordination problems described above (Wolff, personal communication).

Sensorimotor Integration in ACC

Most of the studies of interhemispheric integration have been carried out in the visual modality, using Poffenberger's paradigm (1912). This paradigm makes use of the anatomical connections between a lateralized sensory stimulus and the hand responding to it in a simple reaction time (RT) task (see reviews by Marzi et al., 1991; Milner, 1994). For instance, responses to a flash of light presented in the left visual field are usually faster with the left hand (uncrossed condition) than those with the right hand (crossed condition) and vice versa. The difference in speed is assumed to reflect differences in the length of the trajectory in the two conditions. Thus, in the uncrossed stimulus-response (S-R) condition, the hemisphere receiving the stimulus is the same as the one controlling the responding hand, whereas in the crossed S-R condition, the response originates in the hemisphere opposite the one that receives the sensory stimulus. In the latter condition, some kind of interhemispheric communication is necessary to coordinate sensory input and motor output. The difference between crossed and uncrossed RTs (crossed-uncrossed difference, or CUD) may then be regarded as an indirect estimate of interhemispheric transmission time (ITT).

Interhemispheric transmission times for acallosal subjects generally fall between those of neurologically intact individuals and completely commissurotomized patients. A meta-analysis across 16 studies, conducted by Marzi et al. (1991), concluded to a mean ITT value of 3.8 ms in normal adults, whereas in commissurotomized patients, it may vary between 20 to 96 ms (see Di Stefano et al., 1992; Foster & Corballis, 1998; Marzi et al., 1991; Sergent & Myers, 1985; Tassinari et al., 1994). In subjects with complete absence of the corpus callosum, ITT values vary between 12.8 and 52 ms, with a greater proportion of cases showing an ITT in the 20 ms range. These findings support the assumption that interhemispheric integration of simple visuomotor responses occurs through the corpus callosum in the normal brain.

When unilateral and bilateral responses to lateralized flashes are performed by different effectors (distal, proximal, and axial muscles of the upper limbs), both acallosal and split-brain patients obtain CUD values that are greater for unilateral than for bilateral responses, and both show a decrease in CUDs along a distal-proximal-axial gradient (Aglioti et al., 1993). These results suggest that interhemispheric integration is unnecessary when responses are effected by proximal and axial parts of the motor system that are known to have a greater bilateral distribution (Berlucchi et al., 1995).

Other studies have shown that acallosal subjects differ from normal subjects with regard to the laterality effects obtained under crossed-uncrossed conditions. While normal subjects show a left visual field (right hemisphere) and a right-hand (left hemisphere) advantage in this paradigm, acallosal subjects fail to show any consistent laterality effect (see Marzi et al., 1991). Interestingly, an acallosal boy without associated neural pathology reported by Di Stefano & Salvadori (1998) had considerably longer transmission times when the right hemisphere received the stimulus and the left hemisphere initiated the response than vice versa. This asymmetry would suggest that the left hemisphere is more proficient than the right in controlling the ipsilateral hand. Furthermore, acallosal subjects also have considerably larger CUD values than neurologically intact subjects when they have to respond to lateralized flashes with *both* hands (Jeeves, 1969). This finding suggests that the pathway used in the absence of the corpus callosum is longer, probably involving additional synapses.

Further evidence for the notion that the longer CUDs in callosal agenesis are directly attributable to the absence of the corpus callosum comes from the study of event-related potentials (ERP) on symmetrical points on either side of the scalp while subjects respond to lateralized light flashes. Using this paradigm in normal subjects, Lines et al. (1984) have shown a difference in latency between the early deflections obtained over the visual areas of the two occipital lobes. The difference in the responses over the contralateral hemisphere receiving the visual stimulus and the indirectly stimulated, ipsilateral hemisphere is thought to reflect the interhemispheric transmission time in the normal brain. The ITTs measured under these conditions are between 10 and 15 ms over the occipital regions. When acallosal subjects are tested under the same condition, normal visual ERPs can be demonstrated over the directly stimulated hemisphere but no corresponding deflections are detected over the nonstimulated hemisphere. These findings can be interpreted as supporting the notion that responses to ipsilateral stimulation are normally mediated through the corpus callosum (Rugg et al., 1985).

Although individuals with congenital absence of the corpus show some kind of compensation compared with patients who underwent callosal transection, the fact they that they take longer than normal subjects to make crossed responses points once more to the limitations of the putative pathway or pathways used by these individuals.

Midline Sensory Integration in ACC

Visual Integration   Yet another important role of the corpus callosum is to assure continuity across the entire perceptual field. This is necessary because, as mentioned before, sensory pathways are crossed mainly so that input from each body half and each visual hemifield projects principally to the contralateral hemisphere. This mechanism is less crucial for the auditory system, where the separation of the projections coming from the two ears is less precise (see Lassonde et al., 1995)

Anatomical studies have shown that the vertical meridian is rich in callosal connections (Berlucchi & Rizzolatti, 1968). Receptive fields of neurons from both hemispheres straddle the midline so that information presented to one side of the body, or in one half of the visual or auditory field, excites structures first in one hemisphere and then in the other. Similarly, when a stimulus is presented around the midline, some portions project to one hemisphere and some to the other. This mechanism may also allow for the comparison of depth for stimuli presented near the midline. Binocular depth perception on the midline requires the comparison of disparate images from each retina, and this integration may be achieved via the corpus callosum.

However, the role of the corpus callosum in the processing of depth information is still under debate. Thus, the callosotomized subjects studied by Mitchell and Blakemore (1970) failed to discriminate depth for disparate stimuli presented near the midline but had no problems when the stimuli were presented peripherally (5° from the central fixation point). Similarly, using random dot stereograms, Hamilton and Vermeire (1986) showed midline deficits in two patients with section of all forebrain commissure, whereas Ledoux et al. (1977) found no impairments in patients with sparing of the anterior commissure, suggesting that this commissure is proficient in mediating this function.

This hypothesis was, however, not tenable in the light of a later observation by Hamilton et al. (1987), showing that a patient with complete commissurotomy, including the anterior commissure (patient L.B.), was still able to discriminate stereo patterns in the midline. Hamilton et al. (1987) also noted that the impairments seen in split-brain patients varied with the degree of disparity: deficits were most evident with larger disparities. This led the authors to speculate that the corpus callosum may be principally involved in "coarse" stereopsis, whereas smaller disparities may be handled more efficiently by the optic chiasm or the anterior commissure.

Comparing acallosal subjects and split-brain patients with and without splenial sparing on their ability to judge the distance between two lines, Jeeves (1991) found that all subjects lacking the splenium had difficulties handling uncrossed disparities, thus implicating the corpus callosum in this type of stereopsis. The author speculated that the particular difficulties of the acallosal subjects may be attributed to a reduction of neurons that respond to uncrossed disparities as part of the structural alterations that have been observed in visual cortex of some acallosal subjects (Shoumura et al., 1975). Crossed disparities, on the other hand, were integrated normally by acallosal and callosotomized patients, which tends to make a case for the role of the anterior commissure in this kind of stereopsis (Jeeves, 1991).

All the experiments reported above assessed depth perception essentially on the basis of binocular spatial disparity. There are, however, a number of other cues to depth, some of which may operate even under monocular viewing conditions. One such cue is motion parallax. It is difficult to predict how subjects without corpus callosum would use these cues to compare relative motion between the hemispheres. The first experiment of this kind, carried out by Ramachandran et al. (1986), showed that callosotomized subjects are indeed able to detect the direction of apparent motion produced by alternately flashing spots of light (similar to the phi-phenomenon) presented on either side of the midline. This finding was contested by Gazzaniga (1987), but later partially supported by Naikar and Corballis (1996). The latter showed that the ability of split-brain patients to perceive apparent motion across the midline depends on spatiotemporal parameters. Performance accuracy dropped significantly when these parameters were below a critical

Maryse Lassonde and Hannelore C. Sauerwein

level, which suggests that the compensatory pathway (most probably subcortical) is limited in spatial and temporal resolution.

To test whether callosal agenesis subjects are able to use motion parallax to judge the depth of two stimuli situated on either side of the midline, we designed an experiment where acallosal and IQ-matched subjects viewed two movable plates monocularly or binocularly while either holding their head in a fixed position or moving it from side to side or up and down (Rivest et al., 1994). The results revealed that when binocular spatial disparity was available, the acallosal subjects had no difficulties estimating the relative depth of two stimuli, each presented on one side of the midline. In the fixed-head condition, both groups performed poorly, indicating that the task could not be resolved in the absence of both binocular and monocular depth cues. When horizontal and vertical movements of the head were permitted, performance improved dramatically for the control subjects, but not for the agenesis subjects. We take this as evidence that motion parallax, as a cue for midline depth perception, cannot be integrated interhemispherically in the absence of the corpus callosum.

Somatosensory Integration   As in the visual system, the corpus callosum is important for perceptual continuity in the somatosensory modality. Consequently, callosal pathology should result in functional deficits specific to the midline. To explore this hypothesis, we measured two-point discrimination thresholds in subjects with callosal section or congenital absence of the corpus callosum and normal controls (Schiavetto et al., 1993). As predicted, thresholds in patients lacking the corpus callosum were found to be higher than in normals only in the axial part (trunk area) of the body.

The anatomical structures mediating tactile discrimination probably involve the dorsal-column medial lemniscal system, which is highly lateralized. This may explain why split-brain patients display the typical disconnection deficits on tactile tasks, such as stereognosis, texture discrimination, and cross-localization of touch (Gazzaniga, 1970). As mentioned above, the somatosensory system is also composed of the anterolateral spinothalamic tract, which is less lateralized. Thermal information is transmitted through this tract. To assess the efficiency of this parallel somatosensory pathway in acallosal subjects, we measured thresholds to thermal stimuli for different regions of the body (Lepore et al., 1997). Although the absolute value of the differential thresholds varied from region to region, the acallosals and their controls obtained comparable thresholds for all regions, including the body midline. These results indicate that the corpus callosum is not required for transfer of information in a system that has a relatively large bilateral representation.

Auditory Integration   We also investigated midline fusion in the auditory modality (Poirier et al., 1993). In this experiment, acallosal subjects and matched controls had to point to a fixed auditory target presented on a sound perimeter. It was expected that acallosals would show a comparatively poorer performance at pericentral positions than control subjects. However, contrary to our prediction, both groups were significantly more precise in locating targets in pericentral than in lateral fields, which suggests once more that the corpus callosum is not essential for midline fusion in a system that has a more extensive bihemispheric representation. In fact, we have recently demonstrated that monaural localization is better in acallosals than in neurologically intact individuals, a finding that suggests a greater proficiency of the ipsilateral auditory pathways in acallosal individuals (Lessard et al., 2002).

In sum, the results obtained from studies of midline sensory integration indicate that callosal involvement in midline fusion is important in the visual and lemniscal systems, which are principally subserved by crossed pathways, but it is not essential in the auditory and spinothalamic somatosensory systems, which are largely bilaterally represented. In the latter, there is considerable crossover of information at various levels, especially in the auditory system. Hence, the corpus callosum may contribute little to midline function in these modalities.

CONCLUSION

Agenesis of the corpus callosum has frequently been referred to as a natural model of the split brain, and the majority of studies have focused on the similarities and differences between these two populations deprived of their corpus callosum. The observation that acallosal subjects do not show the typical disconnection symptoms in the visual and tactile modalities found in adult callosotomized patients has given rise to speculations about the compensatory mechanisms that may be operating in a brain that has evolved in the absence of the main interhemi-spheric pathway. Indeed, individuals born without a corpus callosum appear to have access to a number of compensatory mechanisms that are not available to the same extent to patients who have undergone surgical section of the corpus callosum in adulthood.

Most of the earlier research was carried out on patients who were investigated in relation to associated malformations. These patients may show various degrees of cognitive impairment. However, since the introduction of improved imaging techniques, an increasing number of asymptomatic subjects have been detected. Neuropsychological studies of these individuals have shown that acallosal individuals can have normal, even superior, intellectual abilities, thus weakening the hypothesis that the absence of interhemispheric cross talk may result in lower intelligence.

In the same vein, the hypothesis that acallosal individuals may be less lateralized than the normal population, or that lateralized functions, such as language, may be compromised in the acallosal brain, is not tenable in the light of contrary evidence. In fact, laterality research in these subjects suggests not only that the latter show the normal left-right dichotomy for language, motor control, and perceptual functions, but also that they may even be *more* lateralized than callosally intact individuals because of the absence of interhemispheric cross talk would allow for the greater expression of specialized functions in each hemisphere. These findings suggest that, contrary to earlier assumptions, the corpus callosum plays a minor (if any) role in the development of cerebral laterality. This is in line with studies in infants (Entus, 1977; Witelson & Pallie, 1973) which have shown that functional asymmetry is present at birth. It would be interesting to verify whether infants born without the corpus callosum show the same early specialization. Our studies lead us to speculate that they would not differ from normal infants in this respect unless other malformations of the brain coexist.

While earlier studies in acallosals have focused on the absence of disconnection symptoms, recent work has concentrated on testing the limitations of the compensatory mechanisms used by these individuals. One of the major limitations of the compensatory pathway(s) shared, as it seems, by all acallosals concerns the speed of transfer: Acallosal subjects obtain consistently longer response times both in simple reaction time experiments and in tasks involving interhemispheric transfer of more complex material. Furthermore, they are generally slower in tasks requiring bimanual coordination under time stress, although some compensation may occur with time.

Some of the impairments shown by acallosal subjects are similar in nature, albeit not in magnitude, to those observed in split-brain patients. For instance, like callosotomized patients, acallosals are impaired in midline integration of visual and tactile stimulation. Furthermore, like the surgical patients, they show deficits in many tasks involving motor coordination and tactuomotor learning. Thus, acallosals are commonly reported to be clumsy in bimanual operations and they have difficulties effecting bimanual asynchronous movements. There are, however, exceptions, a situation that leads to the evocation of compensatory mechanisms which are not shared by all acallosal individuals.

Acallosals also fail to transfer the locus of a tactile stimulation. Indeed, many of the deficits reported in acallosals appear to be related to activities mediated by the frontal or parietal regions of the brain. This is not surprising, since callosal fibers predominantly connect associative cortex in each hemisphere. Deficits would therefore reflect the limited capacity of extracallosal pathways to mediate this kind of integration.

The most plausible compensatory mechanism for sensorimotor integration is the increased use of ipsilateral pathways of the somatosensory system. Electrophysiological studies suggest that in the absence of the corpus callosum, uncrossed somatosensory connections could take on a greater functional significance, thus allowing for an *intra*-hemispheric exchange of information.

In the motor system, the limitations in intermanual coordination have been attributed to the competition between uncrossed and crossed projections due to the lack of transcallosal inhibition. Indeed, using transcranial magnetic stimulation, both an inhibitory and a facilitatory action of the corpus callosum have been demonstrated in the motor system of neurologically intact subjects. This inhibition was largely absent in callosal agenesis subjects. Nevertheless, fMRI studies in acallosals have failed to point to an enhanced activation of ipsilateral projections during motor tasks.

For visual transfer and integration, the anterior commissure and possibly subcortical commissures, such as the intercollicular commissure, remain the most likely interhemispheric pathways in the absence of the corpus callosum. Furthermore, acallosal individuals may use behavioral strategies (e.g., eye movements) to achieve bilateral representation of the information.

Some of these mechanisms seem to be privileged over others in certain individuals, thus producing different manifestations of the disconnection syndrome. In fact, there appear to be many individual variants of cerebral organization in acallosal patients, and there is no consensus as to which abilities are consistently affected by the absence of the corpus callosum.

In this context, we have suggested that callosal agenesis subjects show deficits in procedural tasks which do not require access to conscious knowledge, but that they may perform normally on certain tests of interhemispheric integration which are accessible to conscious (declarative) experience (De Guise et al., 1999). The use of conscious knowledge would help these individuals to maintain unity of consciousness in the absence of the most important commissural pathway. As pointed out by Sperry (1968b), this unity may further be achieved through bilateral wiring of sensory systems and crossover of information at lower levels of the brain, as well as by the employment of a number of cross-cueing strategies developed as behavioral means of adaptation.

Taken together, the results of the reviewed studies suggest that the corpus callosum is not crucial for the development of cerebral lateralization of cognitive and motor functions. Rather, they indicate that this commissure plays a major role in interhemispheric integration of higher-order information and in coordination of sensory input and motor output from both sides of the body, thus permitting the brain to function as an integrated whole. As the corpus callosum matures, the brain comes to rely more extensively on this large pathway to effect these functions, whereas the acallosal brain has to find other means of interhemispheric communication, which leads to the development of a number of compensatory mechanisms, functional and behavioral, that can mask the presence of a disconnection syndrome in these individuals.

ACKNOWLEDGMENTS

This work was supported by grants from the Québec Formation de Chercheurs et Aide à la Recherche and the Natural Science and Engineering Research Council of Canada awarded to Maryse Lassonde.

REFERENCES

Aglioti, S., Berlucchi, G., Pallini, R., Rossi, G. F., & Tassinari, G. (1993). Hemispheric control of unilateral and bilateral responses to lateralized light stimuli after callosotomy and in callosal agenesis. *Experimental Brain Research, 93,* 51–165.

Aicardi, J., & Chevrie, J. J. (1994). The Aicardi syndrome. In M. Lassonde & M. A. Jeeves (Eds.), *Callosal agenesis. A natural split brain?* (pp. 7–17). New York: Plenum Press.

Allison, J. D., Meador, D. J., Loring, D. W., Figueroa, R. E., & Wright, J. C. (2000). Functional MRI cerebral activation and de-activation during finger movement. *Neurology, 54,* 135–142.

Andermann, E., Andermann, F., Joubert, M., Karpati, G., Carpenter, S., & Melanson, D. (1972). Familial agnesis of the corpus callosum with anterior horn cell disease. A syndrome of mental retardation, areflexia and paraparesis. *Transactions of the American Neurological Association, 97,* 242–244.

Andermann, F., & Andermann, E. (1994). The Andermann syndrome: Agenesis of the corpus callosum and sensorimotor neuropathy. In M. Lassonde & M. A. Jeeves (Eds.), *Callosal agenesis. A natural split brain?* (pp. 19–26). New York: Plenum Press.

Atlas, S. W., Zimmerman, R. A., Bruce, D., Schut, L., Bilaniuk, L. T., Hackney, D. B., Goldberg, H. I., & Grossman, R. I. (1988). Neurofibromatosis and agenesis of the corpus callosum in identical twins: MR diagnosis. *American Journal of Neuroradiology, 9,* 598–601.

Baranzini, S. E., Del Rey, G., Nigro, N., Szijan, I., Chamoles, N., & Cresto, J. C. (1997). Patient with Xp21 contiguous gene deletion syndrome in association with agenesis of the corpus callosum. *American Journal of Medical Genetics, 70*(3), 216–221.

Barkovitch, A. J., Chuang, S. H., & Norman, D. (1988). MR of neuronal migrational anomalies. *American Journal of Roentgenology, 150,* 179–187.

Barr, M. L. (1972). *The human nervous system: An anatomical viewpoint.* New York: Harper & Row.

Bennet, G. L., Bromley, B., & Benacerraf, B. R. (1996). Agenesis of the corpus callosum: Prenatal detection usually is not possible before 22 weeks of gestation. *Radiology, 199,* 447–450.

Berlucchi, G., Agliotti, S., Marzi, C. A., & Tassinari, G. (1995). Corpus callosum and simple visuomotor integration. *Neuropsychologia, 33,* 23–36.

Berlucchi, G., & Rizzolatti, G. (1968). Binocularly driven neurons in visual cortex of split-chiasm cats. *Science, 159,* 308–310.

Bittar, R. G., Ptito, A., Dumoulin, S. O., Andermann, F., & Reutens, D. C. (2000). Reorganization of the visual cortex in callosal agenesis and colpocephaly. *Journal of Clinical Neuroscience, 7,* 13–15.

Bogen, J. E., & Vogel, P. J. (1975). Neurologic status in the long term following cerebral commissurotomy. In F. Michel & E. Schott (Eds.), *Les syndromes de disconnexion calleuse chez l'homme* (pp. 227–251). Lyon: Hôpital Neurologique.

Maryse Lassonde and Hannelore C. Sauerwein

Bremer, F. (1966). Le corps calleux dans la dynamique cérébrale. *Experientia, 22,* 201–208.

Bremer, F. (1967). La physiologie du corps calleux à la lumière de travaux récents. *Laval medical, 38,* 835–843.

Caillé, S., Schiavetto, A., Andermann, F., Bastos, A., De Guise, E., & Lassonde, M. (1999). Interhemispheric transfer without forebrain commissures. *NeuroCase, 5,* 109–118.

Carpenter, S. (1994). The pathology of the Andermann syndrome. In M. Lassonde & M. A. Jeeves (Eds.), *Callosal agenesis. A natural split brain?* (pp. 27–30). New York: Plenum Press.

Chiarello, C. (1980). A house divided? Cognitive functioning with callosal agenesis. *Brain and Language, 11,* 128–158.

Cioni, G., Bartalena, E., & Boldrini, A. (1994). Callosal agenesis: Postnatal sonographic findings. In M. Lassonde & M. A. Jeeves (Eds.), *Callosal agenesis. A natural split brain?* (pp. 69–77). New York: Plenum Press.

Corballis, M. C., & Finlay, D. C. (2000). Interhemispheric visual integration in three cases of familial callosal agenesis. *Neuropsychology, 4,* 60–70.

Corballis, M. C., & Morgan, M. J. (1978). On the biological basis of human laterality. Evidence for a maturational left-right gradient. *Behavioral and Brain Science, 1,* 261–269.

Davidoff, L. M., & Dyke, C. G. (1934). Agenesis of the corpus callosum, its diagnosis by pneumoencephalography, report of three cases. *American Journal of Roentgenology, 32,* 1–10.

De Guise, E., de Pesce, M., Foschi, N., Quattrini, A., Papo, I., & Lassonde, M. (1999). Callosal and cortical contribution to procedural learning. *Brain, 122,* 1049–1062.

Dennis, M. (1976). Impaired sensory and motor differentiation with corpus callosum agenesis. A lack of inhibition during ontogeny? *Neuropsychologia, 14,* 455–469.

Dennis, M. (1977). Cerebral dominance in three forms of early brain disorder. In M. E. Blaw, I. Rapin, & M. Kinsbourne (Eds.), *Topics in child neurology* (pp. 189–212). New York: Spectrum.

Dennis, M. (1981). Language in a congenitally acallosal brain. *Brain and Language, 12,* 33–53.

Di Stefano, M., & Salvadori, C. (1998). Asymmetry of the interhemispheric visuomotor integration in callosal agenesis. *NeuroReport, 9*(7), 1331–1335.

Di Stefano, M. R., Sauerwein, H. C., & Lassonde, M. (1992). Influence of anatomical factors and spatial compatibility on the stimulus-response relationship in the absence of the corpus callosum. *Neuropsychologia, 30*(2), 177–185.

Donnenfeld, A. E., Packer, R. J., Zachai, E. H., Chee, C. M., Sellinger, B., & Emanuel, B. S. (1989). Clinical cytogenic and pedigree findings in 18 cases of Aicardi syndrome. *American Journal of Medical Genetics, 32,* 461–467.

Doty, R. W., Negrao, N., & Yamaga, K. (1973). The unilateral engram. *Acta Neurobiologica Experimentalis* (Warsaw), *33,* 711–728.

Entus, A. (1977). Hemispheric asymmetry in processing of dichotically presented speech and nonspeech stimuli by infants. In S. J. Segalowitz & F. A. Gruber (Eds.), *Language development and neurological theory* (pp. 63–73). New York: Academic Press.

Ettlinger, G., Blakemore, C. B., Milner, A., & Wilson, J. (1972). Agenesis of the corpus callosum: A behavioural investigation. *Brain, 95*, 327–346.

Ferris, G. S., & Dorsen, M. M. (1975). Agenesis of the corpus callosum. Neuropsychological studies. *Cortex, 11*, 95–122.

Fischer, M., Ryan, S. B., & Dobyns, W. B. (1992). Mechanisms of interhemispheric transfer and patterns of cognitive function in acallosal patients of normal intelligence. *Archives of Neurology, 49*, 271–277.

Foster, B., & Corballis, M. C. (1998). Interhemispheric transmission times in the presence and absence of the forebrain commissures: Effects of luminance and equiluminance. *Neuropsychologia, 36*(9), 925–934.

Gazzaniga, M. S. (1970). *The bisected brain*. New York: Appleton-Century-Crofts.

Gazzaniga, M. S. (1987). Perceptual and attentional processes following callosal section in humans. *Neuropsychologia, 25*, 119–133.

Geffen, G. M., Forrester, G. M., Jones, D. L., & Simpson, D. A. (1994). Auditory verbal learning and memory in cases of callosal agenesis. In M. Lassonde & M. A. Jeeves (Eds.), *Callosal agenesis. A natural split brain?* (pp. 247–260). New York: Plenum Press.

Geffen, G. M., Nilsson, J., Simpson, D. A., & Jeeves, M. A. (1994). The development of interhemispheric transfer of tactile information in cases of callosal agenesis. In M. Lassonde & M. A. Jeeves (Eds.), *Callosal agenesis. A natural split brain?* (pp. 185–198). New York: Plenum Press.

Gelot, A., Esperandieu, O., & Pompidou, A. (1998). Histogenesis of the corpus callosum. *Neurochirurgie, 44*, 61–73.

Geoffroy, G. (1994). Other syndromes frequently associated with callosal agenesis. In M. Lassonde & M. A. Jeeves (Eds.), *Callosal agenesis. A natural split brain?* (pp. 55–62). New York: Plenum Press.

Goldstein, M. N., & Joynt, R. J. (1975). The long-term effects of callosal sectioning: Report of a second case. *Archives of Neurology, 32*, 52–53.

Gott, P. S., & Saul, R. E. (1978). Agenesis of the corpus callosum: Limits of functional compensation. *Neurology, 28*, 1272–1279.

Hamilton, C. R., Rodriguez, K. M., & Vermeire, B. A. (1987). The cerebral commissures and midline stereopsis. *Investigative Ophthalmology and Visual Science, 28*, 294.

Hamilton, C. R., & Vermeire, B. A. (1986). Localization of visual functions with partially split-brain monkeys. In F. Lepore, M. Ptito, and H. H. Jaspers (Eds.), *Two hemispheres—one brain: Functions of the corpus callosum* (pp. 315–333). New York: Alan Liss.

Inbar, D., Halpern, G. J., Weitz, R., Sadeh, M., & Shohat, M. (1997). Agenesis of the corpus callosum in a mother and son. *American Journal of Medical Genetics, 69*(2), 152–154.

Jacobson, I., & Jeeves, M. A. (1994). A new syndrome: Familial fronto-nasal dermoid cysts with agenesis of the corpus callosum. In M. Lassonde & M. A. Jeeves (Eds.), *Callosal agenesis. A natural split brain?* (pp. 39–53). New York: Plenum Press.

Jakobson, L., Servos, P., Goodale, M. A., & Lassonde, M. (1994). Control of proximal and distal components of prehension. *Brain, 117,* 1107–1113.

Jeeves, M. A. (1965). Psychological studies of three cases of congenital agenesis of the corpus callosum. In E. G. Ettlinger (Ed.), *Function of the corpus callosum* (pp. 73–94). London: Macmillan.

Jeeves, M. A. (1969). A comparison of interhemispheric transmission times in acallosals and normals. *Psychonomic Science, 16,* 245–246.

Jeeves, M. A. (1979). Some limits of interhemispheric integration in cases of callosal agenesis. In I. S. Russell, M. W. Van Hof, & G. Berlucchi (Eds.), *Structure and function of cerebral commissures* (pp. 449–474). London: Macmillan.

Jeeves, M. A. (1986). Callosal agenesis: Neuronal and developmental adaptations. In F. Lepore, M. Ptito, and H. H. Jaspers (Eds.), *Two hemispheres—one brain: Functions of the corpus callosum* (pp. 403–421). New York: Alan Liss.

Jeeves, M. A. (1991). Stereopsis in callosal agenesis and partial callosotomy. *Neuropsychologia, 29,* 19–34.

Jeeves, M. A. (1994). Callosal agenesis—A natural split-brain: Overview. In M. Lassonde & M. A. Jeeves (Eds.), *Callosal agenesis. A natural split brain?* (pp. 285–300). New York: Plenum Press.

Jeeves, M. A., & Silver, P. H. (1988). The formation of finger grip during prehension in an acallosal patient. *Neuropsychologia, 26,* 153–159.

Jeeves, M. A., Silver, P. H., & Jacobson, I. (1988). Bimanual coordination in callosal agenesis and partial commissurotomy. *Neuropsychologia, 26,* 833–850.

Karnath, H. O., Schumacher, M., & Wallesch, C. W. (1991). Limitations of interhemispheric extracallosal transfer of visual information in calllosal agenesis. *Cortex, 27,* 345–350.

Kinsbourne, M., & Fisher, M. (1971). Latency of crossed and uncrossed reaction in callosal agenesis. *Neuropsychologia, 9,* 472–473.

Laget, P., D'Allest, A. M., Fihey, R., & Lortholary, O. (1977). L'intérêt des potentiels évoqués somesthésiques homolatéraux dans les agénésies du corps calleux. *Revue d'Électroencéphalographie et de Neurophysiologie Clinigue, 7,* 498–502.

Lassonde, M. (1986). The facilitatory influence of the corpus callosum on intrahemispheric processing. In F. Lepore, M. Ptito, and H. H. Jaspers (Eds.), *Two hemispheres—one brain: Functions of the corpus callosum* (pp. 335–350). New York: Alan Liss.

Lassonde, M. (1994). Disconnection syndrome in callosal agenesis. In M. Lassonde & M. A. Jeeves (Eds.), *Callosal agenesis. A natural split brain?* (pp. 275–284). New York: Plenum Press.

Lassonde, M., Bryden, M. P., & Demers, P. (1990). The corpus callosum and cerebral speech lateralization. *Brain and Language, 38*, 195–206.

Lassonde, M., Sauerwein, H. C., Chicoine, A. J., & Geoffroy, G. (1991). Absence of disconnection syndrome in callosal agenesis and early callosotomy: Brain reorganization or lack of structural specificity during ontogeny? *Neuropsychologia, 29*, 481–495.

Lassonde, M., Sauerwein, H., Geoffroy, G., & Décarie, M. (1986). Effects of early versus late transection of the corpus callosum in children. *Brain, 109*, 953–967.

Lassonde, M., Sauerwein, H. C., & Lepore, F. (1995). Extent and limits of callosal plasticity: Presence of disconnection signs in callosal agenesis. *Neuropsychologia, 33*, 989–1007.

Lassonde, M., Sauerwein, H. C., McCabe, N., Laurencelle, L., & Geoffroy, G. (1988). Extent and limits of cerebral adjustment to early section or congenital absence of the corpus callosum. *Behavioural Brain Research, 30*, 165–181.

Ledoux, J. E., Dentsoh, G., Wilson, D. H., & Gazzaniga, M. S. (1977). Binocular depth perception and the anterior commissure in man. *The Psychologist, 20*, 55.

Lepore, F., Lassonde, M., Veillette, N., & Guillemot, J. P. (1997). Interhemispheric differential thresholds for temperature discrimination in acallosal and split-brain subjects. *Neurospychologia, 35*, 1225–1231.

Lessard, N., Lepore, F., Villemagne, J., & Lassonde, M. (2002). Sound localization in callosal agenesis and early callosotomy subjects: Brain reorganization and/or compensatory strategies. *Brain, 125*, 1–15.

Lines, C. R., Rugg, M. D., & Milner, A. D. (1984). The effect of stimulus intensity on visually evoked potential estimates of interhemispheric transmission time. *Experimental Brain Research, 22*, 215–225.

Loeser, J. D., & Alvord, E. C. (1968). Agenesis of the corpus callosum. *Brain, 91*, 553–570.

Martin, A. A. (1985). A qualitative limitation on visual transfer via the anterior commissure. *Brain, 108*, 43–63.

Marzi, C. A., Bisiacchi, P., & Nicoletti, R. (1991). Is interhemispheric transfer of visuomotor information asymmetric? Evidence from a meta-analysis. *Neuropsychologia, 29*, 1163–1177.

Meerwaldt, J. D. (1983). Disturbance of spatial perception in a patient with agenesis of the corpus callosum. *Neuropsychologia, 21*, 161–165.

Melanson, D., & Salazar, A. (1994). CT findings in callosal agenesis. In M. Lassonde & M. A. Jeeves (Eds.), *Callosal agenesis. A natural split brain?* (pp. 77–82). New York: Plenum Press.

Meyer, B.-U., & Röricht, S. (1998). In vivo visualization of the longitudinal callosal fascicle (Probst's bundle) and other abnormalities in an acallosal brain. *Journal of Neurology, Neurosurgery and Psychiatry, 64*, 138–139.

Meyer, B.-U., Röricht, S., Gräfin von Einsiedel, H., Kruggel, F., & Weindl, A. (1995). Inhibitory and excitatory interhemispheric transfers between motor cortical areas in normal humans and patients with abnormalities of the corpus callosum. *Brain, 118*, 429–440.

Meyer, B.-U., Röricht, S., & Niehaus, L. (1998). Morphology of acallosal brains as assessed by MRI in six patients leading a normal daily life. *Journal of Neurology, 245*, 106–110.

Milner, A. D. (1982). Simple reaction times to lateralized visual stimuli in a case of callosal agenesis. *Neuropsychologia, 20*, 411–419.

Milner, A. D. (1994). Visual integration in callosal agenesis. In M. Lassonde & M. A. Jeeves (Eds.), *Callosal agenesis. A natural split brain?* (pp. 171–185). New York: Plenum Press.

Milner, A. D., & Jeeves, M. A. (1979). A review of behavioural studies of agenesis of the corpus callosum. In I. S. Russell, M. W. Van Hof, & G. Berlucchi (Eds.), *Structure and function of cerebral commissures* (pp. 428–448). London: Macmillan.

Milner, A. D., Jeeves, M. A., Silver, P. H., Lines, C. R., & Wilson, J. G. (1985). Reaction times to lateralized visual stimuli in callosal agenesis: Stimulus and response factors. *Neuropsychologia, 23*, 323–331.

Mitchell, D. E., & Blakemore, C. (1970). Binocular depth perception and the corpus callosum. *Vision Research, 10*, 49–54.

Moscovitch, M. (1977). Development of lateralization of language functions and its relations to cognitive and linguistic development: A review and some theoretical speculations. In S. J. Segalowitz & F. A. Gruber (Eds.), *Language development and neurological theory* (pp. 193–211). New York: Academic Press.

Mountcastle, V. B. (1984). Central nervous system mechanisms in mechanoreceptive sensibility. In J. M. Brookhart & V. B. Mountcastle (Eds.), *Handbook of physiology. The nervous system.* Vol. 3, sec. 1, part 2: *Sensory processes* (pp. 789–878). Bethesda, MD: American Physiological Society.

Naikar, M., & Corballis, M. C. (1996). Perception of apparent motion across the retinal midline following commissurotomy. *Neuropsychologia, 34*, 297–309.

Pandya, D. N., & Seltzer, B. (1986). The topography of commissural fibers. In F. Lepore, M. Ptito, and H. H. Jaspers (Eds.), *Two hemispheres—one brain: Functions of the corpus callosum* (pp. 47–73). New York: Alan Liss.

Poffenberger, A. T. (1912). Reaction time to retinal stimulation with special reference to time lost in conduction through nerve centers. *Archiv für Psychologie* (New York), *23*, 1–73.

Poirier, P., Miljours, S., Lassonde, M., & Lepore, F. (1993). Sound localization in acallosal human listeners. *Brain, 116*, 53–69.

Preilowski, B. F. B. (1972). Possible contribution of the anterior forebrain commissures to bilateral motor coordination. *Neuropsychologia, 10*, 267–277.

Rakic, P., & Yakovlev, P. I. (1968). Development of the corpus callosum and cavum septi in man. *Journal of Comparative Neurology, 132*, 45–72.

Ramachadran, V. S., Cronin-Colomb, A., & Myers, J. J. (1986). Perception of apparent motion in commissurotomy patients. *Nature, 320,* 328–359.

Rauch, R. A., & Jinkins, J. R. (1994). Magnetic resonance imaging of corpus callosum dysgenesis. In M. Lassonde & M. A. Jeeves (Eds.), *Callosal agenesis. A natural split brain?* (pp. 83–96). New York: Plenum Press.

Reddy, H., Lassonde, M., Bemasconi, A., Bemasconi, P. M., Mathews, F., Andermann, F., & Amold, D. L. (2000). An fMRI study of the lateralization of motor cortex activation in acallosal patients. *NeuroReport, 11*(11), 2409–2413.

Reddy, H., Lassonde, M., & Mathews, F. (2000). Functional MRI cerebral activation and deactivation during finger movement. *Neurology, 55*(8), 1244.

Reil, J. C. (1812). Mangel des mittleren und freyen Theils des Balkens im Menschengehirn. *Archiv für Physiologie, 11,* 314–344.

Reynolds, M. D., & Jeeves, M. A. (1977). Further studies of tactile perception and motor coordination in agenesis of the corpus callosum. *Cortex, 13,* 257–272.

Rivest, J., Cavanagh, P., & Lassonde, M. (1994). Interhemispheric depth judgment. *Neuropsychologia, 32,* 69–76.

Rugg, M. D., Milner, A. D., & Lines, C. R. (1985). Visual evoked potentials to lateralised stimuli in two cases of callosal agenesis. *Journal of Neurology, Neurosurger and Psychiatry, 48,* 367–373.

Russell, J. R., & Reitan, R. M. (1955). Psychological abnormalities in agenesis of the corpus callosum. *Journal of Nervous and Mental Disease, 121,* 205–214.

Sanders, R. J. (1989). Sentence comprehension following agenesis of the corpus callosum. *Brain and Language, 37,* 59–72.

Sauerwein, H., & Lassonde, M. (1983). Intra- and interhemispheric processing of visual information in callosal agenesis. *Neuropsychologia, 21,* 167–171.

Sauerwein, H., & Lassonde, M. M. (1994). Cognitive and sensori-motor functioning in the absence of the corpus callosum: Neuropsychological studies in callosal agenesis and callosotomized patients. *Behavioral Brain Research, 64,* 229–240.

Sauerwein, H., Lassonde, M., Cardu, B., & Geoffroy, G. (1981). Interhemispheric integration of sensory and motor functions in agenesis of the corpus callosum. *Neuropsychologia, 19,* 445–454.

Saul, R. E., & Sperry, R. W. (1968). Absence of commissurotomy symptoms with agenesis of the corpus callosum. *Neurology, 18,* 307.

Schiavetto, A., Lepore, F., & Lassonde, M. (1993). Somesthetic discrimination thresholds in the absence of the corpus callosum. *Neuropsychologia, 31,* 695–707.

Sergent, J., & Myers, J. (1985). Manual, blowing and verbal simple reactions to lateralized flashes of light in commissurotomized patients. *Perception and Psychophysics, 37,* 571–578.

Serur, D., Jeret, J. S., & Wiesnieswki, K. (1988). Agenesis of the corpus callosum: Clinical, neuroradiological and cytogenic studies. *Neuropediatrics, 19,* 87–91.

Shoumura, K., Ando, T., & Kato, K. (1975). Structural organization of callosal OBg in human corpus callosum agenesis. *Brain Research, 93*, 241–252.

Silver, P. H., & Jeeves, M. A. (1994). Motor coordination in callosal agenesis. In M. Lassonde & M. A. Jeeves (Eds.), *Callosal agenesis. A natural split brain?* (pp. 207–219). New York: Plenum Press.

Sperry, R. W. (1961). Cerebral organization and behavior. *Science, 133*, 1749–1757.

Sperry, R. W. (1968a). Plasticity of neural maturation. *Developmental Biology, Suppl. 2*, 306–327.

Sperry, R. W. (1968b). Hemisphere disconnection and unity in conscious awareness. *American Psychologist, 23*, 723–733.

Sperry, R. W. (1970). Perception in the absence of the neocortical commissures. In *Research Publications—Association for Research in Nervous and Mental Disease*. Vol. 48: *Perception and its disorders* (pp. 123–138). Baltimore: Williams and Wilkins.

Sperry, R. W., Gazzaniga, M. S., & Bogen, J. E. (1969). Interhemispheric relationships: The neocortical commissures; syndromes of hemisphere disconnection. In P. J. Vinken & J. W. Bruyn (Eds.), *Handbook of clinical neurology*. Vol. 4: *Disorders of speech perception and symbolic behaviour* (pp. 273–290). Amsterdam: Elsevier.

Tassinari, G., Aglioti, S., Pallini, R., Berlucchi, G., & Rossi, G. (1994). Interhemispheric integration of simple visuomotor responses in patients with partial callosal defects. *Behavioural Brain Research, 64*, 141–149.

Temple, C. M., & Ilsley, I. (1994). Sound and shapes: Language and spatial cognition in callosal agenesis. In M. Lassonde & M. A. Jeeves (Eds.), *Callosal agenesis. A natural split brain?* (pp. 261–273). New York: Plenum Press.

Vanasse, M., Forest, L. & Lassonde, M. (1994). Short- and middle-latency somatosensory evoked potentials in callosal agenesis. In M. Lassonde & M. A. Jeeves (Eds.), *Callosal agenesis. A natural split brain?* (pp. 199–206). New York: Plenum Press.

Wahlsten, D. (1989). Deficiency of the corpus callosum: Incomplete penetrance and substrain differentiation in BALB/c mice. *Journal of Neurogenetics, 5*, 61–76.

Wahlsten, D., & Bulman-Fleming, B. (1994). Retarded growth of the medial septum: A major gene effect in acallosal mice. *Brain Research Developmental Brain Research, 77*, 203–214.

Wahlsten, D., & Ozaki, H. (1994). Defects of the fetal forebrain in acallosal mice. In M. Lassonde & M. A. Jeeves (Eds.), *Callosal agenesis. A natural split brain?* (pp. 125–133). New York: Plenum Press.

Wisniewski, K., & Jeret, J. S. (1994). Callosal agenesis: Review of clinical, pathological and cytogenetic features. In M. Lassonde & M. A. Jeeves (Eds.), *Callosal agenesis. A natural split brain?* (pp. 7–19). New York: Plenum Press.

Witelson, S. F., & Pallie, W. (1973). Left hemisphere specialization for language in the newborn: Neuroanatomical evidence of asymmetry. *Brain Research, 96*, 641–646.

Zaidel, D., & Sperry, R. W. (1977). Some long-term motor effects of cerebral commissurotomy in man. *Neuropsychologia, 10*, 103–110.

18 Developmental Disorders: Dyslexia

Mark A. Eckert and Christiana M. Leonard

Dyslexia, a specific reading disability that cannot be explained by associated environmental, cognitive, or neurological influences, was originally characterized as a disorder of anomalous cerebral asymmetry and lateralization (Orton, 1937). This conception received support from early reports of temporal and parietal lobe symmetry in dyslexia. These studies suggested the exciting idea that examination of brain scans could contribute to the diagnosis of dyslexia.

Over time and many inconsistent findings, enthusiasm for diagnosing dyslexia with neuroanatomical data has been tempered, but the idea that dyslexia is a disorder of cerebral asymmetry is still popular. Although some predictions about brain asymmetries (planum temporale asymmetry) and dyslexia have not been sustained, there is evidence for anomalous asymmetries and atypical brain structure in dyslexia. In this chapter we review neuroanatomical studies of dyslexia and conclude that dyslexia is associated with a variety of neural risk factors, some of which may involve disregulated development of interhemispheric asymmetry.

CEREBRAL ASYMMETRY AND DYSLEXIA

Cerebral asymmetry is associated with fine motor control in a number of species-specific behaviors. For example, the right eye is dominant for foraging in pigeons (Güntürkün et al., 2000) and chickens (Rogers, 2000), while the left hemisphere controls song production in finches (Nottebohm et al., 1976). In children and adults, structural and functional asymmetries have been associated with good reading and language skills (Eckert et al., 2001; Leonard et al., 1996; Rumsey, Donahue, et al., 1997). Normal readers demonstrate a consistent functional asymmetry in brain activation during phonological processing. In contrast, dyslexic individuals exhibit reduced left hemisphere activation in temporal-parietal (Pugh et al., 2000; Shaywitz et al., 1998) and occipital-temporal regions (Rumsey, Nace, et al., 1997; Salmelin et al., 2000; Simos et al., 2000), and increased right hemisphere activation in these areas (Shaywitz et al., 1998). These findings support the view that cerebral asymmetry of particular brain regions facilitates superior language performance (Galaburda, 1989).

In this context, the repeated failure of modern imaging studies to demonstrate anomalous structural asymmetry in the planum temporale of dyslexics is puzzling (Eckert & Leonard, 2000). In this chapter we will review the literature and propose a possible solution to the dilemma. We conclude that the evidence suggests that anomalous planar asymmetry characterizes individuals who have a global reading and language deficit rather than a specific reading deficit.

For the purpose of this chapter, dyslexia is defined as a reading disability characterized by a specific phonological deficit. This definition distinguishes dyslexia from "garden variety reading disability or specific language impairment," in which comprehension deficits limit reading success (Bishop & Adams, 1990; Stanovich, 1988). Although there has been some debate about the validity of the discrepancy definition (Fletcher et al., 1994), neurobiological evidence supports the distinction between discrepant and nondiscrepant readers (Eckert & Leonard, 2000; Eckert et al., 2001; Leonard, Eckert, Lombardino, Oakland, et al., 2001).

STRUCTURAL HISTORY: PLANAR ASYMMETRY

Early investigators speculated that dyslexia was a language disorder stemming from anomalous asymmetry of temporal lobe structures, in particular the planum temporale (PT). The PT is found on the surface of the temporal lobe, posterior to Heschl's gyrus (figure 18.1). A large postmortem study of 100 brains found that the PT is six times more likely to be larger on the left than on the right (Geschwind & Levitsky, 1968). Since left hemisphere damage is much more likely than right to produce receptive language impairments, Geschwind hypothesized that PT asymmetry is an anatomical correlate for left hemisphere lan-

Mark A. Eckert and Christiana M. Leonard

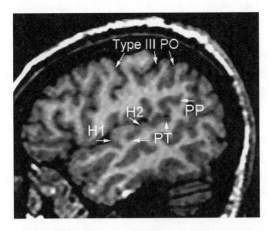

Figure 18.1 The left hemisphere of a dyslexic participant. H1, Heschl's gyrus; H2, duplication of Heschl's gyrus; PT, horizontal ramus of the planum temporale; PP, vertical ramus of the planum temporale; type III PO, Steinmetz type III parietal-operculum classification.

guage dominance. Anomalous asymmetry, defined as symmetry or rightward asymmetry of the planum, was expected to characterize brains with right hemisphere or mixed dominance for language.

In vivo imaging advances in the late 1970s made it possible to examine behavioral correlates for the leftward asymmetry found in postmortem analysis (LeMay & Kido, 1978). The first computerized tomography (CT) study of dyslexia reported parieto-occipital symmetry in 24 poor readers, particularly those with low intelligence (Hier et al., 1978). Sixteen of the poor readers had rightward asymmetry or symmetry of their parieto-occipital area. The ten individuals with rightward asymmetry had significantly lower verbal IQ than those who had leftward asymmetry. A follow-up study also demonstrated anomalous parieto-occipital asymmetry in learning disabled individuals (Rosenberger & Hier, 1980). Another CT study, however, did not find a relation between occipital lobe symmetry and IQ, despite the increased prevalence of symmetrical occipital widths found in the reading-disabled group (Haslam et al., 1981).

The CT studies were followed by Galaburda's groundbreaking series of postmortem studies. These studies had a profound effect on the scientific investigation of learning disabilities and provided strong support for the belief that reading disability is a disorder of cerebral asymmetry (Galaburda, 1989; Galaburda et al., 1978, 1985). Galaburda and his colleagues examined the brains of eight individuals who had been reading disabled. All eight of the brains were reported to have symmetry of the planum temporale due to a larger right planum. This finding was particularly impressive, given the patients' heterogeneous demographic, developmental, and psychiatric histories. Among eight patients were four non-right-handers, four patients with speech and developmental language delay, two with attention deficits, two with a history of seizures, and one with early traumatic brain injury.

Sections of this chapter below show that mixed or left-hand preference (nondominant right-handedness) and language delay are all associated with anomalous planar symmetry, and thus raise the possibility that the association of dyslexia and planar symmetry in the postmortem studies was not specific.

Advances in magnetic resonance imaging (MRI) technology made it possible to examine brain morphology in vivo with much better resolution than CT. Rumsey et al. (1986) used MRI to examine the brains of strongly right-handed subjects with severe phonological impairments and full-scale IQs in the average to superior range. Radiologists evaluated the MRI scans for abnormalities and found symmetrical temporal lobes in nine out of ten individuals. Subsequent studies, however, have produced inconsistent results.

Early studies of the PT and dyslexia supported the idea that dyslexia was associated with anomalous PT asymmetry. Recent work, however, has failed to find this association. These studies have been reviewed extensively (Beaton, 1997; Eckert & Leonard, 2000; Filipek, 1995; Hynd & Semrud-Clikeman, 1989; Morgan & Hynd, 1998). The inconsistencies in early studies can be attributed to differences in diagnostic and measurement criteria, and inadequate control of handedness, sex, and cognitive ability. But as imaging and diagnostic methods have become more standardized, the studies have grown more consistent only in finding that individuals with phonological dyslexia do not exhibit anomalous PT asymmetry (although there is one notable recent exception (Heiervang et al., 2000). In some studies, dyslexic readers actually appear to be less likely than normal readers to exhibit anomalous asymmetry (Leonard, Eckert, Lombardino, Oakland, et al., 2001; Leonard et al., 1993).

Handedness

There is a complex relation between PT asymmetry and hand preference. Normal non-right-handed individuals exhibit reduced or anomalous asymmetry in a variety of brain areas, including the planum temporale, the central sulcus, cerebral hemispheres, and frontal and occipital petalia more often than normal right-handers (Foundas et al., 1995; Steinmetz et al., 1991; Witelson & Kigar, 1992). In studies where a greater percentage of dyslexic individuals had anomalous PT asymmetry than did controls, there was an equally greater percentage of non-right-handed dyslexic individuals among the dyslexic individuals (Hynd et al., 1990; Kushch et al., 1993; Larsen et al., 1990). It is possible that dyslexic individuals in these samples developed reading problems due to a combination of anomalous brain dominance (as revealed by non-right-handedness) and anomalous PT asymmetry. But it is also possible that anomalous planar asymmetry found in these studies is associated with non-right-handedness and is not related to the reading disability.

Intelligence and Language

PT asymmetry also exhibits a significant relation to general cognitive ability or IQ. Because of this relation, interpreting findings of anomalous symmetry becomes difficult when the reading-impaired and control groups differ in IQ. For example, control groups in the Hynd (1990), Semrud-Clikeman (1991), and Kushch (1993) studies had mean full-scale IQs that were at least 15 points higher than the dyslexic groups. Recent structural MRI studies of dyslexia that have controlled for IQ have not found group differences in asymmetry. When the effect of IQ was removed statistically in one recent study (Pennington et al., 1999), the differences in temporal lobe volumes between 75 phonological dyslexic subjects and 22 controls disappeared. It seems possible that PT asymmetry may be more related to general verbal than to specific phonological ability.

Studies of language impairment also support the conclusion that uncontrolled group differences in verbal ability could have been responsible for the positive structural findings in previous studies. Two studies have found that brain size and the surface area of both the left and the right PT are reduced in children with developmental oral language disorder (Gauger et al., 1997; Preis et al., 1998). These findings, together with three other reports of decreased leftward asymmetry in developmental oral language disorders (Jernigan et al., 1990; Plante et al., 1989, 1991), suggest the possibility that small symmetrical temporal lobe structures are found when reading deficits are part of an oral language disorder.

There is suggestive evidence from other studies that PT asymmetry is related to language skills and verbal IQ (Eckert et al., 2001; Heiervang, 2000; Rumsey, Donahue, et al., 1997). In a recent study of a group of sixth grade children from a diverse set of public schools, PT asymmetry was linearly related to verbal ability (Eckert et al., 2001). The structure-function relationship was due to a large right PT in strongly right-handed children with poor comprehension and phonological skills. It is also worth noting that there were three children in the study whose phonological decoding performance was markedly lower than their verbal IQ and passage comprehension; they thus fit a diagnosis of specific reading disability or dyslexia. In these three children PT asymmetry did not predict their reading ability.

We concluded that anomalous PT asymmetry was characteristic of reading disorders in which comprehension and phonological ability were comparable, not discrepant. This conclusion is supported by a recent study by Rumsey and her colleagues. In this study, there was a positive relationship between PT asymmetry and verbal IQ in controls (where comprehension and phonology are assumed to be comparable) but not in dyslexic individuals (where the two skills are discrepant) (Rumsey, Donahue, et al., 1997).

These two studies concur in the finding that PT symmetry does not predict dyslexia when dyslexia is defined as a discrepancy between phonology and other verbal skills, such as comprehension or verbal IQ. Individual differences in PT asymmetry do, however, predict reading skill and comprehension among normal and oral language-impaired individuals who do not exhibit a reading aptitude-achievement discrepancy.

The Planum Parietale

The planum parietale (PP), or ascending ramus of the sylvian fissure, is sometimes included in measures of the PT, and the combined measurement is called PT+. Cytoarchitectural evidence is used as justifi-

Mark A. Eckert and Christiana M. Leonard

cation for combining measurements of structures in the temporal and parietal lobes. Postmortem analysis suggests that the cellular layering and density of the PT and PP are similar (Witelson et al., 1995). It should be remembered, however, that Brodmann did not report cytoarchitectural differences among functionally different subdivisions of area 19 in visual association cortex. Thus it is not clear that cytoarchitectural distinctions in association cortex are necessary for the definition of functional boundaries.

The distribution of PT+ is much less biased toward leftward asymmetry than that of PT because PP is larger on the right in most brains (Steinmetz, Rademacher, et al., 1990). Studies that have measured PT+ have not found an increased incidence of anomalous PT+ asymmetry in dyslexia (Green et al., 1999; Leonard, Eckert, Lombardino, Oakland, et al., 2001; Leonard et al., 1993; Schultz et al., 1994).

Despite the fact that PT+ asymmetry appears normal in dyslexia, there is evidence that the relationship between the asymmetries in the two banks of the planum is disrupted. In most individuals there is an inverse relation between PT and PP asymmetry, in that PT asymmetry tends to be leftward and PP asymmetry tends to be rightward. Leftward asymmetry of both the PT and the PP was not seen in a single case in one database of 200 normal scans (Jäncke, Wunderlich, et al., 1997). Thus it is significant that a number of dyslexic individuals exhibit leftward asymmetry of both PT and PP (Leonard, Eckert, Lombardino, Oakland, et al., 2001; Leonard et al., 1993) (figure 18.2). There is a significant linear relation between PT and PP asymmetry in controls, but not the dyslexics, due in part to a number of dyslexic individuals with leftward PP asymmetry. These findings suggest that the development of PT and PP asymmetry may be more closely regulated in controls than in dyslexics.

Summary

Recent MRI studies support the notion that poor verbal ability, but not dyslexia, is associated with anomalous PT asymmetry. Despite the absence of a specific relation between PT asymmetry and dyslexia, the lack of association between PT and PP asymmetry in dyslexic individuals suggests a divergence or disregulation of PT and PP development. It is possible, furthermore, that the coordinated development of other neural structures also characterizes dyslexia.

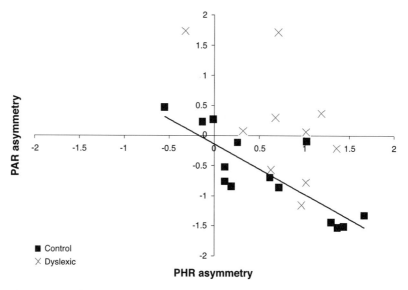

Figure 18.2 Planum temporale and planum parietale asymmetries are linearly related in controls, but not in dyslexic individuals.

DO OTHER BRAIN ASYMMETRIES AND ATYPICAL STRUCTURES CHARACTERIZE DYSLEXIA?

The negative results in studies of planar asymmetry have prompted an examination of other brain regions. For theoretical reasons reviewed below, the parietal lobe, Heschl's gyrus, the corpus callosum, the cerebellum, and the inferior frontal gyrus have become targets for dyslexia research. Despite the shift of focus to other brain regions, an emphasis on disruptions in lateralized structure and function remains a guiding principle.

Perisylvian Anomalies

Heschl's gyrus (HG) is another temporal lobe structure that exhibits a leftward asymmetry in size, although there is a somewhat greater frequency of a second duplicated gyrus in the right hemisphere (Leonard et al., 1998; Musiek & Reeves, 1990; Penhune et al., 1996). The frequency of HG2 varies from sample to sample. Patients with resistance to thyroid hormone (Leonard et al., 1995) and patients with intractable

Mark A. Eckert and Christiana M. Leonard

left hemisphere epilepsy are more likely to exhibit an HG2 (Eckert, unpublished data). In addition, some studies report an elevated incidence of HG2 in dyslexic individuals. In the first study, phonological processing performance decreased as the number of perisylvian anomalies (including HG2) increased (Leonard et al., 1993). In a more recent study, an HG2 was found in the left hemisphere of seven out nine college students with a specific phonological deficit (Leonard, Eckert, Lombardino, Oakland, et al., 2001). Other studies, however, have not found an increased incidence of HG2 in dyslexia (Green et al., 1999).

One possible explanation for these discrepancies is that the relation between HG2 and dyslexia is indirect and modulated by developmental anomalies in other brain regions. One such anomaly is the presence of an extra sulcus in the parietal operculum. In a pioneering anatomical study in postmortem material and sagittal MRI scans, Steinmetz and his colleagues (Steinmetz, Ebeling, et al., 1990) described lateral asymmetries in parietal operculum and sylvian fissure morphology. Four categories of morphological pattern were described. In type I the sylvian fissure bifurcates into an ascending and a descending ramus. This is the most common pattern and is found in a majority of left and right hemispheres. In type II (15% left, 0% right) there is no PP. In type III (20% left, 3% right) there is an extra sulcus between the postcentral sulcus and the termination of the sylvian fissure. In type IV (0% left, 15% right), the PT is very small because the PP rises just behind HG and merges with the postcentral sulcus.

The normal distribution of planar asymmetry is associated with these lateralized morphological asymmetries. Fissures with type II and III patterns tend to be long and found in the left hemisphere, while type IV is short and found predominantly in the right hemisphere. In their paper, Steinmetz and his colleagues suggested that neuropsychological differences might characterize individuals with different morphological patterns.

Two reading disability studies have used the Steinmetz classification system. In the first, the incidence of the type III pattern in the left hemisphere was found to be elevated in both dyslexic individuals and their relatives, and the presence of this pattern contributed to the prediction of poor phonological decoding skills (Leonard et al., 1993). One female control had a type II pattern in the left hemisphere, but no one had a type III pattern in the right hemisphere. The second study found no relation between the incidence of the type III pattern and the diagnosis of dyslexia or performance on reading tests. Children with a type III pattern in the left hemisphere performed more poorly than those with a type I pattern on a test of receptive vocabulary, while a type III pattern in the right hemisphere was associated with poor expressive vocabulary skills. Finally, there were only four children with type II morphology, and all four were dyslexic boys (Hiemenz & Hynd, 2000).

New analyses of our more recent sample of college students confirm that type III patterns predict performance on dimensions of verbal ability regardless of diagnosis. Controls and dyslexic individuals with a type III pattern performed more poorly on a number of verbal measures. They were particularly impaired in a sound-blending task that requires the integration of word parts into a whole word (figure 18.3) (Eckert, unpublished data). Sound-blending performance appears to be depressed in the subjects with a type II pattern as well, but, as in the other two studies, the number of individuals with a type II pattern is too small for statistical analysis.

A final study points to a role for the parietal operculum in the development of dyslexia. Robichon et al. (2000) reported that dyslexic

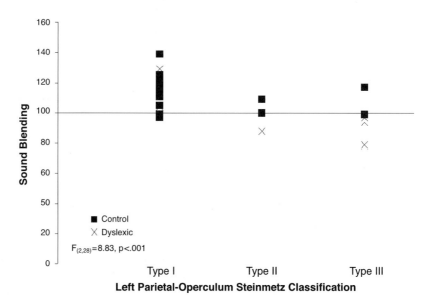

Figure 18.3 Anterior lobe and posterior lobe asymmetries are linearly related in controls, but not in dyslexic individuals.

Mark A. Eckert and Christiana M. Leonard

engineering students have a significantly greater leftward asymmetry of the parietal perisylvian region than do controls. The lengths of the left and right parietal opercula were measured from the central sulcus to the posterior termination of the sylvian fissure. The results of this quantitative study of parietal asymmetry are consistent with the qualitative results described above. The presence of an extra parietal sulcus in the left hemisphere of some members of the dyslexic group would add to the length of the parietal operculum and exaggerate its asymmetry.

Why individuals with extra sulci in their parietal opercula and extra gyri on their temporal planum (HG2) have difficulty with phonological processing is unclear. We and others have proposed that development of these morphological features is associated with misrouted fibers or extra synapses that interfere with efficient processing of phonetic or linguistic information (Hiemenz & Hynd, 2000). The assumption underlying this hypothesis is that gyral and sulcal formations reflect patterns of neuronal connectivity. There is some evidence in primate studies that supports this assumption. Gross neuroanatomical features are frequently associated with cellular and synaptic organization (Rakic, 1991), and it has been proposed that they result from the mechanical tension produced by axons connecting to neighboring structures (Van Essen, 1997). Altered neuronal connectivity could be associated with the anomalous parietal fissures and HG2, and explain different patterns of activation during functional imaging experiments.

Technical improvements in MRI have allowed these hypotheses to be tested. A recent study of dyslexia using diffusion-weighted imaging supports the notion that dyslexia is characterized by anomalous neuronal connectivity. A measure of diffusion anisotropy was bilaterally decreased in the temporoparietal white matter (Klingberg et al., 2000). Diffusion tensor imaging compares the speed of diffusion of water in different directions. More freely moving water indicates that a majority of the axons are oriented in the same direction. The authors interpreted their results as reflecting weakened neuronal connectivity in the arcuate fasciculus that connects Wernicke's and Broca's areas.

Perspectives on Perisylvian Cortex

Cortical morphology has not been analyzed in diffusion tensor and functional imaging studies. It would be interesting to know if weak anisotropy or activation is associated with extra gyri. Such studies could open up a new field of investigation directed at the relation between morphological and functional variation. For example, it is possible that the presence of extra gyri in parietal and temporal cortex might be negatively correlated with accuracy or speed of phonological processing. The current practice of averaging functional activation over individuals with different patterns of cortical morphology may obscure important functional and structural differences between individuals.

These morphological studies have highlighted a possible role for the parietal operculum in the development of dyslexia. But they also have another important message. Studies of dyslexia often identify subsets of individuals with an atypical neuroanatomical feature. Sixty percent of the dyslexic individuals in our first study had a type III pattern (Leonard et al., 1993). Four of the dyslexic individuals from the Hiemenz and Hynd (2000) study had a type II. Only a subset of dyslexic individuals from the Robichon et al. (2000) study had leftward parietal asymmetry. And a majority, but not all, of dyslexic individuals in our latest study had HG2. Hiemenz and Hynd suggest that each of these morphological features may predict a separate behavioral deficit associated with dyslexia. Another perspective, which is not inconsistent with the Hiemenz and Hynd proposal, is that there are multiple neural risk factors for developing dyslexia, and that their cumulative effect increases the probability of a diagnosis of dyslexia.

OTHER MORPHOLOGICAL EXPRESSIONS OF DEVIATIONS IN ASYMMETRY

The Corpus Callosum

Geschwind and Galaburda (1987) proposed that planar symmetry developed as a consequence of altered prenatal hormone levels which increased the size of the right PT. The presence of an enlarged planum in the right hemisphere might be associated with an increased number of axons crossing through the corpus callosum (CC), resulting in a larger CC. In addition, evidence that coordination of motor actions which might require interhemispheric transfer of information is impaired in dyslexia (Moore et al., 1995, 1996) oriented attention to the CC.

There is evidence that CC size is associated with testosterone levels in human (Moffat et al., 1997) and animal models (Nunez & Juraska,

1998). Variation in CC size has also been associated with sex and handedness, although an extensive review of 12 postmortem and 19 in vivo studies failed to find a consistent association of either handedness or sex with variation in CC size (Beaton, 1997). The results from studies examining the shape of the corpus callosum are equally inconsistent. The corpus callosum has been reported to be larger in dyslexic individuals, larger in females only, smaller in dyslexic individuals, or not different in dyslexic individuals and controls.

Why are the findings so inconsistent? These inconsistencies could result from different methods for measuring and subdividing the areas of the CC, definitions of handedness, and the effects of uncontrolled variation in brain size and other individual characteristics (Jäncke, Staiger, et al., 1997; Leonard, 1997).

Measurement Technique

The genu, rostrum, body, isthmus, and splenium of the CC have axons running through them from adjacent cortical regions. The areas of CC subdivisions are assumed to reflect the relative volumes of fibers connecting these regions. Although the gross size of the CC is easily estimated, there is no consensus on how to define these subdivisions. Some studies have attempted to replicate Witelson's (1989) division of the CC into seven areas (Lyoo et al., 1996). Others have divided the CC into sixths (Robichon & Habib, 1998), fifths (Duara et al., 1991; Hynd et al., 1995), or thirds (Pennington et al., 1999; Rumsey et al., 1996).

The differences would be of less concern if the shape of the CC did not vary so greatly from brain to brain. But since there is evidence that the shape of the CC differs in dyslexic individuals (Robichon, Bouchard, et al., 2000; Robichon & Habib, 1998) and females (Allen et al., 1991), it is possible that the number of fibers connecting particular homologous areas is different in CCs with different shapes. The relation between brain and CC size should be investigated in dyslexia to determine if interhemispheric connectivity presents another example of disregulated neural development.

Brain Size

Variation in brain size across a sample is another potential reason for inconsistent findings in studies of the CC. Brain size is controlled in most studies reporting larger sizes in dyslexia (Duara et al., 1991; Njio-kiktjien et al., 1994; Robichon & Habib, 1998; Rumsey et al., 1996). Only Hynd et al. (1995), who did not control for brain size, reported smaller CC volumes in dyslexic individuals than in controls. There is recent evidence that the relation between brain and CC size is not linear. It appears that the positive relationship between CC and brain size plateaus as brain size becomes very large (Jäncke, Staiger, et al., 1997). For this reason, reporting CC sizes that are corrected for brain size would be expected to produce smaller values for subjects with particularly large brains, compared to individuals with average brain size. The relation between brain and CC size should be investigated in dyslexia to determine if it is another example of disregulated neural development.

Demographics

A family history of dyslexia or learning disabilities and non-right-hand preference may interact with diagnosis to contribute to variation in CC size. Njiokiktjien and colleagues (1994) reported that children with a family history of dyslexia had a larger CC (controlling for midsagittal cortical surface area) size than controls of dyslexic individuals with a negative family history. Robichon and Habib (1998) reported a larger CC in dyslexic individuals with a dominant right-hand preference. Future studies should control for all these characteristics.

Summary

Efforts to define characteristics of the CC that distinguish dyslexic individuals have generated mixed results. Dyslexic individuals have been reported to have a larger CC and one that exhibits a greater curvature, with the splenium oriented more ventrally and more posterior than in controls. But studies have also shown dyslexic individuals to have a smaller anterior CC or a normal distribution of CC size. The differences in the findings are probably due to differences in methodology, demographics (diagnosis and handedness), brain size/sex differences, and are driven by subsets of individuals with particular characteristics. The small number of published studies of CC morphology and size in dyslexia is surprising. Although it is easier to obtain reliable measures of the CC than of the PT, there are many more published studies of the PT. The paucity of studies of the CC raises the specter of negative evidence sitting in many desk drawers.

THE CEREBELLUM

The cerebellum, like the cerebral cortex, is functionally lateralized and structurally asymmetric (Snyder et al., 1995). For example, the left cerebellum has been shown to be active during singing, while the right cerebellum is engaged during speech (Riecker et al., 2000). The cerebellum participates in the decoding and expression of articulatory sound patterns and the control of eye movements. A network of brain regions dedicated to decoding text into speech sounds probably includes parts of the oculomotor and articulatory control systems. Furthermore, children with learning disabilities often display motor signs that resemble those seen following cerebellar damage. For these reasons, it has been proposed that disregulation of cerebellar development contributes to a variety of developmental disorders (Diamond, 2000).

In the 1970s and 1980s a series of papers were published that described motor deficits in dyslexia (Levinson, 1988). The motor deficits were attributed to cerebellar dysfunction, and an attempt was made to treat dyslexia with motion sickness drugs. This treatment was rarely successful. There is, however, other evidence for a cerebellar role in the behavioral deficits associated with dyslexia. Nicolson and Fawcett (1990) have been more recent champions of the idea that dyslexic individuals exhibit motor coordination and balance deficits. They initially demonstrated an impairment on dual tasks in which children are required to balance on one foot and perform a supposedly automatized task such as counting backward. In a more recent study, they report that 95% of a large sample of dyslexic children exhibited a deficit of muscle tone or stability (Fawcett et al., 1996). These investigators maintain that every behavioral finding associated with dyslexia can be explained by a cerebellar impairment.

To address the cerebellar deficit hypothesis, we examined asymmetry of the anterior and posterior lobes of the cerebellum. These structures were chosen because the anterior lobe is associated with spinal and brain stem pathways controlling eye movements, balance, and posture, while the posterior lobe, by contrast, acts as a modulator of voluntary cortical activity (Bastian et al., 1999). The dyslexic group was more

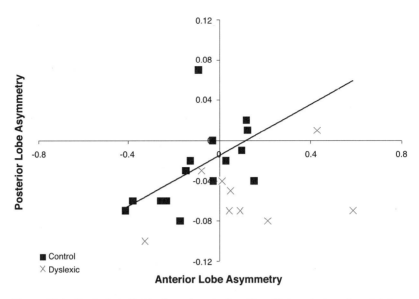

Figure 18.4 Dyslexic individuals and controls with a Steinmetz type I parietal operculum exhibit Woodcock-Johnson sound-blending performance superior to individuals with a type II or type III classification.

likely to have leftward asymmetry of the anterior lobe and rightward asymmetry of the posterior lobe (Leonard, Eckert, Lombardino, Oakland, et al., 2001). A more recent analysis of these data demonstrates a correlation between anterior and posterior lobe asymmetries in the controls, but not in the students with dyslexia (figure 18.4).

Biochemical asymmetries in the cerebellum have also been reported in dyslexia. MR spectroscopy can be used to examine the levels of choline, creatine, and N-acetylaspartate. These measures are thought to reflect cell density, cellular activity, and neuronal density, respectively. One group has reported that the ratio of choline to N-acetylaspartate was significantly lower in the right cerebellar hemisphere of dyslexic individuals compared to controls (Rae et al., 1998). The authors interpret their results as altered patterns of cell density in the right cerebellum.

Finally, results from a functional neuroimaging study also support the role of the cerebellum in dyslexia (Nicolson et al., 1999). A positron emission tomography (PET) study examined the cerebellar activation of dyslexic individuals and controls during motor learning tasks. Activation in the right cerebellar cortex was significantly lower in adult dyslexic individuals than in controls when performing a prelearned finger movement sequence and when learning a new sequence of finger movements.

Summary

Neuroimaging studies suggest altered cerebellar asymmetries in individuals with dyslexia. In some cases, the altered asymmetry is due to a small right cerebellum. The right cerebellum receives and projects information predominantly to the left hemisphere. One question yet to be addressed is whether a small right cerebellum is a unique predictor (phenotype) of dyslexia, or whether structural and functional alterations are a consequence of left hemisphere pathology.

THE FRONTAL LOBE

A few studies have suggested that dyslexia is associated with alterations in frontal lobe control of expressive functions such as rapid naming (Denckla & Rudel, 1976; Wolf, 1997). There are few studies examining frontal lobe structure and function in dyslexia, perhaps because of difficulty in measuring the convolutions of the frontal lobe reliably. An early structural imaging study of dyslexia provided neuroanatomical evidence for the possible involvement of the frontal lobe in dyslexia. Semrud-Clikeman and her colleagues (1991) examined the width of the frontal lobe in 10 controls, 10 dyslexic individuals, and 10 ADD children. A small right frontal width and atypical leftward frontal lobe symmetry were associated with poor passage comprehension and nonword decoding performance.

Structural findings in the frontal lobe have also been reported for children and adults with a history of developmental language disorder (Clarke, 1994; Gauger et al., 1997). Thus it is possible that the findings in the Semrud-Clikeman study reflect an association with language impairment rather than with specific phonological decoding deficits. Each of the three studies measured different structural characteristics of the frontal lobe, however, making comparisons risky.

A recent study has reported that dyslexic individuals were significantly more likely to have rightward asymmetry of Broca's area than were controls (Robichon, Levrier, et al., 2000). In addition the individuals that displayed the best non-word reading performance had leftward Broca's area asymmetry. The findings in this study directly contradict those in the Semrud-Clikeman study, but once again, different selection and measurement criteria could be responsible for the discrepancy.

These two studies are the only ones in the literature that examine frontal lobe anatomy in dyslexic individuals. The conflicting findings on the frontal lobe of dyslexic children and adults force the conclusion that the data are insufficient to determine whether there is a frontal structural signature for dyslexia. The small number of published studies on the frontal lobe probably reflects the difficulty involved in defining reliable anatomical boundaries for frontal gyri, and raise the question, once again, about the number of negative findings that might not have been reported.

IS THE SINGLE STRUCTURE APPROACH CONTRIBUTING DIMINISHING RETURNS?

The expectation that anomalous asymmetry of a single brain structure would characterize a complex behavioral disorder was perhaps somewhat naive. The studies reviewed in this chapter suggest that group differences are frequently influenced by a subset of individuals with a particular anatomical variant. With the exception of the original postmortem studies, no neuroanatomical study has found one atypical structure or anomalous asymmetry that characterizes every member of a diagnosed group.

The variety of neuroanatomical anomalies that identify subsets of dyslexic individuals is consistent with the idea that multiple etiological factors could influence the development of reading ability. Alternatively, the same causative factor could produce a variety of effects on a number of brain regions. For example, enlarged ventricles and white matter abnormalities are common in infants born prematurely (Cooke & Abernethy, 1999; Huppi et al., 1996) and are thought to result from hypoxic ischemia. Enlarged ventricles and white matter abnormalities are also more frequently identified in language-impaired children (Trauner et al., 2000). Together, these studies suggest that a particular event, such as perinatal hypoxia, could induce damage throughout the brain that negatively impacts language function. Whether premature birth or other prenatal and perinatal risk factors are also associated with anomalous asymmetry should be investigated.

It is also probably naive to expect that every neuroanatomical variant identified in dyslexic individuals is directly involved in the deficits associated with dyslexia. Structural anomalies could be a secondary loss or gain in tissue resulting from abnormal development of another brain region. This explanation has been proposed for the unexpected brain structure abnormalities identified in a family with articulation and language deficits (KE family) (Watkins et al., 1999). Affected members of the KE family had small caudate volumes bilaterally, and an elevated number of gray matter pixels in the superior temporal gyrus. Altered connectivity between the temporal lobe and basal ganglia was proposed to explain the altered morphology in the superior temporal gyrus.

MULTIDIMENSIONAL APPROACH TO PREDICTING DYSLEXIA

Genetic studies of dyslexia will probably identify multiple susceptibility genes that put people at risk for developing dyslexia. Each susceptibility gene is likely to have multiple mechanisms for expression. Penetrance (phenotypic expression) may be affected by a number of different specific or nonspecific risk and protective factors. If this argument is valid, it would be astounding if any single neuroanatomical predictor characterized a majority of individuals with dyslexia.

Although a single neuroanatomical marker has not been identified, a number of different brain structures have been implicated in the etiology of dyslexia. While some of these findings could be related to interacting variables such as sex and handedness, it is also possible that these studies have identified subtypes of reading disability.

Two recent studies from our laboratory used a multiple risk factor approach to predict group membership on the basis of the combination of multiple anatomical variables. This approach had proved successful in a study of schizophrenia, where brain volume, third ventricle volume, sylvian fissure length, and the continuity of two frontal sulci predicted diagnosis with 76% accuracy (Leonard et al., 1999). In the study of the dyslexic college students mentioned above, a different set of variables—the size of Heschl's second gyrus, the combined asymmetry of the planum temporale and the planum parietale, cerebral asymmetry, and anterior cerebellar asymmetry—predicted group membership.

When quantitative measures of these variables were normalized and summed, the reading-disabled students with persistent phonological deficits were separated from reading-disabled students whose phonological ability was average or superior (Leonard, Eckert, Lombardino, Oakland, et al., 2001). For each variable, more marked asymmetry characterized the students with a specific phonological impairment.

In a more recent study of 142 children, three additional anatomical variables were found to predict comprehension skill: reduced size of the first Heschl's gyrus, reduced cerebral volume, and rightward planar asymmetry (Leonard, Eckert, Lombardino, Givens, et al., 2001). When seven normalized, weighted anatomical measures of brain size and asymmetry were combined into one anatomical risk factor score, the dyslexic college students clustered on the negative side of the dimension, anatomical phenotype for phonological deficit (PD), while children with developmental language disorders clustered on the positive side, anatomical phenotype for language impairment (LI).

In a new sample of scans from 22 reading-disabled children from Virginia public schools provided by Guinevere Eden and Barbara Givens, the 12 children with an anatomical LI phenotype had significantly lower receptive language scores than the remaining 10 children. Only four of the children in this sample had an anatomical PD phenotype (i.e., anatomical risk factors for a specific reading disability). The disproportionate representation of children with LI phenotypes provides an anatomical validation of the selection criteria in this study, which included evidence of poor oral language skills.

Why would small symmetrical language structures be risk factors for a different type of reading impairment than large asymmetrical structures? We speculate that a small left PT and HG are associated with a smaller surface area for auditory processing, and constitute a risk factor for poor speech perception and subsequent compromised development of receptive language. Marked asymmetries and duplicated gyri may be protective factors that allow the development of lateralized cortical linguistic specializations, but increase the risk for mismatched auditory, visual and motor maps, as well as compromised development of visual-auditory associations and phonological decoding deficits. We feel the congruity of the anatomical evidence from three different samples suggests that specific (discrepant) reading disability and reading disability associated with oral language impairment have different anatomical phenotypes and different etiologies.

Our conclusion is consistent with modern concepts of distributed processing that regard reading and language ability as products of the integrated activity of many diverse processors (Clark, 1997; Elman et al., 1996). In a distributed processing network, one anomalous structure is very unlikely to cause a reading or language impairment, but as the number of anomalies grows, the risk increases. There also appears to be some specificity. Marked asymmetries and duplicated Heschl's gyri affect phonological decoding ability more than comprehension, while reduced volume of the cerebral hemispheres, and auditory structures in the left hemisphere (the first Heschl's gyrus and the planum temporale), affect comprehension more than phonological decoding. There also appears to be an interaction with the environment.

Children from middle-class households who have anomalous brain measurements are less likely to demonstrate reading and language impairments than children with similar measurements who are raised in poverty (Leonard, 2001). Since there is considerable evidence that impoverished families provide a considerably lower number of positive verbal messages to infants and children (Hart & Risley, 1995), we interpret the interaction between poverty and anatomy as support for the hypothesis that early linguistic input can compensate to some extent for anatomical risk factors for reading and language impairment. Such an interaction between environment and anatomical phenotype would provide another reason for inconsistency in anatomical studies of learning disability. If controls are middle-class children whose environment has compensated for their anatomical risk factors, while the experimental group for one reason or another has encountered less protective factors, there might be no anatomical differences found in the two groups. Future anatomical studies should attempt to control for early linguistic experience in reading-disabled and control groups.

SUMMARY

Pigeons with right-eye dominance excel at foraging for grain compared to their unlateralized brethren fowl (Güntürkün et al., 2000). It is possible that dyslexic students resemble left-eyed pigeons and have difficulty foraging for speech sounds in text. In pigeons, prenatal exposure of the right eye to light is the determinant for eye dominance. Perhaps prenatal and perinatal sensory input is one factor influencing the development of dyslexia. The epigenetic factors regulating brain development and the expression of dyslexia present a fascinating unexplored domain.

Recent experimental studies have provided little support for the position that dyslexia is a disorder related to anomalous planar asymmetry. Non-right-handedness and low verbal ability show stronger relations to anomalous planar asymmetry than dyslexia. Dyslexic individuals, in fact, may have a reduced tendency for rightward planar symmetry. Reduced planar symmetry in dyslexia could be an expression of disregulation of inter- and intrahemisphere asymmetry. Altered connectivity among these areas could lead to different and less efficient phonological processing strategies or paths. The presence of extraperisylvian gyri and decreased diffusion anisotropy in the temporoparietal white matter supports this notion.

FUTURE DIRECTIONS

Technological advances in structural and functional MRI studies and molecular approaches to understanding dyslexia are changing the zeitgeist in the world of reading disability. Functional imaging studies, in particular, have made important advances. The frontal lobe is more active, and the posterior temporal lobe less active, in dyslexic individuals than in controls during phonological tasks. The imaging studies do not explain why dyslexic individuals have different activation patterns, or the causal direction between activation and reading.

Functional activation can indicate what areas are active during different tasks, but to date it has been less informative about why areas or individuals differ. Information-processing strategies are likely to influence the areas of brain that are activated during a task (Reichle et al., 2000). The adoption of preferred strategies may be mediated by individual differences in neuroanatomy. A recent study suggests that the location of medial frontal lobe activation during a word generation task is dependent on the presence of a paracingulate sulcus (Crosson et al., 1999). On the basis of this finding, one might also predict that dyslexic individuals have decreased posterior temporal lobe activation due to the presence or absence of a particular neuroanatomical feature. Strangely, no one has investigated the anatomical characteristics of the posterior temporal motion-processing area thought to be disrupted in dyslexia.

Mark A. Eckert and Christiana M. Leonard

The results of the study by Crosson and his colleagues (1999) emphasize the importance of coupling functional and structural neuro-imaging studies. Functional imaging can guide neuroanatomical questions, but structural studies are essential to interpret the functional results. The use of functional and structural MRI has the potential to provide a more detailed understanding of reading and language disabilities.

REFERENCES

Allen, L. S., Richey, M. F., Chai, Y. M., & Gorski, R. A. (1991). Sex differences in the corpus callosum of the living human being. *Journal of Neuroscience, 11,* 933–942.

Bastian, A., Mugnaini, E., & Thach, W. T. (1999). Cerebellum. In M. J. Zigmond, F. E. Bloom, S. C. Landis, J. L. Roberts, & L. R. Squire (Eds.), *Fundamental neuroscience* (pp. 973–992). New York: Academic Press.

Beaton, A. A. (1997). The relation of planum temporale asymmetry and morphology of the corpus callosum to handedness, gender, and dyslexia: A review of the evidence. *Brain and Language, 60,* 255–322.

Bishop, D. V. M., & Adams, C. (1990). A prospective study of the relationship between specific language impairment, phonological disorders and reading retardation. *Journal of Child Psychology and Psychiatry, 31,* 1027–1050.

Clark, A. (1997). *Being there: Putting brain, body, and world together again.* Cambridge MA: MIT Press.

Clarke, G. M. (1994). The genetic basis of developmental stability. I. In T. A. Markow (Ed.), *Developmental instability: Its origins and evolutionary implications* (pp. 17–26). Dordrecht: Kluwer Academic Publishers.

Cooke, R. W., & Abernethy, L. J. (1999). Cranial magnetic resonance imaging and school performance in very low birth weight infants in adolescence. *Archives of Diseases of Children and Fetal Neonatal Education, 81*(2), F116–121.

Crosson, B., Sadek, J. R., Bobholz, J. A., Gokcay, D., Mohr, C., Leonard, C. M., Maron, L., Auerbach, E. J., Browd, S., Freeman, A. J., & Briggs, R. W. (1999). Medial frontal activity during word generation is centered within the paracingulate sulcus: An fMRI study of functional anatomy in 28 individuals. *Cerebral Cortex, 9,* 307–316.

Denckla, M., & Rudel, R. (1976). Rapid "automatized" naming (R.A.N.). Dyslexia differentiated from other learning disabilities. *Neuropsychologia, 14,* 471–479.

Diamond, A. (2000). Close interrelation of motor development and cognitive development and of the cerebellum and prefrontal cortex. *Child Development, 71,* 44–56.

Duara, R., Kuschch, A., Grossglenn, K., Barker, W. W., Jallad, B., Pascal, S., Loewenstein, D. A., Sheldon, J., Rabin, M., Levin, B., & Lubs, H. (1991). Neuroanatomic differences between dyslexic and normal readers on magnetic resonance imaging scans. *Archives of Neurology, 48*, 410–416.

Eckert, M. A., & Leonard, C. M. (2000). Structural imaging in dyslexia: The planum temporale. *Mental Retardation and Developmental Disabilities Research Reviews, 6*, 198–206.

Eckert, M. A., Lombardino, L. J., & Leonard, C. M. (2001). Tipping the environmental playground: Who is at risk for reading failure. *Child Development, 72*, 988–1002.

Elman, J., Bates, E., Johnson, M., Karmiloff-Smith, A., Parisi, D., & Plunkett, K. (1996). *Rethinking innateness: A connectionist perspective on development.* Cambridge MA: MIT Press.

Fawcett, A. J., Nicolson, R. I., & Dean, P. (1996). Impaired performance of children with dyslexia on a range of cerebellar tasks. *Annals of Dyslexia, 46*, 259–283.

Filipek, P. A. (1995). Neurobiological correlates of developmental dyslexia: How do dyslexic brains differ from those of normal readers? *Journal of Child Neurology, 10*, 62–69.

Fletcher, J. M., Shaywitz, S. E., Shankweiler, D. P., Katz, L., Liberman, I. Y., Stuebing, K. K., Francis, D. J., Fowler, A. E., & Shaywitz, B. A. (1994). Cognitive profiles of reading disability: Comparisons of discrepancy and low achievement definitions. *Journal of Educational Psychology, 86*, 1–23.

Foundas, A. L., Leonard, C. M., & Heilman, K. M. (1995). Morphological cerebral asymmetries and handedness: The pars triangularis and planum temporale. *Archives of Neurology, 52*, 501–508.

Galaburda, A. M. (1989). Ordinary and extraordinary brain development: Anatomical variation in developmental dyslexia. *Annals of Dyslexia, 39*, 67–79.

Galaburda, A. M., Sanides, F., & Geschwind, N. (1978). Human brain. Cytoarchitectonic left-right asymmetries in the temporal speech region. *Archives of Neurology, 35*, 812–817.

Galaburda, A. M., Sherman, G. F., Rosen, G. D., Aboitiz, F., & Geschwind, N. (1985). Developmental dyslexia: Four consecutive cases with cortical anomalies. *Annals of Neurology, 18*, 222–233.

Gauger, L. M., Lombardino, L. J., & Leonard, C. M. (1997). Brain morphology in children with specific language impairment. *Journal of Speech, Hearing & Language Research, 40*, 1272–1284.

Geschwind, N., & Galaburda, A. (1987). *Cerebral lateralization: Biological mechanisms, association and pathology.* Cambridge MA: MIT Press.

Geschwind, N., & Levitsky, W. (1968). Human brain: Left-right asymmetries in temporal speech region. *Science, 161*, 186–187.

Green, R. L., Hutsler, J. J., Loftus, W. C., Tramo, M. J., Thomas, C. E., Silberfarb, A. W., Nordgren, R. E., Nordgren, R. A., & Gazzaniga, M. S. (1999). The caudal infrasylvian surface in dyslexia: Novel magnetic resonance imaging-based findings. *Neurology, 53*, 974–981.

Güntürkün, O., Diekamp, B., Manns, M., Nottelmann, F., Prior, H., Schwarz, A., & Skiba, M. (2000). Asymmetry pays: Visual lateralization improves discrimination success in pigeons. *Current Biology, 10*(17), 1079–1081.

Hart, B., & Risley, T. R. (1995). *Meaningful differences*. Baltimore: Paul Brookes.

Haslam, R. H., Dalby, J. T., Johns, R. D., & Rademaker, A. W. (1981). Cerebral asymmetry in developmental dyslexia. *Archives of Neurology, 38*, 679–682.

Heiervang, E. (2000). Personal communication.

Heiervang, E., Hugdahl, K., Steinmetz, H., Inge Smievoll, A., Stevenson, J., Lund, A., Ersland, L., & Lundervold, A. (2000). Planum temporale, planum parietale and dichotic listening in dyslexia. *Neuropsychologia, 38*, 1704–1713.

Hiemenz, J. R., & Hynd, G. W. (2000). Sulcal/gyral pattern morphology of the perisylvian language region in developmental dyslexia. *Brain and Language, 74*, 113–133.

Hier, D. B., LeMay, M., Rosenberger, P. B., & Perlo, V. P. (1978). Developmental dyslexia: Evidence for a subgroup with a reversal of cerebral asymmetry. *Archives of Neurology, 35*, 90–92.

Huppi, P. S., Schuknecht, B., Boesch, C., Bossi, E., Felblinger, J., Fusch, C., & Herschkowitz, N. (1996). Structural and neurobehavioral delay in postnatal brain development of preterm infants. *Pediatric Research, 39*, 895–901.

Hynd, G. W., Hall, J., Novey, E. S., Eliopulos, D., Black, K., Gonzalez, J. J., Edmonds, J. E., Riccio, C., & Cohen, M. (1995). Dyslexia and corpus callosum morphology. *Archives of Neurology, 52*, 32–38.

Hynd, G. W., & Semrud-Clikeman, M. (1989). Dyslexia and brain morphology. *Psychological Bulletin, 106*, 447–482.

Hynd, G. W., Semrud-Clikeman, M., Lorys, A. R., Novey, E. S., & Eliopulos, D. (1990). Brain morphology in developmental dyslexia and attention deficit disorder/hyperactivity. *Archives of Neurology, 47*, 919–926.

Jäncke, L., Staiger, J. F., Schlaug, G., Huang, Y., & Steinmetz, H. (1997). The relationship between corpus callosum size and forebrain volume. *Cerebral Cortex, 7*, 48–56.

Jäncke, L., Wunderlich, G., Schlaug, G., & Steinmetz, H. (1997). A case of callosal agenesis with strong anatomical and functional asymmetries. *Neuropsychologia, 35*, 1389–1394.

Jernigan, T. L., Hesselink, J. R., Sowell, E., & Tallal, P. A. (1990). Cerebral morphology on MRI in language and learning-impaired children. *Archives of Neurology, 48*, 539–545.

Klingberg, T., Hedehus, M., Temple, E., Salz, T., Gabrieli, J. D., Moseley, M. E., & Poldrack, R. A. (2000). Microstructure of temporo-parietal white matter as a basis for reading ability: Evidence from diffusion tensor magnetic resonance imaging. *Neuron, 25*, 493–500. (See comments.)

Kushch, A., Gross-Glenn, K., Jallad, B., Lubs, H., Rabin, M., Feldman, E., & Duara, R. (1993). Temporal lobe surface area measurements on MRI in normal and dyslexic readers. *Neuropsychologia, 31*, 811–821.

Larsen, J. P., Høien, T., Lundberg, I., & Ødegaard, H. (1990). MRI evaluation of the size and symmetry of the planum temporale in adolescents with developmental dyslexia. *Brain and Language, 39*, 289–301.

LeMay, M., & Kido, D. K. (1978). Asymmetries of the cerebral hemispheres on computed tomogram. *Journal of Computer Assisted Tomography, 2,* 471–478.

Leonard, C. M. (1997). Corpus callosum: Sex or size? *Cerebral Cortex, 7,* 1.

Leonard, C. (2001). Structural imaging in children. *Learning Disabilities Quarterly, 42,* 158–176.

Leonard, C. M., Eckert, M. A., Lombardino, L. J., Givens, B. K., & Eden, G. F. (2001). Two anatomical phenotypes for reading impairment. Cognitive Neuroscience Society Annual Meeting Program: A Supplement of the Journal of Cognitive Neuroscience, 22.

Leonard, C. M., Eckert, M. A., Lombardino, L. J., Oakland, T., Kranzler, J., Mohr, C. M., King, W. M., & Freeman, A. J. (2001). Anatomical risk factors for phonological dyslexia. *Cerebral Cortex, 11,* 148–157.

Leonard, C. M., Kuldau, J. M., Breier, J. I., Zuffante, P. A., Gautier, E. R., Heron, D. C., Lavery, E. M., Packing, J., Williams, S. A., & DeBose, C. A. (1999). Cumulative effect of anatomical risk factors for schizophrenia: An MRI study. *Biological Psychiatry, 46,* 374–382.

Leonard, C. M., Lombardino, L. J., Mercado, L. R., Browd, S. R., Breier, J. I., & Agee, O. F. (1996). Cerebral asymmetry and cognitive development in children: A magnetic resonance imaging study. *Psychological Science, 7,* 79–85.

Leonard, C. M., Martinez, P., Weintraub, B. D., & Hauser, P. (1995). Magnetic resonance imaging of cerebral anomalies in subjects with resistance to thyroid hormone. *American Journal of Medical Genetics, 60,* 238–243.

Leonard, C. M., Puranik, C., Kuldau, J. M., & Lombardino, L. J. (1998). Normal variation in the frequency and location of human auditory cortex landmarks. Heschl's gyrus: Where is it? *Cerebral Cortex, 8,* 397–406.

Leonard, C. M., Voeller, K. S., Lombardino, L. J., Morris, M. K., Alexander, A. W., Andersen, H. G., Garofalakis, M. A., Hynd, G. W., Honeyman, J. C., Mao, J., Agee, O. F., & Staab, E. V. (1993). Anomalous cerebral structure in dyslexia revealed with magnetic resonance imaging. *Archives of Neurology, 50,* 461–469.

Levinson, H. N. (1988). The cerebellar-vestibular basis of learning disabilities in children, adolescents and adults: Hypothesis and study. *Perceptual and Motor Skills, 67,* 983–1006.

Lyoo, I. K., Noam, G. G., Lee, C. K., Lee, H. K., Kennedy, B. P., & Renshaw, P. F. (1996). The corpus callosum and lateral ventricles in children with attention-deficit hyperactivity disorder: A brain magnetic resonance imaging study. *Biological Psychiatry, 40,* 1060–1063.

Moffat, S. D., Hampson, E., Wickett, J. C., Vernon, P. A., & Lee, D. H. (1997). Testosterone is correlated with regional morphology of the human corpus callosum. *Brain Research, 767,* 297–304.

Moore, L. H., Brown, W. S., Markee, T. E., Theberge, D. C., & Zvi, J. C. (1995). Bimanual coordination in dyslexic adults. *Neuropsychologia, 33,* 781–793.

Moore, L. H., Brown, W. S., Markee, T. E., Theberge, D. C., & Zvi, J. C. (1996). Callosal transfer of finger localization information in phonologically dyslexic adults. *Cortex, 32,* 311–322.

Morgan, A., & Hynd, G. (1998). Dyslexia, neurolinguistic ability, and anatomical variation of the planum temporale. *Neuropsychology Review, 8,* 79–93.

Musiek, F. E., & Reeves, A. G. (1990). Asymmetries of the auditory areas of the cerebrum. *Journal of the American Academy of Audiology, 1,* 240–245.

Nicolson, R. I., & Fawcett, A. J. (1990). Automaticity: A new framework for dyslexia? *Cognition, 35,* 159–182.

Nicolson, R. I., Fawcett, A. J., Berry, E. L., Jenkins, I. H., Dean, P., & Brooks, D. J. (1999). Association of abnormal cerebellar activation with motor learning difficulties in dyslexic adults. *Lancet, 353*(9165), 1662–1667.

Njiokiktjien, C., de Sonneville, L., & Vaal, J. (1994). Callosal size in children with learning disabilities. *Behavioral Brain Research, 64,* 213–218.

Nottebohm, F. F., Stokes, T. M., & Leonard, C. M. (1976). Central control of song in the canary. *Journal of Comparative Neurology, 165,* 457–486.

Nunez, J. L., & Juraska, J. M. (1998). The size of the splenium of the rat corpus callosum: Influence of hormones, sex ratio, and neonatal cryoanesthesia. *Developmental Psychobiology, 33,* 295–303.

Orton, S. (1937). *Reading, writing, and speech problems in children.* New York: Norton.

Penhune, V. B., Zatorre, R. J., MacDonald, J. D., & Evans, A. C. (1996). Interhemispheric anatomical differences in human primary auditory cortex: Probabilistic mapping and volume measurement from magnetic resonance scans. *Cerebral Cortex, 6,* 661–672.

Pennington, B. F., Filipek, P. A., Lefly, D., Churchwell, J., Kennedy, D. N., Simon, J. H., Filley, C. M., Galaburda, A., Alarcon, M., & DeFries, J. C. (1999). Brain morphometry in reading-disabled twins. *Neurology, 53,* 723–729.

Plante, E., Swisher, L., & Vance, R. (1989). Anatomical correlates of normal and impaired language in a set of dizygotic twins. *Brain and Language, 37,* 643–655.

Plante, E., Swisher, L., Vance, R., & Rapcsak, S. (1991). MRI findings in boys with specific language impairment. *Brain & Language, 41,* 52–66.

Preis, S., Jäncke, L., Schitter, P., Huang, Y., & Steinmetz, H. (1998). Normal intrasylvian anatomical asymmetry in children with developmental language disorder. *Neuropsychologia, 9,* 849–855.

Pugh, K. R., Mencl, W. E., Jenner, A. R., Katz, L., Frost, S. J., Lee, J. R., Shaywitz, S. E., & Shaywitz, B. A. (2000). Functional neuroimaging studies of reading and reading disability (developmental dyslexia). *Mental Retardation and Developmental Disabilities Research Review, 6,* 207–213.

Rae, C., Lee, M. A., Dixon, R. M., Blamire, A. M., Thompson, C. H., Styles, P., Talcott, J., Richardson, A. J., & Stein, J. F. (1998). Metabolic abnormalities in developmental dyslexia detected by 1H magnetic resonance spectroscopy. *Lancet, 351,* 1849–1852.

Rakic, P. (1991). Plasticity of cortical development. In S. Brauth, W. Hall, & R. Dooling (Eds.), *Plasticity of development* (pp. 127–161). Cambridge, MA: MIT Press.

Reichle, E. D., Carpenter, P. A., & Just, M. A. (2000). The neural bases of strategy and skill in sentence-picture verification. *Cognitive Psychology, 40,* 261–295.

Riecker, A., Ackermann, H., Wildgruber, D., Dogil, G., & Grodd, W. (2000). Opposite hemispheric lateralization effects during speaking and singing at motor cortex, insula and cerebellum. *NeuroReport, 11,* 1997–2000.

Robichon, F., Bouchard, P., Demonet, J., & Habib, M. (2000). Developmental dyslexia: Re-evaluation of the corpus callosum in male adults. *European Neurology, 43,* 233–237.

Robichon, F., & Habib, M. (1998). Abnormal callosal morphology in male adult dyslexics: Relationships to handedness and phonological abilities. *Brain and Language, 62,* 127–146.

Robichon, F., Levrier, O., Farnarier, P., & Habib, M. (2000). Developmental dyslexia: Atypical cortical asymmetries and functional significance. *European Journal of Neurology, 7,* 35–46.

Rogers, L. (2000). Evolution of hemispheric specialization: Advantages and disadvantages. *Brain and Language, 73,* 236–253.

Rosenberger, P. B., & Hier, D. B. (1980). Cerebral asymmetry and verbal intellectual deficits. *Annals of Neurology, 8,* 300–304.

Rumsey, J. M., Casanova, M., Mannheim, G. B., Patronas, N., De Vaughn, N., Hamburger, S. D., & Aquino, T. (1996). Corpus callosum morphology, as measured with MRI, in dyslexic men. *Biological Psychiatry, 39,* 769–775.

Rumsey, J. M., Donahue, B. C., Brady, D. R., Nace, K., Giedd, J. N., & Andreason, P. (1997). A magnetic resonance imaging study of planum temporale asymmetry in men with developmental dyslexia. *Archives of Neurology, 54,* 1481–1489.

Rumsey, J. M., Dorwart, R., Vermess, M., Denckla, M. B., Kruesi, M. J., & Rapoport, J. L. (1986). Magnetic resonance imaging of brain anatomy in severe developmental dyslexia. *Archives of Neurology, 43,* 1045–1046.

Rumsey, J. M., Nace, K., Donohue, B. C., Wise, D., Maisog, J. M., & Andreason, P. (1997). A positron emission tomographic study of impaired word recognition and phonological processing in dyslexic men. *Archives of Neurology, 54,* 562–573.

Salmelin, R., Helenius, P., & Service, E. (2000). Neurophysiology of fluent and impaired reading: A magnetoencephalographic approach. *Journal of Clinical Neurophysiology, 17,* 163–174.

Schultz, R. T., Cho, N. K., Staib, L. H., Kier, L. E., Fletcher, J. M., Shaywitz, S. E., Shankweiler, D. P., Katz, L., Gore, J. C., Duncan, J. S., & Shaywitz, B. A. (1994). Brain morphology in normal and dyslexic children: The influence of sex and age. *Annals of Neurology, 35,* 732–742.

Semrud-Clikeman, M., Hynd, G., & Novey, E. S. (1991). Dyslexia and brain morphology: Relationships between neuroanatomical variation and neurolinguistic tasks. *Learning and Individual Differences, 3,* 225–242.

Shaywitz, S. E., Shaywitz, B. A., Pugh, K. R., Fulbright, R. K., Constable, R. T., Mencl, W. E., Shankweiler, D. P., Liberman, A. M., Skudlarski, P., Fletcher, J. M., Katz, L., Marchione, K. E., Lacadie, C., Gatenby, C., & Gore, J. C. (1998). Functional disruption in the organization of the brain for reading in dyslexia. *Proceedings of the National Academy of Sciences, USA, 95,* 2636–2641.

Simos, P. G., Breier, J. I., Fletcher, J. M., Bergman, E., & Papanicolaou, A. C. (2000). Cerebral mechanisms involved in word reading in dyslexic children: A magnetic source imaging approach. *Cerebral Cortex, 10,* 809–816.

Snyder, P. J., Bilder, R. M., Wu, H., Bogerts, B., & Lieberman, J. A. (1995). Cerebellar volume asymmetries are related to handedness: A quantitative MRI study. *Neuropsychologia, 33,* 407–419.

Stanovich, K. (1988). Explaining the differences between the dyslexic and the garden-variety poor reader. *Journal of Learning Disabilities, 21,* 590–604.

Steinmetz, H., Ebeling, U., Huang, Y., & Kahn, T. (1990). Sulcus topography of the parietal opercular region: An anatomic and MR study. *Brain and Language, 38,* 515–533.

Steinmetz, H., Rademacher, J., Jäncke, L., Huang, Y., Thron, A., & Zilles, K. (1990). Total surface of temporoparietal intrasylvian cortex: Diverging left-right asymmetries. *Brain and Language, 39,* 357–372.

Steinmetz, H., Volkmann, J., Jäncke, L., & Freund, H. J. (1991). Anatomical left-right asymmetry of language related temporal cortex is different in left- and right-handers. *Annals of Neurology, 29,* 315–319.

Trauner, D., Wulfeck, B., Tallal, P., & Hesselink, J. (2000). Neurological and MRI profiles of children with developmental language impairment. *Developmental Medicine and Child Neurology, 42,* 470–475.

Van Essen, D. (1997). A tension-based theory of morphogenesis and compact wiring in the central nervous system. *Nature, 385,* 313–318.

Watkins, K. E., Gadian, D. G., & Vargha-Khadem, F. (1999). Functional and structural brain abnormalities associated with a genetic disorder of speech and language. *American Journal of Human Genetics, 65,* 1215–1221.

Witelson, S. F. (1989). Hand and sex differences in the isthmus and genu of the human corpus callosum. A postmortem morphological study. *Brain, 113,* 799–835.

Witelson, S. F., Glezer, I. I., & Kigar, D. L. (1995). Women have greater density of neurons in posterior temporal cortex. *Journal of Neuroscience, 15,* 3418–3428.

Witelson, S. F., & Kigar, D. (1992). Sylvian fissure morphology and asymmetry in men and women: Bilateral differences in relation to handedness in men. *Journal of Comparative Neurology, 323,* 326–340.

Wolf, M. A. (1997). A provisional account of phonological and naming-speed deficits in dyslexia: Implications for diagnosis and intervention. In B. Blachman (Ed.), *Cognitive and linguistic foundations of reading acquisition: Implications for intervention research* (pp. 67–92). Hillsdale, NJ: Lawrence Erlbaum Associates.

19 Structural Correlates of Brain Asymmetry: Studies in Left-Handed and Dyslexic Individuals

Michel Habib and Fabrice Robichon

Although right-hand preference, the best-known example of cerebral dominance, may be traced virtually unchanged through the history of humankind (Coren & Porac, 1977), it was not until the middle of the nineteenth century, with the discovery by Dax and Broca regarding lateralization of language, that the concept of brain asymmetry emerged. Since that time, the concept has gained support from continuing and converging evidence, drawn from sources as varied as brain lesioned patients, split-brain individuals, and experimental investigation in normal subjects, to cite only a few. Today there is hardly a discussion in the field of behavioral neurology where mention is not made of issues of lateralization of function or hemispheric specialization.

Whereas interest in functional asymmetry has caught the scientific eye for a long time, it is only since the 1980s that anatomical and biological associations of cerebral dominance have become a subject of systematic investigation, mainly under the energetic and pioneering impulse of one of the greatest figures of modern neurology, Norman Geschwind. In his quest for the biological underpinnings of cerebral dominance, Geschwind systematically put forward left-handers and dyslexics as two special populations most likely to hold valuable indices as to the mechanisms leading to the brain's asymmetrical functioning (Geschwind & Behan, 1982, 1984; see also Bryden et al., 1994; Hugdahl, 1994). But probably the most remarkable contribution of Geschwind was his apparently trivial idea—which proved to be a genial intuition—that looking at structural asymmetry of the brain may provide crucial information on the origins and intimate mechanisms of brain laterality, an idea that gave rise to hundreds of subsequent investigations which, up to now, have not yet yielded the key of the enigma.

In this chapter, we will review anatomical studies of brain asymmetry carried out following Geschwind's seminal contribution, focusing on these two main populations—left-handers and dyslexics—in the specific perspective of understanding the biological bases of brain lateralization.

ANATOMICAL STUDIES OF ASYMMETRY IN THE NORMAL HUMAN BRAIN

From Broca to Geschwind

While commenting on his discovery of a "center for articulate language" in the left hemisphere of the human brain, Broca stated: "It is quite certain that the two hemispheres of the brain are similar; if cerebral convolutions, indeed, display light and incidental variations from individual to individual, there are none which one could notice between either sides of the encephalon" (Broca, 1865). Yet, not much later, anatomists started studying morphological differences between the hemispheres in more detail. Initially, the weights of the hemispheres were compared (Charpy, 1889; Giacomini & Luys, in Moutier, 1908); some found the left to be heavier and others, the right. Broca himself (1875) had noticed that the right hemisphere was heavier, but others stated that this was the result of decreased right side cortex in the face of excess of white matter (Moutier, 1908). Likewise, the left hemisphere was said to be longer, especially in its posterior pole, as initially found by Cunningham (1892) and then Smith (1907), studying the posterior impressions left by the brain's occipital lobe on the skull inner surface (so-called petalia). Measuring, on coronal slices, the hemispheres' widths in 200 brains, Inglessis (1919) found a larger left frontal lobe in 55% of the brains and a larger left occipital lobe in 89%. Finally, at midcentury, Connolly (1950) measured fetal and infant brains and found a longer left hemisphere in 64%, whereas the reversed asymmetry was present in only 27%. In 1962, the respected anatomist Gerhard von Bonin, assessing asymmetry evidence obtained up until then, concluded that side differences were too small to explain such striking right-left asymmetries as the left hemisphere specialization of language.

Michel Habib and Fabrice Robichon

Geschwind and the Planum Temporale

Paradoxically, the apparently discouraging conclusions of Von Bonin (1962), which seemed to deal a severe blow to any theory linking brain asymmetries to functional lateralization, served to stimulate Norman Geschwind to reexamine the available data. In 1968, he and Walter Levitsky published a short paper in *Science* that acted as a a starter for an impressive scientific endeavor that some have called a "new phrenology," and others, "cognitive neuroanatomy": the search for a structural basis to cerebral dominance. Starting from an earlier report by Pfeifer (1936), a student of the German anatomist Fleischig, Geschwind and Levitsky measured the length of the planum temporale, a region of auditory associative cortex lying on the inner temporal bank of the posterior sylvian fissure, posterior to the primary auditory cortex, or Heschl's gyrus, which forms its anterior border. In 100 autopsy specimens, for which neither sex nor handedness data were available, they found that 65% showed a longer left planum, whereas the right planum was longer in 11% and 24% of the brains showed equal lengths. On the average, the planum proved to be 30% longer on the left hemisphere.[1]

The planum temporale is a triangle-shaped structure thought to be part of the classical Wernicke's area (i.e., one the two regions of the left hemisphere whose role in language has been reliably established). Moreover, available literature on results of sodium amytal intracarotid experiments had solidly established that for a large majority of the population, language functions are lateralized to the left hemisphere. Therefore, Geschwind and Levistky proposed this pattern of morphological asymmetry as the neural substrate of language lateralization.

These results were essentially replicated in several subsequent studies (see table 19.1), some of them providing the important additional information that such asymmetries are also present in fetuses and neonates (see below).

Globally, the anatomical studies summarized in table 19.1 yield a figure of 73% left-sided planum asymmetry, with symmetry or reversed asymmetry roughly equal (respectively 13% and 11.7%).

Other Cortical Asymmetries

Several other investigations carried out during the same period showed the planum asymmetry was but one of the asymmetries demonstrable

Table 19.1 Survey of 14 anatomical studies reporting measurement of planum tempo-rale asymmetry on adult human brains

Studies	Population	L > R (%)	R = L (%)	R > L (%)
Von Economo & Horn, 1930	10	56	33	11
Fukui, 1934	75	75	12	13
Geschwind & Levitsky, 1968	100	65	24	11
Tezner et al., 1972	100	64	26	10
Witelson & Pallie, 1973	16	69	0	31
Wada et al., 1975	100	82	8	10
Rubens et al., 1976	21	67		
Kopp et al., 1977	83	77	1	22
Galaburda et al., 1978	4	75	0	25
Nikkuni et al., 1981	54	83	9	8
Falzi et al., 1982	12	83	0	17
Pieniadz & Naeser, 1984	15	73	20	7
Larsen et al., 1989	10	70	30	
Steinmetz et al., 1990	10	80	20	0

on the neocortical surface, other important one being asymmetry of the sylvian fissures themselves. As early as 1884, Eberstaller had noted that the sylvian fissure was 6.4 mm longer, on average, on the left hemisphere compared to the right. Cunningham (1892) added that the posterior extent of the left sylvian fissure was more horizontal. Connolly (1950) confirmed these early findings in 73 brains, where he found an average greater length of 4.4 mm on the left side.

Sylvian fissure asymmetries have been reevaluated by Yeni-Komshian and Benson (1976), who reported a longer left fissure in 84% of 25 brains. Rubens et al. (1976), in 36 brains, superimposed the course of the left and right fissures and found in one group (25 cases) the standard left > right asymmetry; in the other (11 cases) the brains exhibited either no asymmetry or the reverse pattern. Interestingly, these authors found that this difference was significant only if one considered the horizontal portion of the posterior sylvian fissure; it became nonsignificant if the entire sylvian length was considered. Finally, in the same sample, they found that leftward asymmetry of the planum was present in only 67%. In a preliminary anatomical study designed to serve as

Michel Habib and Fabrice Robichon

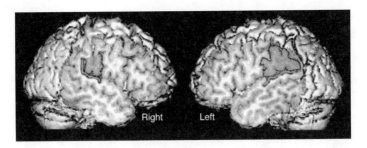

Figure 19.1 Typical asymmetry of the posterior sylvian region on 3D MRI images with superimposed sagittal section. Whereas the planum temporale is roughly symmetrical, the parietal operculum (shaded area within the rounded contours) is clearly larger in the left hemisphere.

reference for subsequent MRI studies, our group (Habib et al., 1984) had already drawn attention to the fact that the shape of the sylvian fissures, whose asymmetry occurs in roughly the same proportion of brains as planum asymmetry, affects the appearance of the whole posterior region of the hemisphere in such a way that in typical cases, the parietal operculum, situated between the central sulcus and the posterior end of the Sylvian fissure, is larger on the left, whereas the adjacent parieto-occipital region, including the supramarginal and angular gyri, is larger on the right, which could be related to the right-hemisphere specialization for attentional and spatial processes (Eidelberg & Galaburda, 1984). This aspect is particularly evident on sagittal cuts of the hemispheres, where the whole extent and direction of the sylvian fissure can be delineated and, as a consequence, the parietal lobes' asymmetry clearly demonstrated (figure 19.1).

More recently, there have been several attempts to classify the individual patterns of posterior sylvian anatomy. In particular, several authors have considered as crucial anatomically the point where the sylvian fissure changes its direction, delimiting an anterior or horizontal segment from a posterior or vertical segment. In several instances, it has been reported that the fissure actually trifurcates at this point, since there is sometimes also a small inferior ramus descending 2 to 5 mm posteriorly and inferiorly. As reported by Witelson and Kigar (1992), Steinmetz et al. (1990), and Aboitiz et al. (1992), a horizontal type of posterior ending of the sylvian fissure is more often observed on left hemispheres, whereas a purely ascending end is more typical of right

Structural Correlates of Brain Asymmetry

hemispheres. Finally, Foundas et al. (1999) confirmed the usual asymmetry of the posterior sylvian fissure and its different effects on the right and left parietal lobes.

The Reliability of Planum Measurements

One important point resulting from these observations is that such global asymmetry of the posterior sylvian region raises some uncertainty about any measurement of the planum temporale, the posterior limit of which, in particular, is subject to discussion (Rubens et al., 1976; Witelson & Kigar, 1988; Steinmetz et al., 1990). Without entering a mostly theoretical and often academic debate about what should be the actual boundaries of the planum temporale, it is important to report here the main objects of the discussion (see Shapleske et al., 1999, and Beaton, 1997 for two recent accounts of this debate). The first point concerns the anterior limit of the planum. As early as 1936, Pfeifer reported hemispheric differences in the anterior border of the planum (i.e., the transverse or Heschl's gyrus). The latter was usually more oblique on the left than on the right hemisphere, which could participate to the usual pattern of a wider left surface of the planum. Probably more problematic for any study of this region is Pfeifer's observation, later confirmed (see, e.g., Campain & Minckler, 1976), that there are often two Heschl's gyri, called first and second transverse gyri, on the right hemisphere and only one on the left. This raises the question of which one of the two must be taken as the anterior limit in measurements of the planum temporale. The consensus is that the second (more posterior) transverse gyrus, when it exists, must be included in the planum surface. This, of course, could artificially increase the degree of asymmetry, since such duplication of the transverse gyrus occurs more often on the right than on the left.

Another, more problematic issue is that of the posterior boundary. In their initial study, Geschwind and Levitsky analyzed postmortem specimens that had been cut "by passing a knife blade along the Sylvian fissure" in order to separate the superior temporal plane from the rest of the hemisphere. It is obvious, even from the original illustrations of Geschwind himself (Geschwind, 1979), that this mode of sectioning the brains may have affected the right and left hemispheres differently, due to differences in orientation of the posterior segment of the Sylvian fissure. If that were the case, then this would weaken the reliability of

Michel Habib and Fabrice Robichon

the initial results, even though they have been replicated with other methodologies (see, e.g., Teszner et al., 1972; Steinmetz et al., 1990).

In this context, further precisions are provided in a re-assessment of these initial data by Galaburda et al. (1987). These authors examined the photographs taken of the brains from the Geschwind and Levitsky study and measured the planum surface using a planimeter. Their illustration of the measurement method (p. 855) dispels any doubt about the validity of the initial results, which are confirmed by this reevaluation. It shows that photographs were in fact taken perpendicular to the plane of the posterior sylvian fissure, whatever its degree of obliquity. However, it is clear, as noticed by Shapleske et al. (1999), that such planimetric measurement cannot take into account all possible irregularities of the planum surface, a problem also raised by Steinmetz et al. (1990, Steinmetz, 1996) who pointed out that the degree of cortical folding is more variable for the right planum than for the left.

Asymmetries of the Inferior Frontal Region

Broca's area in the left inferior frontal region is defined, not without a touch of circular reasoning, as the region that, when damaged, results in Broca's aphasia. Broca himself considered the region that bears his name as including the pars opercularis ("pied de la troisième frontale"), pars triangularis ("cap"), and pars orbitalis, in decreasing order of importance. Stengel (1930) showed that the foot of Broca (pars opercularis) was more developed on the left in 9 of 11 cases, and Falzi et al. (1982), in 12 brains from right-handers, found a greater surface area on the left in nine cases. Galaburda (1980), using photographs of the brains studied by Geschwind and Levitsky (1968), found branching of the ascending limb of the sylvian fissure, which separates the opercular and triangular regions, to be present in 27 out of 102 left hemispheres, but only 13 right hemispheres. On the contrary, Wada et al. (1975) found better development of the right opercular region, but emphasized that if the cortex buried within the sulci were considered, the result could be different. Albanese et al. (1989) found in 24 postmortem specimens that 62.5% showed a left predominance, and 12.5% a right predominance in both weight and cortical surface. Finally, none of the studies published to date has found a strict relationship between asymmetry in the planum temporale and in the frontal operculum, even for those cases with reversed asymmetry.

Cytoarchitectonic Studies

One of the questions raised by the findings of gross anatomical asymmetries was whether they reflected true physiological asymmetries that could be demonstrated at the microscopic level. Therefore, it was asked whether architectonic areas of specific cellular and connectional organization, thus reflecting functional specialization, also exhibited asymmetries in size between the sides. Von Economo and Horn (1930) suggested that planum asymmetry could be the result of the larger extent of auditory cortex on the left temporal lobe, especially areas TB and TA1, which surround the primary auditory cortex TC. Galaburda, Sanides, and Geschwind (1978) carried out a morphometric architectonic study on serially sectioned human brains, which permitted the measurement of the full volume of each architectonic area. They found, in four postmortem specimens, that an area called Tpt, roughly corresponding to Von Economo's area TA1, was larger on the left side in the brains that had a larger left planum temporale. Area Tpt, which lies partly on the planum temporale and partly on the external aspect of the superior temporal gyrus, displays features transitional between those of a specific auditory association cortex and those of the supramodal inferior parietal lobule (Galaburda & Sanides, 1980). An important contribution has been provided by Witelson et al. (1995), who demonstrated that area 22 actually extends beyond the usual boundaries of the planum temporale, namely, on the posterior bank of the parietal ascending ramus of the sylvian fissure. In other words, this observation strongly suggests inclusion of all the intrasylvian cortex, including the ascending ramus when it exists, while measuring asymmetry of the planum temporale. Such a conclusion could invalidate the conclusions of a number of studies published (see below).

Few investigators have tried to approach the structural concomitants of area asymmetry. Galaburda et al. (1990) have shown in a rodent model that two asymmetrical homologous areas are more likely to differ in number of neurons than in their density. Different conclusions have been reached, however, by two important recent works. First, Anderson et al. (1999) have analyzed 16 postmortem brains to compare macroscopic temporal asymmetry (width, height, and length of the planum temporale as well as the total volume of the posterior superior temporal lobe) with structural patterns of the same brains (neuronal density, glial cell volume, and axon diameters). Their conclusion was

Michel Habib and Fabrice Robichon

that asymmetry could be explained neither by neuronal density nor by glial cell volume differences, and that differences in axonal myelination could be the relevant factor. Even more convincingly, Galuske et al. (2000) have shown that asymmetry in area 22 is strongly linked to a different organization of the "intrinsic microcircuitry," a term referring to the regularly spaced clusters of neurons that characterize this cortical area, and the spacing of these clusters. More specifically, a larger area 22 in the left hemisphere is indicative of more interdigitation of the columnar subsystems on the left, and thus more complex functional connectivity. On the other hand, the number of columnar clusters is not increased on the left, and their spacing is not asymmetrical for other areas such as the primary auditory cortex. The authors conclude that these different patterns of connectivity between the two hemispheres could be due in part to use-dependent modifications of circuitry during development, most probably under the influence of early exposure to human language.

Such a conclusion hardly seems compatible with those of the above-reported studies showing that posterior sylvian asymmetries are also present, in similar proportions, on neonate brains and even in fetal brains as early as the 30th gestational week (Teszner et al., 1972; Wada et al., 1975). In other words, it would be very unlikely that asymmetries could arise only under the effect of language learning. More probably the truth lies in between, a genetically predetermined pattern of asymmetry being reinforced under the influence of specific environmental experience. One fascinating hypothesis, suggested by Anderson et al. (1999), is be that larger intracortical connectivity in the left planum temporale, which is reflected in more myelinated fibers, entails more rapid processing, allowing the left hemisphere alone to process rapidly changing auditory stimuli such as those constitutive of the human speech (Tallal et al., 1995).

HANDEDNESS AND BRAIN ASYMMETRY: A CASE FOR A NEW PHRENOLOGY

Central to Geschwind's theory of the biological bases of brain lateralization was the concept of a close relationship between anatomical and functional asymmetry. Specifically, the pattern of morphological asymmetry of the language areas—especially the planum temporale, whose asymmetry has been best documented—would be predictive of the degree of lateralization of language. In vivo brain imaging methods soon appeared ideally suited for this purpose. However, providing evidence of such a relationship necessitates (1) having a good indicator of language laterality and (2) possessing reliable information about both anatomical asymmetry and language dominance in the same subjects. This clearly proved to be beyond early investigators, who had at their disposal only either postmortem brains with few if any indications of the subjects' characteristics, or series of living volunteers explorable only with poorly informative methods of brain investigation, such as carotid angiograms or early CT scans that clearly were unable to yield any accurate information about the morphology of the language cortical areas and, a fortiori, to perform measurements of specific areas (see Witelson, 1992, for a review of these early works). Nevertheless, early investigators initiated a current of thought that can be called "cognitive neuroanatomy" (Witelson & Kigar, 1992) by relating one anatomical index of asymmetry to the most easily accessible manifestation of brain lateralization, the degree and/or type of handedness.

The Rationale for Studying the Handedness/Brain Asymmetries Relationship

Besides studies exploring the relationship of handedness to the motor cortex asymmetries, which will not be reviewed here (see, e.g., Amunts et al., 1996), all studies of this type are based on the postulate of a link between language lateralization and handedness. In theory, the only valid indicator of language lateralization would be language itself. The hemispheric representation of language competence can mainly be assessed in three different ways: the highly invasive Wada (amytal) test, the poorly controllable model of brain lesions causing aphasia, and the sophisticated but methodologically debated dichotic listening procedure. In fact, the well-documented tight statistical link between language lateralization and handedness has encouraged researchers to use dichotic listening as equivalent, though indirectly, to language lateralization.

Rather than a mere indicator of language lateralization, Geschwind considered handedness as the manifestation of an individual belonging to one of two distinct subpopulations: people with "standard dominance" and the population with "atypical (or anomalous) dominance," a typology that has been severely criticized (see, e.g., Annett, 2000).

Michel Habib and Fabrice Robichon

However, beyond a simple way of classifying the population according to a specific behavioral trait, Geschwind attributed a biological relevance to this typology, asserting that strongly right-handers benefit fully from a natural and universal (probably genetic) tendency toward a left hemiphere bias of handedness, language, and planum asymmetry, whereas in left-handers and the ambidextrous, all these variables are randomly distributed, possibly due to the influence of nongenetic factors on the processes leading to brain asymmetry (Geschwind & Galaburda, 1985; see also Bryden et al., 1994 for an in-depth discussion of this theory). From this point of view, handedness, being classified into these two categories, appears as a biologically relevant variable that can usefully stand for the classical accounts of language lateralization.

It is not our purpose here to discuss the validity of handedness as an indicator of brain lateralization. Suffice it to say that two specific topics are the main subjects of debate: (1) the definition and assessment of handedness, either as preferential use of one limb or by comparing the efficiency of right and left hands in specific motor tasks (such as Annett's peg board, for example), with a tendency to consider efficiency as more reliable but a consensus to use preference questionnaires instead, since they are simpler to perform and are strongly correlated (Porac & Coren, 1981); and (2) the mode of classifying subjects according to a preference questionnaire, either as a continuous variable or as a dichotomous one, and, when the latter mode is chosen, the issue of determining an arbitrary cutoff point. All these issues are extensively discussed elsewhere (see, e.g., Annett, 1985; Steenhuis & Bryden, 1989; Witelson & Kigar, 1988; Bryden et al., 1994, as well as in other chapters of this book), and will not be reviewed here.

Magnetic Resonance Imaging: The Ideal Tool

The first anatomically reliable studies in this area appeared with the introduction of magnetic resonance imaging (MRI), so far the only method able to display, with total safety, the cortical anatomy with a precision comparable to postmortem studies. MRI is even superior to macroscopic anatomy from several points: the intactness of the brain, which avoids distorsions often present on postmortem specimens, the simpleness of obtaining any kind of measurement thanks to adequate software, and the easy access to information in several planes simultaneously, with tridimensional imaging and the possibility of surface rendering of the hemispheres' convexity.

In an exploratory anatomical study (Habib et al., 1984), which just preceded the generalization of MRI in neurology, we investigated on cadaver brains the possibility to assess macroscopic asymmetries in different section planes and came to the conclusion that sagittal sections would be best suited to analyzing posterior sylvian anatomy. Moreover, these sections provide a good view of both the temporal surface and the parietal opercular region, allowing the measurement of these two regions with optimal precision and the calculation of an asymmetry coefficient $(L - R/0.5[L + R])$. We began to use this method in 20 young adults (Habib, 1989) in whom the planum temporale was measured (along with the callosal surface; see below). Handedness was assessed with the Edinburgh Handedness Inventory (Oldfield, 1971), classifying subjects into strong right-handers (+80 and more) and nonconsistent right-handers (including left-handers and the ambidextrous). Correlation studies showed that right-handers tended to display a more left-biased asymmetry coefficient, whereas left- and mixed-handers showed, on average, a symmetrical planum area.

In a subsequent study (Habib et al., 1995), the same method was applied to 40 volunteers, with an additional measure of the region of the parietal lobe situated in front of the planum, on the other bank of the sylvian fissure: the parietal operculum. In this study, the parietal measure was obtained by tracing a line from the posterior ending point of the sylvian fissure and projecting orthogonally on the central sulcus. Asymmetry coefficients were then calculated for each measurement, planum and operculum. For both regions, a significantly left-biased asymmetry was observed, more so for the parietal operculum (28/40 = 70%) than for the planum temporale (25/40 = 63%).

Interestingly, no significant correlation emerged between the two anatomical asymmetries, suggesting that they vary independently and may be either convergent or divergent. Finally, the main focus of this study was the distribution of asymmetries according to handedness. As summarized in figure 19.2, the convergence of the two asymmetries toward the left side was strongly predictive of right-handedness, since this pattern was associated with right-handedness in 90% of the cases. When only the Planum was asymmetrical to the left, there were as many non-right-handers as right-handers. Finally, rightward asymme-

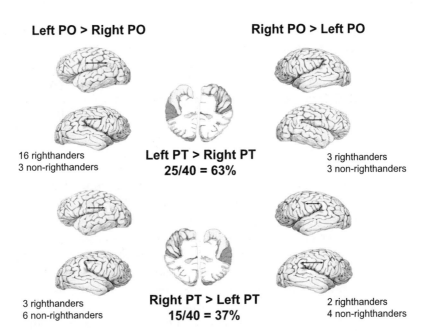

Left PO > Right PO

Right PO > Left PO

16 righthanders
3 non-righthanders

Left PT > Right PT
25/40 = 63%

3 righthanders
3 non-righthanders

3 righthanders
6 non-righthanders

Right PT > Left PT
15/40 = 37%

2 righthanders
4 non-righthanders

Figure 19.2 Symmetry of an MRI study of cortical asymmetries of the planum temporale (PT) and parietal operculum (PO) in 40 volunteers. The conjunction of leftward asymmetry of both indices predicts right-handedness in 90% of the cases. (From Habib et al., 1995.)

try of the planum temporale yielded twice as many non-right-handers as right-handers.

Planum Temporale: The End of a Myth?

Several other groups have carried out similar MRI/handedness studies. Kertesz et al. (1986) were the first to exploit the possibilities of the new method and in 20 subjects found a sharper demarcation of the right posterior sylvian fissure in 60% of right-handers and only 10% of left-handers. Steinmetz et al. (1991) reported a first series of 52 subjects and found no significant difference in planum asymmetry between 26 self-reported right-handers and 26 self-reported left-handers. However, a correlation was found with performance of a dexterity task, those with right-hand advantage more often showing leftward planum asymmetry. One important difference from our own study is thus the mode of measurement of handedness. However, another major methodological point explaining the discrepancies between the two studies is the mode of measurement of the planum temporale: in accordance with our suggestion (Habib et al., 1984), Steinmetz also uses sagittal sections, but his definition of the planum temporale differs, since it excludes any posterior ascendant portion of the sylvian fissure, which in our experience is often indistinguishable from the planum itself, and thus should not be systematically separated (Habib et al., 1995). In a subsequent study, this opposing view is even clearer. Jäncke et al. (1994) proposed the name "planum parietale" for the posterior bank of the posterior ascending ramus of the sylvian fissure, a part that we include in our definition of the planum temporale. However, as often observed (see, e.g., Foundas et al., 1994, 1995, 1996; Moffat et al., 1998, p. 2372 for a typical illustration), the absence of clear demarcation between horizontal and vertical rami leads the investigators to use the "knife cut method," which totally arbitrarily "cuts" the planum along the axis of the sylvian fissure.

As reported above, cytoarchitectonic data provide strong arguments in favor of a continuity between the temporal and "parietal" bank of the posterior infrasylvian cortex, and militates against the suggestion of Jäncke et al. (1994) that the planum parietale is part of the multimodal cortex of area 40 or 39. Instead, it is probable that in cases where the planum temporale is totally absent, as may sometimes occur in right hemispheres, the planum parietale (or posterior bank of the vertical sylvian fissure) comprises association auditory cortex of the area 22 type (Witelson et al., 1995).

In any case, this small region of cortex was found to be asymmetrical toward the right side in a majority of right-handers (Jäncke et al., 1994). This, however, may well be an artifact linked to the more frequent pattern of upward curving of the end of the sylvian fissure in right hemispheres, a typical pattern probably more frequent in right-handers (see figure 19.1). As a consequence, all studies having shown an effect of planum asymmetry on a behavioral measure may in fact have shown a correlation between the behavioral measure and a global pattern of asymmetry of the whole posterior sylvian region. As early as 1976, Rubens et al. noticed that "measures of planum temporale asymmetry alone provide only a partial indication of the anatomic differences underlying functional hemispheric asymmetry." The same authors,

Michel Habib and Fabrice Robichon

examining the classical architectonic studies of Von Economo and Horn (1930), concluded that "gross measurements of planum temporale asymmetry would not be a valid measure of auditory parakoniocortex asymmetry," a conclusion which has since been confirmed by Witelson et al. (1995) and accepted by others (Loftus et al., 1993; Westbury et al., 1999). Finally, these data support the conclusions of Binder et al. (1996), who showed with functional imaging that, contrary to several language areas which responded to speech more than to nonspeech tones, the left planum temporale responds equally to speech and nonspeech. They concluded that "it is the shape rather than the size of the posterior sylvian fissure which is asymmetric."

Finally, it is our opinion, and that of an increasing number of researchers in the field, that in studies thus far carried out on brain asymmetries, the planum temporale has been both overemphasized and often improperly defined (and thus improperly measured), an error that may have originated in the fact that in the influential Geschwind-Levitsky study, all brain tissue above the sylvian fissure had been removed.

Language, Handedness, and Brain Asymmetry

Since handedness, taken as reflecting left lateralization of language, has been found to influence the degree of temporal and parietal asymmetry, one would have expected the few studies that have investigated language asymmetry to find a similar or ever stronger correlation to asymmetry in anatomy. Such was not the case.

In the same population as in the first Steinmetz et al. handedness study, Jäncke and Steinmetz (1993) explored auditory lateralization with four verbal dichotic listening tasks. Surprisingly, none of them proved to be significantly linked to planum asymmetry. One year earlier, Kertesz et al. (1992) had failed to find an association of auditory asymmetry with a more global measure of anatomical asymmetry. Subsequently, Foundas et al. (1994) measured the planum temporale in 12 patients who had undergone Wada amytal testing. Of the 11 with left-hemisphere language, as demonstrated from intracarotid hemispheric inactivation, all had a larger left planum temporale. The only patient with right-hemisphere language (and left-handedness) had rightward asymmetry of the planum temporale. Hellige et al. (1998) examined 27 right-handers and 3 left-handers with a tachistoscopic procedure where subjects had to identify CVC trigrams presented to either hemisphere. A measurement of the sylvian length and planum temporale surface was performed. Of the multiple possible effects, the only significant correlation was found between the length of the right sylvian fissure and the number of errors in trigram identification in the left visual field/right hemisphere. Asymmetry of the planum temporale proved to be unrelated to any behavioral measure.

On the other hand, Moffat et al. (1998) did find significant differences in planum temporale asymmetry, within a group of left-handed males, between those classified as left-hemisphere-dominant for language and those classified as right-hemisphere-dominant on the basis of the Fused Dichotic Words Test, a dichotic listening paradigm where the two simultaneously presented words differ only in the initial consonant. This task had proved to be in close correspondence to speech laterali-zation assessed by the Wada amytal test. The definition of the planum temporale followed Steinmetz's criteria but the measures were taken on a horizontal slice. Left-handed subjects with right-ear advantage (simi-lar to typical right-handers) had a significantly larger left than right planum temporale, whereas no significant asymmetry was found in subjects with left-ear advantage. One of the conclusions of this impor-tant contribution is that reversed speech lateralization is not necessarily accompanied by concomitant reversal of planum asymmetry, adding further evidence to the fact that the link between planum asymmetry and lateralization of language is far from straightforward.[2]

However, the most direct means of exploring language lateraliza-tion is to assess brain activation in various linguistic tasks with brain functional imaging. Karbe et al. (1995) and Binder et al. (1996) have shown dissociations between functional asymmetry as assessed, respec-tively, with PET and functional MRI, and morphological planum asym-metry. Finally, Tzourio et al. (1998), using PET during a story listening task and morphological measures of the planum temporale, found a correlation between activation in the left temporal superior gyrus and left planum size, but not with the degree of planum asymmetry. This result is concordant with several studies in developmentally lan-guage-impaired individuals showing that the left planum, rather than the degree of asymmetry, correlates with behavioral performance (see below).

Michel Habib and Fabrice Robichon

Planum Asymmetry in Musicians: Elucidating the Role of Training and Experience

One of the most remarkable contributions since the mid-1990s to the issue of brain asymmetries undoubtedly was that of Steinmetz's group on professional musicians. Comparing 30 musicians to 30 musically naive controls, Schlaug, Jäncke, Huang, and Steinmetz (1995) first focused on their planum temporale asymmetry, based on the assumption that musically gifted individuals are often suspected to show rightward deviation from the usual pattern of cerebral asymmetry. Actually, the authors' findings were completely the opposite of their expectations, since the planum was found more left-lateralized in musicians than in nonmusicians. Moreover, this effect was found only for musicians with perfect pitch (i.e., a natural aptitude to name any note played to them, without having to refer to a standard pitch for the sake of comparison). However, the authors did not analyze the true nature of perfect pitch, which is no more than a special ability to automatically associate a sound pitch and a specific word, the name of the musical notes. Moreover, it is probable that this aptitude is not an innate characteristic of some musicians, but arises from early intensive learning of this special association. In a later discussion of these results, Steinmetz (1996) considers musicians as biologically representing an extreme form of right-handers, as regards their pattern of planum asymmetry, whereas left-handers and dyslexics (see below) would stand at the other extreme of the continuum. In his conclusion, he states, "it appears tempting to speculate that the processing capacity of certain specialized auditory systems may increase with degree of interhemispheric PT asymmetry."

The issue was reinvestigated by Zatorre et al. (1998), who coupled the use of structural and functional brain imaging to address the question of absolute pitch. Subjects were 20 musically trained young adults, half of whom had verified absolute pitch, and the others had only relative pitch. Besides results of a PET study not relevant to our purpose, the authors report planum temporale measurements obtained on the same subjects: although there was no difference in planum morphometry between the two subgroups of subjects, the 20 subjects as a whole had increased planum size compared to a large reference group. Moreover, for both absolute pitch and relative pitch musicians, they found a correlation between performance on a behavioral task (identify randomly presented notes) and the size of the left planum, but not with an asymmetry index. The authors point out, however, that the planum was never activated in the PET study of the same subjects, suggesting, just as for language, that morphological asymmetries do not necessarily follow functional asymmetries. Finally, the absence of differential effect of absolute pitch versus relative pitch would suggest a general influence of early musical training on planum morphology, rather than the reverse effect of morphology on function. A similar observation on the effect of musical training on callosal morphology (Schaug, Jäncke, Huang, & Steinmetz, 1995) also supports such an interpretation (see below).

ANATOMICAL ASYMMETRIES IN DYSLEXIA: TESTING THE THEORY

The abundant literature on dyslexia reflects a considerable effort of researchers in the field to disclose particularities of the brains of those subjects, adults or children, who experienced specific difficulties in learning to read. Since there is an account of these studies in another chapter of this book, they will not be reviewed here in detail. The reader should consult reviews of the topic by Eckert and Leonard (2000), Habib (2000), Habib and Démonet (2000), Shapleske et al. (1999), Morgan and Hynd (1998), and Beaton (1997). We will only extract from this literature, as summarized in table 19.2, pertinent information on the general issue of the significance of brain structural asymmetries.

The Initial Neuropathological Studies

Norman Geschwind saw dyslexia as an ideal model to test his hypotheses about the biological bases of brain laterality. He and Albert Galaburda therefore initiated a series of neuropathological studies dealing with the careful examination of one, then four, then eight brains of individuals who had died from nonneurological causes and whose personal history was documented with such precision as to ascertain their belonging to the 5–10% group of individuals having suffered from childhood dyslexia, according to now universally admitted diagnosis criteria.

In this context, Galaburda and collaborators (Galaburda & Kemper, 1979; Galaburda et al., 1985; Humphreys et al., 1990; see also Livingstone et al., 1991; Galaburda et al., 1994; Jenner et al., 1999) reported what was to become one tenet of the neurobiology of dyslexia: the absence of the normal asymmetry of language areas. This pattern of symmetry was found in all the brains examined neuropathologically, as well as in the brain of one child who had died from an infectious disease and had been diagnosed as severely language-impaired (Cohen et al., 1989). In their attempt at modeling the causes of dyslexia, Geschwind and Galaburda (1985) referred to the presence, on the same brains, of microscopic malformations suggestive of an anomaly that had occurred during the fetal period, at the postmigrational period when neurons colonizing the developing cortex establish their connections, a process thought to coincide with (and probably to regulate) the physiological death of millions of cortical cells that takes place around the 30th gestational week. Experimental work subsequently carried out in Galaburda's laboratory on a rodent model (see Galaburda et al., 1994) have led this author to conceive asymmetry as the consequence of more cell death on the right hemisphere, and absence of asymmetry, such as in the dyslexic brain, as the consequence of impaired cell death.

Undoubtedly the hypothesis is attractive, but the evidence is quantitatively insufficient to draw firm conclusions about the core of this reasoning (i.e., the absence of asymmetry in dyslexia). Here again, magnetic resonance imaging is the appropriate tool.

Morphological MRI and Brain Asymmetries in Dyslexia

Whereas the first studies dealing with this topic seemed to confirm the general concept of reduced asymmetry in dyslexia, subsequent works changed the initial impression. Of the 20 studies published to date (table 19.2) using MRI for assessing brain asymmetry in dyslexia, only five have yielded unambiguously significant results. However, with improving MRI techniques, the more recent studies failed to confirm these results. In particular, none of the studies published since the mid-1990s have shown the expected reduced asymmetry of the planum temporale. Moreover, virtually all studies having found reduced planum asymmetry have found it as the consequence of a smaller left rather than a

Table 19.2 Morphological MRI investigations of cortical asymmetries in dyslexia

Study	Method	Subjects	Chronological age (sd)
Rumsey et al., 1986	Coronal/axial MRI 0.5T	10 male dyslexics	22.6 (3.34)
Hynd et al., 1990	MRI 0.6T	10 dyslexics (8 males + 2 females)	9.9 (2.04)
		10 ADD/H[a] (8 males + 2 females)	10.0 (3.36)
		10 controls (8 males + 2 females)[a]	11.8 (2.0)
Larsen et al., 1990	Coronal MRI 1.5T	19 dyslexics (ratio: 4 males/1 fem.)	15.1 (0.3)
		17 controls (ratio: 4 males/1 fem.)	15.4 (0.4)
Duara et al., 1991	Axial MRI 1.0T	21 dyslexics (12 males + 9 females)	39.1 (11.0)
		29 controls (15 males + 14 females)	35.3 (10.0)
Jernigan et al., 1991	Axial MRI 1.5T	20 L/LI[b] (13 males + 7 females)	8.9 (0.7)
		12 controls (8 males + 4 females)	9.0 (0.7)
Plante, 1991	Axial MRI 0.5T	8 SLI[c]	5.2
		8 normal MRI scans from male subjects selected from a database	—
Kushch et al., 1993	Coronal MRI 1.5T	17 dyslexics (9 males + 8 females)	26.2 (15.0)
		21 controls (8 males + 13 females)	33.4 (15.0)
Leonard et al., 1993	MRI 1.0T	9 dyslexics (7 males + 2 females)	36 (17.1)
		10 unaffected siblings (4 males + 6 females)	25.7 (20.3)
		12 controls (5 males + 7 females)	37.1 (13.5)
Schultz et al., 1994	Coronal MRI 1.5T	17 dyslexics (10 males + 7 females)	8.68 (0.64)
		14 controls (7 males + 7 females)	8.94 (0.67)
Rumsey et al., 1997	MRI	16 right-handed dyslexic men	18–40 yrs.
		14 matched controls	
Gauger et al., 1997	MRI	11 L/LI and 19 matched controls	5.6–13 yrs.

Anatomical structure measured	Regional asymmetries and/or abnormalities			
	Dyslexics	Controls	Others	p
Lateral ventricles	R < L: 20%			#
Temporal lobes	R > L: 40%			#
	R = L: 90%			#
Length of the planum temporale	R < L: 10%	R < L: 70%	R < L: 70%	*
Length of the insula	R < L	R > L	R < L	**
Width of the frontal lobe	R = L	R > L	R > L	**
Width of occipital lobe	—	—	—	ns
Surface of the planum temporale	R < L: 31.5%	R < L: 70.5%	R = L: 29.5%	*
	R = L: 68.5%			
Postcentral surface	(R > L) ns	(R = L) ns		ns
Posterior surface	R > L***	(R < L) ns		**
"Inf.-Anterior" volume	R > L**			***
"Sup.-Posterior" volume	R < L** ≠			*
"Inf.-Posterior" volume	R < L: 45%			***
	R > L: 50%			
	R = L: 5%			
Perisylvian region	R < L: 25%	R < L: 75%		**
	R > L: 37.5%	R > L: 0		
	R = L: 37.5%	R = L: 25%		
SSTL anterior	(R < L) ns	R < L****		ns
SSTL posterior	(R > L) ns	R < L****		**
SSTL total	(R < L) ns	R < L****		*
Length of the PT	(R < L) ns	(R < L) ns	(R < L) ns	
[T] Temporal length	R < L****	R < L*	R < L**	
[P] Parietal length	R > L**	(R > L) ns	R > L*	
Left intrahemispheric asymmetry	T > P: 78%**	T > P: 100%*****	T > P: 100%*****	
Right intrahemispheric asymmetry	T > P: 44.5% ns	T > P: 100%****	T > P: 50% ns	
Parietal operculum:	*LH RH Bil*	*LH RH Bil*	*LH RH Bil*	
type 3	67%	8%	40%	
type 4	11%	8%		
Multiple Heschl gyri	11%, 22%, 11%		10%	
Surface of PT	(R < L): 76%	(R < L): 71%		ns
Temporal lobe surface	(R < L)	(R < L)		ns
Temporal lobe volume	(R < L)	(R < L)		ns
Supratemporal volume	(R < L)	(R < L)		ns
PT and ascending posterior ramus of SF (planum parietale)	both groups have 70–80% leftward PT asymmetry 50–60% rightward planum parietale asymmetry			
Planum temporale Broca's area (pars triangularis)	• left pars triangularis significantly smaller in SLI children • more incidence of rightward asymmetry of language structures • anomalous morphology in these language areas correlated with depressed language ability			

Table 19.2   (continued)

Study	Method	Subjects	Chronological age (sd)
Hugdahl et al., 1998	MRI 1T	25 dyslexics (20M, 5F) 25 controls (20M, 5F)	11.8 ± 0.4 11.7 ± 0.5
Clark & Plante, 1998	MRI 1.5T	41 normal adults, including 20 parents of LLI children; among these, 15 probable (test-identified) dyslexics. 4 probable dyslexics in the nonparent population	30–51 yrs.
Dalby et al., 1998	Coronal MRI	17 dyslexics, 6 retarded readers, 12 normal controls	Mean 16 yrs.
Best & Demb, 1999	MRI	5 dyslexics (3M, 2F) with documented magnocellular deficit and 5 controls (3M, 2F)	22.2 ± 2.9 26.8 ± 6.1
Pennington et al., 1999	3D-MRI 1.5T	75 RD twin pairs (M/F: 40/35; MZ/DZ: 40/35) 22 control twin pairs (M/F: 11/11; MZ/DZ: 11/11)	17.4 ± 4.3 18.7 ± 3.8
Green et al., 1999	3D-MRI 1.5T	8 male dyslexics 8 male controls	23.5 24
Robichon et al., 2000	Axial/sagittal 1.5T	16 male dyslexics 14 male controls	21.0 ± 0.2 23.6 ± 3.9
Heiervang et al., 2000	Sagittal MRI 1T	20 dyslexics 20 controls	142m (130–149) 141m (126–149)
Hiemenz & Hynd, 2000	Sagittal MRI 0.6T	22 dyslexics 20 ADHD 13 controls	$117m \pm 14$ $119m \pm 13$ $117m \pm 14$

[a] Attention deficit disorder/hyperactivity
[b] Language/learning impaired
[c] Specific language impairment
[d] Total Broca's area includes anterior (BA45) and posterior (BA44) parts

$*p < .05$
$**p < .01$
$***p < .005$
$****p < .001$
$*****p < .0001$

ns not significant
— not reported
p value not reported

Anatomical structure measured	Regional asymmetries and/or abnormalities			P
	Dyslexics	Controls	Others	
Planum temporale area	R < L****	R < L****		ns
Broca's area. 7 types according to gyrification and sulcal patterns	morphological types including an extra sulcus in the inferior frontal gyrus of test-identified dyslexics (both hemispheres combined)			
3 measures of temporal lobes	(R > L)	(R < L)	(R > L)	ns
Depth of SF	R > L: 82%	R < L: 75%	R < L: 67%	*
Temporal lobe 1 area	(R > L)	(R < L)	(R > L)	ns
Temporal lobe 2 area				
PT area	R < L: 100%	R < L: 60%		#
3 methods on sagittal sections	R < L: 60%	R < L: —		#
	R < L: 60%	R < L: 60%		#
Cortical and subcortical structures subdivided into regions:				
Anteriosuperior cortex	RDs < controls			*
Insular cortex	RDs < controls			***
Caudal infrasylvian surface	(R < L) ns	(R < L) ns		*
Inferior frontal gyrus (total Broca's area)[d]	Controls: L > R, dyslexics R > L			*
Broca's sulcal pattern				n.s.
Planum temporale area	L > R (n.s.)			n.s.
Parietal opercular area	Controls L > R, dyslexics L ≫ R*			*
Behavioral measures	Asymmetry in dyslexics correlated with nonword reading and spelling			
Planum temporale and planum parietale, according to Steinmetz	PT: leftward asymmetry in both groups (n.s.) Nonsignificant tendency to smaller left PT			n.s.
CV syllables dichotic listening	PP: rightward asymmetry in both groups, significantly less frequent in dyslexics			*
	Dichotic: No ear x group interaction, no correlation with PT asymmetry			n.s.
Comparison of Steimetz's and Witelson's sulcal types	No sulcal hemispheric differences between the 3 groups except Witelson's H type only in dyslexics (bilaterally and in only 4 subjects) Better correlation of Steinmetz's types with behavioral performance			

larger right planum, as predicted by Galaburda et al. (1987, 1990). On the contrary, the only consistent pattern that seems to emerge from the most recent literature is that of an increase in leftward asymmetry in the parietal region. Thus, Heiervang et al. (2000), in 20 carefully selected dyslexics and 20 matched controls, failed to find significant differences in planum asymmetry, but found a decrease in rightward asymmetry of the so-called planum parietale (i.e., the part of the association auditory cortex situated on the ascending limb, when it exists, of the sylvian fissure). This result is consistent with our own observation (Robichon et al., 2000b) that the parietal rather the temporal bank of the sylvian fissure is the brain region where the singularity of the dyslexic brain must be sought. Likewise, we found that the parietal operculum, measured from the central sulcus along the superior sylvian bank to the posterior end point of the Sylvian fissure, was moderately leftward asymmetrical in controls and significantly more so in dyslexics. This result converges with that of Heiervang et al. in that it globally indicates atypical organization of the sulcal pattern on the parietal rather the temporal bank of the sylvian fissure in dyslexics,[3] whereas the most sophisticated morphometric methods available to date have failed to provide such evidence for the caudal infrasylvian surface (Green et al., 1999).

Indeed, if one considers, as more and more researchers do, that interhemispheric differences in the size of perisylvian cortical structures are the consequence of a difference in sulcal organization, one should address interpretations in terms of global development of the posterior hemisphere and, as suggested by Binder et al. (1996), in terms of the dynamic pressures exerting their effect during brain development. In this respect, valuable information may be derived from observing the developmental characteristics of one privileged witness of these putative forces, the corpus callosum.

The Corpus Callosum: Seeking Clues to Hemispheric Development Rules

It would be out of purpose to review here the enormous literature about callosal anatomy in connection with brain functional asymmetry. The inflation of studies devoted to this brain structure probably results from the unique situation of the callosum, clearly observable and measurable on routine MRI examinations, an open window on the developing brain. We refer the reader to classical reviews by Witelson and

Kigar (1988), Witelson (1985), J. M. Clarke and Zaidel (1994), Aboitiz et al. (1992), and Beaton (1997). The main and most robust finding here is the repeated demonstration that callosal morphology varies consistently with two combined factors: handedness and sex, being larger, in particular, in the isthmus (midposterior) region in male left-handers and, to a lesser degree, in right-handed females (Witelson, 1989; Habib et al., 1991; J. M. Clarke et al., 1993; Cowell et al., 1993). Since this difference probably represents 10 to 30 million interhemispheric fibers, it must have a functional significance that is, however, still very poorly understood (Moffat et al., 1998).

Another related but separate issue is that of the possible developmental mechanisms to explain these sex and handedness differences. The testosterone hypothesis stands as a potentially fruitful lead, in particular after the convincing evidence (Moffat et al., 1997) that there could be a relationship between the morphology of the human callosum and salivary concentration of testosterone. This observation, along with other experimental evidence in animals and developmental studies in humans (Fitch et al., 1987; S. Clarke et al., 1989; see also Habib et al., 1990), suggests a shaping effect of gonadal hormones on the developing corpus callosum during the perinatal period.[4] However, this does not rule out the possibility of a role of environmental factors occurring much later in life (Castro-Caldas et al., 1999; Habib et al., 2000).

Modifications in callosal anatomy have also been found in dyslexic individuals. Robichon and Habib (1998), among others, have documented abnormal callosal connectivity in young male dyslexic adults, with a differential effect of handedness on the size of some callosal subregions. Globally, the callosum was larger in dyslexics, especially in its posterior part and especially in right-handed dyslexics. More recently (Robichon, Bouchard, et al., 2000a) have shown that not only the size but also the shape and position of the callosum may be different in the dyslexic brain. Using a method recently proposed by Oka et al. (1999), who showed a sexual dimorphism in the position of the corpus callosum relative to the brainstem axis, they found a significantly lower posterior callosum in dyslexics compared to controls. The arched aspect of the corpus callosum obviously reflects the telencephalic flexion that characterizes the progressive "closure" of the embryonic brain around its perpendicular axis through the insula. The same movement is also responsible for the formation of the sylvian fissures, whose asymmetry is visible as early as the 16th gestational week (LeMay, 1976, 1992), well before any other sulcus or gyrus becomes visible (see LeMay, 1992 for illustrations). Asymmetry in direction of the posterior sylvian fissure may be the consequence of subtle asymmetry in the process of hemispheric flexion and/or in the level of the axis around which the flexion occurs. This asymmetry probably is genetically determined (and may be universal, as postulated by Geschwind).

The subsequent formation of the sulcal pattern on both sides of the fissure will normally follow the guidelines imposed by this early stage of asymmetry, but remains subject to the influence of multiple environmental factors, including hormonal pre- or perinatal factors, or later shaping by experience and training, at least during the first years of life. However, this would not fundamentally alter the pattern of asymmetry (Preis et al., 1999), but probably would only accentuate it (as in the case of musical training) or, more speculatively, reduce it. This conception of a basic, genetically determined processor of asymmetry that is eventually modifiable by environmental influences is consistent with evidence from twin studies showing conspicuous differences in patterns of planum asymmetry between monozygotic twins (Steinmetz et al., 1995) and evidence that the deep (early) sulci are more strongly genetically determined than superficial sulci (Bartley et al., 1997; Lohmann et al., 1999).

In dyslexia, a neurodevelopmental deviance could interfere with this process, causing both atypical cortical asymmetry and abnormal callosal shape and spatial position. Alternatively, as proposed by Galaburda's group (Rosen et al., 1990), abnormal persistence of ectopic neurons and their interhemispheric connections may explain both callosal and cortical asymmetry abnormalities. However, cases of severe dyslexics with normal callosa and typical asymmetry suggest that neither of the two is critical in these children's difficulties in learning to read. Instead, the complex symptomatic features of this learning disorder (Habib, 2000) can be best understood as resulting from more elementary neural mechanisms, such as the ability to process rapidly changing brief stimuli (Tallal et al., 1995), which is required for most (oral as well as written) language abilities. The above-reported preliminary observations of a specific microscopic organization of the left hemisphere language areas appropriate to process rapid sensory signals, open fascinating perspectives on the use for this purpose of new

Michel Habib and Fabrice Robichon

brain imaging methods, such as magnetic spectroscopy, able to show changes in cell density and biochemical content of specific brain regions (Rae et al., 1998).

NOTES

1. It is important to note here that to reveal the superior temporal region, the authors had dissected each of the 100 brains by removing all brain tissue situated above the plane of the sylvian fissure, including the parietal operculum.

2. Observations of similar asymmetries in chimpanzees (Gannon et al.,1998; Hopkins et al., 1998) are also an argument against a close relationship between anatomical and functional asymmetry of the planum temporale.

3. One extreme form of such atypical sulcal pattern was described by Witelson et al. (1999) on the brain of Albert Einstein, notoriously dyslexic as well as a mathematical genius. The parietal operculum apparently was missing on both sides, which represents an obviously exceptional anatomical configuration. It is, however, difficult to speculate further on the possible link between this unique observation and the anatomical data presented here.

4. The issue of sex variations in brain asymmetry may also be relevant to this discussion, but will not be dealt with here (see Kulynych et al., 1994, and Harasty et al., 1997) for two recent works in the field).

REFERENCES

Aboitiz, F., Scheibel, A. B., & Zaidel, E. (1992). Morphometry of the sylvian fissure and the corpus callosum, with emphasis on sex differences. *Brain, 115*, 1521–1541.

Albanese, E., Merlo, A., Albanese, A., & Gomez, E. (1989). Anterior speech region. Asymmetry and weight-surface correlation. *Archives of Neurology, 46*, 307–310.

Amunts, K., Schlaug, G., Schleicher, A., Steinmetz, H., Dabringhaus, A., Roland, P. E., & Zilles, K. (1996). Asymmetry in the human motor cortex and handedness. *Neuroimage, 4*, 216–222.

Anderson, B., Southern, B., & Powers, R. E. (1999). Anatomic asymmetries of the posterior superior temporal lobes: A postmortem study. *Neuropsychiatry, Neuropsychology and Behavioral Neurology, 12*(4), 247–254.

Annett, M. (1985). *Left, right, hand and brain: The right shift theory*. London: Lawrence Erlbaum Associates.

Annett, M. (2000). Predicting combinations of left and right asymmetries. *Cortex, 36*, 485–505.

Bartley, A. J., Jones, D. W., & Weinberger, D. R. (1997). Genetic variability of human brain size and cortical gyral patteerns. *Brain, 120*, 257–269.

Beaton, A. A. (1997). The relation of planum temporale asymmetry and morphology of the corpus callosum to handedness, gender, and dyslexia: A review of the evidence. *Brain and Language, 60,* 255–322.

Best, M., & Demb, J. B. (1999). Normal planum temporale asymmetry in dyslexics with a magnocellular pathway deficit. *Neuroreport, 10,* 607–612.

Binder, J. R., Frost, J. A., Hammeke, T. A., Rao, S. M., & Cox, R. W. (1996). Function of the left planum temporale in auditory and linguistic processing. *Brain, 119,* 1239–1247.

Broca, P. (1865). Sur le siège du langage articulé. *Bulletin Societé Anthropologie, 6,* 337–393.

Broca, P. (1875). Instructions craniologiques et craniométriques de la Société d'Anthropologie de Paris. *Bulletin Societé Anthropologie, 16,* 534–536.

Bryden, M. P., McManus, I. C., & Bulman-Fleming, M. B. (1994). Evaluating the empirical support for the Geschwind-Behan-Galaburda model of cerebral lateralization. *Brain and Cognition, 26,* 103–187.

Campain, R., & Minckler, J. (1976). A note on the gross configuration of the human auditory cortex. *Brain and Language, 3,* 318–323.

Castro-Caldas, A., Miranda, P. C., Carmo, I., Reis, A., Leote, F., Ribeiro, C., and Ducla-Soares, E. (1999). Influence of learning to read and write on the morphology of the corpus callosum. *European Journal of Neurology, 6*(1), 23–28.

Charpy, A. (1889). *Cours de splanchnologie. Les centres nerveux.* Montauban, France: Guillau.

Clark, M. M., & Plante, E. (1998). Morphology of the inferior frontal gyrus in developmentally language-disordered adults. *Brain and Language, 61,* 288–303.

Clarke, J. M., Lufkin, R. B., & Zaidel, E. (1993). Corpus callosum morphometry and dichotic listening performance: Individual differences in functional interhemispheric inhibition? *Neuropsychologia, 31,* 547–557.

Clarke, J. M., & Zaidel, E. (1994). Anatomical-behavioral relationships: Corpus callosum morphometry and hemispheric specialization. *Behavioral Brain Research, 64,* 185–202.

Clarke, S., Kraftsik, R., Van Der Loos, H., & Innocenti, G. M. (1989). Forms and measures of adult and developing human corpus callosum: Is there sexual dimorphism? *Journal of Comparative Neurology, 280,* 213–230.

Cohen, M., Campbell, R., & Yagmai, F. (1989). Neuropathological abnormalities in developmental dysphasia. *Annals of Neurology, 25,* 567–570.

Connolly, C. J. (1950). *External morphology of the primate brain.* Springfield, IL: Charles C. Thomas.

Coren, S., & Porac, C. (1977). Fifty centuries of right handedness: The historical record. *Science, 198,* 631–632.

Cowell, P. E., Kertesz, A., & Denenberg, V. H. (1993). Multiple dimensions of handedness and the human corpus callosum. *Neurology, 43,* 2353–2357.

Cunningham, D. J. (1892). Contribution to the surface anatomy of the cerebral hemispheres. Cunningham Memoirs, Royal Irish Academy, Dublin.

Dalby, M. A., Elbro, C., & Stodkilde-Jorgensen, H. (1998). Temporal lobe asymmetry and dyslexia: An in vivo study using MRI. *Brain and Language*, *62*, 51–69.

Duara, R., Kushch, A., Gross-Glenn, K., Barker, W. W., Jallad, B., Pascal, S., Loewenstein, D. A., Sheldon, J., Rabin, M., Levin, B. E., & Lubs, H. (1991). Neuroanatomic differences between dyslexic and normal readers on magnetic resonance imaging scans. *Archives of Neurology*, *48*, 410–416.

Eberstaller, O. (1884). Zur oberflachen anatomie des grosshirn hemisphären. *Wien Medical Blatt*, *7*, 479, 642, 644.

Eckert, M. A., & Leonard, C. M. (2000). Structural imaging in dyslexia: The planum temporale. *Mental Retardation Developmental Disorder Research Review*, *6*, 198–206.

Eidelberg, D., & Galaburda, A. M. (1984). Inferior parietal lobule: Divergent architectonic asymmetries in the human brain. *Archives of Neurology*, *41*, 843–852.

Falzi, G., Perrone, P., & Vignolo, L. A. (1982). Right-left asymmetry in anterior speech region. *Archives of Neurology*, *39*, 239–240.

Fitch, R. H., Berrebi, A. S., and Denenberg, V. H. (1987). Corpus callosum: Masculinized via perinatal testosterone. *Social Neuroscience Abstracts*, *13*, 689.

Foundas, A. L., Faulhaber, J. R., Kulynych, J. J., Browning, C. A., & Weinberger, D. R. (1999). Hemispheric and sex-linked differences in sylvian fissure morphology: A quantitative approach using volumetric magnetic resonance imaging. *Neuropsychiatry, Neuropsychology and Behavioral Neurology*, *12*, 1–10.

Foundas, A. L., Leonard, C. M., Gilmore, R., Fennel, E., & Heilman, K. M. (1994). Planum temporale asymmetry and language dominance. *Neuropsychologia*, *32*, 1225–1231.

Foundas, A. L., Leonard, C. M., Gilmore, R. L., Fennel, E. B., & Heilman, K. M. (1996). Pars triangularis asymmetry and language dominance. *Proceedings of the National Academy of Sciences, USA*, *93*, 719–722.

Foundas, A. L., Leonard, C. M., & Heilman, K. M. (1995). Morphologic cerebral asymmetries and handedness. The pars triangularis and planum temporale. *Archives of Neurology*, *52*, 501–508.

Galaburda, A. M. (1980). La région de Broca: Observations anatomiques faites un siècle après la mort de son découvreur. *Revue de Neurologie* (Paris), *36*, 609–616.

Galaburda, A. M., Corsiglia, J., Rosen, G. D., & Sherman, G. F. (1987). Planum temporale asymmetry: Reappraisal since Geschwind and Levitsky, *Neuropsychologia*, *25*, 853–868.

Galaburda, A. M., & Habib, M. (1987). Cerebral dominance: Biological associations and pathology. *Discussions in Neuroscience*, *4*, 1–51.

Galaburda, A. M., & Kemper, T. L. (1979). Cytoarchitectonic abnormalities in developmental dyslexia: A case study. *Annals of Neurology*, *6*, 94–100.

Galaburda, A. M., LeMay, M., Kemper, T. L., & Geschwind, N. (1978). Right-left asymmetries in the brain. Structural differences between the hemispheres may underlie cerebral dominance. *Science, 199,* 852–856.

Galaburda, A. M., & Livingstone, M. S. (1993). Evidence for a magnocellular defect in developmental dyslexia. *Annals of the New York Academy of Sciences, 682,* 70–82.

Galaburda, A. M., Menard, M. T., & Rosen, G. D. (1994). Evidence for aberrant auditory anatomy in developmental dyslexia. *Proceedings of the National Academy of Sciences, USA, 91,* 8010–8013.

Galaburda, A. M., Rosen, G. D., & Sherman, G. F. (1990). Individual variability in cortical organization: Its relationship to brain laterality and implications to function. *Neuropsychologia, 28,* 529–546.

Galaburda, A. M., & Sanides, F. (1980). Cytoarchitectonic organization of the human auditory cortex. *Journal of Comparative Neurology, 190,* 597–610.

Galaburda, A. M., Sanides, F., & Geschwind, N. (1978). Human brain: Cytoarchitectonic left-right asymmetries in the temporal speech region. *Archives of Neurology, 35,* 812–817.

Galaburda, A. M., Sherman, G. F., Rosen, G. D., Aboitiz, F., & Geschwind, N. (1985). Developmental dyslexia: Four consecutive patients with cortical anomalies. *Annals of Neurology, 18,* 222–233.

Galuske, R. A. W., Schlote, W., Bratzke, H., & Singer, W. (2000). Interhemispheric asymmetries of the modular structure in human temporal cortex. *Science, 289,* 1946–1949.

Gannon, P. J., Holloway, R. L., Broadfield, D. C., & Braun, A. R. (1998). Asymmetry of chimpanzee planum temporale: Humanlike pattern of Wernicke's brain language area homolog. *Science, 279*(5348), 220–222.

Gauger, L. M., Lombardino, L. J., & Leonard, C. M. (1997). Brain morphology in children with specific language impairment. *Journal of Speech, Language and Hearing Research, 40*(6), 1272–1284.

Geschwind, N. (1979). Specializations of the human brain. *Scientific American, 241*(3), 158–168.

Geschwind, N., & Behan, P. O. (1982). Left-handedness: Association with immune disease, migraine, and developmental learning disorder. *Proceedings of the National Academy of Sciences, USA, 79,* 5097–5100.

Geschwind, N., & Behan, P. O. (1984). Laterality, hormones, and immunity. In N. Geschwind & A. M. Galaburda (Eds.), *Cerebral dominance: The biological foundations.* Cambridge, MA: Harvard University Press.

Geschwind, N., & Galaburda, A. M. (1985). Cerebral lateralization: Biological mechanisms, associations, and pathology. I. *Archives of Neurology, 42,* 428–459.

Geschwind, N., & Levitsky, W. (1968). Human brain: Left-right asymmetries in temporal speech region. *Science, 161,* 186–187.

Green, R. L., Hutsler, J. J., Loftus, W. C., Tramo, M. J., Thomas, C. E., Silberfarb, A. W., Nordgren, R. E., Nordgren, R. A., & Gazzaniga, M. S. (1999). The caudal infrasylvian surface in dyslexia: Novel magnetic resonance imaging-based findings. *Neurology, 53,* 974–981.

Habib, M. (1989). Anatomical asymmetries of the human cerebral cortex. *International Journal of Neurosciences, 47,* 67–89.

Habib, M. (2000). The neurological basis of developmental dyslexia: Overview and working hypothesis. *Brain, 123,* 2373–2399.

Habib, M., & Démonet, J. F. (2000). Dyslexia and related learning disorders: Recent advances from brain imaging studies. In J. C. Mazziotta, A. W. Toga, & R. S. J. Frackowiak (Eds.), *Brain Mapping: The disorders* (pp. 459–482). San Diego: Academic Press.

Habib, M., & Galaburda, A. M. (1986). Déterminants biologiques de la dominance cérébrale. *Revue de Neurologie* (Paris), *142,* 869–894.

Habib, M., Gayraud, D., Régis, J., Oliva, A., Salamon, G., & Khalil, R. (1991). Effects of handedness and sex on the morphology of the corpus callosum. *Brain and Cognition, 16,* 41–61.

Habib, M., Joanette, Y., Ali-Chérif, A., & Poncet, M. (1983). Crossed aphasia in dextrals: A case report with special reference to site of lesion. *Neuropsychologia, 21,* 413–418.

Habib, M., Renucci, R. L., Vanier, M., Corbaz, J. M., & Salamon, G. (1984). CT assessment of right-left asymmetries in the human cerebral cortex. *Journal of Computer Assisted Tomography, 8,* 922–927.

Habib, M., Robichon, F., Chanoine, V., Démonet, J.-F., Frith, C., & Frith, U. (2000). The influence of language learning on brain morphology: The "callosal effect" in dyslexics differs according to native language. *Brain and Language, 74,* 520–524.

Habib, M., Robichon, F., Levrier, O., Khalil, R., & Salamon, G. (1995). Diverging asymmetries of temporo-parietal cortical areas: A reappraisal of Geschwind/Galaburda theory. *Brain and Langue, 48,* 238–258.

Habib, M., Touze, F., & Galaburda, A. M. (1990). Intrauterine factors of sinistrality: A review. In S. Coren (Ed.), *Left-handedness: Behavioral implications and anomalies* (pp. 99–128). Amsterdam: Elsevier.

Harasty, J., Double, K. L., Halliday, G. M., Kril, J. J., & McRitchie, D. A. (1997). Language-associated cortical regions are proportionally larger in the female brain. *Archives of Neurology, 54,* 171–176.

Heiervang, E., Hugdahl, K., Steinmetz, H., Smievoll, A. I., Stevenson, J., Lund, A., Ersland, L., & Lundervold, A. (2000). Planum temporale, planum parietale and dichotic listening in dyslexia. *Neuropsychologia, 38,* 1704–1713.

Hellige, J. B., Taylor, K. B., Lesmes, L., & Peterson, S. (1998). Relationships between brain morphology and behavioral measures of hemispheric asymmetry and interhemispheric interaction. *Brain and Cognition, 36,* 158–192.

Hiemenz, J. R., & Hynd, G. W. (2000). Sulcal/gyral pattern morphology of the perisylvian language region in developmental dyslexia. *Brain and Language, 74*, 113–133.

Hopkins, W. D., Marino, L., Rilling, J. K., & MacGregor, L. A. (1998). Planum temporale asymmetries in great apes as revealed by magnetic resonance imaging (MRI). *Neuro-Report, 9*, 2913–2918.

Hugdahl, K. (1994). The search continues: Casual relationships among dyslexia, anomalous dominance, and immune function. *Brain and Cognition, 26*, 275–280.

Hugdahl, K., Heiervang, E., Nordby, H., Smievoll, A. I., Steinmetz, H., Stevenson, J., & Lund A. (1998). Central auditory processing, MRI morphometry and brain laterality: Applications to dyslexia. *Scandinavian Audiology, 27* (supp. 49), 26–34.

Humphreys, P., Kaufmann, W. E., & Galaburda, A. M. (1990). Developmental dyslexia in women: Neuropathological findings in three patients. *Annals of Neurology, 28*, 727–738.

Hynd, G. W., Semrud-Clikeman, M., Lorys, A. R., Novey, E. S., & Eliopoulos, D. (1990). Brain morphology in developmental dyslexia and attention deficit disorder/hyperactivity. *Archives of Neurology, 47*, 919–926.

Inglessis, M. (1919). Einiges über seitenventrikel und hirnschwellung. *Archive für Psychologie, 74*, 159–168.

Jäncke, L., Schlaug, G., Huang, Y., & Steinmetz, H. (1994). Asymmetry of the planum parietale. *NeuroReport, 5*, 1161–1163.

Jäncke, L., & Steinmetz, H. (1993). Auditory lateralization and planum temporale asymmetry. *NeuroReport, 5*, 169–172.

Jenner, A. R., Rosen, G. D., & Galaburda, A. M. (1999). Neuronal asymmetries in primary visual cortex of dyslexic and nondyslexic brains. *Annals of Neurology, 46*, 189–196.

Jernigan, T. L., Hesselink, J. R., Sowell, E., & Tallal, P. A. (1991). Cerebral structure on magnetic resonance imaging in language- and learning-impaired children. *Archives of Neurology, 48*, 529–545.

Karbe, H., Wurker, M., Herholz, K., Ghaemi, M., Pietrzyk, U., Kessler, J., & Heiss, W. (1995). Planum temporale and Brodmann's area 22. Magnetic resonance imaging and high-resolution positron emission tomography demonstrate functional left-right asymmetry. *Archives of Neurology, 52*, 869–874.

Kauffmann, W. E., & Galaburda, A. M. (1989). Cerebrocortical microdysgenesis in neurologically normal subjects: A histopathologic study. *Neurology, 39*, 238–244.

Kertesz, A., Black, S. E., Polk, M., & Howell, J. (1986). Cerebral asymmetries on magnetic resonance imaging. *Cortex, 22*, 117–127.

Kertesz, A., Polk, M., Black, S. E., & Howell, J. (1992). Anatomical asymmetries and functional laterality. *Brain, 115*, 589–605.

Koff, E., Naeser, M. A., Pienadz, J. M., Foundas, A. L., & Levine, H. L. (1986). Computed tomographic scan hemispheric asymmetries in right- and left-handed male and female subjects. *Archives of Neurology, 43*, 487–491.

Kopp, N., Michel, F., Carrier, H., Biron, A., & Duvillard, P. (1977). Etude de certaines asymétries hémisphériques du cerveau humain. *Journal of Neurological Science, 34,* 349–363.

Kulynych, J. J., Vladar, K., Jones, D. W., & Weinberger, D. R. (1994). Gender differences in the normal lateralization of the supratemporal cortex: MRI surface-rendering morphometry of Heschl's gyrus and the planum temporale. *Cerebral Cortex, 4,* 107–118.

Kushch, A., Gross-Glenn, K., Jallad, B., Lubs, H., Rabin, M., Feldman, E., & Duara, R. (1993). Temporal lobe surface area measurements on MRI in normal and dyslexics readers. *Neuropsychologia, 31,* 811–821.

Larsen, J. P., Høien, T., Lundberg, I., & Ødegaard, H. (1990). MRI evaluation of the planum temporale in adolescents with developmental dyslexia. *Brain and Language, 39,* 289–301.

LeMay, M. (1976). Morphological cerebral asymmetries of modern man, fossil man, and non-human primate. *Annals of New York Academy of Sciences, 280,* 349–366.

LeMay, M. (1992). Left-right dissymmetry, handedness. *American Journal of Neuroradiology, 13,* 493–504.

Leonard, C. M., Voeller, K. K., Lombardino, L. J., Morris, M. K., Alexander, A. W., Hynd, G. W., Andersen, H. G., Garofalakis, M. A., Honeyman, J. C., Mao, J., Agee, O. F., & Staab, E. V. (1993). Anomalous cerebral structure in dyslexia revealed with magnetic resonance imaging. *Archives of Neurology, 50,* 461–469.

Livingstone, M. S., Rosen, G. D., Drislane, F. W., & Galaburda, A. M. (1991). Physiological and anatomical evidence for a magnocellular defect in developmental dyslexia. *Proceedings of the National Academy of Sciences, USA, 88,* 7643–7647.

Loftus, W. C., Tramo, M. J., Thomas, C. E., Green, R. L., Nordgren, R. A., & Gazzaniga, M. S. (1993). Three-dimensional quantitative analysis of hemispheric asymmetry in the human superior temporal region. *Cerebral Cortex, 3,* 348–355.

Lohmann, G., von Cramon, D. Y., & Steinmetz, H. (1999). Sulcal variability of twins. *Cerebral Cortex, 9,* 754–763.

Moffat, S. D., Hampson, E., & Lee, D. H. (1998). Morphology of the planum temporale and corpus callosum in left-handers with evidence of left and right hemisphere speech representation. *Brain, 121,* 2369–2379.

Moffat, S. D., Hampson, E., Wickett, J. C., Vernon, P. A., & Lee, D. H. (1997). Testosterone is correlated with regional morphology of the human corpus callosum. *Brain Research, 767,* 297–304.

Morgan, A. E., & Hynd, G. W. (1998). Dyslexia, neurolinguistic ability, and anatomical variation of the planum temporale. *Neuropsychology Review, 8,* 79–93.

Moutier F. (1908). *L'aphasie de Broca.* Paris: Steinheil.

Nikkuni, S., Yashima, Y., Ishige, K., Suzuki, S., Ohno, E., & Kumashiro, H. (1981). Left-right hemispheric asymmetry of critical speech zones in Japanese brains. *Brain Nerve, 33,* 77–84.

Oka, S., Miyamuto, O., Janjua, N. A., Honjo-Fujiwara, N., Ohkawa, M., Nagao, S., Kondo, H., Minami, T., Toyoshima, P., & Itano, T. (1999). Re-evaluation of sexual dimorphism in human corpus callosum. *NeuroReport, 10,* 937–940.

Oldfield, R. C. (1971). The assessment and analysis of handedness: The Edinburgh Inventory. *Neuropsychologia, 9,* 97–113.

Pennington, B. F., Filipek, P. A., Lefly, D., Churchwell, J., Kennedy, D. N., Simon, J. H., Filley, C. M., Galaburda, A., Alarcon, M., & DeFries, J. C. (1999). Brain morphometry in reading-disabled twins. *Neurology, 53,* 723–729.

Pfeifer, R. A. (1936). Pathologie der hörstrahlung und der corticalen hörsphäre. In O. Bumke & O. Foersbed (Eds.), *Handbuch der neurologie.* Vol. 6 Berlin: Springer.

Pieniadz, J. M., & Naeser, M. A. (1984). Computed tomographic scan cerebral asymmetries and morphologic brain asymmetries. Correlation in the same cases post mortem. *Archives of Neurology, 41,* 403–409.

Plante, E. (1991). MRI findings in the parents and siblings of specifically language-impaired boys. *Brain and Language, 41,* 67–80.

Porac, C., & Coren, S. (1981). *Lateral preferences and human behavior.* New York: Springer-Verlag.

Preis, S., Jäncke, L., Schittler, P., Huang, Y., & Steinmetz, H. (1998). Normal intrasylvian anatomical asymmetry in children with developmental language disorder. *Neuropsychologia, 36,* 849–855.

Preis, S., Jäncke, L., Schmitz-Hillebrecht, J., & Steinmetz, H. (1999). Child age and planum temporale asymmetry. *Brain and Cognition, 40,* 441–452

Preis, S., Steinmetz, H., Knorr, U., & Jäncke, L. (2000). Corpus callosum size in children with developmental language disorder. *Brain Research Cognitive Brain Research, 10,* 37–44.

Rae, C., Lee, M. A., Dixon, R. M., Blamire, A. M., Thompson, C. H., Styles, P., Talcott, J., Richardson, A. J., & Stein, J. F. (1998). Metabolic abnormalities in developmental dyslexica detected by ^{1}H magnetic resonance spectroscopy. *Lancet, 351,* 1849–1852.

Robichon, F., Bouchard, P., Demonet, J. F., & Habib, M. (2000a). Developmental dyslexia: Re-evaluation of the corpus callosum in male adults. *European Neurology, 43,* 233–237.

Robichon, F., Levrier, O., Farnarier, P., & Habib, M. (2000b). Developmental dyslexia: Atypical cortical asymmetries and functional significance. *European Journal of Neurology, 7,* 35–46.

Robichon, F., & Habib, M. (1998). Abnormal callosal morphology in male adult dyslexics: Relationships to handedness and phonological abilities. *Brain and Language, 62,* 127–147.

Rosen, G. D., Sherman, G. F., & Galaburda, A. M. (1990). Interhemispheric connections differ between symmetrical and asymmetrical brain regions. *Neuroscience, 33,* 525–533.

Rubens, A. B., Mahowald, M. W., & Hutton, J. T. (1976). Asymmetry of the lateral (sylvian) fissures in man. *Neurology, 26,* 620–624.

Rumsey, J. M., Donohue, B. C., Brady, D. R., Nace, K., Giedd, J. N., & Andreason, P. (1997). A magnetic resonance imaging study of planum temporale asymmetry in men with developmental dyslexia. *Archives of Neurology, 54,* 1481–1489.

Rumsey, J. M., Dorwart, R., Vermess, M., Denckla, M. B., Kruesi, M. J. P., & Rapoport, J. L. (1986). Magnetic resonance imaging of brain anatomy in severe developmental dyslexia. *Archives of Neurology, 43*, 1045–1046.

Schlaug, G., Jäncke, L., Huang, Y., Steiger, J. F., & Steinmetz, H. (1995). Increased corpus callosum size in musicians. *Neuropsychologia, 33*, 1047–1056.

Schlaug, G., Jäncke, L., Huang, Y., & Steinmetz, H. (1995) In vivo evidence of structural brain asymmetry in musicians. *Science, 267*, 699–701.

Schultz, R. T., Cho, N. K., Staib, L. H., Kier, L. E., Fletcher, J. M., Shaywitz, S. E., Shankweiler, D. P., Katz, L., Gore, J. C., Duncan, J. S., & Shaywitz, B. A. (1994). Brain morphology in normal and dyslexic children: The influence of sex and age. *Annals of Neurology, 35*, 732–742.

Shapleske, J., Rossell, S. L., Woodruff, P. W., & David, A. S. (1999). The planum temporale: A systematic, quantitative review of its structural, functional and clinical significance. *Brain Research Review, 29*, 26–49.

Smith, G. E. (1907). Asymmetry of the brain and skull. *Journal of Anatomy, 41*, 236.

Steenhuis, R. E., & Bryden, M. P. (1989). Different dimesions of hand preference that relate to skilled and unskilled activities. *Cortex, 25*, 289–304.

Steinmetz, H. (1996). Structure, functional and cerebral asymmetry: In vivo morphometry of the planum temporale. *Neuroscience and Biobehavioral Reviews, 20*, 587–591.

Steinmetz, H., Herzog, A., Schlaug, G., Huang, Y., & Jäncke, L. (1995). Brain (a)symmetry in monozygotic twins. *Cerebral Cortex, 5*, 296–300.

Steinmetz, H., Rademacher, J., Jäncke, L., Huang, Y., Thron, A., & Zilles, K. (1990). Total surface of temporoparietal intrasylvian cortex: Diverging left-right asymmetries. *Brain snd Language, 39*, 357–372.

Steinmetz, H., Volkmann, J., Jäncke, L., & Freund, H. J. (1991). Anatomical left-right asymmetry of language-related temporal cortex is different in left- and right-handers. *Annals of Neurology, 29*, 315–319.

Stengel, E. (1930). Morphologische und cytoarchitektonische studien über den bau der unteren frontalwindung bei normalen und taubstummen. Ihre individuellen und seitenunterschiede. *Zeitung Neurologie und Psychiatrie, 130*, 631–677.

Tallal, P., Miller, S., & Fitch, R. H. (1995). Neurobiological basis of speech: A case for the preeminence of temporal processing. *Irish Journal of Psychology, 16*, 194–219.

Teszner, D., Tzavaras, A., Gruner, J., & Hécaen, H. (1972). L'asymétrie droite-gauche du planum temporale. *Revue de Neurologie* (Paris), *12*, 444–449.

Tzourio, N., Nkanga-Ngila, B., & Mazoyer, B. (1998). Left planum temporale surface correlates with functional dominance during story listening. *NeuroReport, 9*, 829–833.

Von Bonin, G. (1962). Anatomical asymmetries of the cerebral hemispheres. In V. B. Mountcastle (Ed.), *Interhemispheric relations and cerebral dominance*. Baltimore: Johns Hopkins University Press.

Von Economo, C., & Horn, L. (1930). Ueber windungsrelief, masse und rindenarchitekto-nik der supretemporalflésche, ihre individuellen und ihre seite unterschieden. *Zeitschrift für die Gesamte Neurologie und Psychiatrie, 130*, 678–757.

Wada, J. A., Clarke, R., & Hamm, A. (1975). Cerebral hemispheric asymmetry in humans. *Archives of Neurology, 32*, 239–246.

Westbury, C. F., Zatorre, R. J., & Evans, A. C. (1999). Quantifying variability in the planum temporale: A probability map. *Cerebral Cortex, 9*, 392–405.

Witelson, S. F. (1985). The brain connection: The corpus callosum is larger in left-handers. *Science, 229*, 665–668.

Witelson, S. F. (1989). Hand and sex differences in the isthmus and genu of the human corpus callosum. *Brain, 112*, 799–835.

Witelson, S. F. (1991). Cognition et morphologie du cerveau humain: Quelques corréla-tions. *Revue de Neuropsychologie, 1*, 29–54.

Witelson, S. F. (1992). Cognitive neuroanatomy: A new era (editorial). *Neurology, 42*, 709–713.

Witelson, S. F., Glezer, II, & Kigar, D. L. (1995). Women have greater density of neurons in posterior temporal cortex. *Journal of Neuroscience, 15* (pt. 1), 3418–3428.

Witelson, S. F., & Kigar, D. L. (1988). Asymmetry in brain function follows asymmetry in anatomical form. In F. Boller & J. Grafman (Eds.), *Handbook of Neuropsychology*. Vol. 1 (pp. 111–142). Amsterdam: Elsevier.

Witelson, S. F., & Kigar, D. L. (1992). Sylvian fissure morphology and asymmetry in men and women: Bilateral differences in relation to handedness in men. *Journal of Comparative Neurology, 323*, 326–340.

Witelson, S. F., Kigar, D. L., & Harvey, T. (1999). The exceptional brain of Albert Einstein. *Lancet, 353*, 2149–2153.

Witelson, S. F., & Pallie, W. (1973). Left hemisphere specialization for language in the newborn: Neuroanatomical evidence of asymmetry. *Brain, 96*, 641–646.

Yeni-Komshian, G. H., & Benson, D. A. (1976). Anatomical study of cerebral asymmetry in the temporal lobe of humans, chimpanzees and rhesus monkeys. *Science, 192*, 387–389.

Yoshii, F., Barker, W., Apicella, A., Chang, J., Sheldon, J., & Duara, R. (1986). Measure-ments of the corpus callosum on magnetic resonance scans: Effects of age, sex, handed-ness, and decease. *Neurology, 36* (Supp. 1), 133.

Zaidel, E., Aboitiz, F., & Clarke, J. (1995). Sexual dimorphism in interhemispheric rela-tions: Anatomical-behavioral convergence. *Biology Research, 28*, 27–43.

Zatorre, R. J. (1989). Perceptual asymmetry on the dichotic fused words test and cerebral speech lateralization determining by the carotid sodium arnytal test. *Neuropsychologie, 27*, 1207–1219.

Zatorre, R. J., Perry, D. W., Beckett, C. A., Westbury, C. F., & Evans, A. C. (1998). Func-tional anatomy of musical processing in listeners with absolute pitch and relative pitch. *Proceedings of the National Academy of Sciences, USA, 95*, 3172–3177.

VII Psychiatric Disorders

20 Frontal and Parietotemporal Asymmetries in Depressive Disorders: Behavioral, Electrophysiologic, and Neuroimaging Findings

Gerard E. Bruder

My chapter in *Brain Asymmetry*, edited by Davidson and Hugdahl (1995), reviewed findings from behavioral and electrophysiologic studies giving evidence of lateralized hemispheric abnormalities in affective disorders and schizophrenia (Bruder, 1995). Abnormalities of cerebral laterality in depression were shown to be related to the patient's clinical features (i.e., diagnostic subtype and outcome of treatment with antidepressants). An examination of the marked individual differences in laterality data among depressed patients suggested that multiple factors contribute to these abnormalities. The findings were generally supportive of a hypothesis postulating the existence of *both* left frontal and right parietotemporal hypoactivation in depressive disorders (Kinsbourne & Bemporad, 1984). This chapter will focus on recent findings not only from behavioral laterality and electrophysiologic studies, but also from neuroimaging studies, which have provided new evidence of abnormal frontal and parietotemporal asymmetries in depressive disorders. New findings also highlight the importance of taking comorbidity with anxiety disorders into account in studies of brain asymmetry in depression. On a more clinical level, differences in brain asymmetry between responders and nonresponders to antidepressant medications are reviewed for behavioral, electrophysiologic, and neuroimaging measures. The findings suggest the potential value of these measures as predictors of therapeutic responsiveness to treatments for depression.

FRONTAL ASYMMETRIES IN DEPRESSION

Early evidence of left prefrontal hypoactivation in depression was provided by electroencephalographic (EEG) studies of resting alpha asymmetries. Patients having a unipolar major depression (Bell et al., 1998; Henriques & Davidson, 1991) or a bipolar seasonal affective disorder (Allen et al., 1993) showed an abnormal alpha asymmetry indicative of less left frontal activation or greater right frontal activation. Davidson (1992) suggested that this frontal asymmetry identifies a diathesis predisposing individuals to respond predominantly with negative affect. Studies of EEG in infants have revealed that those who cry during maternal separation show less left than right frontal activation when compared to noncriers (Davidson & Fox, 1989; Fox et al., 1992). The hypothesis that left frontal hypoactivation represents a state-independent marker of vulnerability to depression is supported by the presence of this alpha asymmetry in previously depressed adults in a euthymic state (Henrique & Davidson, 1990) and in infants of depressed mothers (Dawson et al., 1997; Field et al., 1995). Some recent EEG studies have not, however, found evidence of decreased left frontal activation in depressed adults (Reid et al., 1998) or adolescents (Kentgen et al., 2000), which has led to a search for possible mediating variables. In addition to methodological issues, such as test-retest reliability and reference electrode site (Debener et al., 2000; Reid et al., 1998), a possible mediating variable discussed below is the presence of comorbid anxiety disorders (Bruder, Fong, et al., 1997).

One of the most consistent findings in neuroimaging studies of depression has been reduced metabolism or regional cerebral blood flow in the left dorsolateral prefrontal cortex (for reviews see George et al., 1994; Grasby, 1999; Videbech, 2000). Reduced metabolism in depressed patients has been found in additional prefrontal regions, including the anterior cingulate (Mayberg, 1994; Drevets et al., 1997). There are, however, other regions of prefrontal cortex (i.e., ventral and orbital regions), in which metabolism was *increased* in depressed patients (Biver et al., 1994; Brody et al., 1999). There is also strong evidence that alterations of prefrontal metabolism in depression are state-dependent. Reduced left dorsolateral prefrontal and anterior cingulate metabolism tends to normalize following clinical recovery from depression (Baxter et al., 1989; Bench et al., 1995). Moreover, normalization of activity in dorsolateral (Mayberg et al., 1999) or ventrolateral prefrontal cortex (Brody et al., 1999) was reported to be even stronger in the right than in the left hemisphere.

Thus, both EEG alpha asymmetry and neuroimaging studies have found evidence of reduced left prefrontal activation in depressed patients. However, it is not clear that these measures converge on a common neurophysiologic deficit in depression. Abnormal prefrontal alpha asymmetry in depression has been hypothesized to be a stable (trait) characteristic, whereas abnormalities of prefrontal metabolism were state-dependent. Studies measuring both EEG alpha asymmetries and glucose metabolism, or other neuroimaging measures (e.g., fMRI), in the same depressed patients and controls are needed to clarify this issue. Further study is also needed to determine how reduced left prefrontal activation impacts on the clinical symptoms and cognitive function of depressed patients.

Davidson and Tomarken (1989) suggested that the abnormal frontal asymmetry in depression reflects a deficit in left prefrontal mechanisms that regulate approach behaviors, which may clinically be manifested in symptoms such as psychomotor retardation and low energy level. This is supported by neuroimaging findings linking left dorsolateral hypoactivation in depression to psychomotor retardation or poverty of speech (Bench et al., 1993; Dolan et al., 1993). In our prior chapter (Bruder, 1995), we presented the results of a principal components analysis (PCA) of event-related brain potential (ERP) and perceptual asymmetry data for depressed patients and controls who were tested on several cognitive tasks. One PCA-derived factor was associated with having longer latency of the P3 potential to auditory stimuli in the right than in the left hemifield and reduced right visual field advantage for perceiving syllables. A slowing of cognitive processing for stimuli in the right hemifield is consistent with the hypothesis of left frontal hypoactivation depression.

PARIETOTEMPORAL ASYMMETRIES IN DEPRESSION

In dichotic listening tasks in which complex tones or musical chords are simultaneously presented to the two ears, healthy adults typically show an advantage for perceiving the stimulus in the left ear. This is thought to reflect the dominance of right temporal cortex for pitch discrimination (Coffey et al., 1989; Sidtis, 1981). Depressed patients have been reported to show reduced left ear (right hemisphere) advantage in nonverbal dichotic listening tasks (Bruder, 1988; Johnson & Crockett, 1982; Overby et al., 1989). Also, Bruder et al. (1995) measured brain ERPs of depressed patients and healthy controls during a dichotic complex tone test. Healthy adults showed the expected left ear advantage for perceiving complex tones, which was associated with having greater P3 amplitude over right than over left hemisphere sites. Depressed patients did not show either this perceptual asymmetry or the associated hemispheric asymmetry of P3, which is consistent with other evidence of right hemisphere dysfunction in depression (Flor-Henry, 1976; Heller et al., 1995; Miller et al., 1995; Liotti et al., 1991). Reduced left ear (right hemisphere) advantage was also found to be related to important clinical features of depression, including diagnostic subtype. Patients having a melancholic depression with pervasive anhedonia and vegetative symptoms such as insomnia, anorexia, or psychomotor retardation had no left ear advantage for complex tones, whereas patients having a nonmelancholic, atypical depression with preserved pleasure capacity and reversed vegetative features showed a normal left ear advantage (Bruder et al., 1989; Bruder, 1995).

Patients having a melancholic depression also had an abnormally large right ear advantage for perceiving dichotic consonant-vowel syllables (Bruder et al., 1989). Accuracy scores indicated that this was due to poorer left ear performance in melancholia, which again points to dysfunction of the right temporal region. Although findings for depressed patients on verbal dichotic listening tests have been inconsistent (for a review, see Bruder, 1988), both adolescents and adults having a major depressive disorder were found to have an abnormally large right ear advantage on the Fused Rhymed Words Test (Pine et al., 2000). This is one of the most reliable and valid dichotic listening tests for assessing hemispheric dominance for language (Wexler & Halwes, 1983; Zatorre, 1989).

A study by Davidson and Hugdahl (1996) suggests that the enhanced right ear advantage may be related to both parietotemporal and prefrontal activational asymmetries. They examined in healthy adults the relationship of right ear advantage for perceiving dichotic consonant vowels and resting EEG alpha asymmetry measured 4 months prior to the dichotic test. As might be expected, individuals with greater activation (less EEG alpha) over left parietotemporal regions had a larger right ear advantage for perceiving dichotic syllables. The larger right ear advantage in depressed patients could therefore stem from greater activation of left than of right parietotemporal regions, which is consistent with the resting alpha asymmetry seen for depressed adults and adolescents in most studies (Davidson et al., 1987; Henriques & Davidson, 1990; Kentgen et al., 2000; Reid et al., 1998; but see Henriques & Davidson, 1991 and Schaffer et al., 1983 for negative findings). Most interestingly, Davidson & Hugdahl (1996) found that alpha asymmetry in the prefrontal region was also related to dichotic listening asymmetry, but in the *opposite* direction. Decreased activation of the left prefrontal region (i.e., the asymmetry seen in depressed adults; Davidson, 1992) and increased activation of the right prefrontal region were associated with greater right ear advantage. Thus, the same pattern of prefrontal and parietotemporal activational asymmetries typically seen in depression were predictive of enhanced right ear advantage for dichotic syllables.

Studies measuring visual field asymmetries for nonverbal stimuli have also found evidence of right parietotemporal dysfunction in patients having a unipolar depressive disorder (Jaeger et al., 1987; Liotti et al., 1991) or bipolar depressive disorders (Bruder et al., 1989, 1992). Moreover, two recent studies measuring brain ERPs to face stimuli have provided direct evidence of right parietal hypoactivation in depressed patients (Deldin et al., 2000; Kayser et al., 2000). Deldin et al. (2000) measured ERPs of depressed patients and healthy controls while they performed a recognition memory task with positive, negative, and neutral face and word stimuli. Amplitude of the N2 potential was reduced in depressed patients, with the greatest reduction over right parietal cortex. This right-lateralized N2 reduction was specific to face stimuli with a positive affective valence.

One of the most consistent findings of ERP studies using emotional stimuli has been the larger amplitude of the late P3 potential to positive or negative affective stimuli when compared to neutral stimuli, and this P3 enhancement was greatest over right parietotemporal sites (see Kayser et al., 1997 for a review). Given the hypothesis of right parietotemporal hypoactivation in depression, Kayser et al. (2000) predicted that depressed patients would be less likely to show an enhancement of late P3 amplitude to emotional stimuli. They measured the ERPs of unmedicated depressed patients and healthy controls to pictures of dermatological patients showing disordered facial areas (negative stimuli) or healed facial areas after cosmetic surgery (neutral stimuli). The pictures were briefly exposed (250 ms) to the right or left visual field so as to directly stimulate the contralateral hemisphere. One of the distinct advantages of this paradigm is that the pictures depicting negative and neutral affective content are highly similar in physical characteristics, so as to reduce the influence of visuospatial processing. Also, no overt response is required to the affective stimuli, thus reducing the influence of cognitive processing and response-related potentials. In agreement with prior studies, healthy adults showed greater late P3 amplitude to the negative than to the neutral pictures, and this was most marked over the right parietotemporal region. In contrast to the healthy adults, depressed patients had a marked reduction of late P3 amplitude and failed to show the enhancement of late P3 to negative as compared to neutral stimuli.

Although these findings are supportive of the hypothesis of right parietotemporal hypoactivation in depression, the depressed patients did show a transient increase of an early P3 subcomponent in response to negative as compared to neutral stimuli, particularly over the right parietal region. The enhancement of this early P3 to negative stimuli in depressed patients and the absence of enhancement of late P3 suggested to Kayser et al. the possibility that early stimulus classification in depressed patients was followed by an inhibition of the later affective processing. In accordance with this suggestion, they found that depressed patients showed the same N2 amplitude and topography as healthy controls, with greatest N2 over the right parietal region. The lack of the N2 reduction seen for depressed patients in the Deldin et al. (2000) study may stem from the different ERP paradigms in these studies. Deldin et al. measured ERPs during a recognition memory task that entails more cognitive and response-related processing than the passive viewing of affective pictures in the Kayser et al. study.

Although neuroimaging studies of depression have focused predominantly on prefrontal regions of interest, there are reports of decreased metabolism in right temporal lobe (Post et al., 1987) and bilaterally in parietal regions (Biver et al., 1994; Cohen et al., 1992). A weakness of most neuroimaging studies of depression has been the failure to control for comorbidity with anxiety disorders. The opposing effects of depression and anxiety or anxious arousal on activational asymmetries in the parietotemporal region could account for why more imaging studies in depressed patients have not reported abnormal asymmetries in this region (Heller et al., 1995). Also, neuroimaging studies often report findings for small samples and generally have not dealt adequately with the issue of diagnostic heterogeneity of depression.

COMORBIDITY OF DEPRESSIVE AND ANXIETY DISORDERS

Anxiety is a common symptom in depressive disorders, and about half of patients having a major depressive disorder exhibit comorbidity with an anxiety disorder (Gulley & Nemeroff, 1993; Zimmerman et al., 2000). This is a potential problem for studies of brain asymmetry in depressive disorders because depression and anxiety appear to be associated with *opposite* abnormalities of lateralized hemispheric function. Findings of reduced left hemifield advantages on visual half-field or dichotic listening tests in depressed patients (Bruder et al., 1989; Jaeger et al., 1987; Overby et al., 1989) or students with high depression scores (Heller et al., 1995) have supported the hypothesis of right hemisphere dysfunction in depression. In contrast, visual hemifield findings suggestive of left hemisphere dysfunction or right hemisphere hyperactivation have been reported for patients having anxiety disorders (Liotti et al., 1991) and for students with high trait anxiety (Heller et al., 1995; Tucker et al., 1981). Similarly, neuroimaging studies have found decreased metabolism or regional cerebral blood flow in the left temporoparietal cortex of patients having a panic disorder (Meyer et al., 2000; Nordahl et al., 1998). A recent study using hierarchical regression analyses of visual perceptual asymmetries for depressed patients and nonpatients has reported further evidence of the opposing patterns of hemispheric asymmetries associated with depression and anxiety (Keller et al., 2000).

The impact of comorbidity of depression and anxiety on regional brain asymmetries was demonstrated in a study in which resting EEG was recorded in depressed patients with or without an anxiety disorder and healthy controls (Bruder, Fong, et al., 1997). Patients with comorbidity of major depressive and anxiety disorders (primarily a panic disorder or social phobia) had the *opposite* alpha asymmetry pattern at parietal sites when compared to patients having a major depression without an anxiety disorder. Patients having an anxious depression showed an alpha asymmetry indicative of greater activation over right than left parietal sites, whereas those having a "pure" depressive disorder showed less activation over right than left parietal sites. This is consistent with the opposite direction of perceptual asymmetries seen in depression and anxiety (Heller et al., 1995; Keller et al., 2000). Depressed patients with an anxiety disorder also showed evidence of greater activation over right than left frontal sites, whereas this was not seen in depressed patients without an anxiety disorder or in healthy controls. Comorbidity of depressive and anxiety disorders may therefore act to heighten the abnormal frontal alpha asymmetry that has been reported to occur in depressive disorders (Davidson, 1992).

Given the relationship of EEG alpha asymmetry at prefrontal and parietotemporal sites to perceptual asymmetry on a dichotic listening task (Davidson & Hugdahl, 1996), we predicted that depressed patients with or without a comorbid anxiety disorder would also differ in their dichotic listening performance (Bruder et al., 1999). Patients having an anxious depression did differ from nonanxious depressed patients and controls in showing a larger left ear (right hemisphere) advantage for complex tones, whereas nonanxious depressed patients differed in showing a larger right ear (left hemisphere) advantage for fused words. An index of characteristic perceptual asymmetry (Levy et al., 1983) indicated that the anxious depressed patients had a bias favoring right hemisphere activation, whereas the nonanxious depressed patients had a bias favoring left hemisphere activation. This difference in characteristic perceptual asymmetry between the anxious and nonanxious depressed patients agrees with the different direction of parietal alpha asymmetries seen for these groups (Bruder, Fong, et al., 1997).

The favoring of right over left hemispheric activation in anxious depression could stem from hyperactivation of right parietotemporal cortex due to anxious arousal (Heller et al., 1995), from left parietotemporal hypoactivation seen in anxiety disorders (Meyer et al., 2000; Nordahl et al., 1998), or from some combination of both. Examination of the absolute accuracy scores indicated that the enhanced left ear advantage of anxious depressed patients was clearly due to their poorer right ear accuracy (Bruder et al., 1999). Given the contralateral nature of the projections from the ear to auditory cortex, this finding may suggest left parietotemporal hypofunction in anxious depression. However, a study of the effects of arousal level on dichotic listening in students suggests an alternative explanation (Asbjörnsen et al., 1992). They observed that a highly arousing negative condition (threat of electric shock) reduced the right ear advantage for perceiving dichotic consonant-vowel syllables, and suggested that threat of a shock not only primes the right hemisphere but also facilitates callosal transfer of the left ear input, and as a result the left ear stimulus interferes with the processing of the right ear stimulus. Thus, heightened right parietotemporal activation in anxious depressed patients may increase left ear stimulus interference with the right ear stimulus and result in reduced right ear accuracy.

A number of studies have reported that the presence of comorbid depressive and anxiety disorders is associated with poorer outcome of treatment with medication or interpersonal therapy (Fava et al., 1997; Feske et al., 2000; Frank et al., 2000), although some studies have not found this relationship (Tollefson et al., 1994). The characteristic perceptual asymmetry observed for depressed patients with a comorbid anxiety disorder (i.e., a favoring of right hemisphere activation) resembles that seen for nonresponders to the antidepressant fluoxetine (Prozac), whereas the opposite asymmetry in patients having a "pure" depressive disorder (i.e., a favoring of left hemisphere activation) resembles that seen for treatment responders (Bruder et al., 1996). Below we review evidence from dichotic listening, EEG, and neuroimaging studies that point to differences in regional brain asymmetry between treatment-responsive and nonresponsive subgroups of depressed patients.

RELATIONS OF BRAIN ASYMMETRY IN DEPRESSION TO TREATMENT OUTCOME

Several studies suggest that individual differences in perceptual asymmetry on dichotic listening tests are related to the therapeutic response to antidepressants or cognitive-behavioral therapy. Our initial study found a difference in pretreatment perceptual asymmetry between subgroups of depressed patients formed on the basis of their subsequent clinical response to a tricyclic antidepressant (Bruder et al., 1990). Patients who showed a favorable response to treatment—a Clinical Global Improvement (CGI) rating of "much improved" or "very much improved"—failed to show the left ear (right hemisphere) advantage for dichotic complex tones seen for both tricyclic nonresponders and healthy controls. This supported our hypothesis that tricyclic responders would show evidence of right hemisphere dysfunction similar to that seen for patients having a melancholic depression, a diagnostic subtype that typically responds well to this type of antidepressant. The findings of this study were, however, only partially replicated in a follow-up study (Stewart et al., 1999). Although there was no difference between tricyclic responders and nonresponders on the complex tone test, there were significant differences between these groups in their left ear accuracy on the dichotic consonant-vowel test. Patients who responded to treatment with a tricyclic antidepressant had poorer left ear accuracy when compared to treatment nonresponders, placebo responders, and healthy controls. Although their poorer left ear accuracy provides evidence of right hemisphere dysfunction in tricyclic responders, the absence of a group difference on the complex tone test weakens this conclusion.

In a multisite study of the selective serotonin reuptake inhibitor (SSRI) fluoxetine, unmedicated depressed patients who subsequently responded to fluoxetine had a greater right ear (left hemisphere) advantage for dichotic fused words and less left ear (right hemisphere) advantage for complex tones when compared to treatment nonresponders (Bruder et al., 1996). There was no change in perceptual asymmetries following treatment, which suggests that these laterality differences between fluoxetine responders and nonresponders represent stable, state-independent characteristics. These findings from two clinical centers support the conclusion that a characteristic perceptual asymmetry favoring greater left than right hemispheric activation during dichotic listening is associated with better outcome of treatment with an SSRI antidepressant.

We also investigated the potential value of dichotic listening tests in predicting outcome of cognitive-behavioral therapy for depression (Bruder, Stewart, et al., 1997). Depressed patients were tested before receiving 16 weekly sessions of standard cognitive therapy. Following treatment, outcome was evaluated, using the CGI scale, by a rater who was unaware of the dichotic listening results. Patients who responded to cognitive therapy had twice the right ear (left hemisphere) advantage compared to nonresponders and healthy controls. Although this resembles the larger right ear advantage observed for fluoxetine responders, the cognitive therapy responders did not show the reduced left ear (right hemisphere) advantage seen for fluoxetine responders. The larger right ear advantage for syllables in cognitive therapy responders was clearly due to their *better* right ear accuracy when compared to nonresponders or healthy controls. This suggests that the abnormal perceptual asymmetry for dichotic syllables in cognitive therapy responders was due to their superior left hemisphere processing of phonetic stimuli, which is likely to involve left parietotemporal activation (Davidson & Hugdahl, 1996). Patients with greater left hemisphere superiority may be better able to use their verbal skills in learning cognitive strategies for relieving depression.

In an ongoing project, we are examining the value of dichotic listening and more direct electrophysiologic measures of hemispheric activation as predictors of response to treatment with an SSRI antidepressive. If differences in perceptual asymmetry observed between fluoxetine responders and nonresponders reflect characteristic, state-independent differences in regional hemispheric activation (Bruder et al., 1996), we predict that these subgroups will also differ in their resting EEG alpha asymmetry patterns. Moreover, perceptual asymmetry scores for these patients should correlate with their alpha asymmetry (Davidson & Hugdahl, 1996). We have also begun to examine whether gender is of importance when studying differences in EEG alpha asymmetry between responders and nonresponders to antidepressants. The greater incidence of depression in women and gender differences in hemispheric asymmetries for cognitive processing underscore the importance of examining the influence of gender in this context (Heller, 1993).

Preliminary dichotic listening and EEG data were analyzed for 34 patients (21 female) who were classified as fluoxetine responders and 19 patients (7 female) who were nonresponders (Bruder et al., 2001). The depressed outpatients in this study were tested during a drug-free phase prior to receiving 12 weeks of treatment with fluoxetine. An independent evaluator, blind to the patient's EEG and dichotic listening data, rated each patient at the end of the 12 weeks of treatment, using the CGI scale. Patients with ratings of "much improved" or "very much improved" were considered to be responders and all other patients were considered as nonresponders. The difference in perceptual asymmetry between treatment responders and nonresponders on the dichotic fused words and complex tone tests replicated those seen in our prior study (Bruder et al., 1996). As can be seen in figure 20.1, there was an overall trend for responders to have a larger right ear (left hemisphere) advantage for words and a smaller left ear (right hemisphere) advantage for complex tones when compared to nonresponders. The differences in asymmetry between responders and nonresponders were, however, dependent on gender. On the words test, female responders showed a markedly larger right ear advantage when compared to female nonresponders, but there was no significant difference between male responders and nonresponders. On the complex tone test, the

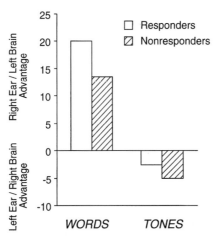

Figure 20.1 Mean perceptual asymmetry for fluoxetine responders and nonresponders on dichotic fused word and complex tone tests. Perceptual asymmetry score = 100 $(R - L)/(R + L)$, where R = right ear score and L = left ear score.

tendency for responders to have a smaller left ear advantage when compared to nonresponders was primarily seen for males.

Analyses of the resting EEG focused on alpha power because of its inverse relation to cortical activation and prior findings of abnormalities of alpha asymmetries in depressed patients (Davidson, 1992). Although there was no significant difference in overall alpha power between fluoxetine responders and nonresponders, these groups did differ in their alpha asymmetry, and this was greatest in the eyes open condition. Figure 20.2 shows the overall alpha asymmetry (averaged over homologous anterior, central and posterior sites) for responders and nonresponders in the eyes open and closed conditions. Positive scores indicate greater activation (less alpha) over the left than the right hemisphere, whereas negative scores indicate greater activation (less alpha) over the right hemisphere. In the eyes open condition, nonresponders showed overall greater activation (less alpha) over the right than the left hemisphere, but responders did not. Further analyses indicated that the difference in alpha asymmetry between responders and nonresponders in the eyes open condition was statistically significant for females but not for males. Also, there was a significant correlation between the perceptual asymmetry for fused words and EEG alpha asymmetry in the eyes open condition for female patients (r = .51,

Gerard E. Bruder

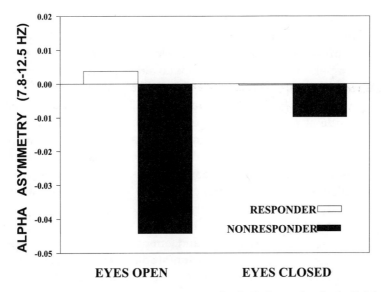

Figure 20.2 Mean EEG alpha asymmetry (log[right hemisphere] − log[left hemisphere]) for fluoxetine responders and nonresponders in the eyes open and eyes closed conditions. Positive scores indicate greater activation (less alpha) over the left than the right hemisphere, and negative scores indicate greater activation (less alpha) over the right than the left hemisphere.

p < .01), but not male patients (r = −.15, ns). Greater activation (less alpha) over the right than the left hemisphere in female patients was associated with smaller left hemisphere advantage for perceiving dichotic words.

The above findings indicate that individual differences among depressed patients in hemispheric asymmetries, as measured by dichotic listening or resting EEG, were related to outcome of treatment with an SSRI antidepressant. In accordance with our prior study (Bruder et al., 1996), patients who responded to fluoxetine differed from nonresponders in favoring left over right hemisphere processing of dichotic stimuli. Also, fluoxetine nonresponders differed from responders in showing an EEG alpha asymmetry indicative of overall greater right than left hemisphere activation. These relationships between hemispheric asymmetries and treatment response were more evident among depressed women than men. However, given the relatively small samples, the influence of gender in this context will need replication.

Neuroimaging studies have also provided preliminary evidence that pretreatment regional brain metabolism is related to response to antidepressants (Little et al., 1996; Mayberg et al., 1997; Ketter et al., 1999). Unipolar depressed patients who subsequently responded to venlafaxine or bupropion had decreased left middle frontal gyral and bilateral prefrontal and temporal metabolism compared to healthy controls (Little et al., 1996). Hypermetabolism of the rostral anterior cingulate was associated with favorable response to treatment with a SSRI, tricyclic antidepressant, or bupropion, whereas hypometabolism was associated with poorer response to these treatments. Interestingly, these anterior cingulate differences tended to be right-lateralized (Mayberg et al., 1997). Most recently, Ketter et al. (1999) found pretreatment frontal and left insular metabolism were differentially related to response to carbamazepine and nimodipine. The large variety of medications used in these imaging studies makes it difficult, however, to compare their findings with those reviewed above for perceptual and electrophysiologic studies.

OVERVIEW AND THEORETICAL INTEGRATION OF BRAIN ASYMMETRY FINDINGS FOR DEPRESSION

EEG measures of alpha asymmetry and neuroimaging measures of regional cerebral metabolism or blood flow in a resting state have provided evidence of left prefrontal hypoactivation in depressive disorders. On the other hand, behavioral laterality tests assessing perceptual asymmetry and brain ERP measures of regional hemispheric activity, and to a lesser extent resting EEG and neuroimaging meaures, have provided evidence of relative hypoactivation of right parietotemporal regions in depressive disorders. The converging evidence from behavioral, electrophysiologic, and neuroimaging studies therefore gives further support to the hypothesis that *both* left prefrontal and right parietotemporal inactivation are involved in depression (Kinsbourne & Bemporad, 1984). Moreover, recent findings confirm that mood disorders following stroke are associated with both left frontal and right posterior lesions (Shimoda & Robinson, 1999).

There is also increasing evidence that individual differences among depressed patients in perceptual, EEG, and ERP asymmetries are related to their clinical features (e.g., diagnostic subtype, comobidity with anxiety disorders, and responsiveness to treatments for depression).

Right parietotemporal dysfunction (e.g., as evidenced by poor left ear accuracy during dichotic listening) is most evident in major depression with melancholia, but is also seen among patients having a non-melancholic depression who respond favorably to treatment with a tricyclic antidepressant. Also, patients having a "pure" major depression show heightened right ear (left hemisphere) advantage for perceiving dichotic fused words and resting EEG alpha asymmetries indicative of greater left than right parietotemporal activation, which is not seen in depressed patients having a comorbid anxiety disorder. This is consistent with evidence that depression and anxiety are associated with opposing patterns of perceptual asymmetry (Heller et al., 1995; Keller et al., 2000), and underscores the need to take comorbidity with anxiety into account in studies of brain asymmetry in depression. Similarly, depressed patients who respond favorably to the SSRI antidepressant fluoxetine (Prozac) show perceptual asymmetries indicative of a characteristic favoring of left over right parietotemporal activation, whereas nonresponders show perceptual and EEG asymmetries indicative of overall greater right than left hemisphere activation. The right hemispheric favoring in fluoxetine nonresponders resembles that seen in depressed adults having a comorbid anxiety disorder, which is of particular interest, given reports of poor treatment outcome in patients having an anxious depression. Also, neuroimaging studies have begun to emerge suggesting that metabolism of right or left prefrontal structures is related to clinical response to antidepressants (Ketter et al., 1999; Mayberg et al., 1997).

Davidson (1992) has proposed that prefrontal asymmetries are related to an approach/withdrawal dimension, with left frontal activation being related to approach behaviors and right frontal activation to withdrawal behaviors. Left frontal hypoactivation could therefore be manifested clinically in symptoms of depression, such as psychomotor retardation, poverty of speech, or absence of motivation, whereas right frontal hypoactivation could be manifested in anxious behaviors or negative affect. This model does not, however, deal with the role of asymmetries in more posterior brain regions. A model developed by Heller (1990) similarly hypothesizes that activity in the frontal region is associated with the valence dimension of emotion and, in addition, proposes that activity in the right posterior region is associated with the arousal dimension of emotion. Low levels of arousal in depression would be associated with decreased activity in right parietotemporal cortex. This model could therefore account for why "pure" depression is accompanied by both left frontal and right parietotemporal hypoactivation. Moreover, as Heller et al. (1995) suggest, panic or other anxious states that increase right parietotemporal activation will act to cancel out the tendency for depression to be associated with decreased right parietotemporal activation. The high incidence of comorbity with anxiety disorders could thereby account for why some EEG and imaging studies have not found evidence of right parietotemporal hypoactivation in depression. These models are, however, limited because they fail to deal with the clinical heterogeneity of depression and its relationship to brain asymmetry.

Several lines of evidence suggest the existence of treatment-responsive and nonresponsive subtypes of depression that differ in brain asymmetry. First, patients who respond to a tricyclic antidepressant show evidence of right parietotemporal dysfunction similar to that seen in major depression with melancholia. Thus, there appears to be a subtype of depression that responds favorably to a tricyclic and shares some of the biologic and clinical features commonly seen in melancholia. Second, patients who respond favorably to an SSRI antidepressant show a characteristic perceptual asymmetry consistent with a favoring of left over right parietotemporal activation. This SSRI responsive subtype includes patients having an "atypical depression" but is less likely to include patients having an "anxious depression" with a comorbid anxiety disorder. Third, patients who do not respond to an SSRI antidepressant show perceptual and electrophysiologic asymmetries consistent with a pervasive favoring of right parietotemporal activation. This SSRI nonresponsive subtype appears to be most common among depressed women and may be characterized by heightened psychological distress and negative affectivity. Depressed patients showing evidence of greater right than left pareitotemporal activation would also be expected to respond poorly to a tricyclic antidepressant (Bruder et al., 1990) or to standard cognitive-behavioral therapy for depression (Bruder, Stewart, et al., 1997), and may therefore represent a general category of treatment-nonresponsive depression.

An important question that needs further research is why right-left brain asymmetries should be related to outcome of treatments for depression. One possibility is that the neurotransmitter systems implicated in depressive disorders and affected by antidepressants may have a lateralized distribution in the brain or may be asymmetrically disrupted in a particular subtype of depression. It has, for instance, been suggested that serotonin pathways are asymmetrically distributed in the brain (Mandell & Knapp, 1979; Tucker & Williamson, 1984), although postmortem studies have not found consistent evidence of asymmetries of serotonin uptake (Arato et al., 1991; Arora & Meltzer, 1991). A study measuring glucose metabolism did find that the serotonin-releasing drug d,l-fenfluramine increased metabolism in left prefrontal cortex and temporoparietal areas, and decreased metabolism in right prefrontal cortex in healthy adults (Mann et al., 1996). Moreover, recent neuroimaging studies have reported lateralized differences in regional brain metabolism between responders and nonresponders to antidepressants (Ketter et al., 1999; Mayberg et al., 1997). Studies that compare treatment responders and nonresponders not only on behavioral laterality and electrophysiologic measures but also on neuroimaging measures are needed to specify the biological basis for the relation of brain asymmetries to treatment outcome.

Further study is also needed to determine the role of gender in abnormalities of brain asymmetry in depression. Given the greater incidence of depression among women, most studies in this area have predominantly tested women. Our initial findings suggest that differences in perceptual asymmetry and EEG alpha asymmetry between fluoxetine responders and nonresponders are more evident among women than men (Bruder et al., 2001). Also, Heller (1993) has speculated on the relation of gender differences in hemispheric organization to gender differences in depression. One of the distinct advantages of behavioral laterality tests and electrophysiologic measures of regional hemispheric activity is that they can be economically administered to relatively large samples, which will be necessary for determining how gender modulates differences in brain asymmetry not only between depressed patients and healthy controls but also between treatment-responsive and nonresponsive subgroups of depression.

ACKNOWLEDGMENTS

Preparation of this chapter was supported in part by grant MH-36295 from the National Institute of Mental Health, National Institute of Health, Bethesda, Maryland. Findings are reviewed for several studies conducted with the collaboration and help of many people at New York State Psychiatric Institute. They include my colleagues in the

Psychophysiology Laboratory: Craig Tenke, Jürgen Kayser, Paul Leite, Barbara Stuart, Nil Bhattacharya, and James Towey, and my collaborators in the Depression Evaluation Service: Jonathan Stewart, Frederic Quitkin, Patrick McGrath, and Deborah Deliyannides.

REFERENCES

Allen, J. J., Iacono, W. G., Depue, R. A., & Arbisi, P. (1993). Regional electroencephalographic asymmetries in bipolar seasonal affective disorders before and after exposure to bright light. *Biological Psychiatry, 33*, 642–646.

Arato, M., Frecska, E., MacCrimmon, D. J., Guscott, R., Saxena, B., Tekes, K., & Tothfalusi, L. (1991). Serotonergic interhemispheric asymmetry: Neurochemical and pharmaco-EEG evidence. *Progress in Neuro-Psychopharmacological & Biological Psychiatry, 15*, 759–764.

Arora, R. C., & Meltzer, H. Y. (1991). Laterality and ^{3}H-imipramine binding: Studies in the frontal cortex of normal controls and suicide victims. *Biological Psychiatry, 29*, 1016–1022.

Asbjørnsen, A., Hugdahl, K., & Bryden, M. P. (1992). Manipulations of subjects' level of arousal in dichotic listening. *Brain and Cognition, 19*, 183–194.

Baxter, L. R., Schwartz, J. M., Phelps, M. E., Mazziotta, J. C., Guze, B. H., Selin, C. E., Gerner, R. H., & Sumida, R. M. (1989). Reduction of prefrontal cortex glucose metabolism common to three types of depression. *Archives of General Psychiatry, 46*, 243–250.

Bell, I. R., Schwartz, G. E., Hardin, E. E., Baldwin, C. M., & Kline, J. P. (1998). Differential resting quantitative electroencephalographic alpha patterns in women with environmental chemical intolerance, depressives, and normals. *Biological Psychiatry, 43*, 376–388.

Bench, C. J., Frackowiak, R. S. J., & Dolan, L. J. (1993). Regional cerebral blood flow (rCFG) in depression, measured by position emission tomography (PET): The relationship with clinical dimensions. *Psychological Medicine, 23*, 570–590.

Bench, C. J., Frackowiak, R. S. J., & Dolan, R. J. (1995). Changes in regional cerebral blood flow on recovery from depression. *Psychological Medicine, 25*, 247–251.

Biver, F., Goldman, S., Delvenne, V., Luxen, A., De Maertelaer, V., Hubain, P., Mendlewicz, J., & Lotstra, F. (1994). Frontal and parietal metabolic disturbances in unipolar depression. *Biological Psychiatry, 36*, 381–388.

Brody, A. L., Saxena, S., Silverman, D. H. S., Alborzian, S., Fairbanks, L. A., Phelps, M. E., Huang, S. C., Wu, H. M., Maidment, K., & Baxter, L. R., Jr. (1999). Brain metabolic changes in major depressive disorder from pre- to post-treatment with paroxetine. *Psychiatry Research: Neuroimaging, 91*, 127–139.

Bruder, G. E. (1988). Dichotic listening in psychiatric patients. In K. Hugdahl (Ed.), *Handbook of dichotic listening: Theory, methods and research* (pp. 527–563). New York: John Wiley & Sons.

Gerard E. Bruder

Bruder, G. E. (1995). Cerebral laterality and psychopathology: Perceptual and event-related potential asymmetries in affective and schizophrenic disorders. In R. Davidson & K. Hugdahl (Eds.), *Brain asymmetry* (pp. 661–691). Cambridge, MA: MIT Press.

Bruder, G. E., Fong, R., Tenke, C. E., Leite, P., Towey, J. P., Stewart, J. W., McGrath, P. J., & Quitkin, F. M. (1997). Regional brain asymmetries in major depression with or without an anxiety disorder: A quantitative electroencephalographic study. *Biological Psychiatry, 41*, 939–948.

Bruder, G. E., Otto, M. W., Stewart, J. W., McGrath, P., Fava, M., Rosenbaum, J. F., & Quitkin, F. M. (1996). Dichotic listening before and after fluoxetine treatment for major depression: Relations of laterality to therapeutic response. *Neuropsychopharmacology, 15*, 171–179.

Bruder, G. E., Quitkin, F. M., Stewart, J. W., Martin, C., Voglmaier, M., & Harrison, W. M. (1989). Cerebral laterality and depression: Differences in perceptual asymmetry among diagnostic subtypes. *Journal of Abnormal Psychology, 98*, 177–186.

Bruder, G. E., Stewart, J. W., Mercier, M. A., Agosti, V., Leite, P., Donovan, S., & Quitkin, F. M. (1997). Outcome of cognitive-behavioral therapy for depression: Relation to hemispheric dominance for verbal processing. *Journal of Abnormal Psychology, 106*, 138–144.

Bruder, G. E., Stewart, J. W., Tenke, C. E., McGrath, P. J., Leite, P., Bhattacharya, N., & Quitkin, F. M. (2001). Electroencephalographic and perceptual asymmetry differences between responders and nonresponders to an SSRI antidepressant. *Biological Psychiatry, 48*, 416–425.

Bruder, G. E., Stewart, J. W., Towey, J. P., Friedman, D., Tenke, C. E., Voglmaier, M. M., Leite, P., Cohen, P., & Quitkin, F. M. (1992). Abnormal cerebral laterality in bipolar depression: Convergence of behavioral and brain event-related potential findings. *Biological Psychiatry, 32*, 33–47.

Bruder, G. E., Stewart, J. W., Voglmaier, M. M., Harrison, W. M., McGrath, P., Tricamo, E., & Quitkin, F. M. (1990). Cerebral laterality and depression: Relations of perceptual asymmetry to outcome of treatment with tricyclic antidepressants. *Neuropsychopharmacology, 3*, 1–10.

Bruder, G. E., Tenke, C. E., Stewart, J. W., Towey, J. P., Leite, P., Voglmaier, M., & Quitkin, F. M. (1995). Brain event-related potentials to complex tones in depressed patients: Relations to perceptual asymmetry and clinical features. *Psychophysiology, 32*, 373–381.

Bruder, G. E., Wexler, B. E., Stewart, J. W., Price, L. H., & Quitkin, F. M. (1999). Perceptual asymmetry differences between major depression with or without a comorbid anxiety disorder: A dichotic listening study. *Journal of Abnormal Psychology, 108*(2), 233–239.

Coffey, C. E., Bryden, M. P., Schroering, E. S., Wilson, W. H., & Mathew, R. J. (1989). Regional cerebral blood flow correlates of a dichotic listening task. *Journal of Neuropsychiatry, 1*, 46–52.

Cohen, R. M., Gross, M., Nordahl, T. E., Semple, W. E., & Oren, D. A. (1992). Preliminary data on the metabolic brain pattern of patients with winter seasonal affective disorder. *Archives of General Psychiatry, 49*, 545–552.

Davidson, R. J. (1992). Anterior cerebral asymmetry and the nature of emotion. *Brain & Cognition, 20*, 125–151.

Davidson, R. J., Chapman, J. P., & Chapman, L. J. (1987). Task-dependent EEG asymmetry discriminates between depressed and non-depressed subjects. *Psychophysiology, 24*, 585.

Davidson, R. J., & Fox, N. A. (1989). Frontal brain asymmetry predicts infants' response to maternal separation. *Journal of Abnormal Psychology, 98*(2), 127–131.

Davidson, R. J., & Hugdahl, K. (Eds.). (1995). *Brain asymmetry.* Cambridge, MA: MIT Press.

Davidson, R. J., & Hugdahl, K. (1996). Baseline asymmetries in brain electrical activity predict dichotic listening performance. *Neuropsychology, 10*, 241–246.

Davidson, R. J., & Tomarken, A. J. (1989). Laterality and emotion: An electrophysiological approach. In F. Boller & J. Grafman (Eds.), *Handbook of neuropsychology* (pp. 419–441). Amsterdam: Elsevier.

Dawson, G., Frey, K., Panagiotides, H., Osterling, J., & Hessl, D. (1997). Infants of depressed mothers exhibit atypical frontal brain activity: A replication and extension of previous findings. *Journal of Child Psychology & Psychiatry, 38*(2), 179–186.

Debener, S., Beauducel, A., Nessler, D., Brocke, B., Heilemann, H., & Kayser, J. (2000). Is resting anterior EEG alpha asymmetry a trait marker for depression? *Neuropsychobiology, 41*, 31–37.

Deldin, P. J., Keller, J., Gergen, J. A., & Miller, G. A. (2000). Right-posterior face processing anomaly in depression. *Journal of Abnormal Psychology, 109*, 116–121.

Dolan, R. J., Bench, C. J., Liddle, P. F., Friston, K. J., Frith, C. D., Grasby, P. M., & Frackowiak, R. S. J. (1993). Dorsolateral prefrontal cortex dysfunction in the major psychoses: Symptom or disease specificity? *Journal of Neurology, Neurosurgery and Psychiatry, 56*, 1290–1294.

Drevets, W. C., Price, J. L., Simpson, J. R., Jr., Todd, R. D., Reich, T., Vannier, M., & Raichle, M. E. (1997). Subgenual prefontal cortex abnormalities in mood disorders, *Nature, 386*, 824–827.

Fava, M., Uebelacker, L. A., Alpert, J. E., Nierenberg, A. A., Pava, J. A., & Rosenbaum, J. F. (1997). Major depressive subtypes and treatment response. *Biological Psychiatry, 42*, 568–576.

Feske, U., Frank, E., Mallinger, A. G., Houck, P. R., Fagiolini, A., Shear, M. K., Grochocinski, V. J., & Kupfer, D. J. (2000). Anxiety as a correlate of response to the acute treatment of bipolar I disorder. *American Journal of Psychiatry, 157*, 956–962.

Field, T., Fox, N. A., Pickens, J., & Nawrocki, T. (1995). Relative right frontal EEG activation in 3- to 6-month old infants of "depressed mothers." *Developmental Psychology, 31*(3), 358–363.

Flor-Henry, P. (1976). Lateralized temporal-limbic dysfunction and psychopathology. *Annals of the New York Academy of Sciences, 280*, 777–795.

Fox, N. A., Bell, M. A., & Jones, N. A. (1992). Individual differences in response to stress and cerebral asymmetry. *Developmental Neuropsychology, 8*(2,3), 161–184.

Frank, E., Shear, M. K., Rucci, P., Cyranoswki, J. M., Endicott, J., Fagiolini, A., Grochocinski, V. J., Houck, P., Kupfer, D. J., Maser, J. D., & Cassano, G. B. (2000). Influence of panic-agoraphobic spectrum symptoms on treatment response in patients with recurrent major depression. *American Journal of Psychiatry, 157*, 1101–1107.

George, M. S., Ketter, T. A., & Post, R. M. (1994). Prefrontal cortex dysfunction in clinical depression. *Depression, 2*, 59–72.

Grasby, P. M. (1999). Imaging strategies in depression. *Journal of Psychopharmacology, 13*(4), 346–351.

Gulley, L. R., & Nemeroff, C. B. (1993). The neurobiological basis of mixed depression-anxiety states. *Journal of Clinical Psychiatry, 54*, 16–19.

Heller, W. (1990). The neuropsychology of emotion: Developmental patterns and implications for psychopathology. In N. Stein, B. L. Leventhal, & T. Trabasso (Eds.), *Psychological and biological approaches to emotion* (pp. 167–211). Hillsdale, NJ: Lawrence Erlbaum Associates.

Heller, W. (1993). Gender differences in depression: Perspectives from neuropsychology. *Journal of Affective Disorders, 29*, 129–143.

Heller, W., Etienne, M. A., & Miller, G. A. (1995). Patterns of perceptual asymmetry in depression and anxiety: Implications for neuropsychological models of emotion and psychopathology. *Journal of Abnormal Psychology, 104*, 327–333.

Henriques, J. B., & Davidson, R. J. (1990). Regional brain electrical asymmetries discriminate between previously depressed and healthy control subjects. *Journal of Abnormal Psychology, 99*, 22–31.

Henriques, J. B., & Davidson, R. J. (1991). Left frontal hypoactivation in depression. *Journal of Abnormal Psychology, 100*, 535–545.

Jaeger, J., Borod, J. C., & Peselow, E. (1987). Depressed patients have atypical hemispace biases in the perception of emotional chimeric faces. *Journal of Abnormal Psychology, 96*, 321–324.

Johnson, O., & Crockett, D. (1982). Changes in perceptual asymmetries with clinical improvement of depression and schizophrenia. *Journal of Abnormal Psychology, 91*, 45–54.

Kayser, J., Bruder, G. E., Tenke, C. E., Stewart, J. W., & Quitkin, F. M. (2000). Event-related potentials (ERPs) to hemifield presentations of emotional stimuli: Differences between depressed patients and healthy adults in P3 amplitude and asymmetry. *International Journal of Psychophysiology, 36*, 211–236.

Kayser, J., Tenke, C., Nordby, H., Hammerborg, D., Hugdahl, K., & Erdmann, G. (1997). Event-related potential (ERP) asymmetries to emotional stimuli in a visual half-field paradigm. *Psychophysiology, 34*(4), 414–426.

Keller, J., Nitschke, J. B., Bhargava, T., Deldin, P. J., Gergen, J. A., Miller, G. A., & Heller, W. (2000). Neuropsychological differentation of depression and anxiety. *Journal of Abnormal Psychology, 109*(1), 3–10.

Kentgen, L. M., Tenke, C. E., Pine, D. S., Fong, R., Klein, R. G., & Bruder, G. E. (2000). Electroencephalographic asymmetries in adolescents with major depression: Influence of comorbidity with anxiety disorders. *Journal of Abnormal Psychology, 109*, 797–802.

Ketter, T. A., Kimbrell, T. A., George, M. S., Willis, M. W., Benson, B. E., Danielson, A., Frye, H. A., Herscovitch, P., & Post, R. M. (1999). Baseline cerebral hypermetabolism associated with carbamazepine response, and hypometabolism with nimodipine response in mood disorders. *Biological Psychiatry, 46*, 1364–1374.

Kinsbourne, M., & Bemporad, B. (1984). Lateralization of emotion: A model and the evidence. In N. A. Fox and R. J. Davidson (Eds.), *The psychobiology of affective development*. Hillsdale, NJ: Lawrence Erlbaum Associates.

Levy, J., Heller, W., Banich, M., & Burton, L. A. (1983). Are variations among right handed individuals in perceptual asymmetries caused by characteristic arousal differences between hemispheres? *Journal of Experimental Psychology: Human Perception and Performance, 9*, 329–359.

Liotti, M., Sava, D., Rizzolatti, G., & Caffarra, P. (1991). Differential hemispheric asymmetries in depression and anxiety: A reaction-time study. *Biological Psychiatry, 29*, 887–899.

Little, J. T., Ketter, T. A., Kimbrell, T. A., Danielson, A., Benson, B., Willis, M. W., & Post, R. M. (1996). Venlafaxine or bupropion responders by not nonresponders show baseline prefrontal and paralimbic hypometabolism compared with controls. *Psychopharmacology Bulletin, 32*, 629–635.

Mandell, A. J., & Knapp, S. (1979). Asymmetry and mood, emergent properties of serotonin regulation. *Archives of General Psychiatry, 36*, 909–916.

Mann, J. J., Malone, K. M., Diehl, D. J., Perel, J., Cooper, T. B., & Mintun, M. A. (1996). Demonstration in vivo of reduced serotonin responsitivity in the brain of untreated depressed patients. *American Journal of Psychiatry, 153*, 174–182.

Mayberg, H. S. (1994). Frontal lobe dysfunction in secondary depression. *Journal of Neuropsychiatry & Clinical Neuroscience, 6*, 428–442.

Mayberg, H. S., Brannan, S. K., Mahurin, R. K., Jerabek, P. A., Brickman, J. S., Tekell, J. L., Silva, A., McGinnis, S., Glass, T. G., Martin, C. C., & Fox, P. T. (1997). Cingulate function in depression: A potential predictor of treatment response. *NeuroReport, 8*, 1057–1061.

Mayberg, H. S., Liotti, M., Brannan, S. K., McGinnis, S., Mahurin, R. K., Jerabek, P. A., Silva, J. A., Tekell, J. L., Martin, C. C., Lancaster, J. L., & Fox, P. T. (1999). Reciprocal limbic-cortical function and negative mood: Converging PET findings in depression and normal sadness. *American Journal of Psychiatry, 156*, 675–682.

Meyer, J. H., Swinson, R., Kennedy, S. H., Houle, S., & Brown, G. M. (2000). Increased left posterior parietal-temporal cortex activation after D-fenfluramine in women with panic disorder. *Psychiatry Research: Neuroimaging, 98*, 133–143.

Miller, E. N., Fujioka, T. A. T., Chapman, L. J., & Chapman, J. P. (1995). Hemispheric asymmetries of function in patients with major affective disorders. *Journal of Psychiatric Research, 29,* 173–183.

Nordahl, T. E., Stein, M. B., Benkelfat, C., Semple, W. E., Andreason, P., Zametkin, A., Uhde, T. W., & Cohen, R. M. (1998). Regional cerebral metabolic asymmetries replicated in an independent group of patients with panic disorders. *Biological Psychiatry, 44,* 998–1006.

Overby, L. A. III, Harris, A. E., & Leck, M. R. (1989). Perceptual asymmetry in schizophrenia and affective disorder: Implications from a right hemisphere task. *Neuropsychologia, 27,* 861–870.

Pine, D. S., Kentgen, L. M., Bruder, G. E., Leite, P., Bearman, K., Ma, Y., & Klein, R. G. (2000). Cerebral laterality in adolescent major depression. *Psychiatry Research, 93,* 135–144.

Post, R. M., DeLisi, L. E., Holcomb, H. H., Uhde, T. W., Cohen, R., & Buchsbaum, M. S. (1987). Glucose utilization in the temporal cortex of affectively ill patients: Positron emission tomography. *Biological Psychiatry, 22,* 545–553.

Reid, S. A., Duke, L. M., & Allen, J. J. B. (1998). Resting frontal electroencephalographic asymmetry in depression: Inconsistencies suggest the need to identify mediating factors. *Psychophysiology, 35,* 389–404.

Schaffer, C. E., Davidson, R. J., & Saron, C. (1983). Frontal and parietal electroencephalogram asymmetry in depressed and nondepressed subjects. *Biological Psychiatry, 18,* 753–762.

Shimoda, K., & Robinson, R. G. (1999). The relationship between poststroke depression and lesion location in long-term follow-up. *Biological Psychiatry, 45,* 187–192.

Sidtis, J. J. (1981). The complex tone test: Implications for the assessment of auditory laterality effects. *Neuropsychologia, 19,* 103–112.

Stewart, J. W., Quitkin, F. M., McGrath, P. J., & Bruder, G. E. (1999). Do tricyclic responders have different brain laterality? *Journal of Abnormal Psychology, 108*(4), 707–710.

Tollefson, G. D., Holman, S. L., Sayler, M. E., & Potvin, J. H. (1994). Fluoxetine, placebo, and tricyclic antidepressants in major depression with and without anxious features. *Journal of Clinical Psychiatry, 55*(2), 50–59.

Tucker, D. M., Stenslie, C. E., Roth, R. S., & Shearer, S. L. (1981). Right frontal activation and right hemisphere performance: Decrement during a depressed mood. *Archives of General Psychiatry, 38,* 169–174.

Tucker, D. M., & Williamson, P. A. (1984). Asymmetric neural control systems in human self-regulation. *Psychological Bulletin, 91,* 185–215.

Videbech, P. (2000). PET measurements of brain glucose metabolism and blood flow in major depressive disorder: A critical review. *Acta Psychiatrica Scandinavica, 101,* 11–20.

Wexler, B. E., & Halwes, T. (1983). Increasing the power of dichotic methods: The fused rhymed words test. *Neuropsychologia, 21,* 59–66.

Zatorre, R. J. (1989). Perceptual asymmetry on the dichotic fused words test and cerebral speech lateralization determined by the carotid sodium amytal test. *Neuropsychologia, 27,* 1207–1219.

Zimmerman, M., McDermut, W., & Mattia, J. I. (2000). Frequency of anxiety disorders in psychiatric outpatients with major depressive disorder. *American Journal of Psychiatry, 157,* 1337–1340.

21 The Laterality of Schizophrenia

Michael F. Green, Mark J. Sergi, and Robert S. Kern

When considering the relative weights of the two hemispheres of the brain, it occurred to me that their ordinary relations to each other in this respect might possibly be reversed by a disease of long standing. It seemed not improbable that the cortical centres which are last organized, which are the most high evolved and voluntary, and which are supposed to be located in the left side of the brain, might suffer first in insanity.
—James Crichton-Browne (1879, p. 42)

In 1879, Crichton-Browne tested his theory of lateralized deficits in insanity by comparing the weights of the left and right hemispheres from 32 cases of "acute insanity." He found a slight but consistent tendency for the left hemisphere to be smaller than the right. Applying caution and appropriate methods, he then weighed the brains from cases without a history of insanity, and found a comparable tendency for the left hemisphere to be smaller. Hence Crichton-Browne failed to find evidence of aberrant laterality associated with insanity. Interest in this question, however, did not fade.

In 1915, E. E. Southard, the pathologist for the State Board of Insanity in Massachusetts, published a detailed examination of brains from 25 patients with dementia praecox, the term for schizophrenia at that time. His conclusions were as bold as they were prophetic. For one, he concluded that schizophrenia (dementia praecox) was a disease of brain structure. "I am disposed to believe that the present work ... goes very far toward *placing dementia praecox in the structural group of mental diseases* (p. 631; italics in original). He goes on to say that "Among the 25 cases systematically studied, there were but two without evidence of cortical atrophy" (p. 632). It is the asymmetric nature of this atrophy that is most relevant to this chapter. He noted that the "atrophies and aplasias, when focal, show a tendency to occur in the left hemisphere (p. 662). Hence, even in 1915 considerable awareness existed that schizophrenia may be a lateralized brain disease.

Although the roots of laterality of schizophrenia date back at least to the 19th century, the modern resurgence of interest can be traced to findings in the 1970s that came from two very different types of methods: phenomenology and psychophysiology. A phenomenological approach was used effectively by Flor-Henry (1976), who made careful observations of patients with lateralized epilepsy. Flor-Henry noticed that epilepsy patients with a left hemisphere focus tended to have schizophrenia-like psychotic features, whereas patients with a right hemisphere focus tended to have more mood-related symptoms. He concluded that abnormal neuronal activity in the dominant temporal lobe was mainly responsible for schizophrenia.

Flor-Henry used a phenomenological approach in which he closely examined the symptoms of patients with lateralized brain damage. Using a similar phenomenological approach, Cutting (1994) examined the symptoms of various neurological conditions and concluded that the evidence favored right hemisphere involvement in schizophrenia. He noted classic schizophrenic symptoms (e.g., disordered self-other boundaries, annihilation of will, and flattened affect) in patients with cerebrovascular accidents in the right hemisphere. That two talented clinical investigators used a similar approach and arrived at opposite sides of the brain probably reflects the limitations of a phenomenological approach.

Another influential observation from the 1970s came from psychophysiology. Gruzelier and Venables (1974) noted that skin conductance was asymmetrical in schizophrenia. Schizophrenic patients tended to show increased skin conductance on the right hand in response to orienting tones. They noted, however, that this effect was labile and seemed to depend on overall levels of arousal. As arousal increased, the R > L difference became more pronounced, and at lower arousal levels this pattern reversed. These early formulations were later elaborated into a model of hemispheric imbalance in schizophrenia. In this model, three clinical subtypes of schizophrenia are considered to have three different types of hemispheric activity. The subgroups are active (behavioral overarousal), negative (withdrawal), and unreality (hallucinations and delusions) (Gruzelier & Raine, 1994; Gruzelier, 1994). The model proposes that each subtype has a characteristic pattern of lateral asymmetry based on neurocognitive and psychophysiological indices. The active group has left > right asymmetry, the negative group has right > left asymmetry, and the unreality group has inconsistent asymmetry.

Following these phenomenological and psychophysiological studies, lateralized performance measures provided a more direct approach to the question of laterality in schizophrenia (Walker & McGuire, 1982). Specialized procedures with lateralized presentation included hemifield tests (in which visual stimuli are presented to one visual field or the other) and dichotic listening tests (in which different auditory stimuli are simultaneously presented to each ear). These tests are ideally suited for the study of schizophrenia because the key measures are within-subject; that is, each subject serves as his or her own control. Schizophrenic patients almost always perform worse than a group of comparison subjects, which sometimes makes inferences difficult. In lateralized performance studies, however, the results are interpretable even in the presence of overall group differences. Likewise, lateralized psychophysiological and electrophysiological studies also provide the ability to interpret lateralized differences against the background of overall group differences. As we will see, the results of these performance studies were often consistent with the notion of a left hemisphere abnormality, possibly due to an overactivation of that hemisphere (Gur, 1978).

As is evident from this discussion, the laterality of schizophrenia is an old story with roots in the 19th century (Petty, 1999). The laterality of schizophrenia can also be considered a new story because the literature has grown dramatically since the mid-1990s. A computerized search of the terms "schizophrenia" and either "laterality" or "asymmetry" produced 380 references between January 1994 and July 2000, roughly the period since the last review by Bruder for the first edition of this volume (Bruder, 1995). As an additional indication of recent interest in the topic, an issue of *Schizophrenia Bulletin* (vol. 25, no. 1, edited by R. E. Gur) was devoted to this topic, as was a series of invited papers in *Cognitive Neuropsychiatry* (vol. 2, no. 3). Since the last review, the literature has shifted in predictable ways to take advantage of newer technologies. For example, there have been comparatively few new data-based studies of handedness (although several conceptual papers have been published on the topic). In contrast, the number of studies on neuroimaging and laterality have grown sharply. In particular, there have been a large number of recent MRI studies of structural asymmetry. In addition to studies of brain structure, functional neuro-imaging studies are starting to emerge, but so far are few in number.

In this review, we will cast a wide net and discuss, admittedly in a cursory manner, some of the major developments since the mid-1990s. This review will be separated according to the assessment methods. Specifically, we will discuss handedness, visual and auditory performance measures, electrophysiological procedures, and neuroimaging. As we discuss these topics, we will also mention factors that could be responsible for inconsistency in this literature, such as gender, symptomatology, and age of onset. We begin our discussion with handedness and schizophrenia.

HANDEDNESS

At first glance, handedness should be a simple and easy way to assess laterality in schizophrenia. However, once one descends into the details, it is neither simple nor easy. The study of handedness in schizophrenia introduces challenges in terms of both concepts and assessment.

Handedness has been used as a marker of cerebral dominance for decades because nearly all right-handers have language represented in the left hemisphere. It is noteworthy that left-handedness does not automatically indicate the reverse relationship (i.e., representation of language in the right hemisphere); approximately two-thirds of non-right-handers have language represented in the left hemisphere. The natural occurrence of left-handedness is primarily tied to genetic factors. Hence, for persons without a family history of left-handedness, such deviations may signal other pathological factors (e.g., perinatal trauma) that could produce the shift. Hence, the examination of handedness can serve as a potentially useful behavioral marker for neurodevelopmental factors in schizophrenia.

Traditionally, handedness has been assessed by asking individuals which hand they use to perform certain common, primarily unimanual, everyday tasks. The methods used to assess handedness vary considerably across studies, ranging from self-report measures to multiple-item questionnaires to demonstration methods. Even within studies that used the same type of method, interpretation is difficult due to differences in the number of tasks included, as well as scoring and classification criteria. Although writing hand has been the most commonly used task, other tasks include throwing, using a pair of scissors, combing hair,

M. F. Green, M. J. Sergi, and R. S. Kern

brushing teeth, eating with a spoon, and using a hammer (Annett, 1970; Oldfield, 1971).

Handedness in Schizophrenia: Is There a Leftward Shift?

If perinatal trauma is an etiological factor for a subgroup of schizophrenic patients, then one would predict a leftward shift in the distribution of handedness in this population. Such a shift has been found in other mental disorders with suspected neurodevelopmental causes (e.g., childhood autism and mental retardation) in which non-right-handedness is pervasive. In a review of the literature on handedness in schizophrenia, Satz and Green (1999) summarized the findings from 23 studies. The results (14 positive, 7 null, and 2 paradoxical) provided some support for a leftward or atypical shift in handedness for persons with schizophrenia. They also examined the data to see whether the shift was due to an increase in left- or mixed-handedness. Mixed-handedness is defined as the nonexclusive use of one hand (either right or left) to perform all handedness tasks within a given inventory (e.g., right hand to write, left hand to comb hair). The vast majority of studies reporting prevalence data found an increase in mixed-handedness. Only two studies reported an increase in left-handedness. Interpretation of these studies requires some consideration of their methodologies.

First, two studies used observed writing hand as the lone item for determining the classification of handedness. Hence, subjects included in these studies could be classified only as right- or left-handed, but not mixed-handed. Second, the criterion used to classify handedness varied across studies. Some studies required that a 100% criterion be met for the classification of handedness (e.g., use of same hand for all items), and others used a less stringent criterion. Third, the items included in the assessment of handedness across studies were not equivalent in terms of their ability to detect lateralized processes. Fourth, the results from studies may differ depending on whether questionnaires or demonstration tests were used.

Though self-report and questionnaire measures are the most frequently used methods for handedness, they have limitations when used to assess handedness in persons with severe mental illness. For example, some persons with severe mental illness may be impaired in the ability to self-reflect, and may not give an accurate account of their true hand preference. In addition, the self-report method is subject to distortion and embellishment, which may be a problem in assessing handedness in some delusional or thought-disordered patients. An alternative method is behavioral observation, which was used to assess handedness in the early 20th century (Durost, 1934). A modern version, the Hand Preference Demonstration Test (HPDT), was developed by investigators from our lab (Soper et al., 1986). In the HPDT, participants demonstrate the use of nine items (presented three times each, in a quasi-random order), which allows for the measurement of within- and between-item consistency. The demonstration method has revealed that a subset of mixed-handers have within-item inconsistency (i.e., failure to use the same hand for all three trials of a given task), a pattern that has been called "ambiguous handedness" (AH).

AH has been observed in studies of other mental disorders with suspected neurodevelopmental pathology, such as autism and mental retardation (Satz et al., 1985; Soper et al., 1986; Soper et al., 1987). The AH subtype has also been found in a subset of hospitalized schizophrenic patients in two separate studies using the HPDT (Green et al., 1989; Nelson et al., 1993). In both studies there was an increased prevalence of mixed handedness in the schizophrenic groups compared to normal controls (approximately 40% compared to 15% in normals), and approximately half of the 40% were subjects with AH. Interestingly, AH is modifiable to some extent, depending on task demands (Nelson et al., 1993). The distribution of AH in schizophrenia could be shifted to the right by making the handedness tasks more complex and, presumably, making greater attentional demands (e.g., requiring a sequence of skilled motor movements, such as putting a penny through a small slit in a can).

Two studies examined whether the leftward shift in handedness in schizophrenia was limited to schizophrenic patients, or if it was also found in first-degree relatives (Clementz et al., 1994; Orr et al., 1999). Clementz et al. examined the prevalence of handedness in groups of patients with schizophrenia, major depression, and bipolar disorder, and their unaffected first-degree relatives and compared the prevalence of handedness in these groups to normal controls. Handedness was assessed using a self-report measure, the 10-item Oldfield Inventory (Oldfield, 1971). The schizophrenic group was significantly more left-handed than the control group, but the results also showed that increased prevalence of left-handedness was specific to schizophrenia. The other psychotic disorder groups did not show this shift away from

M. F. Green, M. J. Sergi, and R. S. Kern

right-handedness. There was no significant difference in the handedness of first-degree relatives of schizophrenic patients and controls, suggesting that atypical handedness may result from nongenetic etiological factors.

Orr et al. (1999) assessed handedness using the Annett Handedness Questionnaire in patients with schizophrenia, affective psychosis, other psychosis, the first-degree relatives of these groups, and normal controls. Like Clementz et al., they found a shift away from right-handedness in the schizophrenia group compared to controls (due mainly to differences between female patients and controls); the other psychotic groups failed to show this leftward shift. In contrast to the Clementz et al., Orr et al. found a trend to an excess of mixed-handedness in the first-degree relatives of schizophrenic patients compared to controls. Like the findings for patients, the excess of mixed-handedness in schizophrenic first-degree relatives was largely due to a greater prevalence in females compared to controls. Excess mixed-handedness was not evident in the first-degree relatives of the other psychotic disorder patients. These investigators also looked at neurodevelopmental correlates of mixed-handedness in schizophrenia to further examine whether the shift in handedness may be due to genetic or to environmental factors. There were no significant associations between mixed-handedness and pregnancy and birth complications, premorbid IQ, or overall premorbid social adjustment among the schizophrenic patients. Overall, the findings of Orr et al. suggest a genetic basis for the shift in handedness in schizophrenia.

Considerations

Because handedness subtypes are believed to reflect differences in cerebral organization, several studies have explored whether handedness in schizophrenia is related to neurocognitive deficits and symptoms. In general, non-right-handed schizophrenic patients have tended to perform more poorly than right-handed patients on neurocognitive tests. Non-right-handed schizophrenic patients have been found to perform more poorly than right-handed patients on measures of executive functioning, nonverbal intellectual functioning, memory, and language functioning (Katsanis & Iacono, 1989; Faustman et al., 1991; Manoach, 1994; Manschreck et al., 1996). In a study from our lab (Hayden et al., 1997), verbal and procedural memory, executive functioning, and manual dexterity were assessed in psychotic inpatients (mainly schizophrenic patients) who had AH (n = 19) and were clearly lateralized (n = 39). The AH group were significantly worse than the lateralized group in terms of verbal memory and manual dexterity, but better in terms of procedural learning. Regarding symptomatology, some studies (Taylor & Amir, 1995) found an association between thought disorder and non-right-handedness. In a large sample (n = 232) of schizophrenic patients, Taylor et al. (1982) found that only one symptom, formal thought disorder, was related to left-handedness and mixed-handedness. Manoach et al. (1988) found a similar relationship between thought disorder and handedness in a study that classified subjects according to writing hand. A later study by Manoach (1994), using a dimensional handedness assessment, yielded similar results. In sum, these findings suggest that atypical forms of handedness in schizophrenia may be associated with a pattern of diffuse neurocognitive deficits and thought disorder.

PERCEPTUAL ASYMMETRY

Few new studies of perceptual asymmetry have been published since the mid-1990s. Not that these procedures have been forgotten; perceptual tasks are starting to be combined with neuroimaging techniques. The literature on performance measures can largely be divided into two types of studies: dichotic listening and visual half field studies.

Dichotic Listening Findings

To study disturbances of left hemisphere processing, investigators have compared the performance of schizophrenic patients and normals on dichotic listening tests using verbal and nonverbal stimuli. Based on a theory of left hemisphere dysfunction in schizophrenia, one would expect schizophrenic patients to be comparable to normals in processing nonverbal stimuli (intact right hemisphere functioning), but show a deficit in processing verbal stimuli (impaired left hemisphere functioning). Studies using nonverbal stimuli, such as tones or clicks, are generally in agreement in showing a left ear advantage (right hemisphere) for schizophrenic patients that is similar to the pattern seen in normal controls (Colbourn & Lishman, 1979; Yozawitz et al., 1979; Overby et al., 1989; Raine et al., 1989). There has been a shift in the findings

M. F. Green, M. J. Sergi, and R. S. Kern

from studies using verbal stimuli on dichotic listening tests, with earlier studies reporting a large right ear (left hemisphere) advantage and more recent ones reporting a reduced or no right ear advantage (see Bruder, 1983, 1988 for a review; Green et al., 1994).

The early studies of dichotic listening tended to include a memory load; for example, a task that required subjects to recall three pairs of digits or words presented to the two ears (e.g., Nachshon, 1980). Most studies using this paradigm showed that schizophrenic patients, or a subgroup with paranoid or positive symptoms, had an abnormally large right ear advantage. The finding was interpreted as left hemisphere overactivation. Unfortunately, the results were confounded by the fact that the task included presentation of stimuli with a heavy memory load. Since six digits were presented on each trial, three to each ear, the order in which items were processed affected performance outcome. If right ear items tend to be reported first, then subjects with memory disturbances were likely to show large right ear advantages for the task because the items presented to the left ear may have been forgotten. Hence, the apparent right hemisphere overactivation might be a by-product of memory deficits (Bruder, 1995).

Subsequent studies have attempted to correct this methodological problem by using "fused" dichotic syllable or word tests, in which subjects perceive only one word or syllable per trial. The majority of studies using fused tests have found reduced or no right ear (left hemisphere) advantage for schizophrenic patients (Bruder et al., 1995; Colbourn and Lishman, 1979; Kiyota, 1987; Løberg et al., 1999; Wexler 1986; Wexler et al., 1991), though the findings are not entirely consistent (Raine et al., 1989; Wexler & Henninger, 1979). Differences in results between studies may be due to other factors, such as the type of stimuli used in the study (e.g., use of real words vs. syllables), the clinical state of the patients (e.g., remitted vs. psychotic state), and whether the patients have a history of hallucinations (Green et al., 1994).

A few recent studies have examined the relationship between symptoms and dichotic listening test performance, the impact of hallucinations, and whether or not ear preference can be modified by introducing an attentional component. Bruder et al. (1995) examined the relationship between symptoms and dichotic listening test performance in a study of 32 schizophrenic patients and 65 patients with major depressive disorder. Subjects were administered the Fused Rhymed

Words Test (Wexler & Hawles, 1983). Laterality Quotient (LQ) scores on the dichotic listening test correlated with PANSS ratings on positive and negative symptoms. A positive LQ indicates a right ear advantage, whereas a negative LQ indicates a left ear advantage. As predicted, there was a general tendency for greater positive symptoms to be associated with less right ear advantage. However, among the symptoms, the association reached statistical significance only for hallucinatory behavior. The results for negative symptoms were less consistent; five subscales yielded a negative relationship and two subscales yielded a positive relationship.

As noted earlier, a reduced right ear advantage could be due to differences in symptom profiles. Using the CV-syllables dichotic listening paradigm developed by Hugdahl (e.g. Hugdahl, 1995), Green et al. (1994) reported that hallucinating psychotic patients showed no right ear (left hemisphere) advantage for dichotic nonsense syllables, whereas nonhallucinating patients had a normal ear advantage. Interestingly, they found no difference in performance when hallucinating patients were retested in a nonhallucinating state. These findings suggest a traitlike characteristic for the abnormality. The study also asked patients to attend to the stimuli presented to one ear versus the other. Neither patient group was able to modify its ear advantage with this attentional manipulation.

A more recent follow-up study focused on the impact of placing attentional demands on dichotic listening test performance (Loberg et al., 1999). Subjects were 33 schizophrenic inpatients and 33 healthy adults matched for handedness, age, and gender distribution. Subjects were administered a consonant-vowel syllables version of the dichotic listening test, and were tested under three conditions: a nonforced attention condition, a forced-right condition, and a forced-left condition. In the latter two conditions, subjects were told to focus on the stimuli presented to the respective ear. The results revealed no right ear advantage for the patients under the nonforced attention condition. Similar to the findings by Green et al. (1994), the patients could not modify their dichotic listening performance under either forced attention condition, although controls could adjust their ear preference with respect to the attentional demands. These findings support a "dual deficit" model of schizophrenia in that patients showed a deficit in both automatic (nonforced attention condition) and controlled (forced attention conditions) levels of processing.

M. F. Green, M. J. Sergi, and R. S. Kern

Visual Field Asymmetry

Studies using tachistoscopic visual hemifield presentation of stimuli have yielded results similar to dichotic listening studies. An early study by Gur (1978) found that schizophrenic patients showed a left field (right hemisphere) advantage for a dot localization task, but no right field (left hemisphere) advantage for a syllable identification task. Subsequent visual hemifield studies involving the assessment of left hemisphere functioning have yielded inconsistent results (Pic'l et al., 1979; Connolly et al., 1979; Magaro & Chamrad, 1983; George & Neufeld, 1987; Merriam & Gardner, 1987; Colbourn & Lishman, 1979; Eaton, 1979), with the more recent studies generally confirming Gur's original finding of no right visual field advantage in the processing of verbal stimuli (Kamali et al., 1991; Min & Oh, 1992). Taken together, the studies suggest that schizophrenic patients are comparable to normal controls in showing a right hemisphere advantage for the processing of nonverbal stimuli. In contrast, the findings for left hemisphere specialization are more equivocal, and suggestive of an abnormality.

A recent study examined hemispheric specialization for the processing of faces and letters in a sample of 15 right-handed schizophrenic outpatients and 14 controls (White et al., 1998). The stimuli (faces and letters) were presented tachistoscopically to one or the other hemifield for 150 ms. Responses followed a go/no-go discrimination such that certain faces/letters were treated as "go" stimuli (requiring a response) and others as "no-go" (requiring no response). The schizophrenic group showed a right field (left hemisphere) advantage on the letter recognition task, but no field advantage for the facial recognition task. The normal controls also showed a (nonsignificant) left hemisphere advantage on the letter task, and the expected right hemisphere advantage on the facial recognition task. This study produced findings contrary to earlier reports of intact right but impaired left hemisphere specialization. It is difficult to reconcile the contrary findings. One possible methodological confound is the degree to which subjects learned the "go/no-go" discrimination for the two tasks. Any delays in their recall for selected stimuli could introduce additional error variance that could explain the lack of an effect for facial processing. Also, the two tasks were not matched for level of difficulty, and the failure to show a significant right visual field (left hemisphere) advantage in normal controls for the processing of letters could be due to the simplicity of the task.

In a study of spatial working memory in schizophrenia, Park (1999) examined hemifield differences in errors. Thirty-three schizophrenic patients and 29 age-matched normal controls were shown a stimulus (a black circle) for 200 ms at one of eight possible target locations about a central fixation point. The task was administered under two conditions (a working memory task with a 10 s delay and a sensory control task). Two types of errors were recorded: those which the subject corrected immediately, and those which were never corrected. Never-corrected errors are believed to reflect a loss of spatial representation of the target, whereas immediately corrected errors reflect intact representation of the target but interference with the output response. Patients made significantly more never-corrected errors when the target was presented in the right visual field than in the left. Interestingly, the same pattern of errors was seen in a sample of "psychosis-prone" university students (as measured by the Perceptual Aberration Scale; Chapman et al., 1978). The results suggest that the loss of spatial representation during a delay period may be more severe for stimuli presented in the right visual field (left hemisphere) for schizophrenic patients and psychosis-prone individuals.

Considerations

Some of the differences in findings for visual hemifield asymmetry in schizophrenia could be related to differences in the clinical syndromes of patients included in these studies. To examine this point, Bustillo et al. (1997) examined covert visuospatial attention in schizophrenic subgroups of patients with "deficit" (n = 17) and "nondeficit" (n = 28) syndromes. Classification of patients with deficit syndrome was determined by the presence of two or more enduring negative symptoms on the Schedule for the Deficit Syndrome (Kirkpatrick et al., 1989). Subjects were instructed to fixate on the center of a computer monitor and respond when a target (an asterisk) appeared. The duration between cue and target was either 100, 200, or 800 ms. Targets appeared on each side of the central fixation point and were preceded by a visual cue that could be neutral, valid, or invalid. Nondeficit patients showed a slower reaction time to targets presented in the right visual field than in the left visual field, but only for the 100 ms cue-target interval. Deficit patients were slowest in overall reaction time but, like normals, showed no asymmetry. The results support the notion of left hemisphere dysfunc-

M. F. Green, M. J. Sergi, and R. S. Kern

tion in the processing of visual information with nondeficit forms of schizophrenia.

ELECTROPHYSIOLOGY AND LATERALITY IN SCHIZOPHRENIA

Event-related potentials (ERPs) provide information about the electrophysiology underlying information-processing deficits in schizophrenia (Pfefferbaum et al., 1995). These methods also provide excellent ways to probe laterality in schizophrenia. Previous studies of P300 (P3) in schizophrenia using an oddball paradigm found an asymmetric left hemisphere amplitude reduction (e.g., Faux et al., 1987, 1990; McCarley et al., 1989, 1993; Strik et al., 1993). Among more recent studies the findings are mixed. Some studies comparing the P3 of persons with schizophrenia and healthy persons have found that patients had reduced P3 amplitude in the left temporal lobe (Salisbury et al., 1998; Turetsky et al., 1998), whereas other studies have found no differences (Egan et al., 1994; Ford et al., 1994).

The disparate findings may be a product of the discriminability of the stimuli. One recent study found that P3 asymmetry in schizophrenia depends on pitch disparity (Weisbrod et al., 1997); P3 amplitude was reduced over the left compared to the right temporal sites in schizophrenic patients when pitch disparity in the oddball paradigm was high (simple discriminability). However, when discriminability was low, the P3 amplitude of patients was similar over the left and right hemispheres. Alternatively, the disparate findings regarding P3 asymmetry in schizophrenia may be a product of the high variability in P3 amplitude in schizophrenia. Hill and Weisbrod (1999) found an association between overall P3 amplitude and P3 asymmetry in a sample of patients: Those with low overall P3 amplitudes showed left hemispheric amplitude reduction in P3, while those with high P3 amplitudes showed right hemispheric amplitude reduction.

Studies of negative ERP components have also produced evidence of atypical laterality in schizophrenia. The N200 (N2) ERP component is associated with initial stimulus classification. In a recent study of the N2 component by Bruder et al. (1999), ERPs were recorded from schizophrenic patients, schizoaffective patients, and healthy controls as they completed a dichotic listening task. Healthy controls showed the expected right ear advantage for dichotic syllables, and their performance was associated with greater N2 amplitude at left relative to right temporoparietal sites. Patients with schizophrenia showed neither the performance nor the N2 asymmetry. The inference was that N2 asymmetry is associated with left hemisphere superiority for language-related processing and that this asymmetry is lacking in schizophrenia, both at the performance and at the electrophysiological level.

Mismatch negativity (MMN), another negative component in auditory ERPs, is believed to index automatic processes involved in verbal sensory (echoic) memory (Näätänen et al., 1978). Recent studies have reported MMN reduction in schizophrenia that is more prominent in the left hemisphere (Hirayasu et al., 1998). Comparing patients with schizophrenia and healthy persons in an auditory oddball task, Hirayasu et al. found that both groups showed an asymmetry (L < R), but this asymmetry was more pronounced in the temporal-parietal region of the patients. The patients' relative reduction of MMN is consistent with abnormalities of primary or adjacent auditory cortex of the left temporal-parietal region, a region involved in verbal sensory (echoic) memory.

Magnetoencephalographic (MEG) studies also provide evidence of atypical electrophysiological asymmetry in schizophrenia. Using 122-channel whole-head MEG and magnetic resonance imaging (MRI), Tiihonen et al. (1998) located the source of auditory ERPs (N100m) to simple tones in patients with schizophrenia (n = 19) and healthy persons (n = 20). Normal controls showed an asymmetry in that the sources were more anterior in the right hemisphere. The sources for the patients were much more variable (dispersed) than for the normal controls, and they tended to show an absence of the normal asymmetry. Such findings, while intriguing, are not always replicated (Hajek et al., 1997).

Considerations

Some of the inconsistency in this literature might be explained by the influence of gender and symptomatology. MEG studies have found gender-related laterality differences in schizophrenia. Psychotic males and females with schizophrenia differ in the 100 ms latency auditory evoked component, M100, with the male patients tending to show more aberrant patterns of activity than the females (Reite and Rojas, 1997; Reite et al., 1997; Rojas et al., 1997). In healthy persons, Heschl's gyrus (the source of M100) is further anterior in the right hemisphere, and this asymmetry is more pronounced in healthy males (Reite et al., 1995). In contrast, schizophrenic men evidenced less laterality for M100, with sources that were relatively anterior in the left hemisphere and posterior in the right. Actively psychotic females showed a source that was further anterior in the right hemisphere, reflecting more asymmetry than normal female controls (Reite and Rojas, 1997; Reite et al., 1997).

Symptoms of schizophrenia are associated with differential patterns of laterality in electrophysiological studies. Starting with the work of Gruzelier and Venables (1974), differences in psychophysiological and electrophysiological asymmetry have been identified with specific symptom clusters. Patients with the active syndrome (raised motor activity, pressured speech, accelerated cognition, positive or labile affect, and affective delusions) tend to display higher activation in the left hemisphere relative to the right hemisphere, whereas patients with the withdrawn syndrome (negative symptoms such as poverty of speech, flattened affect, social and emotional withdrawal, and motor retardation) often display higher activation in the right hemisphere relative to the left hemisphere (Gruzelier et al., 1987, 1988). In a recent study, schizophrenic patients with the active syndrome and withdrawn syndrome were compared on a typical auditory oddball detection task (Gruzelier et al., 1999). Syndrome-related patterns of asymmetry were noted for the N1, N2, and P3 components. The amplitudes for N2 and P3 were reduced in the left hemisphere of active patients, and in the right hemisphere of withdrawn patients. In contrast, the asymmetries for N1 amplitudes were reversed, with higher amplitude in the left for active patients, and higher in the right for withdrawn patients.

NEUROIMAGING AND LATERALITY IN SCHIZOPHRENIA

Although the laterality of brain structure in schizophrenia was explored years ago by Crichton-Browne, Southard, and others, the modern resurgence of interest came from air encephalography, one of the early methods for in vivo neuroimaging. In the lumbar air encephalography procedure, 8 ml of air was injected into the ventricular system through a lumbar puncture. Films of the brain were taken while the subject was placed in different positions (to move the air around). This imaging procedure yields an outline of the lateral ventricles and sometimes of the third ventricle as well. Despite the relative crudeness of the method, it clearly implicated left-side abnormalities in schizophrenia. For example, in one study of air encephalography, 41 chronic psychiatric patients (90% with a diagnosis of schizophrenia) received the procedure. Ten of these patients had ventricular enlargement that was predominantly unilateral—in every instance it was the left hemisphere (Hunter et al., 1968).

The laterality of brain structure and function in schizophrenia can be separated into two different types of questions. One line of research, an extension of the early studies mentioned above, has searched for evidence of left hemisphere abnormality in schizophrenia. A second line of research has looked for an absence of laterality. Instead of exploring whether schizophrenia has abnormal laterality, this line of investigation looks for a *lack* of normal asymmetry. Patients with schizophrenia may have reduced, or even reversed, brain asymmetries compared with controls. We will discuss each of these questions separately.

Are Structural Brain Abnormalities Lateralized in Schizophrenia?

There is no doubt that schizophrenia is associated with structural brain abnormalities, the most replicated finding being enlarged ventricles. The presence of enlarged ventricles in schizophrenia was documented with early forms of the encephalography procedure in the 1930s (Moore et al., 1935). Subsequently findings of enlarged ventricles (the lateral and third ventricles) were established by CT and have been replicated with MRI. Enlarged ventricles in schizophrenia is as solid as imaging findings get for this illness. But is ventricular enlargement symmetric? Several neuroimaging studies (reviewed in Petty, 1999) found the ventricular enlargement to be asymmetrical and larger on the left side. Such ventricular asymmetry has also been found with autopsy studies.

Although ventricular enlargement is a consistent finding in schizophrenia, it is nonspecific and does not implicate a particular brain region. Likewise, asymmetry in ventricular enlargement tells us little about the structures involved. Hence investigators have gone in for a closer look at asymmetry in key brain structures. One region that has received considerable attention is the temporal lobe and its structures. Some studies have reported reduced left temporal lobe volume (Bogerts et al., 1990), and others have found reductions in the left parahippocampal region (Young et al., 1991).

M. F. Green, M. J. Sergi, and R. S. Kern

As the spatial resolution of neuroimaging improves, it becomes possible to visualize more specific areas. One study (Hirayasu et al., 2000) conducted a fine-grained analysis of temporal structures in a sample of 20 first-episode patients with schizophrenia and controls. Patients with schizophrenia had smaller left (but not right) planum temporale volumes than controls. The volume for Heschl's gyrus, which is adjacent, showed bilateral reduction in schizophrenia. These findings are consistent with left-lateralized volume reduction in the posterior superior temporal gyrus in chronic schizophrenic patients. Such findings of asymmetry are not always replicated. For example, a recent MRI study of 53 schizophrenia patients and 29 normal controls found bilateral (not asymmetric) reduction in the superior temporal gyrus, and no reduction in the hippocampus and parahippocampus (Sanfilipo et al., 2000).

One way to make sense of conflicting findings from many studies is to use meta-analyses in which a large number of studies are pooled together to extract general trends. Two meta-analyses of the structural neuroimaging in schizophrenia have been published recently. One of them (Nelson et al., 1998) used data on 522 patients across 18 studies. The focus was on the volume of the hippocampus (sometimes with, and sometimes without, the amygdala). They found bilateral reduction in these structures of about 4%, but no indication of lateralized reduction. A very comprehensive meta-analysis of 58 studies (1588 patients) examined ventricular size, lobe volume, and mesial temporal lobe structures (Wright et al., 2000). Not surprisingly, this meta-analysis found ventricular enlargement (patients' ventricles were about 126% the size of controls'), but no clear lateralized differences. Likewise, the authors found slight reductions in frontal and temporal lobe volume, but without lateralized effects. Similar to the study by Nelson et al., they found bilateral reduction in the hippocampus of 6–7%.

The conclusion is that, despite many reports of lateralized structural findings in schizophrenia, these studies are not always replicated. Applications of meta-analysis raise doubts about whether these lateralized findings are present across a large number of studies. It is entirely possible that lateralized differences are present in some specific brain areas which are missed in the meta-analyses (such as the planum temporale).

The literature on laterality in functional neuroimaging is much smaller than that on structural neuroimaging. But this literature is obviously growing as new technologies become available. Initially, studies used xenon inhalation to measure cerebral blood flow, then positron emission tomography (PET), single photon emission computerized tomography (SPECT), and recently, functional MRI. Gur and Chin (1999) summarized the recent studies in this area—not an easy task, considering that the studies differ in the type of neuroimaging method. In addition, they differ widely in the type of activation task used (e.g., verbal fluency, continuous performance task)—or, indeed, whether any task was used at all (resting). Gur and Chin conclude that "the majority of studies have reported left hemisphere abnormalities, some bilateral abnormalities, and a few primarily right hemisphere effects" (1999, p. 144). The abnormalities are usually reduced activity (metabolism or blood flow), but not always, as we will see. Hence functional neuroimaging may not be any more consistent than structural neuroimaging in implicating a dysfunctional hemisphere for schizophrenia.

One intriguing finding that has been replicated is *increased* activity in the temporal lobe in schizophrenia. For example, a study by Gur et al. (1995) considered metabolism assessed with PET in three groups: neuroleptic naive patients, patients who were previously medicated but were off medications, and a comparison group. The metabolic rates for the three groups were highly comparable across brain regions. An exception was the midtemporal region, in which both patient groups showed relatively increased left/right ratios. This pattern of finding fits with some of the performance studies mentioned above in the section "Perceptual Asymmetry," which suggested a dysfunctional and overactive left hemisphere in schizophrenia.

Do Patients with Schizophrenia Have Normal Asymmetry?

The brains of humans have a predictable asymmetry. For one, the frontal lobe extends further on the right, whereas the occipital lobe extends further on the left. This asymmetry gives the impression that an average brain has been "spun around," and is consequently called "torque." Several studies have considered whether the brains of schizophrenic patients have this torque, or whether the normal asymmetry is lacking, or even reversed. Normal asymmetry can also be detected at the level of individual brain structures. For example, within the superior temporal gyrus, the planum temporale, which is involved in processing speech sounds, is typically larger in the left; and the adjacent region,

M. F. Green, M. J. Sergi, and R. S. Kern

Heschl's gyrus, is typically larger in the right. The reduction or absence of normal laterality in schizophrenia is predicted by Crow's theory of asymmetry and psychosis (Crow, 2000; Crow et al., 1989). This theory, in simplified form, states that schizophrenia is a disorder of the genetic mechanisms which control cerebral asymmetry. It predicts that the greatest structural disturbance should be in regions with the highest degree of asymmetry, and also that the disturbance should be present in first-degree relatives of patients. As we will see, these predictions have received support.

An early study (Luchins & Meltzer, 1983) noted a reversal of the normal asymmetry ($L > R$) in the occipital lobes. Subsequent studies have reported the loss of normal torque, and this has been found in first-episode patients (Bilder et al., 1994). Recent studies have taken advantage of the improved spatial resolution to document the loss of normal asymmetries in highly specific regions. For example, it appears that normal $L > R$ asymmetry in the parietal lobe is reversed in schizophrenia (Niznikiewicz et al., 2000). In this study, the left inferior parietal lobe was 7% larger than the right for the comparison group. But in the patients, it was 6.3% smaller. This finding was largely explained by the absence of an asymmetry in the angular gyrus: In the comparison group, the left was 18.7% larger than the right; in the patients, it was 4.7% smaller.

Even with the impressive developments in neuroimaging, the most exact brain measurements are still obtained on autopsy. Another focused study examined asymmetry of two structures in the medial temporal lobe: the parahippocampal and fusiform gyri (McDonald et al., 2000). Volume measures were obtained for the gray matter of these two gyri in patients and controls. The normal brains had an $L > R$ asymmetry for these gyri, but this asymmetry was significantly reversed for both structures in the brains of patients.

Overall, the evidence for reduced or reversed structural laterality in schizophrenia is rather convincing. If this pattern holds up, it raises a key question: Is it due to the *presence* of the disorder, or is it due to *vulnerability* to the disorder? When differences are found between patients and controls, it is possible to argue that these differences are related to the illness itself (e.g., effects of hospitalization, medications, or the presence of psychosis). On the other hand, it is entirely possible that the brain differences are linked to the predisposition for schizophrenia. If so, then similar abnormalities should be present in the first-degree relatives of schizophrenic patients, even if they have no signs of illness. So far, only a few neuroimaging studies have been conducted with the relatives of schizophrenic patients. One study examined the cerebral asymmetry in patients, their relatives, and normal controls (Sharma et al., 1999). A clever feature of this study was to examine a subgroup of relatives separately. These relatives were considered to be "obligate carriers," nonpsychotic relatives who appeared to be transmitting liability for schizophrenia. For example, the nonpsychotic mother of a schizophrenic patient who has a schizophrenic parent or sibling would be considered an obligate carrier. The study found a lack of normal brain asymmetry in schizophrenia, replicating previous findings. Of interest, the obligate carriers showed the same pattern as the patients, suggesting that the lack of normal asymmetry may be an indicator of vulnerability instead of the presence of illness.

Examinations of absent or reversed laterality are starting to be considered in studies of functional imaging. Spence et al. (2000) assessed three groups of subjects—schizophrenic patients, normal controls, and first-degree relatives who were obligate carriers—on PET during a verbal fluency task. As noted in an invited commentary on the study, one of the most striking findings of the study was that while normal controls activated the left (but not right) dorsolateral prefrontal cortex during the verbal fluency task, patients and obligate carriers activated this region on both left and right (Crow, 2000). Hence, at the level of functional activity, it appears that both patients and obligate carriers had reduced lateralized activation during verbal fluency, again suggesting that the abnormality is associated with vulnerability to illness.

Considerations

Sex differences, symptomatology, and age of onset all appear to be critical variables that moderate the expression of asymmetries in schizophrenia. Gender differences have been observed in studies of structural asymmetry in schizophrenia. For example, male-female differences in brain torque were seven times greater in schizophrenic patients than in healthy persons (Guerguerian & Lewine, 1998). The larger gender difference in brain torque was produced by greater torque in schizophrenic males and reduced torque in schizophrenic females. Differences in the asymmetry of the inferior parietal lobule may be gender-specific (Frederikse et al., 2000). The inferior parietal lobule is involved in visuospatial processing, an area in which males tend to have a performance advantage. Healthy persons show an L > R asymmetry in inferior parietal volume, and this is more pronounced in males (Frederikse et al., 1999). In their study, Frederikse et al. (2000) found that male patients had significantly smaller left inferior parietal volumes than healthy males and showed a reversal of the normal L > R asymmetry. Conversely, females with schizophrenia and healthy females did not differ in left or right inferior parietal lobule volume or in asymmetry. Thus, disruption of the typical L > R asymmetry in the inferior parietal lobe appears to be limited to males with schizophrenia.

In an MRI study of the temporal and frontal lobes, Turetsky et al. (1995) found overall decreases in brain volume in left temporal and right frontal regions. More specifically, the reduced left temporal lobe volume was correlated with ratings of negative symptoms. The suggestion is that consideration of clinical symptoms (or syndromes) might facilitate inferences from a fairly inconsistent literature on structural neuroimaging and laterality.

Age of onset may help to explain the findings of a reduced or reversed structural asymmetry. For example, Maher et al. (1998) used MRI to assess structural asymmetry in schizophrenia and found that low levels of asymmetry in the frontal and temporal areas were strongly associated with early illness onset. Likewise, Fukuzako et al. (1997) reported that early age of onset was related to reduction of the normal asymmetry in the hippocampus.

SUMMARY

Research on the laterality of schizophrenia has gone through at least two major transitions in the past few years: one entirely expected, and one not. The expected transition is that recent studies of laterality in schizophrenia capitalized on new developments, notably powerful neuroimaging techniques. The impressive number of studies in this area since the mid-1990s is a result, in large part, of the proliferation of neuroimaging studies. Also important has been a less obvious transition in the types of questions asked. As typified by the neuroimaging literature, there are two types of theories about lateralization in schizophrenia with subtle, but important differences. Although not mutually exclusive, the two theories search for different underlying abnormalities. One is that schizophrenia involves a primary abnormality of the left hemisphere. Findings in this area are notoriously difficult to replicate, and, sometimes wash out in large meta-analyses. The other theory is that schizophrenia involves an abnormal *lack* of lateralization. Here the story is more consistent and is bolstered with frequent findings of reduced or reversed structural asymmetry. Have we heard such a conclusion before? Indeed, the findings from the most technically complex methods (neuroimaging) converge with the least technically complex (handedness) in suggesting that schizophrenia may involve the failure to establish normal laterality, as opposed to the establishment of an abnormal laterality.

New ways to explore the laterality of schizophrenia have included studies of first-degree relatives. Studies of unaffected first-degree relatives, such as those who are "obligate carriers," are highly informative and help us understand whether abnormal laterality reflects the presence of the illness or vulnerability to the illness. Studies of the laterality of functional neuroimaging that are just starting, and hold promise if (and only if) the activation tasks are well understood. For this reason, studies of lateralized performance measures (such as dichotic listening and visual field asymmetry) should be viewed as prerequisite steps for informed neuroimaging paradigms. Last, careful consideration of several key moderating and/or mediating factors (e.g., gender, symptomatology, and age of onset) may clarify a murky literature.

REFERENCES

Annett, M. (1970). A classification of hand preference by association analysis. *British Journal of Psychology, 61*, 303–321.

Bilder, R. M., Wu, H., Bogerts, B., Degreef, G., Ashtari, M., Alvir, J. M. J., Snyder, P. J., & Lieberman, J. A. (1994). Absence of regional hemispheric volume asymmetries in first-episode schizophrenia. *American Journal of Psychiatry, 151*, 1437–1447.

Bogerts, B., Ashtari, M., Degreef, G., Alvir, J. M. J., Bilder, R. M., & Lieberman, J. A. (1990). Reduced temporal limbic structure volumes of magnetic resonance images in first episode schizophrenia. *Psychiatry Research: Neuroimaging, 35*, 1–13.

Bruder, G. E. (1983). Cerebral laterality and psychopathology: A review of dichotic listening studies. *Schizophrenia Bulletin, 9*, 134–151.

Bruder, G. E. (1988). Dichotic listening in psychiatric patients. In K. Hugdahl (Ed.), *Handbook of dichotic listening: Theory, methods and research* (pp. 527–564). New York: John Wiley & Sons.

Bruder, G. E. (1995). Cerebral laterality and psychopathology: Perceptual and event-related potential asymmetries in affective and scizophrenic disorders. In K. Hugdahl and R. J. Davidson (Eds.), *Brain asymmetry* (pp. 661–691). Cambridge, MA: MIT Press.

Bruder, G., Kayser, J., Tenke, C., Amador, X., Friedman, M., Sharif, Z., & Gorman, J. (1999). Left temporal dysfunction in schizophrenia: Event-related potential and behavioral evidence from phonetic and tonal dichotic listening tasks. *Archives of General Psychiatry, 56,* 267–276.

Bruder, G. E., Rabinowicz, E., Towey, J., Brown, A., Kaufmann, C. A., Amador, X., Malaspina, D., & Gorman, J. M. (1995). Smaller right ear (left hemisphere) advantage for dichotic fused words in patients with schizophrenia. *American Journal of Psychiatry, 152,* 932–935.

Bustillo, J. R., Thaker, G., Buchanan, R. W., Moran, M., Kirkpatrick, B., & Carpenter, W. T., Jr. (1997). Visual information-processing impairments in deficit and nondeficit schizophrenia. *American Journal of Psychiatry, 154,* 647–654.

Chapman, L. J., Chapman, J. P., & Raulin, M. L. (1978). Body-image aberration in schizophrenia. *Journal of Abnormal Psychology, 87,* 399–407.

Clementz, B. A., Iacono, W. G., & Beiser, M. (1994). Handedness in first-episode psychotic patients and their first-degree biological relatives. *Journal of Abnormal Psychology, 103,* 400–403.

Colbourn, C. J., & Lishman, W. A. (1979). Lateralization of function and psychotic illness: A left hemisphere deficit? In J. Gruzelier and P. Flor-Henry (Eds.), *Hemisphere asymmetries of function and psychopathology* (pp. 539–559). Amsterdam: Elsevier/North Holland Biomedical Press.

Connolly, J. F., Gruzelier, J. H., Kleinman, K. M., & Hirsch, S. R. (1979). Lateralized abnormalities in hemisphere-specific tachistoscopic tasks in psychiatric patients and controls. In J. Gruzelier and P. Flor-Henry (Eds.), *Hemisphere asymmetries of function in psychopathology* (pp. 491–509). Amsterdam: Elsevier/North Holland Biomedical Press.

Crichton-Browne, J. (1879). On the weight of the brain and its component parts in the insane. *Brain, 2,* 42–67.

Crow, T. J. (2000). Invited commentary on: Functional anatomy of verbal fluency in people with schizophrenia and those at genetic risk. The genetics of asymmetry and psychosis. *British Journal of Psychiatry, 176,* 61–63.

Crow, T. J., Ball, J., Bloom, S. R., Brown, R., Bruton, C. J., Colter, N., Frith, C. D., Johnstone, E. C., Owens, D. G. C., & Roberts, G. W. (1989). Schizophrenia as an anomaly of development of cerebral asymmetry: A postmortem study and a proposal concerning the genetic basis of the disease. *Archives of General Psychiatry, 46,* 1145–1150.

Cutting, J. (1994). Evidence for right hemisphere dysfunction in schizophrenia. In A. S. David & J. C. Cutting (Eds.), *The neuropsychology of schizophrenia* (pp. 231–242). London: Lawrence Erlbaum Associates.

Durost, W. N. (1934). The development of a battery of objective group tests of manual laterality, with the results of their application to 1300 children. *Genetic Psychological Monographs, 16*, 225–235.

Eaton, E. M. (1979). Hemisphere-related visual information processing in acute schizophrenia before and after neuroleptic treatment. In J. H. Gruzelier and P. Flor-Henry (Eds.), *Hemisphere asymmetries of function in psychopathology* (pp. 511–526). Amsterdam: Elsevier/North Holland Biomedical Press.

Egan, M. F., Duncan, C. C., Suddath, R. L., Kirch, D. G., Mirsky, A. F., & Wyatt, R. J. (1994). Event-related potential abnormalities correlate with structural brain alterations and clinical features in persons with chronic schizophrenia. *Schizophrenia Research, 11*, 259–271.

Ellis, H. D., de Pauw, K. W., Christodoulou, G. N., Papageorgiou, L., Milne, A. B., & Joseph, A. B. (1993). Responses to facial and non-facial stimuli presented tachistoscopically in either or both visual fields by patients with the Capgras delusion and paranoid schizophrenics. *Journal of Neurology, Neurosurgery, and Psychiatry, 56*, 215–219.

Faustman, W. O., Moses, J. A., Ringo, D. L., & Newcomer, H. W. (1991). Left-handedness in male schizophrenia patients is associated with increased impairment on the Luria-Nebraska Neuropsychological Battery. *Biological Psychiatry, 30*, 326–334.

Faux, S. F., McCarley, R. W., Shenton, M. E., Nestor, P. G., Marcy, B., & Ludwig, A. (1990). Preservation of P300 event-related topographical asymmetries in schizophrenia with use of either linked ear or nose reference sites. *Electroencephalographic Clinical Neurophysiology, 75*, 378–391.

Faux, S. F., Torello, M. W., McCarley, R. W., Shenton, M. E., & Duffy, F. H. (1987). P300 topographic alterations in schizophrenia: A replication study. In R. Johnson, J. W. Rohrbaugh, & R. Parasuraman (Eds.), *Current trends in event-related potential research. EEG, supp. 40*, 688–694.

Flor-Henry, P. (1976). Lateralized temporal-limbic dysfunction and psychopathology. *Annals of the New York Academy of Sciences, 280*, 777–795.

Ford, J. M., White, P. M., Csernansky, J. G., Faustman, W. O., Roth, W. T., & Pfefferbaum, A. (1994). ERPs in schizophrenia: Effects of antipsychotic medication. *Biological Psychiatry, 36*, 153–170.

Frederikse, M. E., Lu, A., Aylward, E. H., Barta, P. E., & Pearlson, G. D. (1999). Sex differences in the inferior parietal lobule. *Cerebral Cortex, 9*, 896–901.

Frederikse, M., Lu, A., Aylward, E., Barta, P., Sharma, T., & Pearlson, G. (2000). Sex differences in inferior parietal lobule volume in schizophrenia. *American Journal of Psychiatry, 157*, 422–427.

Fukuzako, H., Yamada, K., Komada, S., Yonezawa, T., Fukuzako, T., Takenouchi, K., Kajiya, Y., Nakajo, M., & Takigawa, M. (1997). Hippocampal volume asymmetry and age of illness onset in males with schizophrenia. *European Archives of Psychiatry and Clinical Neuroscience, 247*, 248–251.

George, L., & Neufeld, R. W. J. (1987). Attentional resources and hemispheric functional asymmetry in schizophrenia. *British Journal of Clinical Psychology, 26,* 35–45.

Green, M. F., Hugdahl, K., & Mitchell, S. (1994). Dichotic listening during auditory hallucinations in patients with schizophrenia. *American Journal of Psychiatry, 151,* 357–362.

Green, M. F., Satz, P., Smith, C., & Nelson, L. (1989). Is there atypical handedness in schizophrenia? *Journal of Abnormal Psychology, 98,* 57–65.

Gruzelier, J., Seymour, K., Haynes, R., Wilson, L., Jolley, T., Flynn, M., & Hirsch, S. (1987). Neuropsychological evidence of hippocampal and frontal impairments in schizophrenia, mania, and depression. In R. Takahashi, P. Flor-Henry, J. Gruzelier, & S. Niwa (Eds.), *Cerebral dynamics, laterality, and psychopathology* (pp. 23–54). Amsterdam: Elsevier Science Publishers.

Gruzelier, J., & Raine, A. (1994). Bilateral electrodermal activity and cerebral mechanisms in syndromes of schizophrenia and the schizotypal personality. *International Journal of Psychophysiology, 16,* 1–16.

Gruzelier, J., Richardson, A., Liddiard, D., Cheema, S., Puri, B., McEvedy, C., & Rippon, G. (1999). Opposite patterns of P300 asymmetry in schizophrenia are syndrome related. *International Journal of Psychophysiology, 34,* 275–282.

Gruzelier, J., Seymour, K., Wilson, L., Jolley, T., & Hirsch, S. (1988). Impairments on neuropsychological tests of temporo-hippocampal and fronto-hippocampal functions and word fluency in remitting schizophrenia and affective disorders. *Archives of General Psychiatry, 45,* 623–629.

Gruzelier, J., & Venables, P. (1974). Bimodality and lateral asymmetry of skin conductance orienting activity in schizophrenics: Replication and evidence of lateral asymmetry in patients with depression and disorders of personality. *Biological Psychiatry, 8,* 55–73.

Gruzelier, J. H. (1994). Syndromes of schizophrenia and schizotypy, hemispheric imbalance and sex differences: Implications for developmental psychopathology. *International Journal of Psychophysiology, 18,* 167–178.

Gruzelier, J. H. (1999). Functional neurophysiological asymmetry in schizophrenia: A review and reorientation. *Schizophrenia Bulletin, 25,* 91–120.

Gruzelier, J. H., Wilson, L., Liddiard, D., Peters, E., & Pusavat, L. (1999). Cognitive asymmetry patterns in schizophrenia: Active and withdrawn syndromes and sex differences as moderators. *Schizophrenia Bulletin, 25,* 349–362.

Guerguerian, R., & Lewine, R. R. J. (1998). Brain torque and sex differences in schizophrenia. *Schizophrenia Research, 30,* 175–181.

Gur, R. E. (1978). Left hemisphere dysfunction and left hemisphere overactivation in schizophrenia. *Journal of Abnormal Psychology, 87,* 226–238.

Gur, R. E., & Chin, S. (1999). Laterality in functional brain imaging studies of schizophrenia. *Schizophrenia Bulletin, 25,* 141–156.

Gur, R. E., Mozley, P. D., Resnick, S. M., Mozley, L. H., Shtasel, D. L., Gallacher, F., Arnold, S. E., Karp, J. S., Alavi, A., Reivich, M., & Gur, R. C. (1995). Resting cerebral glucose metabolism in first-episode and previously treated patients with schizophrenia relates to clinical features. *Archives of General Psychiatry, 52*, 657–667.

Hajek, M., Huonker, R., Boehle, C., Volz, H.-P., Nowak, H., & Sauer, H. (1997). Abnormalities of auditory evoked magnetic fields and structural changes in the left hemisphere of male schizophrenics—A magnetoencephalographic-magnetic resonance imaging study. *Biological Psychiatry, 42*, 609–619.

Hayden, J. L., Kern, R. S., Burdick, N. L., & Green, M. F. (1997). Neurocognitive impairments associated with ambiguous handedness in the chronically mentally ill. *Psychiatry Research, 72*, 9–16.

Hill, H., & Weisbrod, M. (1999). The relation between asymmetry and amplitude of the P300 field in schizophrenia. *Clinical Neurophysiology, 110*, 1611–1617.

Hirayasu, Y., Potts, G. F., O'Donnell, B. F., Kwon, J. S., Arakaki, H., Akdaj, S. J., Levitt, J. L., Shenton, M. E., & McCarley, R. W. (1998). Auditory mismatch negativity in schizophrenia: Topographic evaluation with high-density record montage. *American Journal of Psychiatry, 155*, 1281–1284.

Hugdahl, K. (1995). Dichotic listening: Probing temporal lobe functional integrity. In R. J. Davidson & K. Hugdahl (Eds.), *Brain asymmetry* (pp. 123–156). Cambridge MA: MIT Press.

Hunter, R., Jones, M., & Cooper, F. (1968). Modified lumbar air encephalography in the investigation of long-stay psychiatric patients. *Journal of the Neurological Sciences, 6*, 593–596.

Kamali, D., Galderisi, S., Maj, M., Mucci, A., & DiGregorio, M. (1991). Lateralization patterns of event-related potential and performance indices in schizophrenia: Relationship to clinical state and neuroleptic treatment. *International Journal of Psychophysiology, 10*, 225–230.

Katsanis, J., & Iocono, W. G. (1989). Association of left-handedness with ventricle size and neuropsychological performance. American Journal of Psychiatry, *146*, 1056–1058.

Kiyota, K. (1987). Dysfunction of intra- and interhemispheric complementarity of recognition in schizophrenics hierarchy and laterality. In P. Takahashi, P. Flor-Henry, J. Gruzelier, and S. Niwa (Eds.), *Cerebral dynamics, laterality and psychopathology* (pp. 333–334). Amsterdam: Elsevier.

Kirkpatrick, B., Buchanan, R. W., McKenney, P., Alphs, L. D. et al. (1989). The Schedule for the Deficit Syndrome: An instrument for research in schizophrenia. *Psychiatry Research, 30*, 119–123.

Løberg, E. M., Hugdahl, K., & Green, M. F. (1999). Hemispheric asymmetry in schizophrenia: A "dual deficits" model. *Biological Psychiatry, 45*, 76–81.

Luchins, D. J., & Meltzer, H. Y. (1983). A blind, controlled study of occipital asymmetry in schizophrenia. *Psychiatry Research, 10*, 87–95.

Magaro, P. A., & Chamrad, D. L. (1983). Information processing and lateralization in schizophrenia. *Biological Psychiatry, 18*, 29–44.

Maher, B. A., Manschreck, T. C., Yurgelin-Todd, D. A., & Tsuang, M. (1998). Hemispheric asymmetry of frontal and temporal gray matter and age of onset in schizophrenia. *Biological Psychiatry, 44*, 413–417.

Manoach, D. S. (1994). Handedness is related to formal thought disorder and language dysfunction in schizophrenia. *Journal of Clinical and Experimental Neuropsychology, 16*, 2–14.

Manoach, D. S., Maher, B. A., & Manschreck, T. C. (1988). Left-handedness and thought disorder in the schizophrenias. *Journal of Abnormal Psychology, 97*, 97–99.

Manschreck, T. C., Maher, B. A., Redmond, D. A., Miller, C., & Beaudette, S. M. (1996). Laterality, memory, and thought disorder in schizophrenia. *Neuropsychiatry, Neuropsychology, and Behavioral Neurology, 9*, 1–7.

McCarley, R. W., Faux, S. F., Shenton, M. E., LeMay, M., Cane, M., Ballinger, R., & Duffy, F. H. (1989). CT abnormalities in schizophrenia: A preliminary study of their correlations with P300/P200 electro-physiological features and positive/negative symptoms. *Archives of General Psychiatry, 46*, 698–708.

McCarley, R. W., Shenton, M., O'Donnell, B. F., Faux, S. F., Kikinis, R., Nestor, P. G., & Jolesz, F. A. (1993). Auditory P300 abnormalities and left posterior superior temporal gyrus volume reduction in schizophrenia. *Archives of General Psychiatry, 50*, 190–197.

McDonald, B., Highley, J. R., Walker, M. A., Herron, B. M., Cooper, S. J., Esiri, M. M., & Crow, T. J. (2000). Anomalous asymmetry of fusiform and parahippocampal gyrus gray matter in schizophrenia: A postmortem study. *American Journal of Psychiatry, 157*, 40–47.

Merriam, A. E., & Gardner, E. B. (1987). Corpus callosum function in schizophrenia: A neuropsychological assessment of interhemispheric information processing. *Neuropsychologia, 25*, 185–193.

Min, S. K., & Oh, B. H. (1992). Hemispheric asymmetry in visual recognition of words and motor response in schizophrenic and depressive patients. *Biological Psychiatry, 31*, 255–262.

Moore, M. T., Nathan, D., Elliott, A. R., & Laubach, C. (1935). Encephalographic studies in mental disease. *American Journal of Psychiatry, 92*(1), 43–67.

Näätänen, R., Gaillard, A. W., & Mantysalo, S. (1978). Early selective-attention effect on evoked potential reinterpreted. *Acta Psychologica, 42*, 313–329.

Nachshon, I. (1980). Hemispheric dysfunctioning in schizophrenia. *Journal of Nervous and Mental Disease, 168*, 241–242.

Nelson, L. D., Satz, P., Green, M. F., & Cicchetti, I. (1993). Re-examining handedness in schizophrenia: Now you see it—now you don't. *Journal of Clinical and Experimental Neuropsychology, 15*, 149–158.

Nelson, M. D., Saykin, A. J., Flashman, L. A., & Riordan, H. J. (1998). Hippocampal volume reduction in schizophrenia as assessed by magnetic resonance imaging: A meta-analytic study. *Archives of General Psychiatry, 55*, 433–440.

Niznikiewicz, M., Donnino, R., McCarley, R. W., Nestor, P. G., Iosifescu, D. V., O'Donnell, B., Levitt, J., & Shenton, M. (2000). Abnormal angular gyrus asymmetry in schizophrenia. *American Journal of Psychiatry, 157*, 428–437.

Oldfield, R. C. (1971). The assessment and analysis of handedness. *Neuropsychology, 9*, 97–111.

Orr, K. G. D., Cannon, M., Gilvarry, C. M., Jones, P. B., & Murray, R. M. (1999). Schizophrenic patients and their first-degree relatives show an excess of mixed-handedness. *Schizophrenia Research, 39*, 167–176.

Overby, L. A. III, Harris, A. E., & Leck, M. R. (1989). Perceptual asymmetry in schizophrenia and affective disorder: Implications from a right hemisphere task. *Neuropsychologia, 27*, 861–870.

Park, S. (1999). Hemispheric asymmetry of spatial working memory deficit in schizophrenia. *International Journal of Psychophysiology, 34*, 313–322.

Petty, R. G. (1999). Structural asymmetries of the human brain and their disturbance in schizophrenia. *Schizophrenia Bulletin, 25*, 121–139.

Pfefferbaum, A., Roth, W. T., & Ford, J. M. (1995). Event-related potentials in the study of psychiatric disorders. *Archives of General Psychiatry, 52*, 559–563.

Pic'l, A. K., Magaro, P. A., & Wade, E. A. (1979). Hemispheric functioning in paranoid and nonparanoid schizophrenia. *Biological Psychiatry, 14*, 891–903.

Raine, A., Andrews, H., Sheard, C., Walder, C., & Manders, D. (1989). Interhemispheric transfer in schizophrenics, depressives, and normals with schizoid tendencies. *Journal of Abnormal Psychology, 98*, 35–41.

Reite, M., & Rojas, D. (1997). MEG correlates of psychoses: Anomalous lateralization and abnormal memory function. In H. White, U. Zwiener, B. Schack, & A. Doering (Eds.), *Quantitative and topographical EEG and MEG analysis*. Jena and Erlangen, Germany: Druckhaus Mayer Verlag.

Reite, M., Sheeder, J., Teale, P., Adams, M., Richardson, D., Simon, J., Jones, R. H., & Rojas, D. C. (1997). Magnetic source imaging evidence of sex differences in cerebral lateralization in schizophrenia. *Archives of General Psychiatry, 54*, 433–440.

Reite, M., Sheeder, J., Teale, P., Richardson, D., Adams, M., & Simon, J. (1995). MEG based brain laterality: Sex differences in normal adults. *Neuropsychologia, 33*, 1607–1616.

Rojas, D. C., Teale, P., Sheeder, J., Simon, J., & Reite, M. (1997). Sex-specific expression of Heschl's gyrus functional and structural abnormalities in paranoid schizophrenia. *American Journal of Psychiatry, 154*, 1655–1662.

Salisbury, D. F., Shenton, M. E., Sherwood, A. R., Fischer, I. A., Yurgelin-Todd, D. A., Tohen, M., & McCarley, R. W. (1998). First-episode schizophrenic psychosis differs from

M. F. Green, M. J. Sergi, and R. S. Kern

first-episode affective psychosis and controls in P300 amplitude over left temporal lobe. *Archives of General Psychiatry, 55,* 173–180.

Sanfilipo, M., Lafargue, T., Rusinek, H., Arena, L., Loneragan, C., Lautin, A., Feiner, D., Rotrosen, J., & Wolkin, A. (2000). Volumetric measure of the frontal and temporal lobe regions in schizophrenia: Relationship to negative symptoms. *Archives of General Psychiatry, 57,* 471–480.

Satz, P., & Green, M. F. (1999). Atypical handedness in schizophrenia: Some methodological and theoretical issues. *Schizophrenia Bulletin, 25,* 63–78.

Satz, P., Orsini, D. L., Saslow, E., & Henry, R. (1985). The pathological left-handedness syndrome. *Brain and Cognition, 4,* 27–46.

Sharma, T., Lancaster, E., Sigmundsson, T., Lewis, S., Takei, N., Gurling, H., Barta, P., Pearlson, G., & Murray, R. (1999). Lack of normal pattern of cerebral asymmetry in familial schizophrenic patients and their relatives: The Maudsley Family Study. *Schizophrenia Research, 40,* 111–120.

Soper, H. V., Satz, P., Orsini, D. L., Henry, R. R., Zvi, J. C., & Shulman, M. (1986). Handedness patterns in autism suggest subtypes. *Journal of Autism and Developmental Disorders, 16,* 155–167.

Soper, H. V., Satz, P., Orsini, D. L., van Gorp, W. G., & Green, M. F. (1987). Handedness distribution within severe to profound mental retardation. *American Journal of Mental Deficiency, 92,* 94–102.

Southard, E. E. (1915). On the topographical distribution of cortex lesions and anomalies in dementia praecox with some account of their functional significance. *American Journal of Insanity, 71,* 603–671.

Spence, S. A., Liddle, P. F., Stefan, M. D., Hellewell, J. S. E., Sharma, T., Friston, K. J., Hirsch, S. R., Frith, C. D., Murray, R. M., Deakin, J. F. W., & Grasby, P. M. (2000). Functional anatomy of verbal fluency in people with schizophrenia and those at genetic risk: Focal dysfunction and distributed disconnectivity reappraised. *British Journal of Psychiatry, 174,* 52–60.

Strik, W. R., Dierks, T., Franzek, E., Maurer, K., & Beckmann, H. (1993). Differences in P300 amplitudes and topography between cycloid psychosis and schizophrenia in Leonhard's classification. *Acta Psychiatrica Scandinavica, 87,* 179–183.

Taylor, P., & Amir, N. (1995). Left-handedness in schizophrenia and affective disorder. *Journal of Nervous and Mental Disease, 183,* 3–9.

Taylor, P., Dalton, R., & Fleminger, J. J. (1982). Handedness and schizophrenic symptoms. *British Journal of Medical Psychology, 55,* 287–291.

Tiihonen, J., Katila, H., Pekkonen, E., Jaaskelainen, I. P., Huotilainen, M., Aronen, H. J., Ilmoniemi, R. J., Rasanen, P., Virtanen, J., Salli, E., & Karhu, J. (1998). Reversal of cerebral asymmetry in schizophrenia measured with magnetoencephalography. *Schizophrenia Research, 30,* 209–219.

Turetsky, B., Cowell, P. E., Gur, R. C., Grossman, R. I., Shtasel, D. L., & Gur, R. E. (1995). Frontal and temporal lobe brain volumes in schizophrenia: Relationship to symptoms and clinical subtype. *Archives of General Psychiatry, 52,* 1061–1070.

Turetsky, B. I., Colbath, E. A., & Gur, R. E. (1998). P300 subcomponent abnormalities in schizophrenia, I: Physiological evidence for gender and subtype specific differences in regional pathology. *Biological Psychiatry, 43,* 84–96.

Walker, E., & McGuire, M. (1982). Intra- and interhemispheric information processing in schizophrenia. *Psychological Bulletin, 92*(3), 701–725.

Weisbrod, M., Winkler, S., Maier, S., Hill, H., Thomas, C., & Spitzer, M. (1997). Left lateralized P300 amplitude deficit in schizophrenic patients depends on pitch disparity. *Biological Psychiatry, 41,* 541–549.

Wexler, B. E. (1986). Alterations in cerebral laterality during acute psychotic illness. *British Journal of Psychiatry, 149,* 202–209.

Wexler, B. E., Giller, E. L., Jr., & Southwick, S. (1991). Cerebral laterality, symptoms, diagnosis in psychotic patients. *Biological Psychiatry, 29,* 103–116.

Wexler, B. E., & Hawles, T. (1983). Increasing the power of dichotic methods: The Fused Rhymed Words Test. *Neuropsychologia, 21,* 59–66.

Wexler, B. E., & Henninger, G. R. (1979). Alterations in cerebral laterality during acute psychotic illness. *Archives of General Psychiatry, 6,* 278–288.

White, M. S., Maher, B. A., & Manschreck, T. C. (1998). Hemispheric specialization in schizophrenics with perceptual aberration. *Schizophrenia Research, 32,* 161–170.

Wright, I. C., Rabe-Hesketh, S., Woodruff, P. W. R., David, A. S., Murray, R. M., & Bullmore, E. T. (2000). Meta-analysis of regional brain volumes in schizophrenia. *American Journal of Psychiatry, 157,* 16–25.

Yozawitz, A., Bruder, G., Sutton, S., Sharpe, L., Gurland, B., Fleiss, J., & Costa, L. (1979). Dichotic perception: Evidence for right hemisphere dysfunction in affective psychosis. *British Journal of Psychiatry, 135,* 224–237.

Young, A. H., Blackwood, D. H., Roxborough, H., McQueen, J. K., Martin, M. J., & Kean, D. (1991). A magnetic resonance imaging study of schizophrenia: Brain structure and clinical symptoms. *British Journal of Psychiatry, 158,* 158–164.

Contributors

John J. B. Allen
Department of Psychology
University of Arizona
Tucson, Arizona

Marie T. Banich
Department of Psychology
University of Colorado
Boulder, Colorado

Alan A. Beaton
Department of Psychology
University of Wales
Swansea, U.K.

Craig W. Berridge
Psychology Department
University of Wisconsin—
Madison
Madison, Wisconsin

Gerard E. Bruder
Department of Biopsychology
New York State Psychiatric
Institute and Department of
Psychiatry
College of Physicians and
Surgeons
Columbia University
New York, New York

Christopher F. Chabris
Nuclear Magnetic Resonance
Center
Department of Radiology
Massachusetts General Hospital
and Harvard Medical School
Boston, Massachusetts

James A. Coan
Department of Psychology
University of Arizona
Tucson, Arizona

Richard J. Davidson
Laboratory for Affective
Neuroscience
Department of Psychology
University of Wisconsin—
Madison
Madison, Wisconsin

Mark A. Eckert
Department of Neuroscience
McKnight Brain Institute
University of Florida
Gainesville, Florida

Rodrigo A. España
Psychology Department
University of Wisconsin—

Madison
Madison, Wisconsin

John J. Foxe
Cognitive Neuroscience and
Schizophrenia Program
Nathan Kline Institute for
Psychiatric Research
Orangeburg, New York

Karl J. Friston
The Wellcome Department of
Cognitive Neurology
Institute of Neurology
London, U.K.

Michael F. Green
Department of Psychiatry and
Biobehavioral Sciences
UCLA
Los Angeles, California

Onur Güntürkün
Biopsychologie
Fakultät für Psychologie
Ruhr-Universität Bochum
Bochum, Germany

Michel Habib
Department of Neurology,
CHU Timone
Marseilles, France

Wendy Heller
Department of Psychology and
Beckman Institute
University of Illinois at Urbana-
Champaign
Champaign, Illinois

Kenneth Hugdahl
Department of Biological and

Medical Psychology
University of Bergen
Bergen, Norway

Lutz Jäncke
Institute of General Psychology
Otto-von-Guericke-University
Magdeburg
Magdeburg, Germany

Robert S. Kern
Department of Psychiatry and
Biobehavioral Sciences
UCLA
Los Angeles, California

Stephen M. Kosslyn
Department of Psychology
Harvard University
Cambridge, Massachusetts

Nancy S. Koven
Department of Psychology and
Beckman Institute
University of Illinois at Urbana-
Champaign
Champaign, Illinois

Bruno Laeng
Department of Psychology
University of Tromsø
Tromsø, Norway

Maryse Lassonde
Groupe de Recherche en
Neuropsychologie Expérimentale
Département de Psychologie
Université de Montréal
Montréal, Canada

Christiana M. Leonard
Department of Neuroscience

McKnight Brain Institute
University of Florida
Gainesville, Florida

Gregory A. Miller
Department of Psychology and
Beckman Institute
University of Illinois at Urbana-
Champaign
Champaign, Illinois

Daniel S. O'Leary
University of Iowa Hospitals and
Clinics
Mental Health Clinical Research
Center
Iowa City, Iowa

Alvaro Pascual-Leone
Laboratory for Magnetic Brain
Stimulation
Beth Israel Deaconess Medical
Center
Boston, Massachusetts

Diego Pizzagalli
Laboratory for Affective
Neuroscience and W. M. Keck
Neuroimaging Laboratory
University of Wisconsin—
Madison
Madison, Wisconsin

Fabrice Robichon
LEAD, Université de Bourgogne
Dijon, France

Clifford D. Saron
Cognitive Neuroscience and
Schizophrenia Program
Nathan Kline Institute for

Psychiatric Research
Orangeburg, New York

Hannelore C. Sauerwein
Groupe de Recherche en
Neuropsychologie Expérimentale
Département de Psychologie
Université de Montréal
Montréal, Canada

Charles E. Schroeder
Cognitive Neuroscience and
Schizophrenia Program
Nathan Kline Institute for
Psychiatric Research
Orangeburg, New York

Mark J. Sergi
Department of Veterans Affairs,
VISN 22
Mental Illness Research,
Education, and Clinical Center
Department of Psychology
California State University at
Northridge
Northridge, California

Alexander J. Shackman
Laboratory for Affective
Neuroscience and W. M. Keck
Neuroimaging Laboratory
University of Wisconsin—
Madison
Madison, Wisconsin

Thomas A. Stalnaker
Psychology Department
University of Wisconsin—
Madison
Madison, Wisconsin

Helmuth Steinmetz
Department of Neurology
Johann Wolfgang Goethe-
University Frankfurt am Main
Frankfurt, Germany

Akaysha C. Tang
Department of Psychology
University of New Mexico
Albuquerque, New Mexico

Herbert G. Vaughan, Jr.
Department of Neuroscience
Albert Einstein College of
Medicine
Bronx, New York

Vincent Walsh
Department of Psychology
University of Oxford
Oxford, U.K.

Robert J. Zatorre
Montreal Neurological Institute
McGill University
Montreal, Canada

Author Index

Please note that only first authors are listed.

Barlow, D. H., 540
Barnard, R. O., 291
Barneoud, P., 41
Barnes, C., 43
Barnsley, R. H., 109
Barr, M. L., 629
Bartels, A., 523–527
Bartley, A. J., 706
Bartres-Faz, D., 242, 243
Bashore, T. R., 341, 343
Bastian, A., 665
Baxter, L. R., 720
Beamont, J. G., 314
Bean, R. B., 210
Beaton, A. A., 107, 111, 120–121, 131, 138, 200, 443, 654, 663, 686, 698, 705
Beaulieu, S., 83
Behrmann, M., 308
Belger, A., 273, 280, 290, 295
Belin, P., 421, 430, 431
Bell, I. R., 720
Bell, J., 118
Bellini, L., 292
Bem, D. J., 570
Benavidez, D. A., 292
Benca, R. M., 590
Bench, C. J., 546, 720, 721
Bennet, G. L., 620
Benton, A. L., 108, 110
Berger, B., 76
Bergson, C., 76
Berlin, C. I., 479, 480
Berlucchi, G., 266, 341, 346, 349, 627,630, 634, 635
Berrebi, A. S., 212
Berridge, C. W., 71–72, 74, 78–80, 89
Berridge, K. C., 88, 92
Best, M., 702
Bhatia, K. P., 134
Biederman, I., 306, 320
Bilder, R. M., 761
Binder, J. R., 423, 426, 444, 695, 696, 704
Binggeli, R. L., 4
Bishop, D. V. M., 107, 110, 125–126, 131, 652
Bishop, K. M., 210, 441

Bisiacchi, P., 138, 345
Bittar, R. G., 623
Biver, F., 720, 724
Blackhart, G. C., 590
Bleier, R., 131
Bliss, T., 43
Blood, A. J., 524
Boecker, H., 136
Bogen, J. E., 627
Bogerts, B., 758
Bol, P., 105
Bolhuis, J., 20
Bonanno, G. A., 551
Boroojerdi, B., 347, 348
Borowsky, B., 87
Bouchard, T. J., 218
Boussaoud, D., 349
Bracha, H. S., 132
Brackenridge, C. J., 118
Bradley, P. M., 19
Bradshaw, J. L., 308
Braun, C. M., 343, 345, 349, 364
Bredenötter, M., 19
Bremer, F., 631
Brindley, G. S., 358, 392
Brinkman, J., 135
Broca, P., 3, 682
Brodmann, K., 199, 517
Brody, A. L., 720
Brog, J. S., 72
Brooks, D. J., 134–135
Brown, H., 61
Brown, M. W., 20
Brown, W. S., 263, 269, 345, 364
Brozoski, T. J., 86
Bruder, G. E., 578, 719–723, 725–729, 731, 734, 735, 745, 751, 755
Bruyer, R., 317, 322
Bryden, M. P., 105, 107, 109, 122, 199, 314, 322, 446, 447, 451, 459, 460, 569, 681, 691
Braak, H., 194
Bubser, M., 86
Buchanan, A., 112, 119
Buchanan, T. W., 195
Burnod, Y., 329

Cunningham, D. J., 188–189, 682, 684
Curt, F., 105, 109–110
Cutting, J., 744

Dalby, M. A., 702
Damasio, A. R., 535, 545, 550
Damasio, H., 313
Damsma, G., 92
D'Angio, M., 79
Dantzer, R., 82–83
Dassonville, P., 137
Davatzikos, C., 205, 208
Davey, N. J., 383
David, A. S., 291, 292
Davidoff, L. M., 622
Davidoff, R. A., 44, 136
Davidson, R., 44
Davidson, R. J., 86, 269, 343, 441, 448, 511,
    513, 514, 516, 522, 524, 526, 528, 534, 536,
    550, 565, 567, 570–572, 574, 575, 578, 584–
    586, 588, 589, 590, 594, 600, 603, 605, 606,
    719–723, 726–730, 733
Davis, A., 118
Davis, M., 83
Dawson, G., 571, 577, 578, 590, 603, 720
Dawson, M. E., 291
Day, B. L., 233
De Agostini, M., 105
De Guise, E., 631, 641
de Kloet, E., 40, 55, 61
De Lacoste M. C., 204, 209, 210, 217, 266,
    294
De Lacoste M. C., 209, 210, 217, 266, 294
De Lacoste-Utamsing, M. C., 204, 210
De Renzi, E., 123, 313, 326
De Souza, E. B., 576
de Toledo-Morell, L., 44
Debener, S., 570, 578, 584, 720
deCharms, R. C., 433
Deecke, L., 362
Deiber, M. P., 136, 369
Deldin, P. J., 544, 723, 724
Delgado, M. R., 520
Delis, D. C., 311
Dellatolas, G., 110, 120, 127
Démonet J.-F., 424, 426

Denckla, M., 667
Denenberg, V., 37–38, 46, 55, 61, 204, 205
Deng, C., 8, 15, 17–18
Dennis, M., 624, 625, 628, 631, 632
Depy, D., 327, 328
Derbyshire, S. W. G., 545
Desimone, R., 484, 486–488
Deutch, A. Y., 73–74, 88
Deutsch, D., 420
Devinsky, O., 545
DeYoe, E. A., 358, 392
Di Lazzaro, V., 347
Di Steffano, M., 343, 349, 633
Di Virgilio, G., 375
Diamond, A., 665
Diamond, I., 417
Diaz, J., 89
Diekamp, B., 7
Diorio, D., 75, 87
Dittrich, W. H., 11
Dodrill, C. B., 109
Doherty, M. D., 88
Dolan, R. J., 544, 721
Donders, F. C., 353
Donnenfeld, A. E., 622
Dorion, A. A., 209
Doty, R. W., 5, 625
Downhill, J. E., 294
Dreher, B., 316
Drevets, W. C., 544, 545, 720
Driesen, N. R., 131
Duara, R., 663, 664, 700
Duffy, S., 43, 47
Dum, R. P., 362, 365, 376, 391
Dunn, A. J., 71
Durost, W. N., 748
Duzel, E., 247

Earnest, C., 580
Eaton, E. M., 753
Eberstaller, O., 187, 188, 684
Eckert, M. A., 651, 652, 654, 656, 659, 660,
    698
Economo, C., 187, 192, 194
Efron, R., 322
Egan, M. F., 775

Eggermont, J., 433
Ehlers, A., 543
Eichenbaum, H., 40, 43
Eidelberg, D., 685
Ekman, P., 566, 567, 589, 590, 594, 603
Elbert, T., 120, 133
Elchisak, M. A., 89
Elliot, R., 534, 544
Elliott, D., 108
Ellis, L., 128
Ellsworth, P. C., 533, 534
Elman, J., 671
Emmerton, J., 4
Emmorey, K., 322
Endo, H., 350
Engel, A. K., 268
Engelage, J., 13
Entus, A., 639
Epstein, C. M., 242
Erdler, M., 368
Ettlinger, G., 625, 627, 628, 630
Evarts, E. V., 413
Everling, S., 383
Eysenck, M. W., 542

Fadiga, L., 349
Falek, A., 110
Fallon, J. H., 75
Falzi, G., 684, 687
Farah, M., 308
Faustman, W. O., 749
Faux, S. F., 755
Fava, M., 727
Fawcett, A. J., 665
Ferbert, A., 347
Ferman, T. J., 293
Ferrera, V. P., 350
Ferris, G. S., 632
Fersen, L., 5, 6
Feske, U., 727
Field, T., 570, 577, 580, 583, 720
Fiez, J. A., 195
Filipek, P. A., 654
Finlay, J. M., 74, 90–91
Fischer, M., 628
Fitch, R., 38, 46, 130, 705

Flechsig, P., 187
Fleishman, E. A., 109
Fletcher, J. M., 652
Flitman, S. S., 244
Flor-Henry, P., 722, 744
Foa, E. B., 543
Fodor, J., 61
Fogassi, L., 349
Foong, J., 294
Foote, S. L., 76
Ford, J. M., 755
Forster, B., 343, 345, 346, 393, 633
Foundas, A. L., 192, 195–196, 443, 655, 686,
   694, 695
Fox, N. A., 569, 571, 572, 575, 576, 580, 585,
   586, 589, 590, 594, 603, 720
Fox, R., 4
Frank, E., 727
Frederiksen, M. E., 762, 763
Friedman, A., 271
Friedman, B. H., 594
Friston, K. J., 164, 165, 171, 179, 182
Frith, C. D., 465
Fudge, J. L., 83
Fuente-Fernández, R., 134
Fukuzako, H., 763
Fuller, R. W., 87
Funahashi, S., 350, 388
Funnell, M. G., 267

Gainotti, G., 313, 537
Galaburda, A. M., 121–122, 194, 199–200,
   442, 652, 654, 662, 684, 687, 688, 699,
   704
Galuske, R., 194, 689, 435
Gangestad, S. W., 117–118
Gannon, P. J., 189, 707
Gardner, R. A., 109
Garris, P. A., 76
Gaspar, P., 76
Gaston, K. E., 5
Gauger, L. M., 656, 667, 700
Gazzaniga, M., 124, 135, 137, 264, 313, 327,
   442, 624, 629, 636, 637
Geffen, F., 266
Geffen, G. M., 138, 630, 631

Gelot, A., 620
Geoffroy, G., 621, 622
George, M. S., 235–236, 544, 720, 753
Gerloff, C., 368
Gersh, F., 124
Gerstein, G. L., 180
Geschwind, N., 120–125, 130, 132, 188, 195, 266, 322, 443, 652, 662, 681, 684, 686–687, 691, 699
Giedd, J. N., 213
Gilbert, D. B., 23
Gilbert, D. G., 592
Gillbert, A. N., 107, 109, 118, 592
Glick, S., 57, 131
Goel, V., 329, 524
Goldberg, T. E., 292
Goldenberg, G., 124
Goldman-Rakic, P. S., 75–76, 86
Goldstein, L. E., 71, 83
Goldstein, M. N., 627, 632
Gonon, F., 76
Gooddy, W., 137
Goodglass, H., 325
Goodmann, N., 304
Gordon, H., 125
Gorynia, I., 138
Gotlieb, I. H., 568, 577, 580, 603
Gott, P. S., 630, 632
Gottlieb, Y., 420
Gozales, C., 83
Grady, C. L., 500
Grafman, J., 247
Grafton, S., 170
Grasby, P. M., 720
Gray, J. A., 571
Gray, P. M., 411
Graziano, M. S., 349
Green, M. F., 465
Green, R. L., 657, 659, 702, 704, 747, 748, 751, 752
Griffiths, T. D., 424–426, 486
Grimshaw, G. M., 122
Groenwegen, H. J., 71
Gross, J., 551
Gruzelier, J., 744, 757
Guerguerian, R., 762

Guiard, Y., 108
Gulley, L. R., 725
Gur, R. C., 219, 293
Gur, R. E., 745, 753, 760
Güntürkün, O., 4–5, 8, 11–15, 17–18, 24–26, 651, 671

Habib, M., 122, 195, 207, 685, 692–694, 698, 705, 706
Habley, J. W., 4
Hagelthorn, K. M., 289
Hagemann, D., 566, 570, 572, 586, 588, 592, 597, 599, 603, 604
Hager, F., 543
Haier, R. J., 542
Hajek, M., 756
Halpern, A. R., 427, 429
Hamilton, C. R., 327, 635, 636
Hanes, D. P., 353, 354, 382, 383, 391
Hannay, H. L., 325
Hansen, J. C., 481
Harastay, J., 707
Hardy, O., 14
Harik, D. I., 88
Harmon-Jones, E., 541, 556, 570, 571, 572, 574, 575, 592, 594, 595, 600, 603
Haroutunian, V., 88
Harrington, A., 303
Harris, L., 105, 112, 125–126
Hart, B., 671
Hart, N. S., 7
Haslam, R. H., 653
Hasnain, M. K., 358, 392
Hasselmo, M., 40, 44
Hatta, T., 109
Haxby, J. V., 484, 485
Hayden, J. L., 749
Healey, J. M., 109
Hedreen, J. C., 375
Heffner, H. E., 413
Heiervang, E., 220, 654, 656, 702, 704
Heilmann, K., 119, 123, 313, 329, 536
Heimer, L., 71, 73
Heinen, F., 238
Heinze, H. J., 484, 485
Helleday, J., 122

Joels, M., 40
Johnson, L. E., 263
Johnson, M. H., 20
Johnson, O., 721
Johnsrude, I. S., 415–417, 420, 431
Johnston, A. N. B., 20, 26
Johnston, D., 37, 43
Jones, C. A., 83
Jones, G. V., 115
Jones, N. A., 570, 572, 580, 583, 592, 594
Jones, R. D., 137
Jänke, L., 134, 195, 196, 199, 208, 210, 215, 443, 448, 657, 663, 664, 694, 695

Kaczmarek, L., 40
Kahneman, D., 512
Kaiser, J., 368
Kalin, N. H., 572, 576
Kalivas, P. W., 74
Kaluzny, P., 349
Kamali, D., 753
Kang, D. H., 572
Kapp, B. S., 83
Karbe, H., 696
Karnath, H. O., 214, 630
Karreman, M., 88
Katsanis, J., 749
Kauranen, K., 109
Kawamichi, H., 350
Kawasaki, H., 524
Kawashima, R., 137
Kayser, J., 723
Keller, J., 539, 544, 725, 733
Kemmerer, D., 326
Kennedy, D. N., 358
Kennedy, H., 375
Kentgen, L. M., 720, 723
Kertesz, A., 135–136, 208, 216, 693, 695
Kesler, M. L., 490, 495, 497
Ketter, T. A., 732, 733, 735
Keysers, C., 12, 14
Kilshaw, D., 109, 113
Kim, S. G., 136, 365, 369
Kimchi, R., 286
Kimura, D., 109, 123–124, 136, 446, 447, 468, 478

King, G. D., 109
Kinney, H. C., 212
Kinsbourne, M., 348, 349, 351, 352, 385, 470, 478, 719, 732
Kirby, L. G., 71
Kirkpatrick, B., 754
Kitchen, I., 87
Kitterle, F., 311
Kiyota, K., 751
Klar, A. J., 114
Klein, E., 236
Kline, J. P., 566, 572, 575, 592, 607
Klingberg, T., 661
Koch, H., 106–108, 111, 120
Koenig, O., 318, 322
Koepp, M. J., 513, 519, 520
Kogure, T., 317, 318
Komssi, S., 346, 348
Kooistra, C. A., 131
Kopp, N., 684
Kosslyn, S. M., 37, 303, 305, 307–319, 322, 324, 328, 329, 331, 332, 427
Kujirai, T., 232
Kulynych, J. J., 196, 707
Kuo, Z. Y., 24
Kurata, K., 385
Kushch, A., 655, 700
Künig, G., 521

LaBar, K.S., 515
Laeng, B., 309, 318–323, 325, 326, 328, 330–332
Laget, P., 629
Laland, K. N., 115–116
Lalumiére, M. L., 118
LaMantia, A. S., 212, 268, 344, 346, 348
Lane, R. D., 523
Lang, P. J., 522, 523, 534, 545, 557
Larsen, J. P., 535, 536, 655, 684, 700
Larson, E. B., 269
Lassonde, M., 343, 625–628, 630–632, 635
Laumire, M. L., 118
Lausberg, H., 124–125
Lavenex, P., 44
Lavielle, S., 74–75, 83
Lawrence, D. G., 135

Oertel, D., 344
Ogle, W., 119, 123
Öhman, A., 534
Oka, S., 705
Oke, A., 41
Okuda, B., 134
Oldfield, R. C., 110, 464, 692, 747, 748
Oliveri, M., 232, 251, 252, 351
Orr, K. G. D., 748, 749
Orton, S., 651
Otto, M. W., 544
Overby, L. A., 721, 725, 750

Palmer, A. R., 116
Palmer, R. E., 111
Pandya, D. N., 213, 265, 347, 620
Papousek, I., 138, 582
Pardo, J. V., 514, 546
Park, S., 754
Parlow, S. E., 138
Parrot, M., 317
Parson, B. S., 112
Parsons, C. H., 14
Pascual-Leone, A., 231, 232, 234–236, 238,
    241, 243, 251, 383
Passarotti, A. M., 275, 295
Patel, S. N., 22
Patterson, T. A., 23
Paus, T., 250, 432
Pavlov, I. P., 516
Payne, M. A., 105
Pelizzari, C. A., 495
Pelletier, J., 291
Penhune, V. B., 415, 423, 434, 435, 658
Pennington, B. F., 655, 663, 702
Peoples, R. W., 83
Perelle, I. B., 119
Peretz, I., 419
Perrin, F., 355
Perry, D. W., 418, 421, 424, 429
Peters, M., 105, 107–108, 110, 116, 127, 134,
    136, 214
Petersen, S. E., 170, 465
Petrides, M., 350, 420, 423
Petruzello, S. J., 582
Petty, R. G., 745

Pfefferbaum, A., 755
Pfeifer, R. A., 187, 192, 683
Philips, A. G., 92
Phillips, C. G., 162
Phillips, D. P., 430, 433
Piaget, J., 304
Pic'l, A. K., 753
Pierce, R. C., 72
Pine, D. S., 722
Pipe, M. E., 125
Pizzagalli, D., 545
Plante, E., 122, 656, 700
Poffenberger, A. T., 341, 342, 345, 349, 352,
    392, 633
Poirier, P., 638
Pollmann, S., 447, 468
Polster, M. R., 285
Pontieri, F. E., 72
Porac, C., 109, 118, 120, 138, 691
Posner, M. I., 483, 484, 489, 463, 465, 551,
    554
Post, R. M., 724
Potter, S. M., 138
Powls, A., 128
Preilowski, B., 269, 631
Preis, S., 201, 656, 700
Preuss, T. M., 75
Previc, F. H., 125, 127, 131–132, 322
Price, C. J., 170, 432
Prior, H., 7
Provins, K. A., 110, 119
Praamstra, A. T., 361, 363, 368
Pugh, K. R., 652
Pujol, J., 212, 213
Pulvirenti, L., 72
Purves, D., 133, 201
Pycock, C. J., 77, 88
Pye-Smith, P. H., 106

Quinn, K., 289

Rademacher, J., 413
Rae, C., 666, 707
Rager, G., 4
Raine, A., 750, 751
Raiteri, M., 83

Raiteri, M. S., 83
Rajendra, S., 16
Rakic, P., 212, 620, 661
Ramachandran, V. S., 636
Ramón y Cajal, S., 13
Ramsdell, A. F., 27
Rao, S. M., 291
Rapcsack, S. Z., 124
Rashid, N., 8
Ratinckx, E., 344
Rauch, S. L., 86
Rausch, R. A., 620, 622, 623, 628
Rauschecker, J. P., 25
Raye, C. L., 290
Rayman, J., 280
Raymer, A. M., 124, 125
Reddy, H., 632
Reep, R. L., 75
Reeves, B., 592
Regan, D., 355
Reggia, R., 37, 39
Reichle, E. D., 672
Reid, P. D., 235
Reid, S. A., 569, 577, 582, 585, 606, 720, 723
Reil, J. C., 619
Reiman, E. M., 523, 526
Reinarz, S. J., 208
Reinvang, I., 441, 465, 469
Reite, M., 756, 757
Remy, M., 8, 11, 17
Rengachary, S. S., 467
Reuter- Lorenz, P. A., 290
Reynholds, M. D., 138, 632
Riddoch, M. J., 123
Riecker, A., 665
Riehle, A., 349
Rigal, R. A., 108–109
Ringo, J. L., 61, 207, 212, 216, 348
Risch, N., 116
Risse, G. L., 5, 267, 294
Rivest, J., 637
Rizzolatti, G., 350, 488
Robert, F., 14
Roberts, R. J., 447
Robertson, L. C., 285, 311

Robichon, F., 208, 660, 662–664, 667, 702, 704, 705
Robin, D. A., 415
Robinson, T. E., 88
Rochon-Duvigneaud, A., 4
Rogers, L. J., 15–18, 24, 38, 651
Rogers, R. D., 520
Rojas, D. C., 756
Roland, P. E., 133
Rolls, E. T., 43–44, 519, 525
Romanski, L., 420
Rose, S. P. R., 22–23
Rosen, G. D., 48, 138, 207, 706
Rosenberger, P. B., 653
Rosenfeld, J. P., 582, 595
Rosenweig, M., 47
Ross, G., 128–129
Roth, E. C., 317
Roth, R. H., 71, 89
Rothi, L. J. G., 123
Rothwell, J. C., 232
Rouiller, E. M., 137,368, 376, 385, 391
Roy, E. A., 123
Rubens, A. B., 188, 684, 686, 694
Rubin, N., 322
Rugg, M. D., 266, 345, 346, 635
Rumelhart, D., 37, 39
Rumsey, J. M., 651, 652, 654, 656, 663, 664, 700
Russel, J. A., 534, 557, 632
Rybash, J. M., 317, 318

Sabatini, B. L., 344
Sabotka, S. S., 592
Sackeim, H. A., 236
Sadato, N. V., 136
Sagar, H. J., 466
Saint-Cyr, J. A., 466
Salamone, J. D., 92
Salamy, A., 289
Salenius, S., 361, 362, 379–381
Salinska, E. J., 22
Salisbury, D. F., 755
Salmelin, R., 368, 652
Salmond, C., 177
Samson, S., 415, 419

Sanders, G., 109
Sanders, R. J., 625
Sanfilipo, M., 759
Sarnat, H. B., 27
Saron, C. D., 342, 343, 345, 346, 349, 350,
    354, 356, 359, 364, 367, 373, 374, 379, 382,
    390
Satz, P., 120–121, 125, 747–748
Sauerwein, H., 624–628, 630–632
Saul, R. E., 624, 627
Scaffer, C. E., 568, 576
Scarrone, S., 291
Schachter, S. C., 122
Schaeffer, A. A., 132
Schaffer, C. E., 582, 723
Schall, J. D., 349, 350, 353
Scheibel, A., 133
Scheirs, J. G. M., 122
Scherer, K. R., 594
Schiavetto, A., 637
Schlaug, G., 131, 197, 213, 697–698
Schmahmann, J. D., 219
Schmidt, L. A., 566, 572, 574, 576, 603
Schmidt, S. L., 108
Schnitzler, A., 347
Schoenemann, P. T., 219
Schouten, J., 413
Schreiber, H., 292
Schultz, R. T., 657, 700
Schultz, W., 77, 519
Schulze, H. A. F., 194
Schwartz, G. E., 575
Schwartz, M., 127
Schwarz, I. M., 17
Schaafsma, A., 238
Searleman, A., 127
Seldon, H. L., 194, 435
Selye, H., 70
Semal, C., 420
Semendeferi, K., 217
Semrud-Clikeman, M., 655, 667
Sergent, J., 263, 264, 311, 315, 317, 326, 343,
    394, 633
Serur, D., 622
Servos, P., 318
Sesack, S. R., 75–76

Shallice, T., 308
Shannon, R. V., 430
Shapiro, K., 244–247
Shapleske, J., 199, 200, 686–687, 698
Sharma, T., 762
Shaywitz, S. E., 652
Shenker, J. I., 287, 295
Shepard, R. N., 318
Sherman, S. M., 25
Shettleworth, S. J., 8
Shevtsova, M., 39
Shibasaki, H., 136
Shimizu, T., 11
Shimoda, K., 732
Shoumura, K., 623, 636
Shtyrov, Y., 444
Sidtis, J. J., 415, 447, 721
Silver, P. H., 632
Simon, J. H., 291
Simos, P. G., 652
Skolnick, P., 88
Smart, J. J. C., 303
Smiley, J. F., 76
Smith, G. E., 120 682
Snyder, P. J., 105, 134, 202, 665
Solomonia, R. O., 20
Soper, H. V., 126, 748
Southard, E. E., 743
Sparks, R., 447
Speigler, B. J., 105
Spellacy, F., 478
Spence, S. A., 762
Sperry, R. W., 261, 264, 619, 624, 626, 629,
    641
Spreen, O., 465
Springer, S., 308, 443
Spydell, J. D., 606
Squire, L., 40, 43–44
St. John, R., 267, 341, 343
Stančák, A., 369, 370
Stanfield, B. B., 27
Stanovitch, K., 652
Starkmann, S. P., 467
Steele, R. J., 22, 133
Steenhuis, R. E., 107–110, 691
Stein, J. F., 134

Subject Index

Acallosal individuals, 635, 639
Across-hemisphere advantage, 290
Across-hemisphere condition, 294
Across-hemisphere processing, 289
Affective chronometry, 522, 605
Affective neuroscience, 511, 534
American Sign Language, 322
Amygdala, 83, 517, 528, 535
Anterior cingulate, 133, 174, 720
Anterior commissure, 262, 263
Antidepressant medication, 732
Anxiety, 93, 533, 537, 539, 540, 542, 566,
  725
Anxiety Symptom Questionnaire, 552
Approach behavior, 553, 565
Apraxia, 124, 125
Arachnoid cysts, 467
Arousal, 556, 733
Asymmetry coefficient, 692
Attention, 138, 252, 265, 284, 291, 311, 384,
  451, 459, 460, 477, 480, 485, 488, 533, 542
Attention network, 252
Auditory cortex, 413, 417, 430, 726
Auditory integration, 638
Auditory lateralization, 197, 441, 442
Autonomic modulation, 533

Basal ganglia, 131
Behavioral activation systems (BAS), 571
Behavioral inhibition systems (BIS), 571
Benzodiazepines, 90
Bergen Dichotic Listening Database, 451

Binaural listening, 500
Binocular seeing, 11, 13
Birth stressor, 127, 128
Blood oxygen level-dependent (BOLD),
  522, 525
Bottom-up processing, 37, 60, 485
Brain imaging, 293
Brain size, 215, 218, 663
Brain stem, 75
Broca's area, 174, 191, 245, 331, 543, 667
Brodmann area, 248, 331

Callosal axons, 212
Callosal connectivity, 266
Callosal interaction, 262, 271
Callosal transfer, 214, 341, 469
Categorical encoding, 306
Categorical spatial relations, 304, 311, 317,
  325
Cerebellar deficit hypothesis, 665
Cerebellum, 134, 174, 202, 535, 665
Cerebral hemispheres, 263
Chimeric Faces Task (CFT), 537
Chronometry, 233, 253
Cognitive neuroanatomy, 683
Cognitive neuroscience, 219, 534
Cognitive subtraction, 169
Commissures, 4, 261, 628
Commissurotomy, 124
Commissural pathway, 641
Computerized tomography (CT), 231, 653,
  758

Congenital adrenal hyperplasia (CAH), 122
Conjunction, 169, 174
Connectivity, 162, 163
Consonant-vowel syllables (CV), 444, 477, 722
Consonant-vowel-consonant syllables (CVC), 477, 495
Coordinate spatial relations, 304, 311, 318
Corpus callosum, 129, 130, 138, 204, 211, 265, 292, 619, 620, 630, 632, 640, 662, 704
Corpus callosum agenesis, 622
Cortex, 133, 162, 202
Corticospinal projection, 241
Corticosterone, 52, 87
Cross-cueing, 629
Crossed/uncrossed difference (CUD), 341, 345, 634
Current source density (CSD), 355
Cytoarchitectonic, 194, 668

Depression, 235, 533, 537, 539, 543, 550, 556, 566, 577, 721, 724, 725
Developmental language disorders, 199
Dichotic listening (DL), 208, 275, 441, 446, 447, 451, 477, 728, 729, 745, 750, 751
Diffusion tensor imaging, 266
Disconnection syndrome, 641
Divided attention, 292
Divided visual field, 314
Dizygotic twins, 582
Dopamine (DA), 69, 132, 519
Dorsolateral prefrontal cortex (DLPFC), 176, 177, 183, 236, 331, 497, 521, 720
Dyslexia, 208, 652, 654, 658, 662, 665, 669, 699

EEG asymmetry, 448, 595, 720, 731
Electroencephalography (EEG), 136, 231, 250, 266, 535, 539, 565
Emotion, 511, 514, 526, 533–535, 545, 565, 585, 594, 733
Emotion regulation, 512, 533, 551
Emotional states, 528
Endocrine modulation, 533
Event-related potentials (ERP), 269, 345, 346, 368, 480, 634, 723, 755

Event-related functional magnetic resonance (efMRI), 512, 524, 551, 640
Experimental design, 161
Explicit memory, 543
Eye dominance, 138

Fear, 534
Fear conditioning, 516, 517
Forced-left attention, 457
Forced-right attention, 456
Frontal cortex, 244, 248
Frontal EEG asymmetry, 565, 570, 577, 582, 606
Frontal lobe, 667
Functional asymmetry, 651
Functional brain imaging, 161
Functional imaging, 253, 417
Functional magnetic resonance imaging (fMRI), 161, 165–167, 294, 329, 350, 369, 485
Functional neuroanatomy, 324
Functional segregation, 163
Functional specialization, 162
Fused dichotic words test (FDWT), 197, 722, 751

GABA, 77, 86
Gender differences, 209, 210, 453
General linear model, 165
Genetic, 112, 123, 189

Habituation, 517
Hallucinations, 751
Hand preference, 109
Handedness, 38, 41, 105, 109, 114, 119, 123, 131, 132, 135, 202, 209, 214, 236, 453, 458, 655, 689, 745, 746, 748
Hemiplegia, 126
Hemispatial bias, 537
Hemisphere interaction, 162, 515
Hemodynamic response, 170
Heschl's gyrus (HG), 187, 413, 416, 425, 434, 443, 658, 670, 759
Heschl's sulcus, 192
Hippocampus, 37, 38, 40, 43, 54, 59, 61, 219

Hormones, 120, 130
Hypothalamus, 535

Imprinting, 20, 26
Inerhemispheric connectivity, 209
Interheimspheric differences, 187
Interheimspheric interaction, 287
Interhemispheric commissures, 124
Interhemispheric communication, 626
Interhemispheric integration, 295, 270, 275, 295, 468
Interhemispheric interaction, 290
Interhemispheric processing, 262
Interhemispheric transfer, 138
Interhemispheric transfer time (IHHT), 268, 341, 345
International Affective Picture Series (IAPS), 522
Isthmus, 209

Kinsbourne's attention model, 351

Language, 243, 244, 655
  impairment (LI), 670
  lateralization, 625
Laterality index, 455
Left ear advantage (LEA), 447, 452, 454, 478, 722
Left visual field (LFV), 269, 270, 359, 363
Left-handedness, 105, 107, 111, 131, 746
Left-hemisphere overactivation, 293
Limbic structures, 75
Long-term potentiation (LTP), 43, 50, 51

Magnetic resonance imaging (MRI), 136, 188, 192, 207, 217, 231, 691, 696
Magnetoencephalography (MEG), 231, 368, 444
Magnocellular pathway, 316
Melancholic depression, 722
Memory, 5, 247, 290, 465, 544
Mini Mental State (MMS) test, 466
Mismatch negativity, 481
Mixed-handedness, 107
Monocular deprivation, 7, 9, 25
Monozygotic twins, 189, 198, 582, 706

Mood disorders, 511, 552
Morphology, 187, 190, 209, 212
Morphometry, 209, 210, 217, 219
Motor cortex, 233, 242, 252, 369, 387
Multiple sclerosis (MS), 292
Music, 411
Musical imagery, 426

Neuronal network, 248
Nucleus accumbens, 79

Occipital cortex, 553
Oddball task, 757
Oldfield Inventory, 748
Olfactory stimuli, 525
Orbitofrontal cortex, 545, 550

PANSS, 752
Parietal region, 486
Parvocellular pathway, 316
Pathological left-handedness (PLH), 125, 126
Pavlovian conditioning, 516
Personality traits, 571
Phonetic processing, 209
Phonological deficit, 244, 652
Phonological processing, 652
Planum parietale (PP), 192, 193, 199, 215, 656
Planum temporale (PT), 120, 121, 138, 188, 189, 192, 200, 215, 443, 444, 652, 683, 688, 693
Poffenberger paradigm, 266, 342, 351
Positive and Negative Affect Scale (PANS), 552
Positron emission tomography (PET), 134, 136, 161, 167, 231, 328, 369, 418, 484, 490, 666, 696, 760
Posterior commissure, 262
Postmortem studies, 207
Prefrontal cortex (PFC), 69, 248
Premotor area, 133, 369
Processing, 519
Prozac, 733
Psychosis, 761
PT asymmetry, 197

rCBF, 487, 490, 496
Reaction times (RT), 341, 520, 553
Reading disability, 669
Receptive language impairment, 652
Receptive visual fields, 309
Reward, 519
Right ear advantage (REA), 447, 452, 454, 478, 722
Right visual field (RFV), 269, 270, 363
Right-handedness, 105, 107, 111, 131, 137, 201, 252

Schizophrenia, 199, 291, 462, 490, 743, 744, 748, 755, 758
Selective attention, 292, 488
Sensorimotor integration, 633
Serotonin (5-HT), 82
Serotonin reuptake inhibitor (SSRI), 728, 734
Sex differences, 16, 123, 210, 762
Single photon emission computerized tomography (SPECT), 760
Somatosensory areas, 206
Spatial encoding, 306
Speech, 411
  areas, 191
  arrest, 241, 242
  dominance, 106
  lateralization, 197
Splenium, 204
Split-brain patients, 262, 263, 264, 265, 636
State frontal asymmetry, 596
Statistical parametric mapping (SPM), 161, 164, 166, 175, 183
Stereotaxic space, 204
Stress, 69, 70
Striatum, 79, 519
Stroop task, 287, 546, 547, 550, 551
Structural asymmetry, 651
Superior temporal gyrus (STG), 423, 424, 425, 428, 496
Sylvian fissure (SF), 187, 188, 190, 200, 684, 685

Temporal lobe, 120
Testosterone, 121, 130

Thalamus, 174
Top-down processing, 37, 485
Trait frontal asymmetry, 585, 596
Transcranial magnetic stimulation (TMS), 132, 137, 231, 236, 244, 247

Ventricular enlargement, 758
Verbal fluency, 192
Vigilance, 459
Visual areas, 234
Visual cortex, 316, 387
Visual field asymmetry, 753
Visuoconstructive deficits, 630
Wada test, 241, 695
WAIS-R, 217
Wernicke's area, 244
White matter fibers, 266
Within-hemisphere processing, 289, 294
Working memory, 86, 247, 412, 420, 421